# Advanced Reconstruction
## Elbow 2



AAOS
American Academy of Orthopaedic Surgeons

# ADVANCED RECONSTRUCTION
## Elbow 2

**Edited by**

David Ring, MD, PhD
Associate Dean for Comprehensive Care
Dell Medical School
The University of Texas at Austin
Austin, Texas

Scott P. Steinmann, MD
Professor of Orthopedic Surgery
Department of Orthopedic Surgery
Mayo Clinic
Rochester, Minnesota

American Shoulder and Elbow Surgeons

AAOS
AMERICAN ACADEMY OF ORTHOPAEDIC SURGEONS

## Staff

Ellen C. Moore, *Chief Education Officer*

Hans Koelsch, PhD, *Director, Department of Publications*

Lisa Claxton Moore, *Senior Manager, Book Program*

Laura Goetz, *Managing Editor*

Courtney Dunker, *Editorial Production Manager*

Abram Fassler, *Publishing Systems Manager*

Michelle Wild, *Associate Senior Editor*

Suzanne O'Reilly, *Graphic Designer*

Susan Morritz Baim, *Production Coordinator*

Karen Danca, *Permissions Coordinator*

Charlie Baldwin, *Digital and Print Production Specialist*

Hollie Muir, *Digital and Print Production Specialist*

Emily Douglas, *Page Production Assistant*

Rachel Winokur, *Editorial Coordinator/Copy Editor*

Genevieve Charet, *Editorial Coordinator*

Brian Moore, *Manager, Electronic Media Programs*

Katie Hovany, *Digital Media Specialist*



Published 2016 by the
American Academy of Orthopaedic Surgeons
9400 West Higgins Road
Rosemont, IL 60018



Library of Congress Control Number: 2016937868

ISBN 978-1-62552-546-8

Printed in the USA

# Acknowledgments

Explore the full portfolio of AAOS educational programs and publications across the orthopaedic spectrum for every stage of an orthopaedic surgeon's career, at www.aaos.org. The AAOS, in partnership with Jones & Bartlett Learning, also offers a comprehensive collection of educational and training resources for emergency medical providers, from first responders to critical care transport paramedics. Learn more at www.aaos.org/ems.

# Contributors

**Julie E. Adams, MD**
*Associate Professor*
*Department of Orthopaedic Surgery*
*Mayo Clinic*
*Austin, Minnesota*

**Christopher S. Ahmad, MD**
*Orthopaedic Surgeon*
*Center for Shoulder, Elbow, and Sports Medicine*
*Columbia University Medical Center*
*New York, New York*

**April D. Armstrong, BSc(PT), MD, MSc, FRCSC**
*Professor*
*Department of Orthopaedics*
*Penn State Milton S. Hershey Medical Center*
*Hershey, Pennsylvania*

**George S. Athwal, MD, FRCSC**
*Associate Professor*
*Roth | McFarlane Hand & Upper Limb Centre*
*St. Joseph's Health Care London*
*Western University*
*London, Ontario, Canada*

**Donald S. Bae, MD**
*Associate Professor of Orthopaedic Surgery*
*Harvard Medical School*
*Boston Children's Hospital*
*Boston, Massachusetts*

**Gregory I. Bain, MBBS, FRACS, FAOrthA, PhD**
*Professor of Upper Limb and Research*
*Department of Orthopaedic Surgery*
*The Flinders University of South Australia*
*South Australia, Australia*

**Joshua A. Baumfeld, MD**
*Associate Director of Sports Medicine*
*Department of Orthopaedic Surgery*
*Lahey Hospital and Medical Center*
*Burlington, Massachusetts*
*Assistant Professor*
*Boston University Graduate School of Medicine*
*Boston, Massachusetts*

**Ryan P. Calfee, MD, MSc**
*Associate Professor*
*Department of Orthopaedic Surgery*
*Washington University School of Medicine*
*St. Louis, Missouri*

**Michael J. Carroll, MD, FRCSC**
*Clinical Fellow*
*Department of Orthopaedic Surgery*
*Roth | McFarlane Hand & Upper Limb Centre*
*St. Joseph's Health Care London*
*Western University*
*London, Ontario, Canada*

**Neal C. Chen, MD**
*Assistant in Orthopaedic Surgery*
*Department of Orthopaedic Surgery*
*Hand and Upper Extremity Service*
*Massachusetts General Hospital*
*Boston, Massachusetts*

**Emilie V. Cheung, MD**
*Associate Professor*
*Department of Orthopaedic Surgery*
*Stanford University*
*Redwood City, California*

**Mark S. Cohen, MD**
*Professor*
*Director, Hand and Elbow Section*
*Director, Orthopaedic Education*
*Department of Orthopaedic Surgery*
*Rush University Medical Center*
*Chicago, Illinois*

**Aaron Daluiski, MD**
*Assistant Professor of Clinical Orthopaedic Surgery*
*Department of Orthopaedic Surgery*
*Hospital for Special Surgery*
*New York, New York*

**Reid W. Draeger, MD**
*Assistant Professor*
*Department of Orthopaedics*
*University of North Carolina School of Medicine*
*Chapel Hill, North Carolina*

**Thomas R. Duquin, MD**
*Assistant Professor*
*Department of Orthopaedic Surgery*
*University at Buffalo*
*Buffalo, New York*

**Kenneth J. Faber, MD, MHPE, FRCSC**
*Associate Professor*
*Roth | McFarlane Hand & Upper Limb Centre*
*St. Joseph's Health Care London*
*Western University*
*London, Ontario, Canada*

**Varun Kashyap Gajendran, MD**
*Hand Surgery Fellow*
*Department of Orthopaedic Surgery*
*Cleveland Clinic Foundation*
*Cleveland, Ohio*

**Hill Hastings II, MD**
*Clinical Professor of Orthopedic Surgery*
*Department of Orthopedics*
*Indiana University Medical Center*
*Indianapolis, Indiana*

**Michael R. Hausman, MD**
*Lippmann Professor of Orthopaedic Surgery*
*Chief of Hand and Elbow Surgery*
*Department of Orthopaedic Surgery*
*Mount Sinai Medical Center*
*New York, New York*

**John P. Haverstock, MD, FRCSC**
*Fellow*
*Roth | McFarlane Hand & Upper Limb Centre*
*St. Joseph's Health Care London*
*Western University*
*London, Ontario, Canada*

**Jonah Hebert-Davies, MD, FRCSC**
*Fellow*
*Department of Orthopaedics*
*Washington University School of Medicine*
*St. Louis, Missouri*

**David L. Helfet, MD**
*Director*
*Orthopaedic Trauma Service*
*Hospital for Special Surgery*
*New York Presbyterian Hospital*
*New York, New York*

**Justin L. Hodgins, MD**
*Clinical Fellow*
*Center for Shoulder, Elbow and Sports Medicine*
*Columbia University*
*New York, New York*

**Robert N. Hotchkiss, MD**
*Orthopaedic Hand and Upper Extremity Service*
*Hospital for Special Surgery*
*New York, New York*

**Jeffery S. Hughes, MBBS, FRACS**
*Orthopaedic Consultant*
*Sydney Orthopaedic and Arthritis*
*North Shore Private Hospital*
*Sydney, New South Wales, Australia*

**Claudius D. Jarrett, MD**
*Assistant Professor of Orthopaedic Surgery*
*Department of Orthopaedic Surgery*
*Emory University School of Medicine*
*The Emory Orthopaedic Center*
*Atlanta, Georgia*

**Jesse B. Jupiter, MD**
*Hansjorg Wyss/AO Professor*
*Massachusetts General Hospital*
*Boston, Massachusetts*

**H. Mike Kim, MD**
*Assistant Professor*
*Department of Orthopaedics and Rehabilitation*
*Penn State Milton S. Hershey Medical Center*
*Hershey, Pennsylvania*

**Graham J.W. King, MD, MSc, FRCSC**
*Director, Roth | McFarlane Hand & Upper Limb Centre*
*Professor, Department of Orthopaedics and Biomedical Engineering*
*Western University*
*London, Ontario, Canada*

**Peter Kloen, MD, PhD**
*Director of Orthopaedic Trauma*
*Department of Orthopaedic Surgery*
*Academic Medical Centre*
*Amsterdam, Netherlands*

**L. Scott Levin, MD, FACS**
*Paul B. Magnuson Professor of Bone and Joint Surgery, Chairman*
*Department of Orthopaedic Surgery*
*Perelman School of Medicine*
*University of Pennsylvania*
*Philadelphia, Pennsylvania*

 

**Michael J. O'Brien, MD**
*Associate Professor*
*Department of Orthopaedic Surgery*
*Tulane University School of Medicine*
*New Orleans, Louisiana*

**Shawn William O'Driscoll, MD, PhD**
*Professor of Orthopedic Surgery*
*Department of Orthopedic Surgery*
*Mayo Clinic College of Medicine*
*Rochester, Minnesota*

**Joideep Phadnis, MBChB, MRCS, FRCS (TR & Orth)**
*Upper Limb Fellow*
*Department of Orthopaedics*
*Flinders Medical Centre*
*Adelaide, South Australia*

**Marc Prud'homme-Foster, MD, FRCSC**
*Lecturer*
*Department of Orthopaedic Surgery*
*University of Ottawa*
*Ottawa, Ontario, Canada*

**David Ring, MD, PhD**
*Associate Dean for Comprehensive Care*
*Dell Medical School*
*The University of Texas at Austin*
*Austin, Texas*

**Felix H. Savoie III, MD**
*Professor and Vice Chairman*
*Department of Orthopaedic Surgery*
*Tulane University School of Medicine*
*New Orleans, Louisiana*

**Christopher C. Schmidt, MD**
*Director of Shoulder Surgery*
*Department of Orthopaedic Surgery*
*University of Pittsburgh Medical Center*
*Pittsburgh, Pennsylvania*

**William H. Seitz, Jr, MD**
*Professor of Orthopaedic Surgery*
*Cleveland Clinic Lerner College of Medicine of Case Western Reserve University*
*Chairman, Orthopaedic Surgery Letterman Hospital*
*Cleveland Clinic Orthopaedic & Rheumatologic Institute*
*Cleveland, Ohio*

**Xavier C. Simcock, MD**
*Upper Extremity Fellow*
*Cleveland Clinic Foundation*
*Orthopaedic & Rheumatologic Institute*
*Cleveland, Ohio*

**David Stanley, MBBS, BSc, FRCS**
*Consultant Shoulder Elbow Surgeon*
*Orthopaedic Department*
*Sheffield Teaching Hospitals*
*Sheffield, England*

**Scott P. Steinmann, MD**
*Professor of Orthopedic Surgery*
*Department of Orthopedic Surgery*
*Mayo Clinic*
*Rochester, Minnesota*

**Milan Stevanovic, MD**
*Professor of Orthopaedic Surgery*
*Department of Orthopaedic Surgery*
*Keck School of Medicine*
*University of Southern California*
*Los Angeles, California*

**Eric T. Tolo, MD**
*Director, Hand and Upper Extremity Fellowship*
*Department of Orthopaedic Surgery*
*Lahey Hospital and Medical Center*
*Burlington, Massachusetts*

**Steve W. Wang, MD**
*Hand Surgeon*
*Department of Orthopedic Surgery*
*Hawaii Permanente Medical Group*
*Honolulu, Hawaii*

**Jennifer Moriatis Wolf, MD**
*Associate Professor*
*Department of Orthopaedic Surgery*
*University of Connecticut Health Center*
*Farmington, Connecticut*

**Ken Yamaguchi, MD, MBA**
*Sam & Marilyn Fox Distinguished Professor of Orthopaedic Surgery*
*Department of Orthopaedic Surgery*
*Washington University School of Medicine*
*St. Louis, Missouri*

# Preface

Welcome to the second edition of ***Advanced Reconstruction Elbow***, a joint venture of the American Shoulder and Elbow Surgeons and the American Academy of Orthopaedic Surgeons. We are indebted to our gifted surgeon-authors for volunteering their time, efforts, and knowledge to this book.

The second edition features surgical videos, technique sections in a bulleted format, and learning objectives to enhance reader comprehension and learning. The group of elbow enthusiasts is relatively small, and we enjoy substantial camaraderie and much alignment in opinion. Nevertheless, we edited our colleagues' chapters with care to highlight the areas of current debate, the range of opinion, and the type of data that would help inform patient and surgeon decision-making.

We would also like to thank the team that made us surgeons look good in print: Director Hans Koelsch; editors Lisa Claxton Moore, Laura Goetz, Michelle Wild, and Rachel Winokur; Katie Hovany for helping with the video; and the production staff—Courtney Dunker, Abram Fassler, Suzanne O'Reilly, Karen Danca, Susan Morritz Baim, Charlie Baldwin, Hollie Muir, and Emily Douglas. Most importantly, we thank our families for their support and patience with all our endeavors.

We hope you get as much out of this book as we did.

David Ring, MD, PhD
Scott P. Steinmann, MD

# Table of Contents

# Video Index

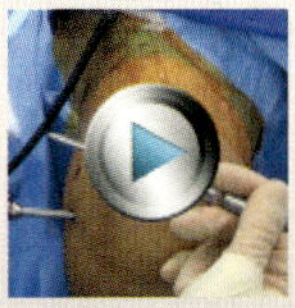

**Video 1.1** The Stiff Elbow: Arthroscopic Management of Elbow Arthritis and Elbow Arthrofibrosis. Scott P. Steinmann, MD (18 min)

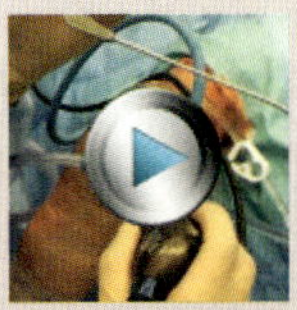

**Video 2.1** Arthroscopic Treatment of Osteochondritis Dissecans. Christopher S. Ahmad, MD; Lauren H. Redler, MD (16 min)

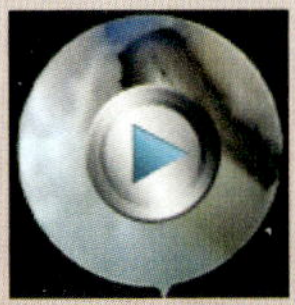

**Video 3.1** Arthroscopic Radial Head Excision. Felix H. Savoie III, MD (2 min)

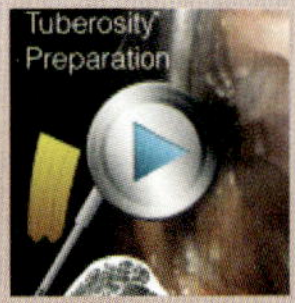


**Video 9.1** Anatomic Distal Biceps Repair: Two Intramedullary Buttons or Modified Trough Technique and Chronic Distal Biceps Repair With Achilles Tendon Allograft. Christopher C. Schmidt, MD (12 min)

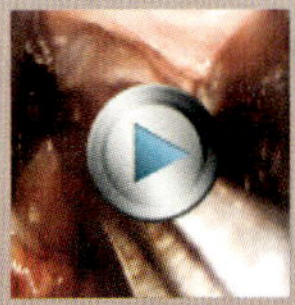

**Video 10.1** Anatomic Distal Biceps Tendon Repair. Joideep Phadnis, MBChB, MRCS, FRCS (Tr & Orth) (5 min)

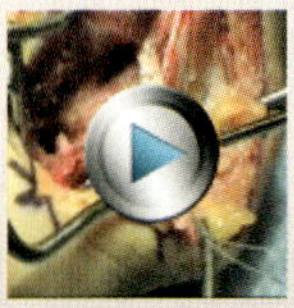

**Video 12.1** Hybrid Technique for Reconstruction of the Medial Collateral Ligament of the Elbow. J. Michael Bennett, MD; Thomas L. Mehlhoff, MD; Rodney K. Baker (6 min)

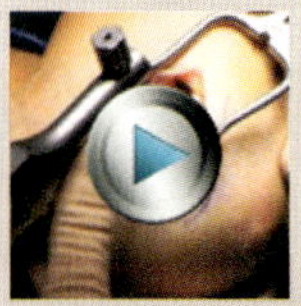

**Video 16.1** Radiocapitellar Arthroplasty of the Elbow: Surgical Technique. Matthias Vanhees, MD; Frederik Verstreken, MD; Roger P. van Riet, MD, PhD (12 min)

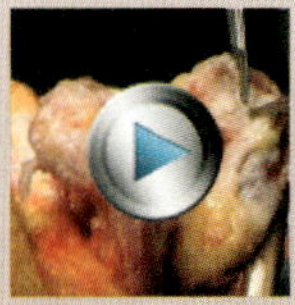

**Video 18.1** Total Elbow Arthroplasty in a Rheumatoid Elbow. Hill Hastings II, MD (4 min)

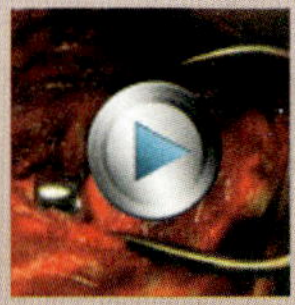

**Video 25.1** Radial Head Arthroplasty. Graham J.W. King, MD (17 min)

SECTION 1
# Elbow Arthroscopy

# Chapter 1

# Basic Elbow Arthroscopy

*Julie E. Adams, MD*

**Learning Objectives**

- Identify indications for and contraindications to elbow arthroscopy.
- Understand and describe safe and effective methods for performing elbow arthroscopy.

## Indications

The indications for elbow arthroscopy continue to expand with increased understanding of elbow pathology, surgeons' increased comfort with arthroscopy of the elbow, and improved instrumentation and setup. Current indications for elbow arthroscopy include rheumatoid arthritis, osteoarthritis, hemophilic arthritis, septic elbow arthritis, select fractures and instabilities, osteochondral defects, loose body extraction, contracture release, tennis elbow, and diagnosis.

## Contraindications

Elbow arthroscopy involves the risk of neurovascular injury, which can be devastating and permanent. This risk is higher in the elbow than in other joints because of the proximity of neurovascular structures to arthroscopy portals in the surgical field. Elbow arthroscopy is best reserved for surgeons who have arthroscopic training or arthroscopic experience in other joints, a high level of comfort with the anatomy of the elbow, and facility with open elbow surgery. Other contraindications may be considered based on diagnosis or the extent of pathology. Some conditions may be better managed with open procedures. For example, patients with advanced elbow arthritis and pain throughout the arc of motion may be better served by interposition or prosthetic arthroplasty.

It may be very difficult to safely or adequately perform elbow arthroscopy in patients who have little elbow motion. Prior trauma or surgical procedures about the elbow may distort normal bony and soft-tissue anatomy and may represent a relative contraindication to arthroscopy. Although previous subcutaneous transposition of the ulnar nerve is not necessarily a contraindication, the nerve should be definitively identified and protected. Prior submuscular or intramuscular transposition of the ulnar nerve is generally considered a contraindication because it places the ulnar nerve directly adjacent to the anterior elbow capsule.

## Alternative Treatments

Open procedures are a good alternative to arthroscopy in many patients. Few studies involving a comparison between open and arthroscopic procedures about the elbow have been published; the results of those that do exist demonstrate variable and modest differences. No definitive evidence to date demonstrates superiority of arthroscopy for any procedure; however, both patients and surgeons appreciate the several advantages it offers. The joint is easily and well visualized from several perspectives and orientations. Intra-articular pathology can be diagnosed and treated. Patients appreciate the smaller incisions and decreased pain with the arthroscopic approach.

## Results

The results of arthroscopic procedures for the elbow depend on the procedure being performed. Results of select studies are noted in **Table 1**. In general, however, high rates of satisfactory outcomes

---

*Dr. Adams or an immediate family member has received royalties from Arthrex and Biomet; is a member of a speakers' bureau or has made paid presentations on behalf of Arthrex; and serves as a board member, owner, officer, or committee member of the American Association for Hand Surgery, the American Shoulder and Elbow Surgeons, the American Society for Surgery of the Hand, the Arthroscopy Association of North America, and the Minnesota Orthopaedic Society.*

**Table 1** Results of Elbow Arthroscopy

| Authors (Year) | Number of Patients | Procedure or Approach | Mean Patient Age in Years | Mean Follow-up in Months | Success Rate (%) | Results | Level of Evidence |
|---|---|---|---|---|---|---|---|
| Cohen et al (2000) | 44 | Open (18 patients) or arthroscopic (26 patients) débridement for osteoarthritis | 55 (open), 46 (arthroscopic) | 35.3 | NR | Better pain relief in the arthroscopic group and better motion in the open group | II |
| Adams et al (2008) | 41 (42 elbows) | Arthroscopic débridement for osteoarthritis | NR | 40 (minimum, 24) | 81 (good to excellent results) | — | III |
| Grewal et al (2009) | 36 | Arthroscopic tennis elbow release | 45.3 ± 7.0 (range, 29-61) | 42 (range, 19-74) | 83.3 | 30 patients improved<br>Mayo Elbow Performance Index scores were good to excellent in 22 patients, fair in 9, and poor in 5 | II |
| Wada et al (2009) | 18 (20 elbows) | Arthroscopic lateral epicondylitis surgery | 54 (range, 42-71) | 28 (range, 24-40) | 100 | 14 of 20 elbows were much better postoperatively, and 6 were better | III |

NR = not reported.

have been reported across series. Risks associated with elbow arthroscopy include devastating and permanent neurovascular injury, recurrent or residual symptoms, synovial cutaneous fistula, and heterotopic ossification (which, although rare, is possible). Each susceptible nerve about the elbow has been reported as injured, and more than one nerve may be injured in a single procedure.

**Video 1.1** The Stiff Elbow: Arthroscopic Management of Elbow Arthritis and Elbow Arthrofibrosis. Scott P. Steinmann, MD (18 min)

## Techniques

### Setup/Exposure

- If examination under anesthesia is required, the patient is placed supine, and the examination is completed before the patient is positioned for the elbow arthroscopy.
- The patient is placed in the lateral decubitus, prone, or supine position, based on surgeon preference. The author of this chapter prefers the lateral decubitus position.
- If the lateral decubitus position is used, then the patient is placed on a beanbag and secured with safety straps, taking care to ensure that all bony prominences are padded.
- The patient's arm is placed into an arm holder and positioned such that free access to the elbow is maintained during the procedure and elbow flexion and extension are possible intraoperatively. Ideally, the arm is positioned to avoid any impingement of the soft tissues in the antecubital fossa and ensure that the elbow is slightly higher than the shoulder (**Figure 1**).

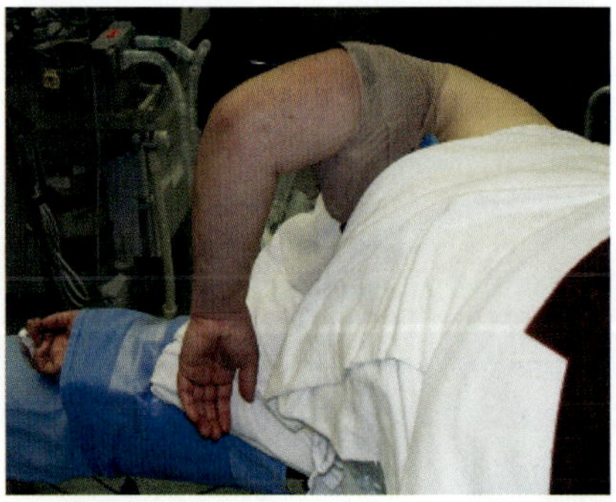

**Figure 1** Preoperative photograph shows the setup of a patient for elbow arthroscopy in the lateral decubitus position. (Courtesy of Scott P. Steinmann, MD, Rochester, MN.)

- A sterile or nonsterile tourniquet may be applied to the upper arm.

### Instruments/Equipment/Implants Required

- A dedicated arm holder may be used; alternatively, a knee holder may be used.

 

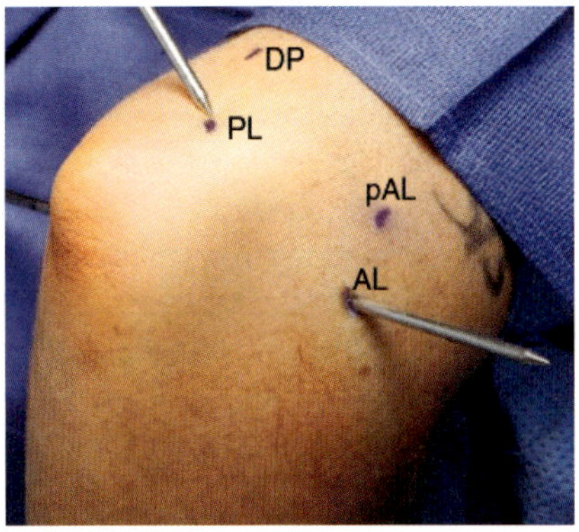


**Figure 2** Intraoperative photograph shows the portals for elbow arthroscopy. The switching stick is protruding through the anterolateral (AL) and anteromedial portals, and the free switching stick points to the posterolateral (PL) portal. The proximal anterolateral portal (pAL) is seen just above the AL portal, and the direct posterior portal (DP) is visualized medial and proximal to the PL portal. (Reproduced with permission from the Mayo Foundation for Medical Education and Research, Rochester, MN.)

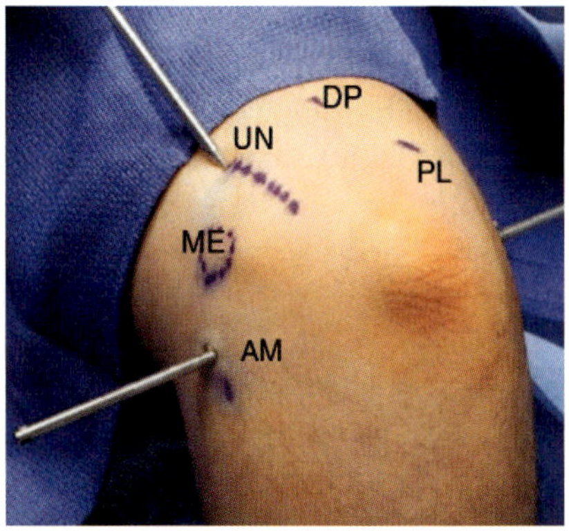


**Figure 3** Intraoperative photograph shows the portals for elbow arthroscopy. The switching stick is protruding through the anterolateral and anteromedial (AM) portals, and the free switching stick points to the path of the ulnar nerve (UN). The circular outline represents the medial epicondyle (ME). DP = direct posterior portal, PL = posterolateral portal. (Reproduced with permission from the Mayo Foundation for Medical Education and Research, Rochester, MN.)

- Standard knee arthroscopy equipment can be used, typically a 4.0- or 4.5-mm arthroscope and a cannula.
- Nontrephinated cannulas should be used because trephinations allow egress of fluid out of the joint capsule and into the subcutaneous tissues.
- A variety of arthroscopic burrs, shavers, graspers, and retractor devices can be used, in addition to simple Freer elevators or Howarth elevators for retraction and small osteotomes for osteophyte removal.

## Procedure

- After the patient is secured on the surgical table in the lateral decubitus position and the arm is placed in an arm holder, the patient is prepped and draped in the usual manner, and the upper arm tourniquet is applied.
- The bony and soft-tissue landmarks are identified and marked with a skin scribe. The medial and lateral epicondyles, radial head, olecranon, intermuscular septum, and ulnar nerve are marked. The ulnar nerve is examined to ensure that there is no subluxation. The intended portal sites are identified and marked.
- The arm is elevated, and the tourniquet is inflated.
- The elbow joint is insufflated with 25 to 30 mL of saline infused through the direct lateral portal, the direct posterior portal, or the intended anterolateral portal site. The arm will extend as the capsule is inflated, confirming correct placement of fluid into the joint.
- Depending on the pathology to be addressed and the surgeon's experience, the procedure may begin in either the anterior or posterior joint, and the initial portal may be medial, lateral, or posterior. Typically, the author of this chapter begins with an anterolateral portal, unless the patient's pathology dictates otherwise.
- The anterolateral portal is made just anterior to the radiocapitellar joint (**Figure 2**). This portal places the posterior interosseous nerve at risk, so the author of this chapter prefers to create this portal at the start of the procedure before any soft-tissue distension alters the landmarks. A No. 15 blade is used to incise the skin only, and blunt dissection down to the capsule is performed with a hemostat. A sudden egress of fluid confirms articular entry.
- The blunt trocar and cannula are placed into the joint. With experience, the surgeon can confirm intra-articular placement by feel in most patients, driving the cannula and the trocar to the medial side of the joint and tenting the skin and soft tissues to create the anteromedial portal (**Figure 3**).
- Alternatively, and as recommended for surgeons who are less experienced with arthroscopy, the trocar is withdrawn after placement, and visualization proceeds through the anterolateral portal.
- The anteromedial portal is located 1 to 2 cm distal and anterior to the medial epicondyle, and it may be created with either an inside-out technique or in the usual manner.
- A cannula is placed for instrumentation.
- The author of this chapter typically begins the procedure by visualizing through the anterolateral portal and using the anteromedial portal as the working portal.
- A shaver is introduced to remove any synovitis and improve visualization. The suction tubing is intentionally left off the shaver to avoid suction of soft tissue into the jaws of the shaver. However, the suction tubing is used to trap a loose body (if present) against the humerus to shave it away.
- Loose bodies are removed with a grasper or a shaver. Sometimes, it

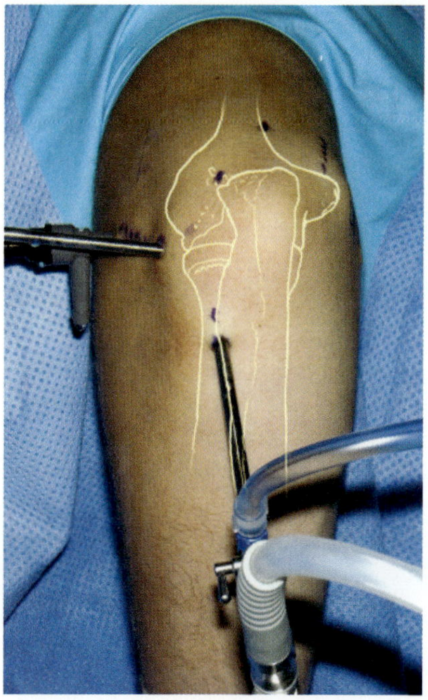

**Figure 4** Intraoperative photograph shows use of the distal ulnar portal to visualize osteochondral lesions. The arthroscope is in the distal ulnar portal, and the shaver is in the direct lateral (soft-spot) portal. (Reproduced with permission from the Mayo Foundation for Medical Education and Research, Rochester, MN.)

is helpful to trap any loose bodies with a spinal needle against the humerus and break them into smaller fragments with the shaver.

- Usually, bony work is completed before soft-tissue work because after the capsule is breached, fluid escapes from the joint into the surrounding soft tissues and limits the time available to complete the procedure. In the setting of contracture releases, it may be necessary to incise the joint capsule, elevate it (for capsulotomy), or remove it (for capsulectomy). Complete capsulectomy typically is avoided because of the dangers it poses to neurovascular structures.
- Retraction portals are created as needed. For example, the proximal anterolateral portal is created approximately 1 to 2 cm proximal and 1 cm anterior to the lateral epicondyle, and the proximal anteromedial portal is created approximately 2 cm proximal to the medial epicondyle and directly anterior to the medial intermuscular septum (**Figure 2**).
- The so-called soft-spot portal is made at the center of a triangle between the radial head, the lateral epicondyle, and the tip of the olecranon. This portal often is helpful to address pathology about the radial head (such as excision of the plica or the radial head) or about the capitellum (such as osteochondral lesions).
- Movement of the plica over the radial head on elbow flexion and extension is visualized arthroscopically through the direct lateral (soft-spot) portal. The plica is resected using a shaver in the anterolateral portal; a second direct lateral portal or a posterolateral portal can facilitate removal of the plica. A probe or blunt trocar may be used to manipulate the thickened plica away from the radial head. The plica is resected with an arthroscopic shaver and/or biter. Similar to open excision, care should be taken to avoid resection of the posterolateral ligamentous structures, which could lead to posterolateral rotatory instability.
- After plica resection, elbow range of motion is assessed, ensuring that no remaining plical fold can be impinged, which would result in persistent symptoms.
- The distal ulnar portal is ideal for addressing osteochondral lesions on the posterior capitellum (**Figure 4**). The skin incision for this portal is made 3 to 4 cm distal to the radiocapitellar joint, and a blunt trocar and sleeve are passed proximally along the lateral border of the ulna to enter the joint.
- The direct posterior portal is placed 2 to 3 cm proximal to the proximal edge of the olecranon (**Figures 2** and **3**). This portal passes through the triceps, so the knife must pass through skin, subcutaneous tissue and muscle, and capsule down to bone.
- A trocar is placed through the direct posterior portal, and the so-called cup of the olecranon is abraded to remove olecranon fat and synovial tissue, which creates space for visualization.
- Taking care to orient the instrument away from the region of the ulnar nerve, a shaver is placed and used to blindly shave synovial tissue and fat to facilitate visualization of the joint and create a working space.
- After the working space has been created, the posterolateral portal is made (**Figures 2** and **3**). This portal, which is created nearly level with the proximal edge of the olecranon on the posterolateral surface, is used mostly for visualization. The posterolateral portal has a high margin of safety away from the named neurovascular structures.

### Wound Closure

- To avoid creating a synovial cutaneous fistula, portal sites are closed with sutures rather than thin adhesive strips alone.

## Postoperative Regimen

The postoperative regimen depends on the pathology addressed. Details regarding specific postoperative regimens are discussed elsewhere in this publication in the chapters dedicated to the particular arthroscopic procedures.

## Limiting Adverse Events

The published literature describes injuries associated with elbow arthroscopy involving each major peripheral nerve about the elbow. Nerve injury is more common in patients who have distortion of normal bony and soft-tissue anatomy, such as those who have rheumatoid arthritis, posttraumatic conditions, and preoperative joint contracture. The surgeon should be aware of the risks associated with these conditions. To avoid inadvertently pulling tissue into the jaws of the shaver, suction tubing should not be used in conjunction with a shaver. To decrease the risk of persistent drainage from the joint or the development of synovial cutaneous fistulae, portals should be sutured (not bound with thin adhesive tapes).

## Bibliography

Adams JE, King GJW, Steinmann SP, Cohen MS: Elbow arthroscopy: Indications, techniques, outcomes, and complications. *J Am Acad Orthop Surg* 2014;22(12):810-818.

Adams JE, Steinmann SP: Nerve injuries about the elbow. *J Hand Surg Am* 2006;31(2):303-313.

Adams JE, Wolff LH III, Merten SM, Steinmann SP: Osteoarthritis of the elbow: Results of arthroscopic osteophyte resection and capsulectomy. *J Shoulder Elbow Surg* 2008;17(1):126-131.

Cohen AP, Redden JF, Stanley D: Treatment of osteoarthritis of the elbow: A comparison of open and arthroscopic debridement. *Arthroscopy* 2000;16(7):701-706.

Grewal R, MacDermid JC, Shah P, King GJ: Functional outcome of arthroscopic extensor carpi radialis brevis tendon release in chronic lateral epicondylitis. *J Hand Surg Am* 2009;34(5):849-857.

Kelly EW, Morrey BF, O'Driscoll SW: Complications of elbow arthroscopy. *J Bone Joint Surg Am* 2001;83(1):25-34.

Ruch DS, Papadonikolakis A, Campolattaro RM: The posterolateral plica: A cause of refractory lateral elbow pain. *J Shoulder Elbow Surg* 2006;15(3):367-370.

Savoie FH III: Guidelines to becoming an expert elbow arthroscopist. *Arthroscopy* 2007;23(11):1237-1240.

Steinmann SP: Elbow arthroscopy: Where are we now? *Arthroscopy* 2007;23(11):1231-1236.

Steinmann SP: Elbow arthroscopy. *J Am Soc Surg Hand* 2003;3(4):199-207.

Verhaar J, van Mameren H, Brandsma A: Risks of neurovascular injury in elbow arthroscopy: Starting anteromedially or anterolaterally? *Arthroscopy* 1991;7(3):287-290.

Wada T, Moriya T, Iba K, et al: Functional outcomes after arthroscopic treatment of lateral epicondylitis. *J Orthop Sci* 2009;14(2):167-174.

Yeoh KM, King GJW, Faber KJ, Glazebrook MA, Athwal GS: Evidence-based indications for elbow arthroscopy. *Arthroscopy* 2012;28(2):272-282.

## Video Reference

Steinmann SP: The stiff elbow: Arthroscopic management of elbow arthritis and elbow arthrofibrosis, in Field LD, Steinmann SP, eds: *Arthroscopic Surgical Techniques: Elbow Arthroscopy* [DVD]. Rosemont, IL, American Academy of Orthopaedic Surgeons, 2013.

# Chapter 2

# Surgery for Osteochondritis Dissecans of the Capitellum

*John P. Haverstock, MD, FRCSC*

*Robert N. Hotchkiss, MD*

*George S. Athwal, MD, FRCSC*

**Learning Objectives**

- Understand the indications for surgical and nonsurgical management of osteochondritis dissecans.
- Understand the prognostic factors for osteochondritis dissecans.
- Review classic and landmark studies on the management of osteochondritis dissecans.
- Understand surgical decision making and treatment options for patients with osteochondritis dissecans.

## Indications

Osteochondritis dissecans (OCD) of the capitellum is a disorder that can result in separation of the subchondral bone and formation of loose bodies. OCD of the capitellum typically occurs in adolescent athletes, most often baseball players, gymnasts, and other athletes who place repetitive loads across the capitellum. OCD of the capitellum should be differentiated from Panner's disease, which affects the entire capitellum in children younger than 10 years and is self-limiting with few long-term consequences. Symptoms of OCD of the capitellum include pain, locking, catching, and elbow stiffness.

Early-stage OCD lesions in skeletally immature adolescents are typically managed with limitation of athletic activity. However, higher-grade lesions in older children that progress and remain symptomatic may benefit from surgery. Surgical management for OCD of the capitellum is indicated in patients who have a symptomatic loose body, who are dissatisfied with the results of nonsurgical treatment, who have a symptomatic OCD lesion in an elbow with a closed capitellar physis, or who have a limited ability to heal after nonsurgical treatment. Arthroscopy is most frequently used to manage OCD of the capitellum; however, arthrotomy may be required for patients who have larger or more advanced lesions.

*Dr. Hotchkiss or an immediate family member has received research or institutional support from Auxilium Pharmaceuticals. Dr. Athwal or an immediate family member has received royalties from Imascap and Tornier; serves as a paid consultant to DePuy Synthes, Smith & Nephew, and Tornier; and has received research or institutional support from DePuy Synthes, Exactech, Smith & Nephew, Tornier, and Zimmer Biomet. Neither Dr. Haverstock nor any immediate family member has received anything of value from or has stock or stock options held in a commercial company or institution related directly or indirectly to the subject of this chapter.*

## Contraindications

Patients with an open capitellar physis, near–full elbow range of motion (ROM) (<20° limitation), and an early radiographic appearance of capitellar flattening or radiolucency have an early OCD lesion (often referred to as "stable") and may have good outcomes after nonsurgical treatment. In patients who have early OCD lesions, the avoidance of sporting activities and limited weight bearing results in healing in 70% of patients with an open capitellar physis and only 9% of patients with a closed physis, as reported in a 2007 prognostic study. Patients who have early OCD lesions and do not avoid provocative sports have a higher likelihood of disease progression and poorer outcomes.

## Classifications

Baumgarten et al created an arthroscopic classification system for capitellar OCD lesions based on a classification system for talar OCD lesions that was described by Ferkel and Chang. A grade 1 OCD lesion of the capitellum has smooth, soft articular cartilage. A grade 2 OCD lesion of the capitellum has fibrillations or fissuring of the articular cartilage. A grade 3 OCD lesion of the capitellum has exposed bone with a fixed osteochondral fragment. A grade 4 OCD lesion of the

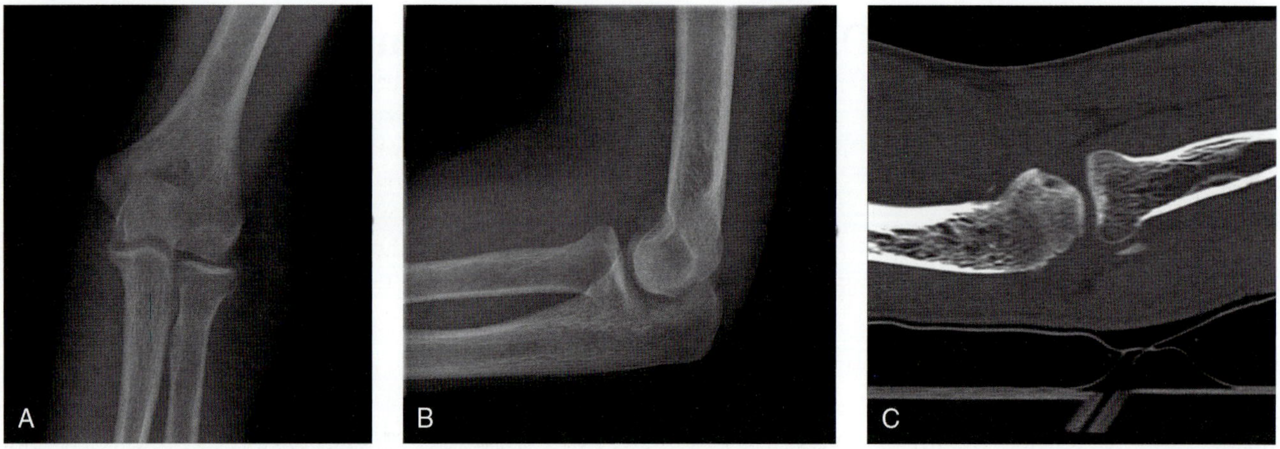


**Figure 1** **A,** AP radiograph of an elbow demonstrates a capitellar osteochondritis dissecans (OCD) lesion with notable lucency and flattening of the capitellum. **B,** Lateral radiograph of an elbow demonstrates anterior loose bodies proximal to the capitellum. **C,** Sagittal CT reconstruction of an elbow demonstrates an OCD defect in the subchondral bone of the capitellum with surrounding sclerosis and a loose body proximal to the capitellum.

capitellum has a loose but nondisplaced fragment. A grade 5 OCD lesion of the capitellum has a displaced fragment that becomes one or more loose bodies.

The International Cartilage Repair Society (ICRS) also developed an arthroscopic classification system for capitellar OCD lesions. Stable OCD lesions of the capitellum that have a continuous but softened area covered by intact cartilage are classified as ICRS grade I. OCD lesions of the capitellum with partial discontinuity that are stable if probed are classified as ICRS grade II. OCD lesions of the capitellum with complete discontinuity that remain contained within the crater are classified as ICRS grade III. Empty defects or OCD lesions of the capitellum with a dislodged or a loose fragment are classified as ICRS grade IV.

Takahara et al reviewed a large series of patients and created a simple classification system for capitellar OCD lesions. OCD lesions of the capitellum were classified as stable (indicating a good prognosis after nonsurgical management) in patients who had an open capitellar physis, localized flattening or radiolucency of the subchondral bone, and near-normal elbow ROM. Capitellar OCD lesions in all other patients, including those who had a closed physis, fragmentation (**Figure 1**), or elbow ROM that was restricted more than 20°, were classified as unstable (indicating a worse prognosis after nonsurgical management).

## Alternative Treatments

The goals of treatment are to address a patient's symptoms (pain, stiffness, or locking) and, ideally, allow the capitellar OCD lesion to heal. A healed, aligned fragment with a patient's native articular cartilage is optimal. Management options for fragments deemed to have a poor chance of healing include débridement with stimulation of fibrocartilage and articular cartilage reconstruction.

### Stable Capitellar OCD Lesions

Arthroscopic techniques have become standard for the management of capitellar OCD. Arthroscopy can be used to assess, débride, and microfracture or drill OCD lesions. Advantages of arthroscopy include the capacity to assess the entire elbow joint, the ability to remove loose bodies, and the minimally invasive nature of the procedure.

Surgical options for patients who are unsatisfied after nonsurgical management of stable capitellar OCD lesions (that is, lesions unlikely to progress after nonsurgical management) include fluoroscopic-assisted drilling into the fragment to stimulate healing as well as fragment internal fixation (arthroscopic or open). Drilling can be accomplished from posterior to anterior through the intact humerus using Kirschner wires (K-wires) under arthroscopic or fluoroscopic guidance. Multiple passes are made with the K-wires to stimulate healing and create channels for blood flow. Internal fixation can be accomplished with small screws (**Figure 2**), bone spicules, sutures, or bioabsorbable tacks or darts. The anconeus muscle-splitting approach with the elbow in hyperflexion is used for open reduction and internal fixation (**Figure 3**).

### Unstable Capitellar OCD Lesions

Unstable capitellar OCD lesions can be reduced and fixed or excised. After excision, microfracture is intended to stimulate the growth of fibrocartilage; alternatively, these lesions can be reconstructed with osteochondral autograft. These techniques can be accomplished via all-arthroscopic, arthroscopic-assisted, or open surgery. Realignment osteotomies of the distal humerus to offload the capitellum also have been described in the literature.

## Results

OCD of the capitellum is relatively uncommon, and most of the evidence is limited to case series (**Table 1**). A study of patients who underwent nonsurgical treatment or loose-body removal reported that approximately one-half of the patients had stiffness and pain with activity postoperatively. Another study of patients who underwent nonsurgical or surgical treatment reported that poorer outcomes were associated with advanced lesions at the time of presentation. Seven of the 14 patients who were treated nonsurgically and 18 of the 39 patients who were treated surgically had elbow symptoms with activities of daily living.

Although numerous studies have reported the short-term and midterm outcomes of loose-body excision and microfracture, fewer studies report the outcomes of fragment fixation and osteochondral grafting. A study of patients who were treated for capitellar OCD lesions reported that near-complete healing was seen in 7 of 10 patients with an open physis and in 1 of 11 patients with a closed physis who complied with a nonsurgical treatment regimen of rest. The outcomes of patients who continued to subject the elbow to stress were significantly worse with respect to radiographic findings ($P < 0.05$) and the formation of loose bodies ($P < 0.05$) compared with the outcomes of the patients who complied with the nonsurgical rest regimen. Patients with an open physis who continued to subject the elbow to stress had worse outcomes with respect to pain ($P < 0.05$), radiographic findings ($P < 0.05$), and healing ($P < 0.01$) compared with those patients with an open physis who complied with the nonsurgical rest regimen. Among the patients who underwent surgical treatment, pain intensity was significantly lower in the patients who underwent fragment fixation or reconstruction of the articular surface compared with those who underwent fragment excision alone ($P < 0.05$). Better pain and radiographic scores were reported in patients

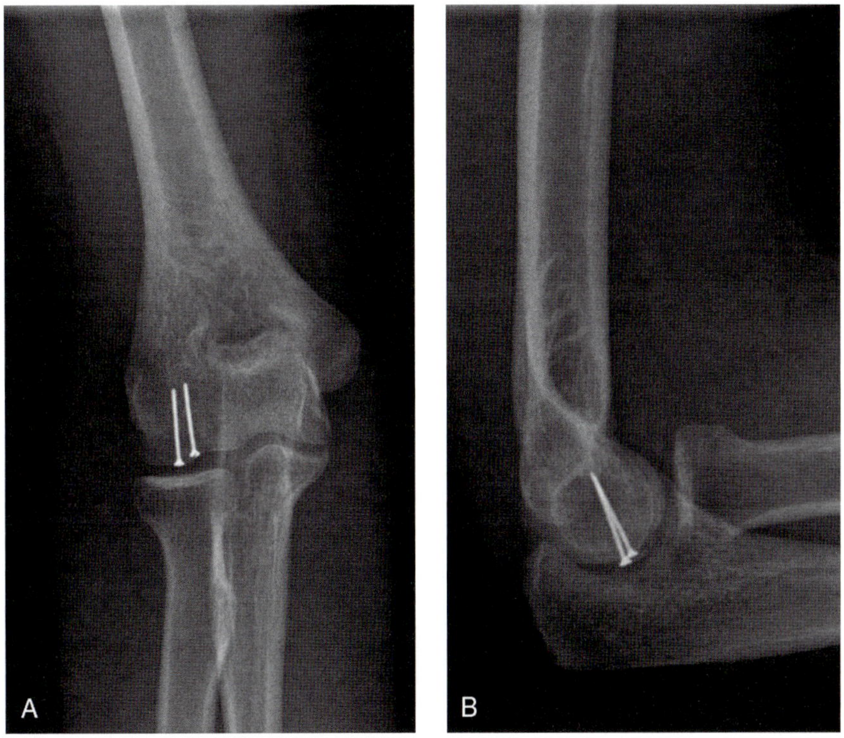


**Figure 2** AP (**A**) and lateral (**B**) radiographs of an elbow demonstrate an unstable osteochondritis dissecans lesion of the capitellum that was fixed with countersunk screws. (Courtesy of Graham J.W. King, MD, London, ON, Canada.)

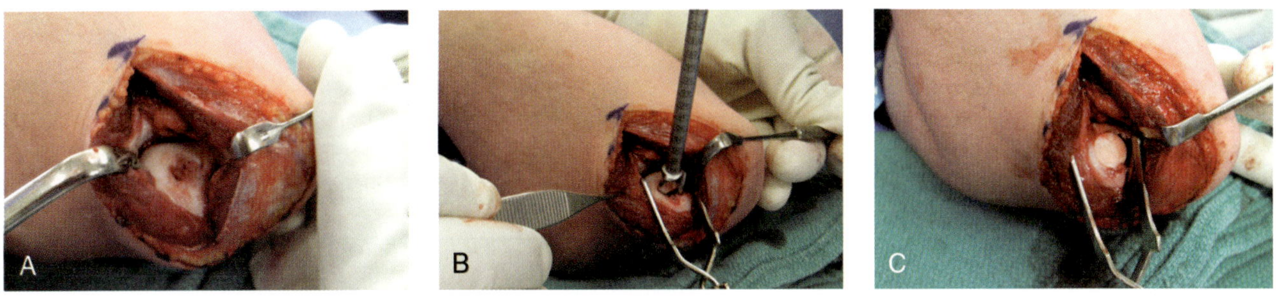


**Figure 3** Intraoperative photographs of an elbow show the anconeus muscle-splitting approach, which is used to access a posterior capitellar osteochondritis dissecans lesion (**A**). With the elbow in hyperflexion, orthogonal access is permitted for recipient site preparation with a reamer (**B**) and for autologous osteochondral grafting with a 10-mm diameter plug (**C**).

**Table 1** Results of Treatment for Osteochondritis Dissecans (OCD)

| Authors (Year) | No. of Patients | Procedure or Approach | Mean Patient Age in Years (Range) | Mean Follow-up in Months (Range) | Results | Level of Evidence |
|---|---|---|---|---|---|---|
| Bauer et al (1992) | 31 | 23 treated surgically with débridement of loose bodies | 20 (14-57) | 276 (132-420) | At follow-up, 13 elbows were symptomatic: reduced ROM in 11, pain on effort in 5<br>Degenerative changes seen on 19 of 31 elbow radiographs | IV |
| Takahara et al (1999) | 53 | Nonsurgical treatment (14), excision (39) | 16.6 (10-34) | 151.2 (36-300) | Poor outcome at long-term follow-up in 32% of patients who had early lesions and 50% of patients who had advanced lesions<br>Residual elbow symptoms in 50% of patients who were treated nonsurgically and 46% of patients who were treated surgically | III |
| Iwasaki et al (2006) | 8 | Autologous osteochondral mosaicplasty from lateral femoral condyle | 14 (11-16) | 24 (14-42) | Radiographic healing in all patients<br>Mean Timmerman and Andrews score improved from 140 to 183 points<br>7 patients were free from elbow pain, and 1 patient had occasional elbow pain<br>6 patients returned to competitive baseball | IV |
| Takahara et al (2007) | 106 | Fragment excision (55), fragment fixation/grafting (12), osteochondral graft plugs (3), nonsurgical treatment (36) | 15.3 (10-34) | 86.4 (6-300) | Stable OCD lesions with open capitellar physis and preserved ROM had good outcomes<br>Better outcomes achieved in patients with unstable lesions who underwent surgical treatment<br>6 of 7 patients with stable lesions who were treated with rest healed spontaneously | II |
| Jones et al (2010) | 21 (22 elbows) | Arthroscopic treatment (10) with mini-arthrotomy for removal of loose bodies and bone grafting (12) | 13.1 (10-17) | 48 (21-83) | Mean SANE score was 87%<br>ROM improved 17° in extension and 10° in flexion<br>87% of patients returned to preinjury level of sport | IV |

NA = not available, ROM = range of motion, SANE = Single Assessment Numeric Evaluation.

 

**Table 1** Results of Treatment for Osteochondritis Dissecans (OCD) (*continued*)

| Authors (Year) | No. of Patients | Procedure or Approach | Mean Patient Age in Years (Range) | Mean Follow-up in Months (Range) | Results | Level of Evidence |
|---|---|---|---|---|---|---|
| Miyake and Masatomi (2011) | 106 | Arthroscopic débridement of the capitellum | 15 (12-18) | 13 (8-46) | Clinically important ROM was unchanged<br>89 patients had no pain, 15 had mild pain, and 2 had severe pain<br>85% of patients returned to preinjury level of sport | V |
| Bojanić et al (2012) | 9 | Arthroscopic débridement and microfracture | 15 (12-19) | 63.6 (24-108) | 8 patients had excellent results and 1 patient had a good result | IV |
| Shi et al (2012) | 42 (43 elbows) | Arthroscopic treatment for removal of loose bodies (22), drilling (32), internal fixation (6): 60 procedures in 43 elbows | 14.2 (11.2-18.2) | 19.5 (3.5-63.6) | Uncontained lesions had larger postoperative flexion contracture and higher rates of effusion<br>17% of patients required revision surgery for pain or mechanical symptoms | IV |
| Shimada et al (2012) | 26 | Cylindrical costal osteochondral autograft | 16 (12-43) | 36 (24-51) | Mean Timmerman and Andrews score improved from 11 to 180 points<br>All patients returned to former activities and sports participation | IV |
| Tis et al (2012) | 12 | Arthroscopic treatment for removal of loose bodies (3), drilling and chondroplasty (9) | 13.1 (10.8-14.6) | 23.4 (2-60) | 67% of patients reported no pain, and 33% of patients reported occasional pain<br>9 patients were successfully treated<br>3 patients eventually underwent revision surgery | NA |
| Wulf et al (2012) | 10 | Arthroscopic microfracture | 13.9 (10.8-18.5) | 42 (27-54) | Extension improved from 20.4° to −2.2°<br>6 of the 8 patients who were involved in athletics preoperatively returned to their preinjury level of sport<br>67% of patients had no pain<br>33% of patients had occasional pain<br>83% of patients reported no locking or catching<br>17% of patients reported occasional locking or catching | IV |

NA = not available, ROM = range of motion, SANE = Single Assessment Numeric Evaluation.

who underwent fragment excision of defects that were less than one-half the width of the capitellum.

**Video 2.1** Arthroscopic Treatment of Osteochondritis Dissecans. Christopher S. Ahmad, MD; Lauren H. Redler, MD (16 min)

# Techniques

## Arthroscopic Treatment

### SETUP/EXPOSURE

- The authors of this chapter prefer the lateral decubitus position with the patient secured using a beanbag with an axillary roll.
- An arm holder is positioned at the anterior midhumerus to allow for unrestricted elbow flexion and extension.
- The lateral decubitus position allows for the anconeus muscle-splitting approach, if necessary.

### INSTRUMENTS/EQUIPMENT/IMPLANTS REQUIRED

- A standard 4.0-mm 30° arthroscope is used in most patients.
- A 2.4-mm arthroscope should be available for patients who have smaller elbows or tighter joint spaces.
- An arthroscopic shaver can be used for débridement and synovectomy.
- An 18-gauge needle is used to template the positions of the required portals to allow for appropriate access to the lesion.
- A variety of sizes of pituitary graspers is useful for removing loose bodies.
- Angled and straight ring curets for débridement and an angled microfracture awl should be available.
- A drill or K-wire driver may be used for retrograde drilling.
- Fixation can be accomplished with sutures, headless screws, absorbable pins, or cortical bone plugs.

### PROCEDURE

- The bony landmarks are palpated and marked, and the tourniquet is inflated.
- Diagnostic arthroscopy is begun, with initial portal locations made according to preoperative imaging. If loose bodies are suspected or noted in the anterior compartment on preoperative imaging, arthroscopy should begin anteriorly. If no anterior loose bodies are suspected or noted on preoperative imaging, arthroscopy should begin in the posterior compartment. The entire elbow joint, however, should be arthroscopically examined by the conclusion of the procedure to identify occult loose bodies and other potential pathologies.
- The elbow is insufflated with 15 to 20 mL of normal saline.
- The ulnar nerve is confirmed as stable within its groove.
- Anterior compartment arthroscopy is initiated at the anteromedial portal. Typically, only the skin is incised, and the anteromedial portal is established with a blunt switching stick. The arthroscope is inserted over the switching stick.
- Laterally, the anterolateral portal is established under direct visualization with the use of a spinal needle for localization.
- Diagnostic arthroscopy is begun, and loose bodies are removed with the use of a large pituitary grasper.
- The posterior compartment is accessed via the posterior central portal and the midposterolateral portal. The midposterolateral portal is established proximally enough to allow for visualization of the tip of the olecranon and the medial gutter. The midposterolateral portal also is used to view the distal lateral gutter and the posterior radiocapitellar joint.
- Loose bodies are often found in the posterior compartment and the posterolateral recess between the lateral ulna, the radial head, and the distal humerus. To improve visualization, a shaver is used to remove the synovial tissue that usually occupies this space.
- The posterior capitellum is visualized with the arthroscope, and the portal is located in the lateral soft spot with the use of a spinal needle. One or two portals are safely established in the posterolateral elbow sharply with a No. 11 blade scalpel; enough room should be maintained to maneuver in this small space.
- Depending on the size and position of the lesion, an assistant can flex the elbow to improve visualization and access.
- In addition to the standard posterolateral viewing portals, a distal ulnar portal can be used to view the capitellum head on.
- After the capitellar OCD lesion is fully visualized, the size of the lesion and the status of the cartilage are assessed.
- Lesions that have intact cartilage are managed with transhumeral drilling to keep the cartilage intact and stimulate healing of the underlying subchondral bone. Fluoroscopy is used to guide K-wire placement.
- Loose osteochondral fragments that have a healthy cancellous bed and are large enough to accept fixation are fixed with intraosseous sutures, bone pegs, chondral darts, or headless compression screws. This can be accomplished via all-arthroscopic, arthroscopic-assisted, or open surgery via the anconeus muscle-splitting approach.
- Unstable osteochondral fragments that are smaller than approximately one-half of the width of the capitellum and have little chance of healing or holding fixation are débrided to a stable margin and then managed with microfracture

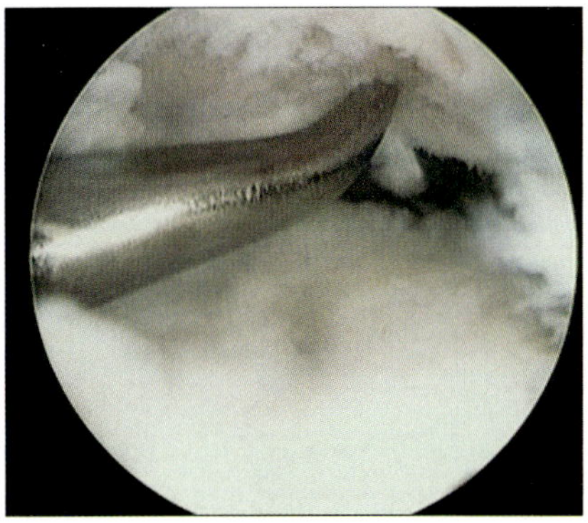

**Figure 4** Arthroscopic image of an elbow shows microfracture of an osteochondritis dissecans lesion of the capitellum after initial débridement, which was performed with a motorized shaver.

to stimulate fibrous cartilage healing (**Figure 4**). Microfracture is accomplished with an angled, sharp-tipped awl, which is used to penetrate from the sclerotic bone to the underlying cancellous bone to allow the egress of blood.

- In compliant patients, unstable osteochondral fragments or OCD defects larger than approximately one-half of the width of the capitellum—especially uncontained lesions at the lateral capitellum that articulate with the radial head—are reconstructed with osteochondral autograft from the femoral condyle.

#### WOUND CLOSURE

- The portals are sutured closed to minimize the likelihood of synovial fistula (especially in the lateral portal).
- A soft bandage is applied, and the patient is encouraged to move the elbow as tolerated.

#### POSTOPERATIVE REGIMEN

After 1 to 3 days postoperatively, the initial bulky gauze dressing is removed and portals are covered with smaller bandages. Typically, ROM normalizes without formal physical therapy within 3 to 4 weeks postoperatively. Patients are instructed to gently conduct stretching and ROM exercises of the elbow. If stiffness is present, formal stretching exercises are initiated under the supervision of a physical therapist. Joint loading in the form of throwing, weight lifting, and athletic activities must be avoided until signs of radiographic healing are noted.

## Osteochondral Autograft

#### PREOPERATIVE PLANNING

- The diameter and depth of the lesion should be estimated preoperatively.
- If the lesion is even with or posterior to the midaxis of the capitellum, a posterior approach (anconeus muscle-splitting approach) is used.
- If there is concern that placing a perfectly aligned graft will not be possible because of inadequate exposure, a lateral approach, in which the origin of the lateral collateral ligament is released and subluxation of the joint is used to allow orthogonal access, may be done.
- If prior microfracture or drilling procedures have been unsuccessful, there is no need to perform arthroscopy before arthrotomy and grafting.
- If there is a clear line of delamination, defect, and detachment, arthroscopy is of little benefit.

#### SETUP/EXPOSURE

- The patient is placed in the supine position and the contralateral knee is draped.
- If arthroscopy is to be performed first, the arm is suspended in a traction device to facilitate arthroscopic access to the posterior elbow and allow osteochondral autograft harvest from the contralateral knee. If the lateral decubitus position is preferred, the elbow is placed over an arthroscopic positioner, and the ipsilateral knee is used as the donor.
- A skin incision is made over and slightly posterior to the lateral epicondyle. Typically, the length of the incision is approximately 7 cm.
- The bony landmarks are confirmed, and the common extensor muscles and anterior capsule are divided in the midline of the capitellum.
- The anterior joint is exposed, and the lesion is visualized.
- If required for exposure, the origin of the lateral collateral ligament is detached sharply from the distal humerus, permitting subluxation of the joint. A small piece of bone or epicondylar cartilage is included in the reflected tissue to ensure accurate repositioning for the repair (**Figure 5, A**).
- If the defect can be visualized with hyperflexion of the elbow, the posterior approach is simpler than the lateral approach. A posterior skin incision is made and the anconeus muscle is split to provide a direct path to the defect. The anterior margin of the defect must be visualized. The rest of the procedure, including sizing, excavation, and graft placement, is identical to that performed with the lateral approach, except that the lateral collateral ligament is not detached and, therefore, will not require repair.

#### INSTRUMENTS/EQUIPMENT/ IMPLANTS REQUIRED

- Many commercially available systems for the harvest of osteochondral autografts exist. Ideally, the system should include graft sizes that range from 6 to 10 mm in diameter.
- In preparing the recipient site, the authors of this chapter prefer a reamer technique to excavate bone rather than a punch. The reamer provides controlled incremental bone removal, which is preferred in the limited visual field of the capitellum.

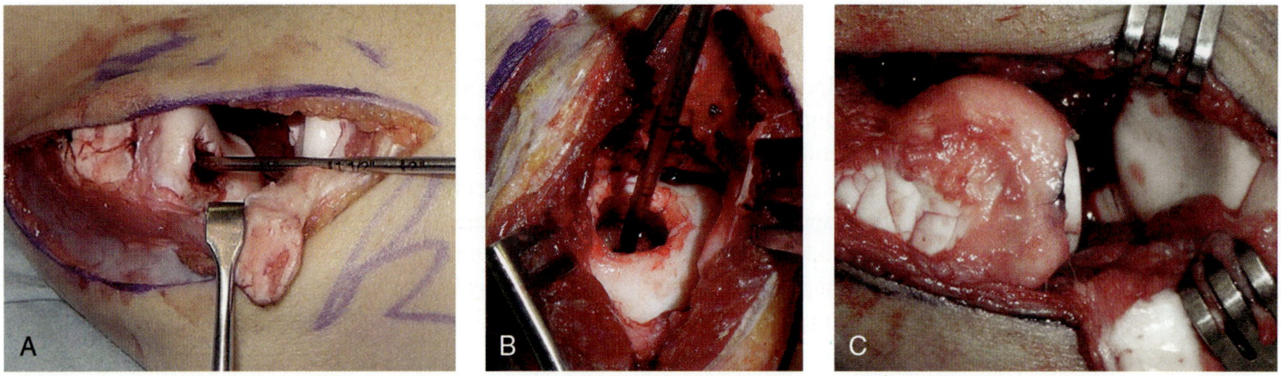

**Figure 5** Intraoperative photographs of an elbow show treatment of an osteochondritis (OCD) defect with the use of an osteochondral autograft. **A,** Photograph shows the OCD defect after takedown of the lateral ligament complex. Note the small piece of bone located just off the lateral epicondyle; this bone is used to help restore the proper origin of the lateral collateral ligament during later reattachment. **B,** Photograph taken after the OCD defect was reamed to the measured depth. The bed is ready for the autograft plug. **C,** Photograph shows the osteochondral autograft plug, which matches the curvature of the capitellar lesion.

**PROCEDURE**

- If there is any question regarding the size of the defect, the authors of this chapter recommend increasing the diameter of the recipient site to the next larger harvester size.
- Because the growth plates may still be open, it is necessary to gently excise the subchondral bone but not penetrate beyond 8 to 10 mm in depth. Therefore, the authors of this chapter use a 2.4-mm centering pin to ensure that alignment is orthogonal to the cartilage surface. The depth of the pin should be slightly greater than the depth of the excavation.
- A reamer of the proper diameter is placed over the guide pin, and the defect is carefully excavated, using power, down to bleeding bone (**Figure 5, B**). In the experience of the authors of this chapter, a 1.0-cm diameter graft is the most common graft size used.
- The location of the donor site is determined with the aid of preoperative MRI. The lateral-superior anterior surface of the femoral trochlea is a safe zone that provides a closely matching curvature in all planes for replacement of the diseased and damaged tissue. The bone of an adolescent femur is quite hard, and retrieving a graft from it can be a challenge. A rapid twisting movement is often necessary to free the plug.
- The plug is harvested from the femur, and the graft is sized for depth so that it can be gently impacted but not countersunk into place. Ideally, the cartilage should be absolutely flush with the surrounding native cartilage of the capitellum; however, 1 mm or less of prominence also is acceptable.
- The depth of the defect should be measured before the graft is seated. The graft should be equal to the depth of the defect. Removal of bone from the base of the plug may be required.
- The insertion alignment of the osteochondral plug should be closely observed, making certain that the cylinder of the graft is aligned with the walls of the defect. Any angular misalignment will cause the graft to wedge and prevent full insertion.
- The graft is seated in the defect. No supplemental fixation is required if the graft is stable (**Figure 5, C**).
- The contact of the joint against the graft is assessed with the elbow in flexion-extension and pronation-supination.

**WOUND CLOSURE**

- If the lateral approach was used, the origin of the lateral ligament must be accurately restored.
- With the posterior anconeus approach, the anconeus fascia should be closed to minimize muscle herniations.

**POSTOPERATIVE REGIMEN**

The elbow is placed in a resting splint in 90° of elbow flexion and neutral forearm rotation for approximately 4 to 6 weeks postoperatively. The patient begins active ROM within 1 week postoperatively. If the ligament origin was detached and repaired, varus stress is avoided for the first 4 to 6 weeks postoperatively. In patients who have stiffness that persists beyond 6 weeks postoperatively, static progressive flexion and extension splinting is initiated under the guidance of a physical therapist.

## Limiting Adverse Events

To enhance visualization of a capitellar OCD lesion, an AP radiograph of the elbow in 45° of flexion as well as CT and MRI should be obtained preoperatively. Although MRI can help surgeons appreciate the position, depth, and size of a capitellar OCD lesion, it provides poor visualization of the depth and quality of the subchondral bone that remains on the fragment. Therefore, the authors of this chapter prefer to use CT to assess the bony composition of a capitellar OCD fragment. In addition, three-dimensional CT allows for excellent visualization of the position of an OCD lesion on the capitellum.

Although loose bodies are most often found in the recess between the posterior radial head and the ulna, they can be found anywhere in the elbow. The failure to locate and remove all loose bodies can result in persistent mechanical symptoms.

Good early results have been reported in patients who underwent débridement alone; however, patients who have larger lesions may have better long-term outcomes with reconstruction of the articular surface. Throwers who have lateral capitellar lesions that articulate with the radial head and adaptive medial collateral ligament laxity should be strongly considered for reconstructive procedures to restore hyaline cartilage. Poor long-term outcomes have been reported in patients who underwent excision alone; however, these patients were older and often had advanced lesions. There are no long-term follow-up data on patients who underwent the more modern treatment strategies described in this chapter.

## Bibliography


Bauer M, Jonsson K, Josefsson PO, Lindén B: Osteochondritis dissecans of the elbow: A long-term follow-up study. *Clin Orthop Relat Res* 1992;(284):156-160.

Baumgarten TE, Andrews JR, Satterwhite YE: The arthroscopic classification and treatment of osteochondritis dissecans of the capitellum. *Am J Sports Med* 1998;26(4):520-523.

Bojanić I, Smoljanović T, Dokuzović S: Osteochondritis dissecans of the elbow: Excellent results in teenage athletes treated by arthroscopic débridement and microfracture. *Croat Med J* 2012;53(1):40-47.

Brittberg M, Winalski CS: Evaluation of cartilage injuries and repair. *J Bone Joint Surg Am* 2003;85(suppl 2):58-69.

Davis JT, Idjadi JA, Siskosky MJ, ElAttrache NS: Dual direct lateral portals for treatment of osteochondritis dissecans of the capitellum: An anatomic study. *Arthroscopy* 2007;23(7):723-728.

Iwasaki N, Kato H, Ishikawa J, Saitoh S, Minami A: Autologous osteochondral mosaicplasty for capitellar osteochondritis dissecans in teenaged patients. *Am J Sports Med* 2006;34(8):1233-1239.

Jones KJ, Wiesel BB, Sankar WN, Ganley TJ: Arthroscopic management of osteochondritis dissecans of the capitellum: Mid-term results in adolescent athletes. *J Pediatr Orthop* 2010;30(1):8-13.

Mihara K, Tsutsui H, Nishinaka N, Yamaguchi K: Nonoperative treatment for osteochondritis dissecans of the capitellum. *Am J Sports Med* 2009;37(2):298-304.

Miyake J, Masatomi T: Arthroscopic debridement of the humeral capitellum for osteochondritis dissecans: Radiographic and clinical outcomes. *J Hand Surg Am* 2011;36(8):1333-1338.

Shi LL, Bae DS, Kocher MS, Micheli LJ, Waters PM: Contained versus uncontained lesions in juvenile elbow osteochondritis dissecans. *J Pediatr Orthop* 2012;32(3):221-225.

Shimada K, Tanaka H, Matsumoto T, et al: Cylindrical costal osteochondral autograft for reconstruction of large defects of the capitellum due to osteochondritis dissecans. *J Bone Joint Surg Am* 2012;94(11):992-1002.

Takahara M, Mura N, Sasaki J, Harada M, Ogino T: Classification, treatment, and outcome of osteochondritis dissecans of the humeral capitellum. *J Bone Joint Surg Am* 2007;89(6):1205-1214.

Takahara M, Mura N, Sasaki J, Harada M, Ogino T: Classification, treatment, and outcome of osteochondritis dissecans of the humeral capitellum: Surgical technique. *J Bone Joint Surg Am* 2008;90(suppl 2 pt 1):47-62.

Takahara M, Ogino T, Sasaki I, Kato H, Minami A, Kaneda K: Long term outcome of osteochondritis dissecans of the humeral capitellum. *Clin Orthop Relat Res* 1999;(363):108-115.

Takeba J, Takahashi T, Hino K, Watanabe S, Imai H, Yamamoto H: Arthroscopic technique for fragment fixation using absorbable pins for osteochondritis dissecans of the humeral capitellum: A report of 4 cases. *Knee Surg Sports Traumatol Arthrosc* 2010;18(6):831-835.

Tis JE, Edmonds EW, Bastrom T, Chambers HG: Short-term results of arthroscopic treatment of osteochondritis dissecans in skeletally immature patients. *J Pediatr Orthop* 2012;32(3):226-231.

van den Ende KI, McIntosh AL, Adams JE, Steinmann SP: Osteochondritis dissecans of the capitellum: A review of the literature and a distal ulnar portal. *Arthroscopy* 2011;27(1):122-128.

Wahegaonkar AL, Doi K, Hattori Y, Addosooki A: Technique of osteochondral autograft transplantation mosaicplasty for capitellar osteochondritis dissecans. *J Hand Surg Am* 2007;32(9):1454-1461.

Wulf CA, Stone RM, Giveans MR, Lervick GN: Magnetic resonance imaging after arthroscopic microfracture of capitellar osteochondritis dissecans. *Am J Sports Med* 2012;40(11):2549-2556.

## Video Reference

Ahmad CS, Redler LH: Arthroscopic treatment of osteochondritis dissecans, in Field LD, Steinmann SP, eds: *Arthroscopic Surgical Techniques: Elbow Arthroscopy* [DVD]. Rosemont, IL, American Academy of Orthopaedic Surgeons, 2013.

 

# Chapter 3

# Arthroscopic Radial Head Excision

*Felix H. Savoie III, MD*
*Michael J. O'Brien, MD*

**Learning Objectives**

- Recognize the appropriate indications for arthroscopic radial head excision.
- Appreciate the visualization and surgical portals needed for arthroscopic radial head excision.
- Recognize the risks as well as the short- and long-term complications of arthroscopic radial head excision.

## Indications

Arthroscopic radial head excision is indicated to manage arthritis and/or deformity about the radiocapitellar joint in which most of the pathology is on the radial head side of the joint, with resultant pain and limitation of motion sufficient to warrant surgery. Evidence suggests that injuries to the lateral column may lead to further deterioration of the entire elbow joint, and radial head excision mitigates that risk. In patients in whom the elbow and forearm ligaments are stable, excision of the radial head is a reasonable treatment option.

## Contraindications

Radial head excision is contraindicated in patients with an abnormal interosseous ligament of the forearm and in those with medial or lateral instability of the elbow. In these patients, excision of the radial head will result in increased instability.

## Alternative Treatments

Alternatives to radial head excision include radial head replacement and total elbow arthroplasty. Radial head replacement is a satisfactory alternative if additional ligament reconstruction is planned and in patients with a dysfunctional interosseous ligament with risk of proximal migration of the radius. Total elbow arthroplasty is an excellent option for the older, sedentary individual with preexisting arthritis of the ulnohumeral articulation.

## Results

Published results of arthroscopic radial head excision are summarized in **Table 1**. Limited data are available, but in general the results of arthroscopic radial head excision are comparable to, if not better than, those of open resection. In four studies evaluating a total of 64 patients treated arthroscopically, the average success rate was 95%. The primary complications were stiffness (one patient) and difficulty with heavy activities (number of patients not reported). In most patients, additional arthroscopic procedures were performed simultaneously because of the improved visualization and access afforded by the arthroscopic technique.

**Video 3.1** Arthroscopic Radial Head Excision. Felix H. Savoie III, MD (2 min)

*Dr. Savoie or an immediate family member has received royalties from Exactech; is a member of a speakers' bureau or has made paid presentations on behalf of Mitek Sports Medicine and Smith & Nephew; serves as an unpaid consultant to Biomet, Exactech, Mitek Sports Medicine, Rotation Medical, and Smith & Nephew; has received research or institutional support from Mitek Sports Medicine; and serves as a board member, owner, officer, or committee member of the American Shoulder and Elbow Surgeons and the Arthroscopy Association of North America. Dr. O'Brien or an immediate family member serves as a paid consultant to Smith & Nephew; has received research or institutional support from Mitek Sports Medicine; has received nonincome support (such as equipment or services), commercially derived honoraria, or other non–research-related funding (such as paid travel) from DePuy Synthes, Mitek Sports Medicine, and Smith & Nephew; and serves as a board member, owner, officer, or committee member of the Association of American Medical Colleges and the Arthroscopy Association of North America.*

**Table 1** Results of Arthroscopic Radial Head Excision

| Authors (Year) | No. of Patients | Mean Patient Age in Years (Range) | Mean Follow-up in Months (Range) | Success Rate (%) | Results | Level of Evidence |
|---|---|---|---|---|---|---|
| Lo and King (1994) | 1 | 48 | 6 | 100 | Flexion from 30°-135°<br>Pronation and supination unrestricted<br>Pain decreased to 60% of the preoperative level | V |
| Menth-Chiari et al (2001) | 12 | 38 (17-55) | 39 (12-97) | 91.7 | 7 excellent<br>4 good<br>1 poor | IV |
| McLaughlin et al (2006) | 36 | 45.7 (26-68) | 52 (18-91) | 94.4 | Results were better after early excision than after delayed excision | IV |
| Wijeratna et al (2012) | 15 | 49.6 (34-73) | 20 (5-47) | 100 | Mean VAS pain score, 1.7 (range, 0-4)<br>Mean QuickDASH score, 24.7 (range, 7-44) | IV |

DASH = Disabilities of the Arm, Shoulder and Hand; VAS = visual analog scale.

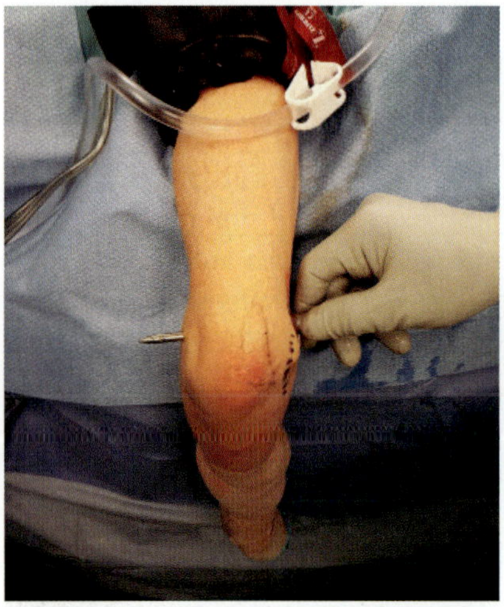

**Figure 1** Intraoperative photograph of the elbow with the patient in the prone position, which allows multiple entry points for cannula placement. The dashed line indicates the location of the ulnar nerve. (Copyright Felix H. Savoie III, MD, New Orleans, LA.)

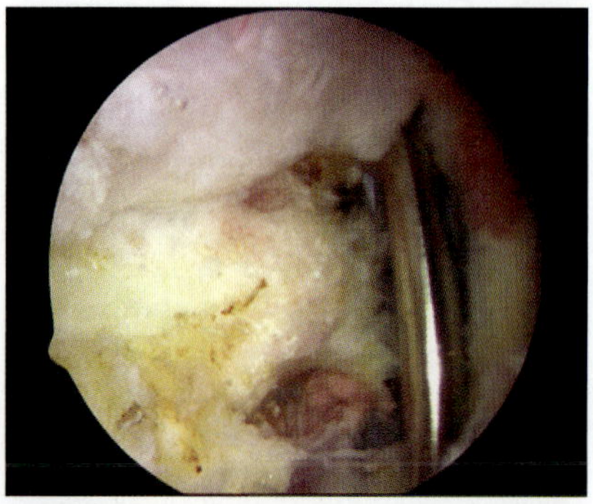

**Figure 2** Arthroscopic view from the proximal anterolateral portal demonstrates a posttraumatic radiocapitellar joint with painful, limited motion. The joint is essentially destroyed. (Copyright Felix H. Savoie III, MD, New Orleans, LA.)

# Technique

## Setup/Exposure

- The patient is placed in the prone or lateral decubitus position with the affected upper arm supported by a small bolster or arm holder (**Figure 1**).
- General or regional anesthesia is administered.
- The elbow is insufflated via a posterior central portal.
- The ulnar nerve and landmarks are marked on the affected elbow.
- The arthroscope is inserted via a proximal anteromedial portal to visualize the radiocapitellar joint (**Figure 2**).

## Instruments/Equipment/Implants Required

- The authors of this chapter prefer a standard 4-mm arthroscope using a bridge system to allow easy movement of the arthroscope and instruments from portal to portal.
- A standard soft-tissue shaver and hooded burr are used for the resection.

## Procedure

- After the preoperative decision to excise the arthritic or deformed radial head has been confirmed, a proximal anterolateral portal is placed to allow instrumentation to the anterior radial head.
- A hooded burr is used to remove the anterior aspect of the radial head to the predetermined depth. The width of the shaver can be useful in helping to judge the amount of bone resected (**Figure 3**).

 

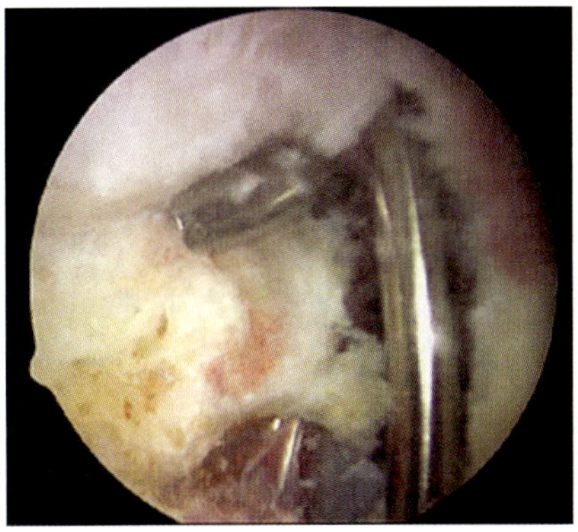

**Figure 3** Arthroscopic view from the proximal anteromedial portal demonstrates the initial step in arthroscopic radial head excision. The anterior aspect of the radial head is resected while staying inside the ring of the annular ligament. (Copyright Felix H. Savoie III, MD, New Orleans, LA.)

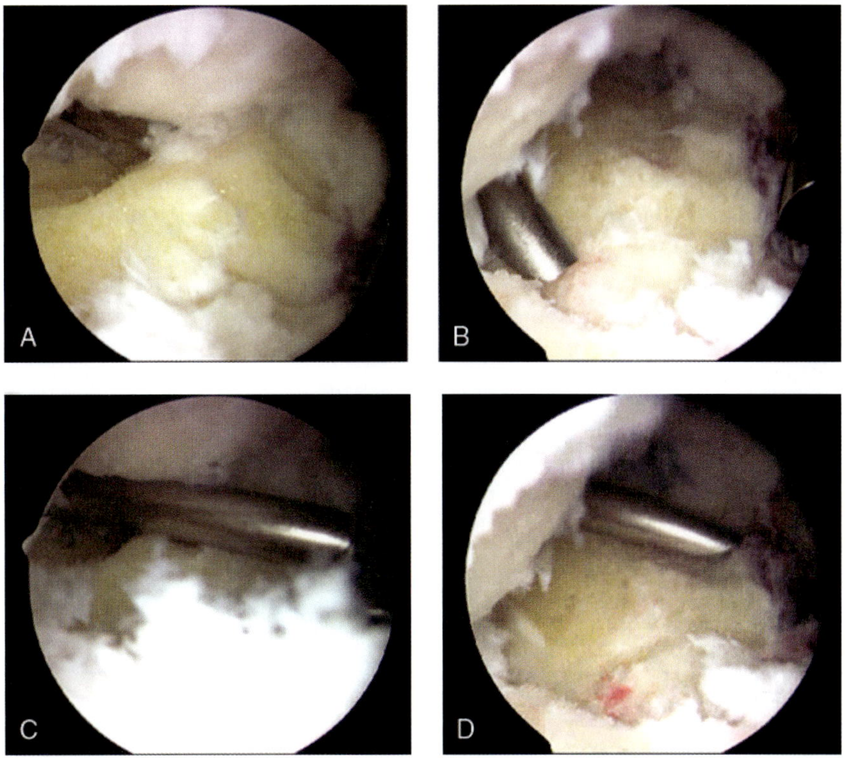


**Figure 4** Arthroscopic images demonstrate the sequential steps in radial head excision. **A,** A spinal needle is used to localize the correct angle and placement of the soft-spot portal. **B,** The anterior cannula is positioned to act as a retractor and protect the radial nerve. **C,** The shaver is used to resect the radial head from the posterior soft-spot portal. **D,** The completed radial head resection. (Copyright Felix H. Savoie III, MD, New Orleans, LA.)

- A spinal needle is placed through the soft-spot portal to confirm proper angulation (**Figure 4, A**). Creation of the skin incision slightly more distal than normal is helpful to enable adequate coplaning.
- A cannula is inserted across the radiocapitellar joint into the anterior compartment.
- A blunt trocar is inserted into the anterolateral cannula and placed inside the annular ligament to act as a retractor and protect the radial nerve (**Figure 4, B**).
- The hooded burr is introduced into the soft-spot portal, and the remainder of the radial head is resected until it is level with the anterior resection (**Figure 4, C**).
- The radial neck is coplaned until the appropriate amount has been excised (**Figure 4, D**).
- The forearm is pronated and supinated to confirm adequate resection. The soft-tissue shaver is used in the anterolateral and soft-spot portals to remove any loose fragments.
- The arthroscope is moved to the posterocentral portal, and the medial and lateral gutters are evaluated for loose bodies and other pathology. The area of resection is also visualized from this portal to confirm adequate radial head resection (**Figure 5**).

### Wound Closure

- The lateral portals are closed with a 3-0 nylon suture.
- The posterior and medial portals are left open for drainage.

## Postoperative Regimen

A soft dressing is placed over the incisions and the patient undergoes cryocompression therapy and stretching for the first 72 hours postoperatively. Physical therapy is started within 1 week postoperatively in patients who had substantial loss of range of motion

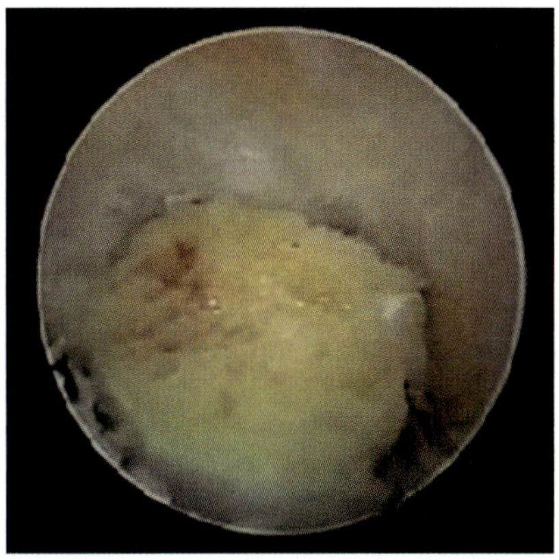

**Figure 5** Arthroscopic view from the posterior portal shows the final step. The resection of the radial head is evaluated to ascertain the accuracy of the resection. (Copyright Felix H. Savoie III, MD, New Orleans, LA.)

preoperatively. Patients are encouraged to begin strengthening exercises and return to normal activity as soon as possible.

## Limiting Adverse Events

Elbow arthroscopy may be fraught with complications. A thorough understanding of the anatomy is essential before attempting arthroscopic management of the radial head. To limit problems, it is important to begin by establishing a proximal anteromedial portal for visualization, using a retractor to protect the radial nerve at all times. In patients with anteriorly displaced fractures that have penetrated the capsule, it is necessary to identify the posterior interosseous nerve before initiating the arthroscopy. Standard precautions of marking the neurovascular structures and insufflating the elbow are common to any elbow arthroscopy. In patients with posttraumatic elbows, the anatomy may be substantially altered and arthroscopy should be halted immediately if there is a lack of orientation during the procedure.

## Bibliography

Desloges W, King GJ: Arthroscopic radial head resection and open radial head replacement, in Savoie FH, Field LD, Steinmann SP, eds: *The Elbow and Wrist: AANA Advanced Arthroscopic Surgical Techniques.* Thorofare, NJ, Slack, 2016, pp 109-126.

Lo IK, King GJ: Arthroscopic radial head excision. *Arthroscopy* 1994;10(6):689-692.

McLaughlin RE II, Savoie FH III, Field LD, Ramsey JR: Arthroscopic treatment of the arthritic elbow due to primary radiocapitellar arthritis. *Arthroscopy* 2006;22(1):63-69.

Menth-Chiari WA, Ruch DS, Poehling GG: Arthroscopic excision of the radial head: Clinical outcome in 12 patients with post-traumatic arthritis after fracture of the radial head or rheumatoid arthritis. *Arthroscopy* 2001;17(9):918-923.

Petterson SC, Stelma S, Plancher KD: Arthroscopic radial head resection in Savoie FH, Field LD, Steinmann SP, eds: *The Elbow and Wrist: AANA Advanced Arthroscopic Surgical Techniques.* Thorofare, NJ, Slack, 2016, pp 127-136.

Wijeratna M, Bailey KA, Pace A, Tytherleigh-Strong G, Van Rensburg L, Kent M: Arthroscopic radial head excision in managing elbow trauma. *Int Orthop* 2012;36(12):2507-2512.

## Video Reference

Savoie FH III: Video. *Arthroscopic Radial Head Excision.* New Orleans, LA, 2015.

 

# Chapter 4
# Arthroscopic Management of Osteoarthritis of the Elbow

*Scott P. Steinmann, MD*

**Learning Objectives**

- Understand and identify indications for arthroscopic débridement to manage elbow osteoarthritis.
- Understand techniques for arthroscopic management of elbow arthritis.

## Indications

Patients with primary elbow arthritis who have notable limitation of motion and pain at the end range of motion are candidates for arthroscopic débridement of osteophytes. Most patients with posttraumatic contracture have heterotopic ossification, errant implants, ulnar neuropathy, or malunion and will benefit from open surgery to gain motion. However, a small subset of these patients who do not present with these complications but do have posttraumatic osteoarthritis may benefit from arthroscopic treatment.

## Contraindications

Patients with implants that block motion and who have undergone previous ulnar nerve transposition may be best treated with an open procedure. In some patients with prior ulnar nerve transposition, the nerve can be localized and protected using palpation or ultrasonography in an effort to reduce the risks associated with placement of medial portals. Patients who previously underwent submuscular transposition should be treated with open surgery.

## Alternative Treatments

In patients with pain through the entire arc of motion, arthroscopic débridement of osteophytes may not result in improvement. Resurfacing procedures should be considered in such patients. Because of the modest and temporary gains achieved with surgical treatment and its attendant risks, discomforts, and inconveniences, each patient should consider a course of nonsurgical management such as intra-articular steroid injections and oral NSAIDs.

*Dr. Steinmann or an immediate family member has received royalties from Arthrex, Zimmer Biomet, and Innovative Medical Device Solutions; serves as a paid consultant to Arthrex, Zimmer Biomet, and Elsevier; and serves as a board member, owner, officer, or committee member of the American Shoulder and Elbow Surgeons and the American Society for Surgery of the Hand.*

## Results

Arthroscopic and open débridement of osteophytes for osteoarthritis of the elbow produce similar motion and pain relief as well as a similar rate of adverse events (**Table 1**). The risk of neurologic injury cannot be eliminated even when the procedure is performed by an expert surgeon.

## Technique

### Setup/Exposure

- Preoperative radiographs as well as two- and three-dimensional CT reconstructions are useful in surgical planning.
- The author of this chapter prefers to administer general anesthesia so that nerve injuries are apparent during the hospital stay.
- The author of this chapter prefers to place the patient in the lateral decubitus position (**Figure 1**).
- Use of an arm holder that elevates the elbow and is not bulky allows substantial flexion and limits interference from the patient's body.
- A nonsterile tourniquet is applied to the upper arm.
- The arm is secured to the arm holder with a light bandage.
- The arm is washed with antibacterial solution and sterile drapes are applied.
- A compressive wrap is applied from

**Table 1** Results of Débridement of Osteophytes to Manage Osteoarthritis[a]

| Authors (Year) | Number of Patients (Elbows) | Procedure or Approach | Mean Patient Age in Years (Range) | Mean Follow-up in Months (Range) |
|---|---|---|---|---|
| Antuña et al (2002) | 45 (46) | Open | 48 (30-74) | 80 (24-164) |
| Wada et al (2004) | 32 (33) | Open | 50 (23-83) | 121 (25-199) |
| McLaughlin et al (2006) | 36 (36) | Arthroscopic | 45.7 (26-68) | 52 (18-91) |
| Krishnan et al (2007) | 11 (11) | Arthroscopic | 36 (23-47) | 26 (24-29) |
| Adams et al (2008) | 41 (42) | Arthroscopic | 53 (20-73) | 44 (26-68) |
| Hattori et al (2011) | 31 (31) | Open | 59 (40-75) | 19 (12-36) |
| MacLean et al (2013) | 20 (21) | Arthroscopic | 42 (22-79) | 66 (24-144) |
| Lim et al (2014) | 43 (43) | Arthroscopic | 51.4 (33-69) | 38 (18-77) |
| Miyake et al (2014) | 20 | Arthroscopic | 38 (19-55) | 25 (24-29) |

[a] All studies are level IV evidence.
[b] Good-to-excellent results reported unless otherwise noted.
[c] Success rates based on pain relief and satisfaction with procedure.

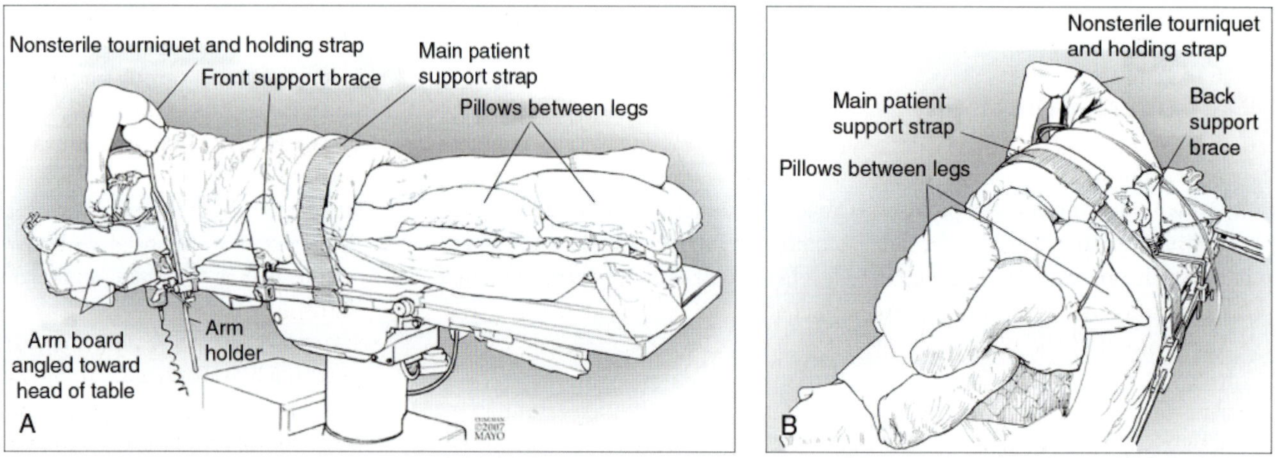


**Figure 1** Illustrations show side (**A**) and end-on (**B**) views of a patient placed in the lateral decubitus position in preparation for elbow arthroscopy. (Reproduced with permission from the Mayo Foundation for Medical Education and Research, Rochester, MN.)

 

**Table 1** Results of Débridement of Osteophytes to Manage Osteoarthritis[a] *(continued)*

| Success Rate (%)[b] | Results | Comments |
|---|---|---|
| 74 | Mean flexion-extension arc of motion improved from 79° to 101°<br>Pain was nonexistent or mild in 35 elbows (76%) and moderate or severe in 11 (24%)<br>13 patients had ulnar neuropathy | — |
| 85 | Mean total range of motion improved from 70° to 94°<br>Pain was nonexistent in 28 elbows (85%) and mild in 5 (15%) | 19 elbows were followed for >10 yr<br>Revision surgery was performed on 3 elbows |
| 100 (radial head excision alone)<br>93 (radial head excision and ulnohumeral arthroplasty)[c] | Total arc of motion increased 62° after radial head excision alone and 46° after radial head excision and ulnohumeral arthroplasty | 8 patients underwent radial head excision alone, and 28 patients underwent radial head excision with ulnohumeral arthroplasty<br>2 patients who underwent both procedures subsequently underwent revision |
| Not reported | Mean total arc of motion improved from 60° to 133°<br>Mean subjective pain level improved from 9.2 to 1.7 (10 indicates worst pain, 0 indicates no pain) | — |
| 81 | Mean flexion arc of motion improved from 117.3° to 131.6° | Heterotopic ossification developed in 1 elbow<br>Ulnar neuropathy occurred in 1 elbow |
| 100 | Elbow motion improved in all patients | Hematoma developed in 3 elbows |
| 76 | No notable improvement in mean flexion arc | — |
| 79 | Pain decreased in 38 patients (88%)<br>Mean flexion arc increased from 103° to 116° | 5 patients underwent revision surgery<br>Ulnar neuropathy developed in 3 of 4 patients with persistent pain and limited motion |
| 100 | Mean flexion improved from 121° to 130°<br>Pain decreased or resolved in all patients | — |

[a] All studies are level IV evidence.
[b] Good-to-excellent results reported unless otherwise noted.
[c] Success rates based on pain relief and satisfaction with procedure.

the hand to the proximal forearm to limit distal swelling.

- The patient's body is oriented 20° toward the surgeon to limit pressure in the antecubital fossa.
- All bony landmarks are palpated and marked, including the medial and lateral epicondyles, capitellum, radial head, and olecranon process.
- The location of the ulnar nerve is noted and marked.
- The ulnar nerve is examined for subluxation with flexion.

## Instruments/Equipment/Implants Required

- A standard 4.0- to 4.5-mm arthroscope with 30° angulation is used.
- A low-pressure (20 to 30 mm Hg), low-flow saline pump is needed.
- A shaver (4.0 to 5.5 mm) and burr (4.0 to 5.0 mm) are used.
- A radiofrequency probe is used, but not around the ulnar or radial nerve.
- Standard arthroscopy instruments such as graspers are used.

## Procedure

- In patients with preoperative ulnar neuropathy, an in situ decompression of the ulnar nerve is performed.
- Surgery is begun through the medial or the lateral portal on either the anterior or the posterior side of the joint.
- Starting the procedure posterior is preferred in patients with the greatest number of osteophytes on the posterior aspect of the joint and for whom increased terminal extension is a primary goal of the surgery.

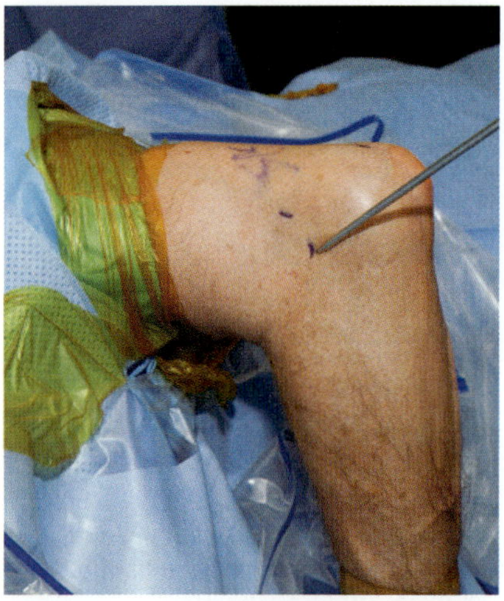

**Figure 2** Intraoperative photograph of an elbow shows a switching stick identifying the anterolateral portal.

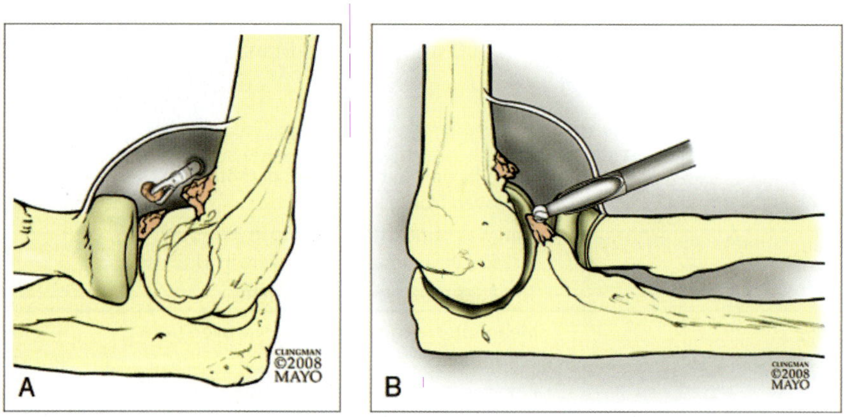


**Figure 3** **A,** Illustration of an elbow shows removal of loose bodies with a grasper placed through the anteromedial portal. The capsule is intact. The area is depicted as it would be seen through the anterolateral portal. **B,** Illustration of the medial view of the surgical site shows removal of osteophytes with a shaver placed through the anterolateral portal. The capsule is intact. (Reproduced with permission from the Mayo Foundation for Medical Education and Research, Rochester, MN.)

- The joint is insufflated with 20 mL of saline through an 18-gauge needle.
- The author of this chapter prefers to create the initial portal on the anterolateral side (**Figure 2**).
- The anterolateral portal is established at the radiocapitellar joint.
- An incision is made in the skin, the soft tissues are spread, and a blunt trocar is directed through the capsule to the center of the coronoid fossa.
- The anteromedial portal is established using an inside-out technique. The anteromedial portal is safer to work through than the anterolateral portal because there is more distance between the median nerve and the capsule on the medial side than between the radial nerve and the capsule on the lateral side.
- The site of portal placement is visualized, the camera and cannula are advanced to the capsule (to be sure that the correct site has been reached), the camera is removed from the cannula, and a switching stick is driven through the capsule and subcutaneous tissues to the skin.
- The skin is incised with a knife.
- An outflow cannula is placed over the switching stick.
- The cannulas are centered in the joint, the switching stick is removed, and the camera is inserted.
- Retractor portals are added proximal to the medial and lateral sides as needed.
- A switching stick, a Freer elevator, or a specially designed instrument can be used as a retractor.
- To improve visualization, it is better to add a retractor than to use increased fluid flow or pressure.
- The surgical site is visualized through the anterolateral portal, and the shaver and burr are inserted through the anteromedial portal for removal of loose bodies, osteophytes excision, and removal of the contracted capsule (**Figure 3, A**).
- An effort is made to keep the capsule intact while débriding the osteophytes to avoid extravasation of fluid into the soft tissues, which limits access and visibility (**Figure 3, B**).
- Release of the humeral attachment of the capsule is often sufficient to improve elbow extension. Suction can increase the risk of neurologic injury and is not recommended in the anterior elbow compartment.
- Suction is unnecessary when using a shaver in the anterior joint. Typically, gravity flow through the shaver is sufficient to remove debris when the shaver is held horizontal to the floor.
- To address the lateral half of the joint, the arthroscope is moved to the medial portal and the shaver and burr are moved to the lateral portal.
- The radial and posterior interosseous nerves are at risk during resection of the capsule over the radial head and anterolateral elbow (**Figure 4**).
- The posterior interosseous nerve lies in the fat pad that is often encountered just anterior to the radial head after the capsule is resected.
- The first posterior portal to be placed is the posterolateral portal located just lateral to the tip of the olecranon.
- The working portal for the shaver and burr is the direct posterior portal located centrally at the proximal part of the olecranon fossa (**Figure 5**).
- To improve visualization, a shaver is used to remove the fat pad from

 

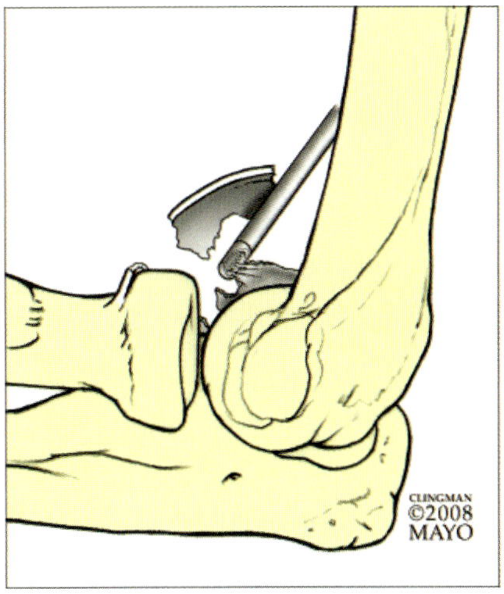


**Figure 4** Lateral illustration of the elbow shows the appearance of the portion of the capsule left intact over the area of the posterior interosseous nerve. (Reproduced with permission from the Mayo Foundation for Medical Education and Research, Rochester, MN.)

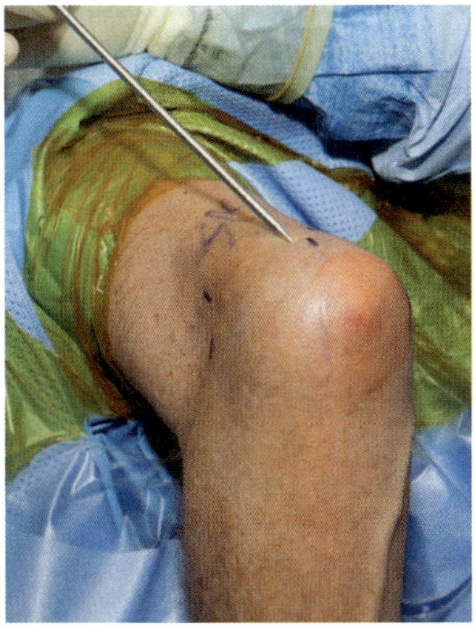

**Figure 5** Intraoperative photograph of an elbow shows the switching stick identifying the direct posterior working portal.

the posterior fossa.

- Osteophytes on the medial and lateral aspects of the olecranon are removed with a burr or high-speed rasp.
- If an in situ release of the ulnar nerve was performed, the nerve is visualized and protected throughout the procedure.
- In a patient with mild neuropathy, an expert surgeon may attempt an all-arthroscopic release of the nerve to resolve symptoms.

### Wound Closure

- The author of this chapter prefers to close portals with nylon simple sutures in the skin.
- Medial portals may drain, and it is important to close these adequately.
- In situ ulnar nerve release can be closed with a running nylon suture.

## Postoperative Regimen

A soft compressive dressing is applied from midarm to the wrist before the tourniquet is released. The patient is discharged on the day of surgery. Use of the elbow for activities of daily living is encouraged. The patient is taught to do active, self-assisted stretching exercises beginning after postoperative day 2 when the dressing is removed. Patients who can, on the second postoperative day, move the treated elbow through an arc of motion measuring at least 45° are prescribed a hinged static progressive splint to aid in stretching. For the small number of patients in whom pain is too severe for them to move and exercise the elbow themselves, a brachial plexus catheter and continuous passive motion machine can be used for the first 48 hours postoperatively. Manipulation under anesthesia can be done 2 to 3 weeks postoperatively if progress is slow. Manipulation later than 1 month postoperatively is rarely successful.

## Limiting Adverse Events

Heterotopic ossification may develop at the site of osteophyte removal. If the bone blocks motion, a second surgery may be needed to remove the bone. Some patients experience persistent pain postoperatively, and additional surgery may be required.

The ulnar, median, and radial nerves at the level of the elbow are at risk intraoperatively. Neurologic injury is more common in patients with abnormal joint architecture, such as patients with posttraumatic injuries and those who have undergone previous procedures on the elbow. Ulnar neuropathy is often managed with a second surgery to release the nerve.

## Bibliography

Adams JE, Steinmann SP: Nerve injuries about the elbow. *J Hand Surg Am* 2006;31(2):303-313.

Adams JE, Wolff LH III, Merten SM, Steinmann SP: Osteoarthritis of the elbow: Results of arthroscopic osteophyte resection and capsulectomy. *J Shoulder Elbow Surg* 2008;17(1):126-131.

Antuña SA, Morrey BF, Adams RA, O'Driscoll SW: Ulnohumeral arthroplasty for primary degenerative arthritis of the elbow: Long-term outcome and complications. *J Bone Joint Surg Am* 2002;84(12):2168-2173.

Hattori Y, Doi K, Sakamoto S, Hoshino S, Dodakundi C: Capsulectomy and debridement for primary osteoarthritis of the elbow through a medial trans-flexor approach. *J Hand Surg Am* 2011;36(10):1652-1658.

Kovachevich R, Steinmann SP: Arthroscopic ulnar nerve decompression in the setting of elbow osteoarthritis. *J Hand Surg Am* 2012;37(4):663-668.

Krishnan SG, Harkins DC, Pennington SD, Harrison DK, Burkhead WZ: Arthroscopic ulnohumeral arthroplasty for degenerative arthritis of the elbow in patients under fifty years of age. *J Shoulder Elbow Surg* 2007;16(4):443-448.

Lim TK, Koh KH, Lee HI, Shim JW, Park MJ: Arthroscopic débridement for primary osteoarthritis of the elbow: Analysis of preoperative factors affecting outcome. *J Shoulder Elbow Surg* 2014;23(9):1381-1387.

MacLean SB, Oni T, Crawford LA, Deshmukh SC: Medium-term results of arthroscopic debridement and capsulectomy for the treatment of elbow osteoarthritis. *J Shoulder Elbow Surg* 2013;22(5):653-657.

McLaughlin RE II, Savoie FH III, Field LD, Ramsey JR: Arthroscopic treatment of the arthritic elbow due to primary radiocapitellar arthritis. *Arthroscopy* 2006;22(1):63-69.

Miyake J, Shimada K, Oka K, et al: Arthroscopic debridement in the treatment of patients with osteoarthritis of the elbow, based on computer simulation. *Bone Joint J* 2014;96(2):237-241.

Ogilvie-Harris DJ, Gordon R, MacKay M: Arthroscopic treatment for posterior impingement in degenerative arthritis of the elbow. *Arthroscopy* 1995;11(4):437-443.

Ruch DS, Poehling GG: Anterior interosseus nerve injury following elbow arthroscopy. *Arthroscopy* 1997;13(6):756-758.

Steinmann SP, King GJ, Savoie FH III; American Academy of Orthopaedic Surgeons: Arthroscopic treatment of the arthritic elbow. *J Bone Joint Surg Am* 2005;87(9):2114-2121.

Wada T, Isogai S, Ishii S, Yamashita T: Débridement arthroplasty for primary osteoarthritis of the elbow. *J Bone Joint Surg Am* 2004;86(2):233-241.

 

# Chapter 5
# Arthroscopic Posteromedial Decompression for Valgus Extension Overload

*Christopher S. Ahmad, MD*
*Justin L. Hodgins, MD*

**Learning Objectives**

- Recognize the history, physical examination maneuvers, and radiographic findings consistent with valgus extension overload.
- Discuss patient selection for posteromedial decompression, identify relative contraindications to the procedure, and demonstrate knowledge of alternative treatments.
- Demonstrate knowledge of surgical setup, portal placement, and identification of pathology during diagnostic arthroscopy.
- Identify techniques to avoid injury to the ulnar nerve during olecranon osteophyte removal.
- Discuss postoperative care and rehabilitation after surgical management of valgus extension overload.

## Indications

Valgus extension overload is a type of elbow arthritis that results from repetitive valgus stress in throwing athletes. High compression and shear forces are experienced when the posteromedial olecranon contacts the trochlea, resulting in posteromedial impingement (PMI). Patients have a history of throwing or repetitive overhead activity, and symptoms are often preceded by a decrease in pitch velocity, a decrease in control, and early fatigability. In patients with isolated valgus extension overload, elbow pain is localized to the posteromedial aspect of the olecranon when the elbow reaches terminal extension just after ball release in the deceleration phase of throwing. Patients may experience limited extension, which results from posterior osteophyte impingement, or locking and catching, which results from the presence of loose bodies or chondral injury. Patients may have ulnar collateral ligament (UCL) or flexor-pronator insufficiency as well as ulnar neuritis or subluxation.

Because many throwing athletes adapt to degenerative changes in the shoulder and elbow, appropriate management depends on the identification of pathophysiology directly correlated to symptoms on physical examination, thorough history, and imaging. Physical examination may reveal tenderness over the posteromedial olecranon and a loss of extension with a firm end point. The extension impingement test elicits pain localized to the posterior compartment when the elbow is snapped into terminal extension. During the arm bar test, the patient's shoulder is positioned at 90° of forward flexion and full internal rotation and the patient's hand is placed on the examiner's shoulder. When the examiner pulls down on the olecranon to simulate forced extension, reproduction of pain is considered a positive result. The authors of this chapter find that the patient is typically more relaxed when in a supine position with the elbow held off the edge of the examining table. With the patient in this position, the examiner can perform the arm bar test by resting the posterior part of the patient's elbow on the examiner's knee and applying manual stress to the wrist or forearm.

Axillary, AP, lateral, and oblique radiographs of the elbow may demonstrate posteromedial olecranon osteophytes and/or loose bodies (**Figure 1**). CT with two-dimensional sagittal and coronal reconstructions and three-dimensional surface rendering can demonstrate loose bodies and osteophyte formation (**Figure 2**). Bony hypertrophy, ligament ossification, and osteophyte fracture may be observed. The use of MRI can be helpful to assess UCL integrity and identify osteochondral damage, synovial plicae, bony edema, and stress fractures of the olecranon.

Surgical decompression is an option for patients with valgus extension overload in whom symptoms of PMI are bothersome and limiting despite nonsurgical management.

*Dr. Ahmad or an immediate family member serves as a paid consultant to Arthrex and has received research or institutional support from Arthrex, Major League Baseball, and Stryker. Neither Dr. Hodgins nor any immediate family member has received anything of value from or has stock or stock options held in a commercial company or institution related directly or indirectly to the subject of this chapter.*

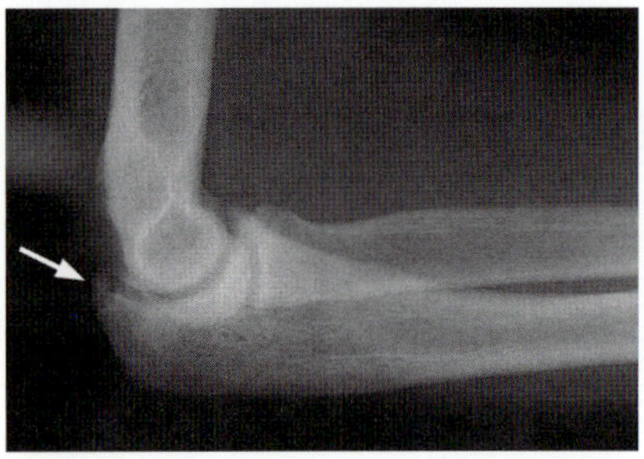

**Figure 1** Lateral radiograph demonstrates a fractured osteophyte (arrow) on the posterior olecranon.

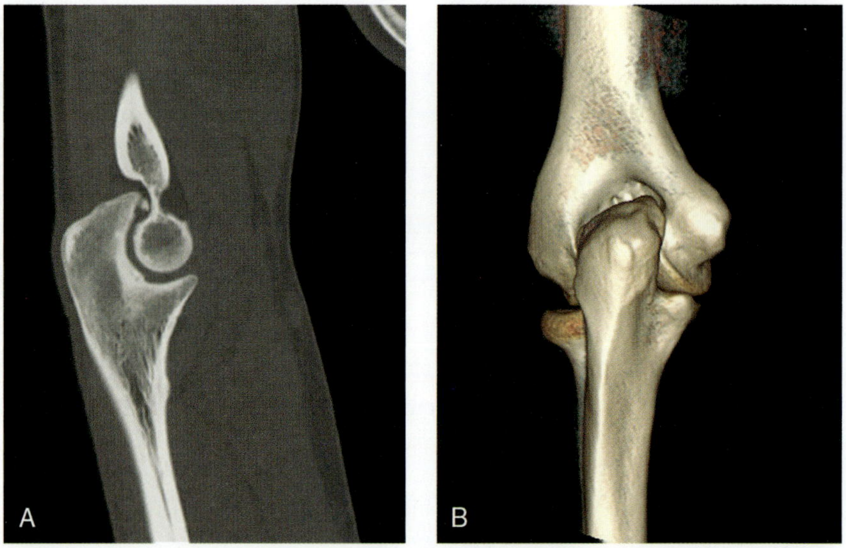


**Figure 2** Sagittal CT scan (**A**) and three-dimensional coronal CT reconstruction (**B**) demonstrate an osteophyte on the posteromedial aspect of the olecranon.

## Contraindications

Posteromedial decompression is not indicated in patients with negative provocative testing on physical examination, even if olecranon abnormalities are observed on radiographs or advanced imaging, because these abnormalities are commonly found in the absence of symptoms. In one study, researchers found that 13 of 16 professional baseball players with asymptomatic elbows had MRI findings consistent with PMI. Patients with UCL insufficiency are unlikely to benefit from olecranon osteophyte débridement alone. The authors of a cadaver study found that resection of the posteromedial olecranon beyond 3 mm increased strain on the UCL during flexion and valgus testing. They concluded that resection beyond 3 mm may exacerbate attenuation of the UCL. In a different study, UCL insufficiency was found to result in alterations of contact area and pressure in the posteromedial compartment that may cause symptomatic chondrosis and reactive osteophyte formation that manifests as valgus extension overload syndrome. This finding suggests that valgus extension overload with symptomatic PMI and valgus instability resulting from UCL insufficiency are related. In fact, posteromedial decompression may exacerbate UCL insufficiency. The senior author of this chapter (C.S.A.) recommends combined treatment to address both the UCL insufficiency and the valgus extension overload in patients with substantial UCL insufficiency (gap ≥3 mm between the coronoid process and the medial trochlea when a valgus stress is manually applied to the elbow in 70° of flexion).

## Alternative Treatments

Nonsurgical palliative treatment options include acetaminophen, NSAIDs, and intra-articular corticosteroid injections. Pitching instruction can help the patient identify mechanics that create greater valgus stress on the elbow and modifications that might improve comfort and effectiveness. For example, strengthening of the flexor-pronator mass may improve control during arm deceleration. After a rest period, the patient should undertake a progressive throwing program under the supervision of experienced therapists and trainers before returning to play.

An alternative to arthroscopic débridement of posteromedial osteophytes is open débridement through a small posteromedial incision. An open approach may pose less risk to the ulnar nerve than arthroscopy would and is indicated in patients with prior ulnar nerve transposition and patients with substantial heterotopic ossification. However, the smaller incisions required for arthroscopy may facilitate recovery, and arthroscopy offers a more thorough intra-articular diagnostic assessment of the elbow than an open approach.

## Results

The goal of posteromedial decompression is to decrease pain resulting from PMI, allowing throwing athletes to return to their desired level of performance. Posteromedial decompression is associated with 85% to 95% satisfaction and 68% to 100% return to sport in several studies (**Table 1**). One study demonstrated excellent or good short-term outcomes in 85% of patients who underwent arthroscopic decompression, with a complication rate of 1.6%. However, the authors of a different study reported that 25% of professional baseball players who underwent posteromedial decompression had subsequent UCL reconstruction. In high-level throwing athletes, the effectiveness of débridement

 

**Table 1** Results of Posteromedial Decompression for Valgus Extension Overload[a]

| Authors (Year) | No. of Elbows | Procedure or Approach | Mean Patient Age in Years (Range) | Mean Follow-up in Months (Range) | Success Rate (%) | Results |
|---|---|---|---|---|---|---|
| Wilson et al (1983) | 5 | Open decompression | 24 (NR) | 12 (NR) | 100 | All patients returned to throwing for 1 season |
| Rosenwasser and Steinmann (1991) | 9 | Arthroscopic decompression | 30.2 (13-45) | 26 (NR) | 83 | 83% of patients returned to sports 6 mo postoperatively |
| Andrews and Timmerman (1995) | 34 | Arthroscopic decompression | 24.2 (NR) | 42 (24-72) | 65 | 68% of patients returned to play<br>41% of patients underwent revision surgery |
| Hepler et al (1998) | 28 | Arthroscopic decompression | 29 (15-45) | 54 (24-108) | 95 | No reported complications |
| Reddy et al (2000) | 96 | Arthroscopic decompression[b] | 30 (10-64) | 42 (7-115) | 85 | 85% of patients returned to their preoperative level of competition |

NR = not reported.

[a] All studies are level IV evidence.

[b] Study included patients with multiple diagnoses, and procedures were not limited to posteromedial decompression for valgus extension overload.

compared with that of UCL reconstruction or nonsurgical treatment is unclear.

## Technique

### Setup/Exposure

- Anesthesia and patient positioning vary depending on surgeon preference. The patient may be placed in the supine, prone, or lateral decubitus position.
- When concomitant UCL reconstruction is planned, the supine position may be preferred to avoid the need to reposition the patient after the arthroscopy. Alternatively, the patient may be placed in the lateral decubitus position for the arthroscopy and then repositioned, prepped, and draped for UCL reconstruction.
- The authors of this chapter prefer to position the patient in the lateral decubitus position, perform anterior compartment diagnostic arthroscopy, and then perform posterior compartment decompression and débridement.
- A tourniquet is applied proximal to the surgical field and set at 250 mm Hg.
- Anatomic landmarks (including the ulnar nerve) and portals are appropriately marked on the patient's skin (**Figure 3**).
- To distend the joint, the elbow is injected with 15 to 20 mL of normal saline using a 60-mL syringe attached to an 18-gauge needle introduced into the soft-spot lateral portal.

### Instruments/Equipment/Implants Required

- A 4.0-mm arthroscope, shavers, burrs, and arthroscopic grasping instruments are required.
- Small straight and curved osteotomes are necessary.
- A curved 3.2-mm articulating retractor is required (**Figure 4**).
- A mini C-arm is necessary for intraoperative imaging.

### Procedure

- A superficial incision is made at the proximal medial portal.
- Soft-tissue blunt dissection is performed to avoid injury to neighboring neurovascular structures. A blunt-tipped trocar is introduced into the anterior compartment. The trocar should slide along the anterior side of the humerus and toward the radiocapitellar joint.
- Diagnostic arthroscopy is performed systematically to identify loose bodies, osteochondral lesions of the anterior radiocapitellar joint, osteophytes at the coronoid tip and fossa, and chondral lesions of the trochlea.
- The proximal lateral portal of the anterior compartment is established

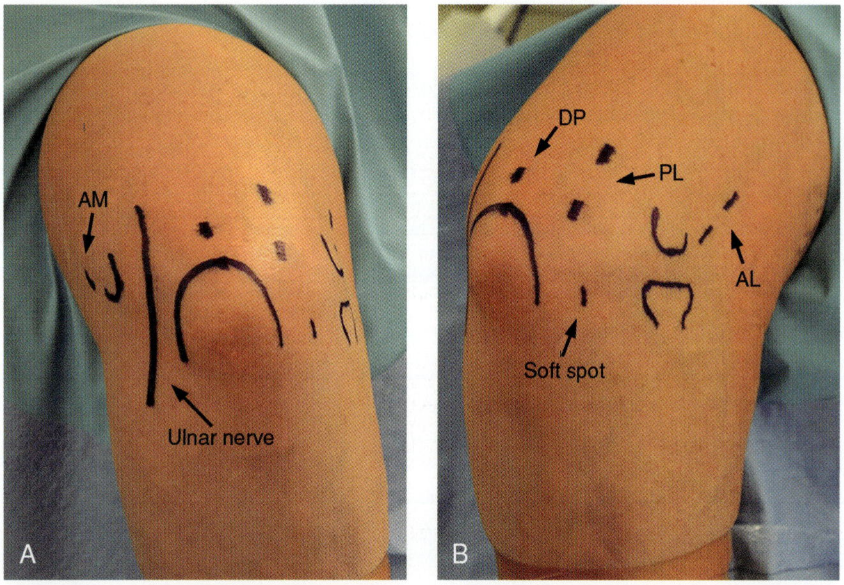


**Figure 3** Preoperative photographs show external skin markings for portal placement on the medial (**A**) and lateral (**B**) sides of the elbow. AL = anterolateral, AM = anteromedial, DP = direct posterior, PL = posterolateral.

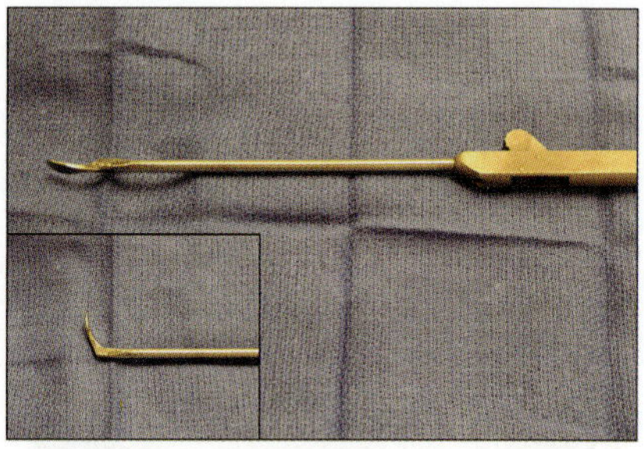

**Figure 4** Photograph of a 3.2-mm articulating retractor in the extended position. This retractor is used to protect the ulnar nerve during posteromedial resection with a motorized shaver. The inset shows the retractor in the flexed position.

under direct visualization with the assistance of a spinal needle.

- The arthroscope is inserted into the proximal lateral portal to allow the surgeon to visualize the medial compartment and assess UCL integrity. A common threshold for UCL reconstruction is a gap of 3 mm or more between the coronoid process and the medial trochlea when a valgus stress is manually applied to the elbow in 70° of flexion.
- A posterolateral viewing portal is established.
- A direct posterior working portal is established through the triceps tendon.
- Posterior diagnostic arthroscopy is performed to evaluate for the presence of loose bodies, osteophytes on the posteromedial aspect of the olecranon, and evidence of chondromalacia (**Figure 5**).
- If intra-articular synovitis is observed, the affected tissue can be removed with the use of an ablation device or a shaver.
- The posterior aspect of the radiocapitellar joint is examined for loose bodies. If loose bodies are identified, an accessory midlateral portal can be created through the lateral soft spot to facilitate removal.
- The ulnar nerve is located superficial to the capsule in the posteromedial gutter and is vulnerable to damage when motorized instruments and cautery are used. To protect the nerve and improve visualization, a curved retractor may be placed through an accessory posterolateral portal to retract the medial capsule and soft tissues (**Figure 6**). Suction should be removed from the shaver to avoid inadvertent suctioning of the capsule and nerve. Débridement within the posteromedial gutter should be performed cautiously and only by a surgeon highly experienced in elbow arthroscopy.
- Olecranon osteophytes are removed with the use of a small osteotome that is inserted through the direct posterior portal and placed at the margin of the osteophyte and the normal olecranon. A motorized shaver introduced through either the posterior portal or the posterolateral portal may be used to further contour the olecranon tip (**Figure 7**). The ulnar nerve is at risk during all of these maneuvers.
- A lateral radiograph may be obtained intraoperatively to ensure that adequate bone has been removed and that no bone debris remains within the soft tissues surrounding the elbow. The authors of this chapter attempt to remove only osteophytes and maintain the normal olecranon to limit strain on the UCL during valgus loading. Because posteromedial contact is necessary in throwing athletes, the surgical goal is not to decrease posteromedial contact but to reduce discomfort.
- Osteophytes in the olecranon fossa and on the posteromedial distal humerus are addressed. Any loose chondral flaps on the trochlear cartilage are débrided. Microfracture is considered if a well-shouldered, contained chondral lesion is present.

## Wound Closure

- After the arthroscopic procedure has been completed, the fluid is evacuated from the posterior

 

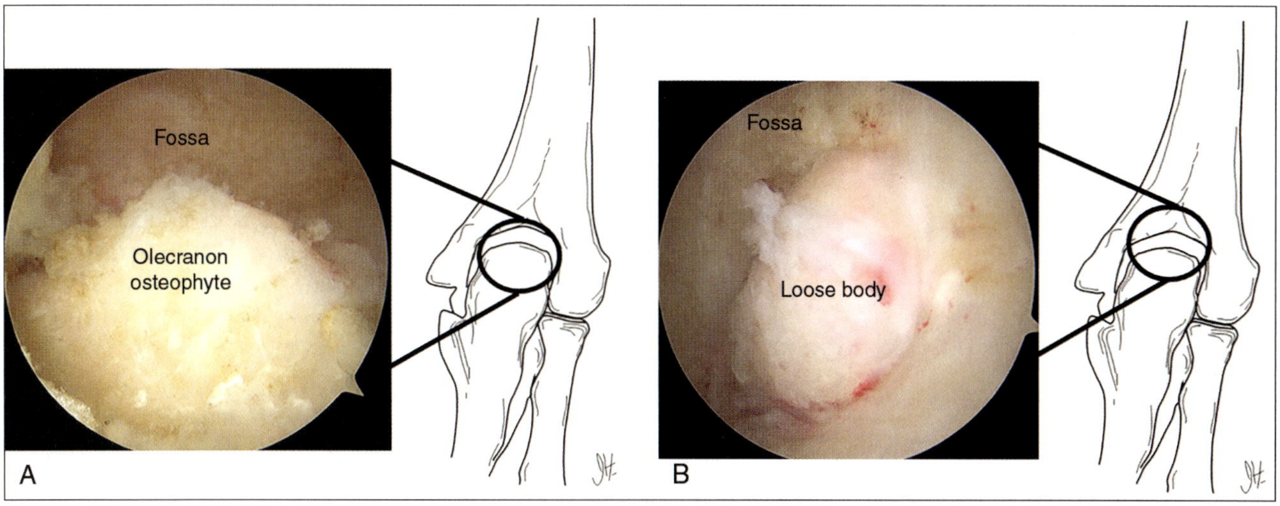


**Figure 5** Arthroscopic images viewed through the posterior portal during diagnostic arthroscopy demonstrate an osteophyte on the posteromedial aspect of the olecranon (**A**) and a loose body encased in soft tissue within the olecranon fossa (**B**). Illustrations indicate the region of the elbow demonstrated in the arthroscopic images.

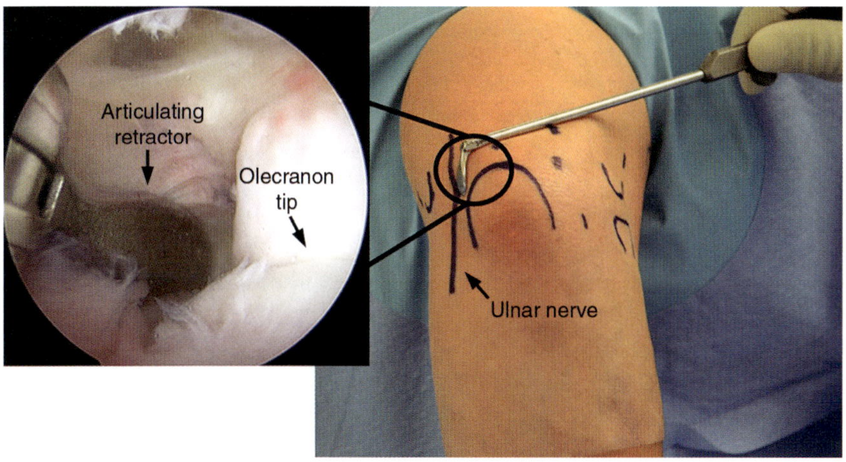


**Figure 6** Photograph and corresponding arthroscopic image viewed through the posterior portal demonstrate placement of an articulating retractor to protect the ulnar nerve in the region of the posteromedial aspect of the olecranon.

cannulas, and the portals are closed with simple interrupted 3-0 nylon sutures.

- If concomitant UCL reconstruction is planned, it is performed at this time. As noted previously, if the arthroscopy was performed with the patient in the lateral decubitus position, the patient must be repositioned in the supine position and prepped and draped for the UCL reconstruction.

## Postoperative Regimen

A compressive dressing is applied to the elbow, and the arm is placed in a simple sling postoperatively. The dressing is removed the day after the surgical procedure to facilitate movement. The sling is discontinued after 1 week. Active elbow flexion/extension exercises are started the day after the procedure. Emphasis is placed on restoring flexor-pronator strength and maintaining rotator cuff and periscapular muscle strength. At 6 weeks postoperatively, a progressive throwing program is initiated. A plyometric exercise program, neuromuscular training, and an endurance exercise program also are initiated at 6 weeks and are progressed to increase muscle performance. Return to competition is typically attempted 3 to 4 months postoperatively. Criteria for return to play include the return of preoperative range of motion, lack of pain or tenderness on stress testing and palpation, and full strength of the involved elbow and ipsilateral shoulder.

## Limiting Adverse Events

Joint distention with normal saline at the beginning of the procedure facilitates the introduction of the trocar and separates neurovascular structures from the bone, decreasing the risk of nerve injury.

Débridement in the posteromedial gutter places the ulnar nerve at risk. Suction should be disconnected from shavers or burrs when the surgeon is

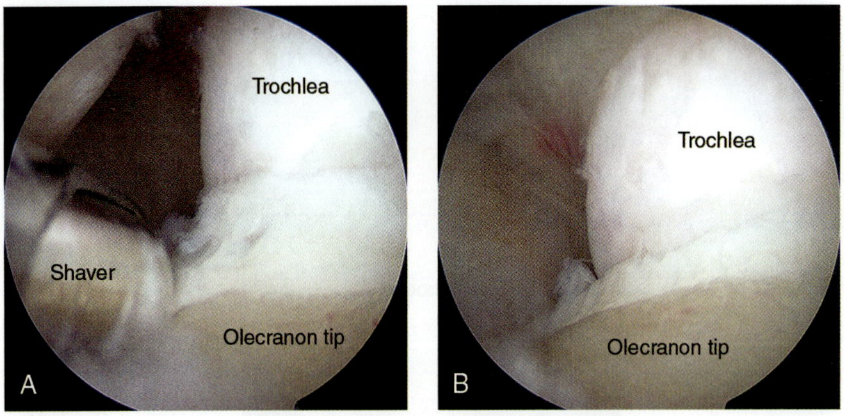


**Figure 7** Arthroscopic images viewed through the posterior portal demonstrate olecranon resection with the use of a motorized shaver introduced through the posterolateral portal (**A**) and the contoured olecranon tip after resection (**B**).

working in this area. A shaver is preferable for posteromedial débridement because a burr can siphon soft tissues by means of the Bernoulli-Venturi effect. A curved retractor inserted through an accessory posterolateral portal can be used to protect the ulnar nerve and improve visualization. If visualization is poor, osteophytes are close to the nerve, or the surgeon is not experienced in arthroscopic techniques, the nerve should be explored through an open incision and protected during débridement.

Prior to surgical treatment, ulnar nerve subluxation should be noted on physical examination and taken into account when incisions are made and portals are created. If ulnar neuropathy with intrinsic muscle weakness is identified, ulnar nerve transposition should be performed through an open approach.

## Bibliography

Ahmad CS, Conway JE: Elbow arthroscopy: Valgus extension overload. *Instr Course Lect* 2011;60:191-197.

Ahmad CS, Park MC, ElAttrache NS: Elbow medial ulnar collateral ligament insufficiency alters posteromedial olecranon contact. *Am J Sports Med* 2004;32(7):1607-1612.

Andrews JR, Timmerman LA: Outcome of elbow surgery in professional baseball players. *Am J Sports Med* 1995;23(4):407-413.

Field LD, Altchek DW: Evaluation of the arthroscopic valgus instability test of the elbow. *Am J Sports Med* 1996;24(2):177-181.

Hepler MD, Steinman S, Rosenwasser M: Abstract: Elbow arthroscopy in the treatment of posterior olecranon impingement. *Arthroscopy* 1998;14(4):430-431.

Kamineni S, ElAttrache NS, O'Driscoll SW, et al: Medial collateral ligament strain with partial posteromedial olecranon resection: A biomechanical study. *J Bone Joint Surg Am* 2004;86(11):2424-2430.

Kamineni S, Hirahara H, Pomianowski S, et al: Partial posteromedial olecranon resection: A kinematic study. *J Bone Joint Surg Am* 2003;85(6):1005-1011.

Kooima CL, Anderson K, Craig JV, Teeter DM, van Holsbeeck M: Evidence of subclinical medial collateral ligament injury and posteromedial impingement in professional baseball players. *Am J Sports Med* 2004;32(7):1602-1606.

O'Driscoll SW: Valgus extension overload and plica, in Levine WN, ed: *The Athlete's Elbow.* Rosemont, IL, American Academy of Orthopaedic Surgeons, 2008, pp 71-83.

 

Reddy AS, Kvitne RS, Yocum LA, ElAttrache NS, Glousman RE, Jobe FW: Arthroscopy of the elbow: A long-term clinical review. *Arthroscopy* 2000;16(6):588-594.

Rosenwasser MP, Steinmann SP: Abstract: Elbow arthroscopy in the treatment of posterior olecranon impingement. *Arthroscopy* 1991;7(3):327-328.

Wilson FD, Andrews JR, Blackburn TA, McCluskey G: Valgus extension overload in the pitching elbow. *Am J Sports Med* 1983;11(2):83-88.

# Chapter 6
# Arthroscopic Synovectomy of the Elbow

*Marc Prud'homme-Foster, MD, FRCSC*
*Graham J.W. King, MD, MSc, FRCSC*

**Learning Objectives**

- Identify elbow conditions and pathologies that can benefit from elbow arthroscopic synovectomy.
- Understand the risks and benefits of elbow arthroscopic synovectomy and expected outcomes.

## Indications

Arthroscopic synovectomy is a well-established technique to manage inflammatory synovitis, but it requires advanced technical skills in elbow arthroscopy. Synovectomy of the elbow is indicated for inflammatory arthritis that persists despite medical management and that is associated with pain, stiffness, and loss of function. In general, the best results of arthroscopic surgery are obtained in patients with some remaining articular cartilage and mild bony deformity (Mayo grades I and II). Although the outcomes of arthroscopic synovectomy generally are not as reliable in the setting of more advanced joint damage, the concern regarding the longevity of total elbow arthroplasty makes arthroscopic débridement and synovectomy a reasonable option in younger patients with more advanced articular and bony destruction (Mayo grade III).

Synovectomy also is indicated in the management of psoriatic arthritis of the elbow that does not demonstrate acceptable clinical improvement despite the application of medical therapy. Response to medical treatment can be assessed using criteria such as the 28-joint Disease Activity Score and the European League Against Rheumatism classification. Patients with hemophilia who have recurrent elbow hemarthroses even after factor replacement also should be considered for arthroscopic synovectomy. Hemophilic synovitis with synovial hypertrophy develops in these patients, and this condition eventually leads to joint contracture. Patients with synovial osteochondromatosis are commonly treated with loose body removal and arthroscopic synovectomy.

Arthroscopic synovectomy also can be used to treat patients with acute septic arthritis. Acute onset of joint pain, warmth, effusion, and decreased range of motion are suggestive of septic arthritis. Elevated preoperative white blood cell count, erythrocyte sedimentation rate, C-reactive protein level, joint fluid analysis (white blood cell count >50,000/μL with or without neutrophils >90%), and Gram staining are used to support the clinical diagnosis of septic arthritis.

Improved instrumentation and techniques have contributed to increased interest in arthroscopic synovectomy. The advantages of arthroscopic synovectomy include smaller incisions and better visualization of the elbow. Synovitis typically is most evident as boggy swelling posterolaterally. The location and function of the ulnar nerve should be assessed. Preoperative ulnar nerve dysfunction is an indication for in situ decompression or transposition at the time of arthroscopy.

A previous ulnar nerve transposition precludes safe percutaneous anteromedial portal placement. Even if the ulnar nerve is palpable, limited open portal placement is recommended to prevent iatrogenic nerve injury.

A soft end point of elbow flexion and extension is consistent with soft-tissue swelling, synovitis, and effusion. In patients with loss of forearm rotation, the distal radioulnar joint also should be examined and radiographs obtained to determine the contribution of the proximal and distal articulations to forearm stiffness. Radial head excision should be reserved for patients with articular deformity of the radial head that impedes rotation in the presence of a competent medial collateral ligament. Radial head excision can be performed arthroscopically at the time of synovectomy. Osteophyte removal and capsulectomy also can be performed arthroscopically concomitant with the synovectomy to improve motion and relieve pain. In patients with secondary osteoarthritis, CT is recommended to visualize the location and severity of the impinging osteophytes, which aids the surgeon in locating and removing the osteophytes.

---

*Dr. King or an immediate family member has received royalties from and serves as a paid consultant to Wright Medical Technology and Tornier. Neither Dr. Prud'homme-Foster nor any immediate family member has received anything of value from or has stock or stock options held in a commercial company or institution related directly or indirectly to the subject of this chapter.*

## Contraindications

The primary contraindication to arthroscopic synovectomy is inexperience of the treating surgeon. Patients with greater stiffness and deformity are more challenging to treat arthroscopically because of diminished capsular volume, which reduces the available space to work in the elbow, thereby increasing the risk of nerve injury. Surgeons with less arthroscopic experience are advised to treat these patients with open surgery. Concomitant radial head excision is contraindicated in patients with valgus instability because the loss of this secondary stabilizer often exacerbates preexisting instability. Inadequate medical management of inflammatory arthritis is an important contraindication to arthroscopic synovectomy because recurrent synovitis can be expected. The nonsurgical management of rheumatoid arthritis has markedly improved in recent years with the development and more aggressive use of conventional disease-modifying antirheumatic drugs, such as methotrexate and hydroxychloroquine, and so-called biologic disease-modifying antirheumatic drugs, such as infliximab and etanercept. Intra-articular injections of steroids into the elbow provide short-term relief of acute disease exacerbations; however, such injections may not be desirable because of the detrimental effects of steroids on articular cartilage. Low-demand patients with advanced articular destruction and bony deformity may be better treated with total elbow arthroplasty.

## Alternative Treatments

Alternative surgical treatment options include open synovectomy, interposition arthroplasty, and total elbow arthroplasty. Numerous studies document the beneficial effects of open radial head excision and synovectomy in patients with early to moderate rheumatoid arthritis. Although open synovectomy is successful in most patients, as with arthroscopic débridement, the effectiveness of the procedure decreases with time. Open procedures with longer incisions have the additional risk of wound dehiscence and delayed early range of motion. Open synovectomy should be considered in patients with severe stiffness because of the increased risk associated with arthroscopic management of severe stiffness. Although some surgeons may consider concomitant ulnar nerve transposition to be a relative contraindication to open synovectomy, the authors of this chapter prefer to use arthroscopy because of improved visualization of synovium in all areas of the joint. Furthermore, medial portal placement is simplified after ulnar nerve transposition, which increases the safety of arthroscopy. Results deteriorate more rapidly in a subgroup of patients with valgus instability after radial head excision, likely because radial head excision concentrates stress on the lateral portion of the ulnohumeral articulation and thereby potentially accelerates degenerative wear. The potential downsides of radial head resection may be outweighed by the potential gains in forearm rotation among patients with severe radial head deformity. Interposition arthroplasty has a limited role in inflammatory arthritis because it seems less predictable than total elbow arthroplasty. Interposition arthroplasty is indicated in young patients with pauciarticular inflammatory arthritis associated with cartilage loss, mild bony deformity, and persistent pain. Total elbow arthroplasty remains the procedure of choice for patients with advanced rheumatoid arthritis who have low activity demands.

## Results

Few data exist on the results of arthroscopic synovectomy for rheumatoid arthritis, and even less information is available on the use of this procedure for other conditions. The outcomes and complications may depend on the arthroscopic experience of the surgeon. Published studies suggest that the outcome of arthroscopic synovectomy is dependent on the severity of the arthritis present, with better results expected in elbows without substantial osseous destruction and some remaining articular cartilage (**Table 1**; **Figures 1** and **2**). Patients maintained on concomitant disease-modifying antirheumatic drugs are likely to have a lower incidence of recurrent synovitis and a better long-term outcome. Transient nerve paresthesias, recurrent synovitis, persistent pain, and subsequent total elbow arthroplasty are reported complications.

Early reports suggested that the arthroscopic technique resulted in incomplete synovectomy, and results deteriorated more rapidly than after an open procedure. In a study published in 1997, 93% good to excellent results were reported initially, but these results deteriorated to 57% by 42 months postoperatively. In a study published in 2002, 71% good to excellent results were reported at 2-year follow-up but deteriorated to 43% by 8 years postoperatively. However, if only those elbows without advanced cartilage loss and bony deformity were analyzed, the results in the 2002 study were 100% and 71% good or excellent at 2 and 8 years, respectively. This finding suggests that arthroscopic synovectomy was a durable procedure in a subset of patients.

In a 2006 study in which the outcomes of open synovectomy and arthroscopic synovectomy were compared, no significant difference was found in the overall clinical results. Slightly better outcomes were noted after arthroscopy

 

**Table 1** Results of Arthroscopic Synovectomy of the Elbow to Manage Rheumatoid Arthritis[a]

| Author(s) (Year) | Number of Elbows | Mean Patient Age in Years (Range) | Mean Follow-up in Months (Range) | Success Rate (%) | Results |
|---|---|---|---|---|---|
| Lee and Morrey (1997) | 14 | NA | 42 (24-84) | 57 | Flexion improved slightly<br>Rotation improved slightly<br>Pain improved initially but improvement decreased across time<br>Complications included 1 radial and 1 transient ulnar nerve paresthesia<br>4 elbows in 4 patients were converted to total elbow arthroplasty<br>Recurrent synovitis occurred in 6 elbows |
| Horiuchi et al (2002) | 21 | 51 (19-71) | 97 (42-160) | 43 | Patients demonstrated radiographic changes of Larsen grade 1, 2, 3, or 4<br>Flexion and pain improved<br>No change in rotation occurred<br>Joint arthritic damage increased across time<br>Best results occurred in patients with preserved joint space and those on disease-modifying antirheumatic drugs<br>Complications included 3 transient ulnar nerve paresthesias<br>Recurrent synovitis occurred in 5 elbows |
| Nemoto et al (2004) | 11 | 54 (38-68) | 37 (15-39) | 66 | Patients demonstrated radiographic changes of Larsen grade 1, 2, 3, or 4<br>Flexion and pain improved<br>No change in rotation occurred<br>Joint arthritic damage increased across time<br>Recurrent synovitis and pain occurred in 1 elbow, requiring 1 repeat synovectomy |
| Tanaka et al (2006) | 23 | 51 (31-64) | 156 (120-216) | 48 | Patients demonstrated radiographic changes of Larsen grade 1 or 2<br>Flexion and pain improved<br>Arthroscopic synovectomy resulted in less loss of elbow motion<br>Complications consisted of transient neurapraxia of the ulnar nerve in 1 patient and transient neurapraxia of the radial nerve in 1 patient |
| Kang et al (2010) | 26 | 46 (27-57) | 34 (13-68) | 85 | Patients demonstrated radiographic changes of Larsen grade 1, 2, or 3<br>Flexion and pain improved<br>No complications were reported<br>Unsuccessful in 4 elbows because of recurrent synovitis and pain |

NA = not available.

[a] All studies are level IV evidence.

Adapted from King GJW: Arthroscopic synovectomy of the elbow, in Yamaguchi K, King GJW, McKee MD, O'Driscoll SWM, eds: *Advanced Reconstruction: Elbow*. Rosemont, IL, American Academy of Orthopaedic Surgeons, 2007, pp 69-75.

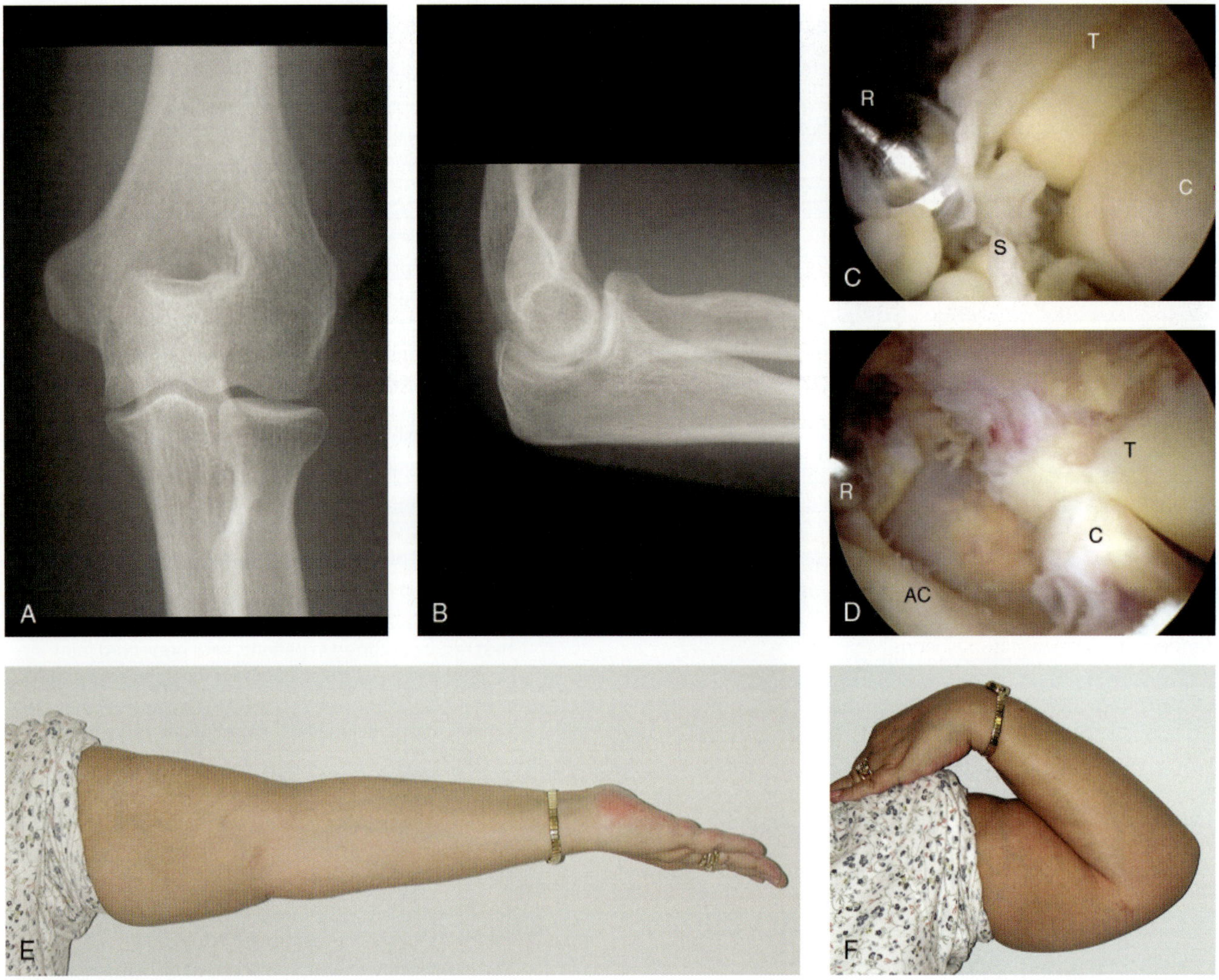


**Figure 1** Images from a 60-year-old woman who had intractable synovitis of the left elbow, mild cartilage damage, and a flexion arc of motion of 30° to 125° and was treated with arthroscopic synovectomy. **A,** Preoperative AP radiograph demonstrates preserved joint space. **B,** Preoperative lateral radiograph demonstrates mild periarticular osteopenia. **C,** Arthroscopic image from the proximal anterolateral portal demonstrates the appearance of the trochlea (T) and the coronoid (C) as well as removal of the florid synovitis (S) using a full radius shaver (R). **D,** Arthroscopic image obtained after synovectomy with the shaver (R) demonstrates the improved visualization of the articular cartilage of the trochlea (T) and the coronoid (C). The integrity of the anterior capsule (AC) has been maintained. Clinical photographs show improved elbow extension (**E**) and flexion (**F**) 4 months postoperatively. At that time, the patient also reported minimal pain. (Reproduced from King GJW: Arthroscopic synovectomy of the elbow, in Yamaguchi K, King GJW, McKee MD, O'Driscoll SWM, eds: *Advanced Reconstruction: Elbow.* Rosemont, IL, American Academy of Orthopaedic Surgeons, 2007, pp 69-75.)

in patients with a preoperative flexion arc of less than 90°. The authors of that study suggested that an arthroscopic procedure provided better balance between pain relief and postoperative improvement in range of motion (ROM). Patients with preoperative elbow stiffness who underwent open synovectomy had a higher risk of decreased ROM after surgery. In a study published in 2010, successful results (that is, no recurrence) were reported after arthroscopic synovectomy to manage rheumatoid arthritis in 22 of 26 elbows; no complications were reported.

Few data have been published on arthroscopic management of elbow joint involvement in patients with acute septic arthritis (**Table 2**). A study published in 1995 reported on two septic elbows successfully treated with arthroscopic débridement and lavage. Studies published in 2012 and 2014 describe low recurrence rates of infection, infrequent reoperation, good function, and limited pain in a total of 23 patients.

 

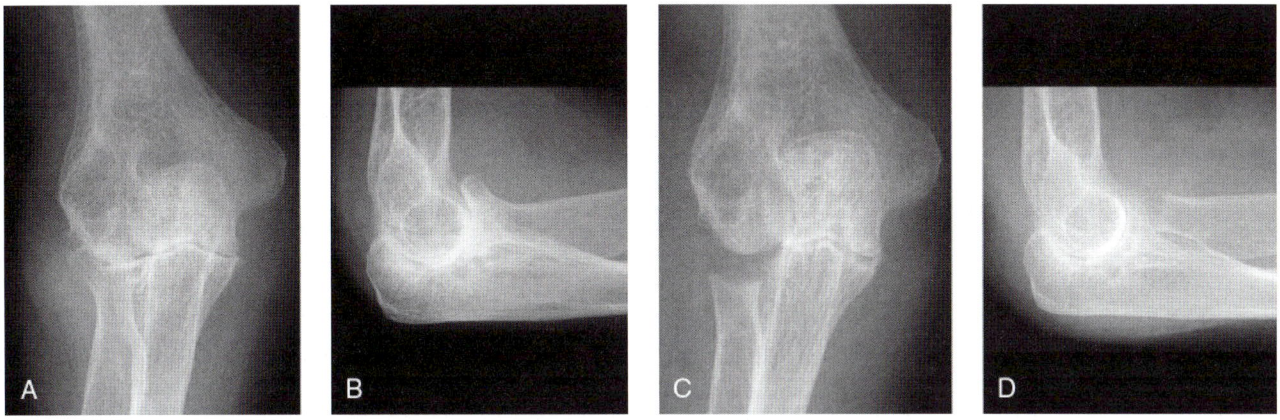


**Figure 2** Images from an active 65-year-old woman with intractable synovitis of the left elbow who was treated with arthroscopic synovectomy and radial head excision. Her preoperative flexion arc of motion was 45° to 135°, and rotation was limited to 50° of pronation and 50° of supination with painful crepitus. **A,** Preoperative AP radiograph demonstrates joint space narrowing and deformity of the radial head. **B,** Preoperative lateral radiograph demonstrates an absence of joint space. **C,** Postoperative AP radiograph obtained after radial head excision, which was done just distal to the radial notch of the ulna to avoid impingement postoperatively. **D,** Postoperative lateral radiograph confirms adequate excision of the radial head. The patient's rotational pain resolved, flexion improved to 20° to 140°, and supination and pronation increased to 70° and 80°, respectively. (Reproduced from King GJW: Arthroscopic synovectomy of the elbow, in Yamaguchi K, King GJW, McKee MD, O'Driscoll SWM, eds: *Advanced Reconstruction: Elbow.* Rosemont, IL, American Academy of Orthopaedic Surgeons, 2007, pp 69-75.)

# Technique

## Setup/Exposure

- Standard elbow arthroscopic positioning, equipment, and instruments are used.
- General anesthesia is typically used.
- In patients with more severe stiffness and advanced articular damage, a continuous brachial plexus block can be considered for postoperative pain control and to facilitate early elbow motion exercises.
- The authors of this chapter prefer to place the patient in the lateral decubitus position on a beanbag with careful cervical spine control, axillary roll, and padding of all bony prominences.

## Instruments/Equipment/Implants Required

- A 4.0-mm arthroscope is used for visualization, and a 4.5-mm full radius resector is used for the synovectomy.
- The shaver is typically used with the outflow open to the floor rather than using suction because suction may increase the risk of nerve injury.
- Retractors (typically a Howarth elevator) can be used to push away the joint capsule or muscles to improve visualization.

## Procedure

- In patients with extensive synovitis, the initial view after scope insertion often is poor. The surgeon should proceed cautiously with minimal débridement until the intra-articular position of the arthroscope can be confirmed, carefully gaining an improved view with synovial resection while avoiding nerve injury.
- The joint synovium is removed first while preserving the joint capsule.
- The anterior, posterior, and posterolateral compartments are sequentially débrided using as many portals as required—typically five—but more may be needed if retractors are used.
- Extra caution should be used when removing synovium anterior to the radial head in the region of the radial nerve and in the posteromedial gutter near the ulnar nerve.
- Osteophytes that are impeding joint motion are removed with a 5.5-mm hooded burr.
- The radial head is removed with a burr only if it is deformed and impedes forearm rotation.
- The joint capsule is removed last if substantial restriction of elbow flexion or extension is present.

## Wound Closure

- Portal sites are sutured to reduce the incidence of synovial fistulae.

# Postoperative Regimen

Postoperative management depends on the extent of the arthroscopic surgery. If only a synovectomy is performed,

**Table 2** Results of Arthroscopy to Manage Septic Arthritis

| Author(s) (Year) | Number of Elbows | Mean Patient Age in Years (Range) | Mean Follow-up in Months (Range) | Success Rate (%) | Results | Comments | Level of Evidence |
|---|---|---|---|---|---|---|---|
| Jerosch et al (1995) | 2 | 16 (4-28) | NA | 100 | Immediate postoperative decrease in fever and pain relief was indicative of a successful result<br>Final outcome of painless joint and full ROM was achieved in all patients<br>Complications were not reported | At the end of the procedure, an intra-articular gentamicin collagen fleece was placed, and intravenous antibiotics were administered | III |
| van den Ende and Steinmann (2012) | 12 | 63 (34-81) | 39 (5-80) | 100 | Good outcomes were achieved in elbows without a previous history of problems that were managed within 2 days of the onset of clinical symptoms<br>One patient had repeat arthroscopy for persistent infection and died within 1 wk of hospitalization | Patients were administered intravenous antibiotics tailored to the organism cultured | IV |
| Moon et al (2014) | 11 | 45 (7-83) | 31 (12-54) | 91 | Good outcomes with only 1 reoperation<br>Flexion contractures of 10°-20° were achieved in 4 patients | Patients were administered intravenous antibiotics tailored to the organism cultured | IV |

NA = not available, ROM = range of motion.

patients are usually discharged to home with a light dressing and are encouraged to do early active ROM exercises on postoperative day 1. Patients who undergo a more extensive débridement with capsulectomy are admitted to the hospital for 2 days. In these patients, the authors of this chapter prefer a continuous passive motion machine and a continuous brachial plexus block for postoperative pain control, followed by the use of a nighttime extension splint for 12 weeks to retain extension.

## Limiting Adverse Events

Arthroscopic synovectomy of the elbow is more challenging than standard elbow arthroscopic procedures because the reduced capsular volume reduces the available viewing space; the presence of synovitis impedes visualization; and the thin, often deficient capsule increases the risk of neurologic injury. The joint capsule should be expanded using a syringe with a large-gauge needle to inject 20 mL of irrigation solution into the posterior fossa before inserting the arthroscopic instruments. The authors of this chapter prefer to start the synovectomy in the anterior compartment.

 

The proximal anterolateral portal is established first, with the capsule distended by fluid. The proximal anteromedial portal is established next under direct visualization. A proximal posterocentral portal is used as an outflow portal with a drainage cannula. The viewing and working portals are exchanged using a switching stick to complete the anterior synovectomy. If the view is insufficient, a mid anterolateral or mid anteromedial portal can be established, and a retractor (typically a Howarth elevator) is inserted to retract the capsule.

One review of the complications of elbow arthroscopy found that nerve injuries (all transient) were more common following arthroscopic procedures for rheumatoid arthritis compared with other procedures. Other studies have reported permanent nerve injuries.

Sufficient arthroscopic experience with other elbow procedures should be developed before performing arthroscopy of the rheumatoid elbow. Conversion to an open procedure should be performed if the view is inadequate to proceed safely or if technical challenges slow progression of the arthroscopy. The ulnar nerve should be decompressed or transposed if the patient has clinical signs or symptoms of ulnar neuritis or neuropathy preoperatively. Patients with less than 110° of elbow flexion should be considered for prophylactic ulnar nerve in situ release or transposition because increased postoperative motion can cause ulnar neuropathy. Careful fluid management and low inflow pressures should be used to avoid excessive joint swelling.

## Bibliography

Dunn AL, Busch MT, Wyly JB, Sullivan KM, Abshire TC: Arthroscopic synovectomy for hemophilic joint disease in a pediatric population. *J Pediatr Orthop* 2004;24(4):414-426.

Ferlic DC, Patchett CE, Clayton ML, Freeman AC: Elbow synovectomy in rheumatoid arthritis: Long-term results. *Clin Orthop Relat Res* 1987;(220):119-125.

Gallay SH, Richards RR, O'Driscoll SW: Intraarticular capacity and compliance of stiff and normal elbows. *Arthroscopy* 1993;9(1):9-13.

Gendi NS, Axon JM, Carr AJ, Pile KD, Burge PD, Mowat AG: Synovectomy of the elbow and radial head excision in rheumatoid arthritis: Predictive factors and long-term outcome. *J Bone Joint Surg Br* 1997;79(6):918-923.

Hahn M, Grossman JA: Ulnar nerve laceration as a result of elbow arthroscopy. *J Hand Surg Br* 1998;23(1):109.

Horiuchi K, Momohara S, Tomatsu T, Inoue K, Toyama Y: Arthroscopic synovectomy of the elbow in rheumatoid arthritis. *J Bone Joint Surg Am* 2002;84(3):342-347.

Jerosch J, Hoffstetter I, Schröder M, Castro WH: Septic arthritis: Arthroscopic management with local antibiotic treatment. *Acta Orthop Belg* 1995;61(2):126-134.

Kahlenberg JM, Fox DA: Advances in the medical treatment of rheumatoid arthritis. *Hand Clin* 2011;27(1):11-20.

Kamineni S, O'Driscoll SW, Morrey BF: Synovial osteochondromatosis of the elbow. *J Bone Joint Surg Br* 2002;84(7):961-966.

Kang HJ, Park MJ, Ahn JH, Lee SH: Arthroscopic synovectomy for the rheumatoid elbow. *Arthroscopy* 2010;26(9):1195-1202.

Kelly EW, Morrey BF, O'Driscoll SW: Complications of elbow arthroscopy. *J Bone Joint Surg Am* 2001;83(1):25-34.

Lee BP, Morrey BF: Arthroscopic synovectomy of the elbow for rheumatoid arthritis: A prospective study. *J Bone Joint Surg Br* 1997;79(5):770-772.

Ljung P, Jonsson K, Larsson K, Rydholm U: Interposition arthroplasty of the elbow with rheumatoid arthritis. *J Shoulder Elbow Surg* 1996;5(2 pt 1):81-85.

Lonner JH, Stuchin SA: Synovectomy, radial head excision, and anterior capsular release in stage III inflammatory arthritis of the elbow. *J Hand Surg Am* 1997;22(2):279-285.

Mäenpää HM, Kuusela PP, Kaarela K, Kautiainen HJ, Lehtinen JT, Belt EA: Reoperation rate after elbow synovectomy in rheumatoid arthritis. *J Shoulder Elbow Surg* 2003;12(5):480-483.

Menth-Chiari WA, Ruch DS, Poehling GG: Arthroscopic excision of the radial head: Clinical outcome in 12 patients with post-traumatic arthritis after fracture of the radial head or rheumatoid arthritis. *Arthroscopy* 2001;17(9):918-923.

Moon JG, Biraris S, Jeong WK, Kim JH: Clinical results after arthroscopic treatment for septic arthritis of the elbow joint. *Arthroscopy* 2014;30(6):673-678.

Nemoto K, Arino H, Yoshihara Y, Fujikawa K: Arthroscopic synovectomy for the rheumatoid elbow: A short-term outcome. *J Shoulder Elbow Surg* 2004;13(6):652-655.

Savoie FH III, O'Brien MJ, Field LD: Arthroscopy for arthritis of the elbow. *Hand Clin* 2011;27(2):171-178, v-vi.

Studer A, Athwal GS: Rheumatoid arthritis of the elbow. *Hand Clin* 2011;27(2):139-150, v.

Tamurian RM, Spencer EE, Wojtys EM: The role of arthroscopic synovectomy in the management of hemarthrosis in hemophilia patients: Financial perspectives. *Arthroscopy* 2002;18(7):789-794.

Tanaka N, Sakahashi H, Hirose K, Ishima T, Ishii S: Arthroscopic and open synovectomy of the elbow in rheumatoid arthritis. *J Bone Joint Surg Am* 2006;88(3):521-525.

van den Ende KI, Steinmann SP: Arthroscopic treatment of septic arthritis of the elbow. *J Shoulder Elbow Surg* 2012;21(8):1001-1005.

Woods DA, Williams JR, Gendi NS, Mowat AG, Burge PD, Carr AJ: Surgery for rheumatoid arthritis of the elbow: A comparison of radial-head excision and synovectomy with total elbow replacement. *J Shoulder Elbow Surg* 1999;8(4):291-295.

 

# Chapter 7

# Arthroscopic Reduction and Internal Fixation of Elbow Fractures

*Michael R. Hausman, MD*

*Steve W. Wang, MD*

**Learning Objectives**

- Understand possible indications for arthroscopy in the management of elbow trauma.
- Learn the basic steps and principles of arthroscopically assisted treatment of elbow fractures.

## Indications

Endoscopic and arthroscopic techniques afford unparalleled exposure while minimizing surgical trauma and nociception. Although the evolution of elbow arthroscopy is in its early stages, several trauma-related applications are promising. The slow adoption of arthroscopically assisted fixation of elbow fractures may be the result of surgeons' lack of familiarity with elbow arthroscopy and lack of experience with elbow trauma in general.

Arthroscopic elbow procedures range in difficulty from simple to challenging. Diagnostic arthroscopy and simple loose body removal are relatively straightforward. Next in the hierarchy of difficulty and risk are débridement, such as for the management of lateral epicondylitis (tennis elbow); arthroscopic reduction and internal fixation of elbow fractures; and osteocapsular arthroplasty for the management of arthritis. Posttraumatic contracture release, rheumatoid synovectomy, and the management of severe contracture requiring an extra-articular approach are the most challenging and risky procedures. Although elbow arthroscopy for trauma might seem difficult and risky, more often it is an intermediate challenge and risk because, unlike a severe, posttraumatic contracture, the fractured elbow was normal prior to the trauma. Thus, the capsule is normal, thin, and pliant, and the joint is distended by hematoma. Therefore, entry into the elbow is relatively easy and safe, and all work on the fracture is done within the capsule, thereby maintaining a barrier between it and the neurovascular structures.

In the management of elbow fractures, arthroscopy facilitates adequate exposure for accurate diagnosis, precise reduction of fracture fragments, and correct orientation and sizing of implants. Arthroscopy has been useful in pediatric patients and in the management of capitellum-trochlea and lateral condyle fractures, simple distal humerus fractures, coronoid fractures, posterolateral rotatory instability, radial head fractures, pediatric supracondylar malunion, and osteonecrosis. Patients with elbow trauma often can benefit from arthroscopy because exposure of elbow fractures typically involves detachment of muscles and sometimes requires detachment of ligaments.

In the management of pediatric lateral condyle fractures, the advantages of arthroscopic techniques compared with open approaches include accuracy of reduction, which is difficult to assess with arthrography; easier placement of fixation pins in the secondary ossification center rather than in cartilage; and limited soft-tissue dissection to minimize the risk of osteonecrosis.

In patients with capitellar fractures, which frequently involve the lateral trochlea, the lateral epicondyle is often fractured. The posterior part of the lateral column and the posterior trochlea may be fractured but stable. A bent or impacted posterior wall hinders reduction of the capitellum and anterior trochlea. Although good exposure of the lateral trochlea can be difficult depending on the extent of a limited lateral approach, this area is easily seen through the arthroscope.

*Dr. Hausman or an immediate family member has received royalties from Smith & Nephew; is a member of a speakers' bureau or has made paid presentations on behalf of TriMed; serves as a paid consultant to Stryker; serves as an unpaid consultant to Checkpoint Surgical, NDI Medical, SPR Therapeutics, and Flower Orthopedics; and has stock or stock options held in Checkpoint Surgical, NDI Medical, and SPR Therapeutics. Neither Dr. Wang nor any immediate family member has received anything of value from or has stock or stock options held in a commercial company or institution related directly or indirectly to the subject of this chapter.*

 

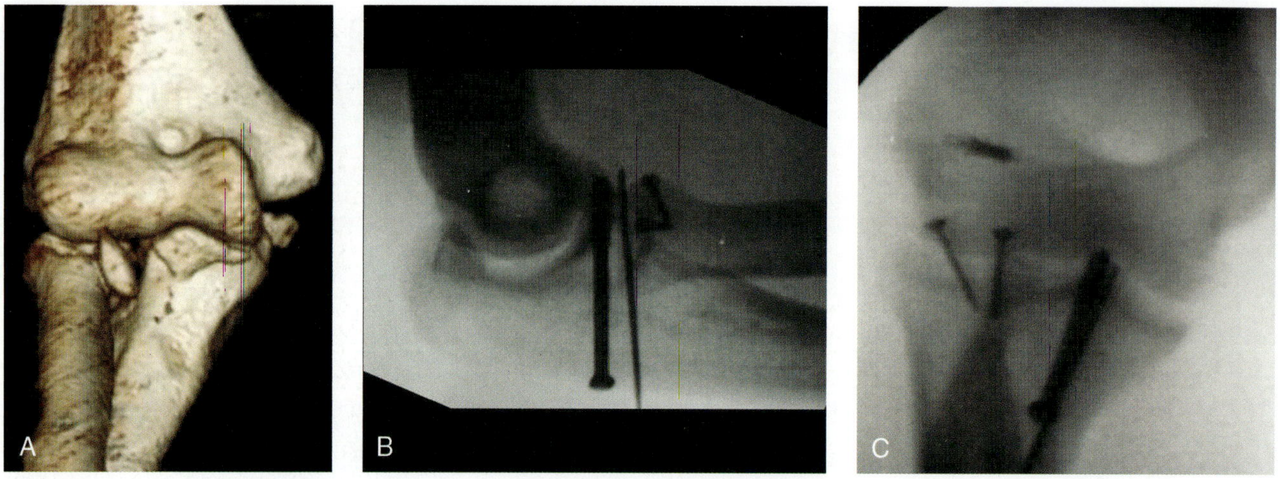


**Figure 1** **A,** Three-dimensional CT reconstruction of an elbow demonstrates a terrible triad injury, with a salvageable radial head and a type II coronoid fracture. The patient has posterolateral and posteromedial instability. Final lateral (**B**) and AP (**C**) fluoroscopic images demonstrate the arthroscopically assisted reduction and fixation with a coronoid screw and a supplemental threaded pin. The open reduction and internal fixation (ORIF) of the radial head was performed through a limited Kaplan interval approach. ORIF of the coronoid would have required a much more extensive exposure. The lateral ulnar collateral ligament is repaired with an anchor.

The management of unicondylar, intra-articular distal humerus fractures is a logical extension of the technique used in the management of capitellar fractures. A hybrid arthroscopic/open approach is used to reduce the joint surface and place a plate on the supracondylar ridge. The use of plates designed for medial or lateral placement obviates the need for soft-tissue dissection. The hybrid arthroscopic/open approach eliminates the need for an olecranon osteotomy or a paratricipital approach while affording an excellent view of the articular surface.

Although the indications for repair of coronoid fractures continue to evolve, the association between even small coronoid fractures and instability is well established. Regan-Morrey type I and II coronoid fractures are frequently associated with ligament and soft-tissue injuries and ultimately, elbow instability. Modifications of the classification have shown the association of medial coronoid facet fractures (Mayo type II) with varus instability. This fracture pattern is also associated with posteromedial rotatory instability. Transverse coronoid tip and anterolateral coronoid facet fractures (Mayo type I) can be associated with medial collateral ligament rupture and/or posterolateral rotatory instability.

The advantages of open reduction versus arthroscopic reduction and internal fixation of coronoid fractures are not clear. A medial coronoid facet fracture is usually a crush injury best treated with a buttress plate, which requires an open approach. Anterolateral fractures and coronoid transverse tip or anterolateral fractures are shearing injuries and are amenable to arthroscopic reduction and fixation. Most coronoid tip fractures are part of a terrible triad injury (dislocation with fractures of the radial head and coronoid). If the radial head must be replaced, access to the coronoid from an open lateral approach is straightforward. Patients with a coronoid tip fracture with posterolateral instability and a reparable radial head fracture might benefit from arthroscopically assisted fixation of the coronoid to avoid the need for proximal extension of a lateral approach or a substantial medial approach in order to work around the radial head (**Figure 1**).

Coronoid fractures are frequently associated with rupture of the lateral ulnar collateral ligament (LUCL). Arthroscopic suture plication of the LUCL has been described for the management of posterolateral rotatory instability of the elbow. Repair to the anatomic origin using a suture anchor is also possible.

Arthroscopically assisted reduction and fixation of radial head fractures has been reported. Arthroscopic techniques may have fewer advantages in the management of radial head fractures than in the management of other fracture types. Visualization is frequently limited as a result of synovitis and soft-tissue trauma, and radial head fractures are often firmly impacted and difficult to realign. An open approach through the Kaplan interval (between the extensor digitorum communis and the extensor carpi radialis brevis) affords sufficient exposure through a small incision to disimpact and fix the fracture. In contrast, arthroscopic management of pediatric radial neck fractures may offer advantages. The Métaizeau technique is widely used but can damage the growth plate. Arthroscopic examination of the elbow from the anteromedial portal shows the angulated radial head incarcerated by an anterolateral fold of capsule (**Figure 2**). The use of a Freer elevator placed through the anterolateral portal to lift or pry the capsule over the radial head will allow the head to pop back into position with its capitellar articulation. If the reduction is not stable, percutaneous pins may be placed under arthroscopic visualization. In addition to facilitating management of the radial neck fracture, arthroscopy allows for evaluation of associated chondral injuries and coronoid or LUCL injury, which are not visible radiographically.

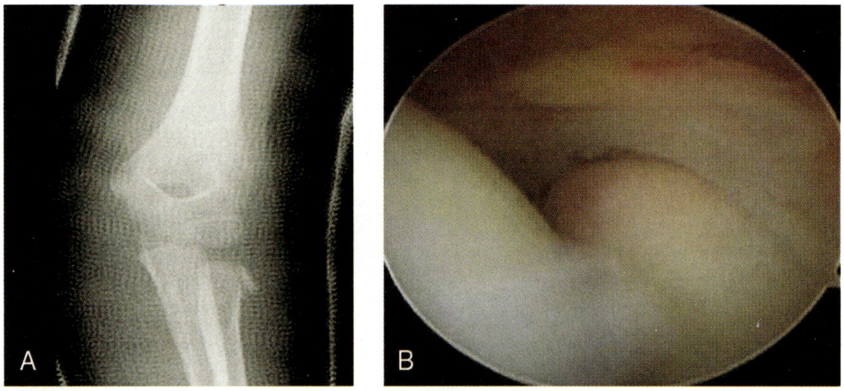

**Figure 2** **A,** AP radiograph of an elbow demonstrates an angulated radial neck fracture with failure of closed reduction. **B,** Arthroscopic image of the elbow from the anteromedial portal demonstrates immediate reduction of the radial head from the recess lateral to the capsular fold. In this patient, the reduction is stable because of the presence of an intact periosteal hinge.

Malunion is a well-recognized complication of pediatric supracondylar humerus fractures. The results of corrective osteotomies vary, and complication rates as high as 40% have been reported. Furthermore, the osteotomy typically requires an extensile posterior or lateral approach with considerable soft-tissue dissection. The use of an arthroscopic supracondylar osteotomy to correct malunion has been described. In addition to the limitation of flexion that occurs when a supracondylar fracture heals in extension, this type of malunion results in an incongruent motion of the radial head on the capitellum (**Figure 3**). Although it has not been well described, the long-term consequences of this incongruent motion are unknown, and this fact alone may suggest an advantage of corrective osteotomy.

The frequency of osteonecrosis after lateral condyle and supracondylar fractures is unknown (**Figure 4**). The consequences of this complication include pain and limited range of motion. Fragmentation of the secondary ossification center with ovoid deformity of the capitellum and secondary flattening of the radial head can result in progressively impeded elbow motion. Formation of a physeal bar that tethers growth is also common and can affect the capitellum or the lateral trochlea, resulting in the characteristic fishtail deformity. Due to the unfavorable prognosis, the approach to these complications has been relatively nihilistic because no reliable treatment option exists. Epiphyseal recontouring is a feasible option, and arthroscopy affords excellent exposure for this procedure because of the magnification. However, the utility of this procedure has yet to be established.

After a lateral condyle fracture, osteonecrosis of the lateral condyle can result in softening and flattening of the capitellum and reciprocal, adaptive so-called mushrooming of the radial head. The flattening of the capitellum blocks elbow flexion. Motion helps to mold the damaged bone and cartilage into a more normal shape. The proposed treatment involves resecting the physeal bar and narrowing the lateral column, as viewed in the sagittal plane, to restore the shape of the capitellum, while fixing and uniting the anterior capitellar fragment to the posterior wall in much the same way that a capitellum fracture is fixed. In this scenario, arthroscopy offers excellent visualization and a high degree of precision in executing a complex reconstruction while minimizing soft-tissue dissection, particularly around the tenuous soft-tissue connection to the capitellar fragment. Postoperatively, the elbow is immobilized, and healing is prioritized. Because the elbow was stiff before the surgical treatment, simultaneous release and open reduction and internal fixation offers no advantage and carries the risk of nonunion. After the capitellum has healed as demonstrated on MRI, a staged, arthroscopic contracture release can be performed to restore elbow motion.

## Contraindications and Alternative Treatments

The elbow is relatively easy to enter arthroscopically, but visualization may be difficult. If visualization remains poor, arthroscopy should be abandoned and the procedure converted to a conventional, open approach.

Arthroscopy currently has no role in the management of olecranon fractures. Although arthroscopy has been described for radial head fractures, arthroscopic techniques do not offer advantages over conventional open techniques in the management of this injury. As with any arthroscopic procedure, if adequate visualization and working space cannot be created with gentle, conservative evacuation of the hematoma, the procedure should be converted to conventional open treatment to avoid accidental injury to the neurovascular structures.

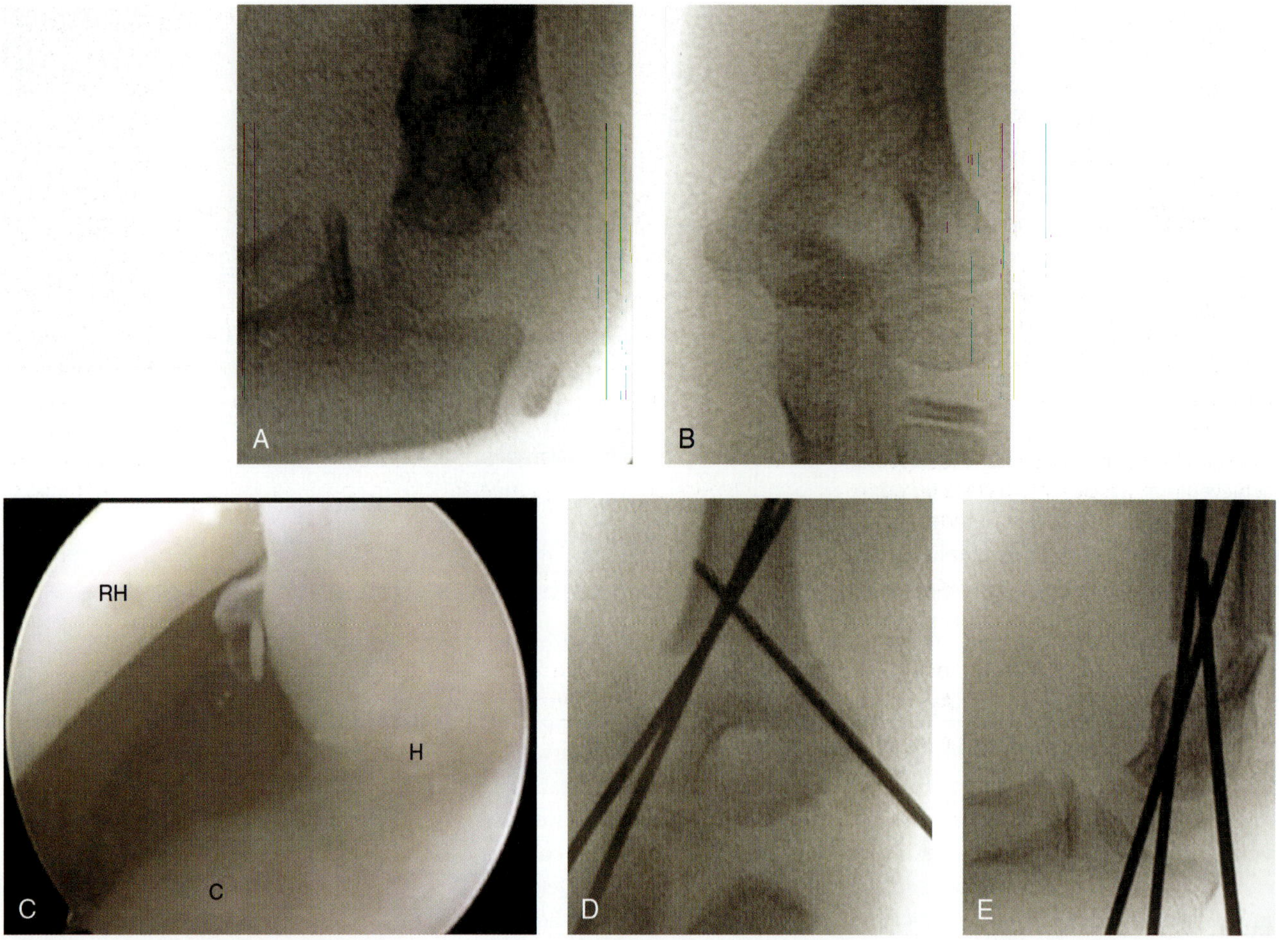


**Figure 3** Lateral (**A**) and AP (**B**) fluoroscopic images demonstrate a supracondylar humerus fracture in a pediatric patient. The fracture has healed in extension, blocking flexion at 90°. **C,** Arthroscopic image viewed through the proximal anteromedial portal demonstrates the often unappreciated incongruent radial capitellar motion that involves the radial head (RH) translating or "wiping" across the capitellum in flexion, rather than gliding congruently. AP (**D**) and lateral (**E**) fluoroscopic images demonstrate fixation with Steinmann pins provisionally placed in the distal fragment. After the pins were provisionally placed, the distal fragment was flexed with the surgeon's thumbs to deform the posterior cortex to reduce the distal fragment and restore the proper angle. The pins were advanced to fix the osteotomy. C = capitellum, H = humerus.

## Results

Studies of arthroscopic reduction and internal fixation of elbow fractures are summarized in **Table 1**. This technique has become increasingly popular, with promising results in preliminary studies.

## Techniques

### Setup/Exposure

- A lateral decubitus position is commonly used for arthroscopy.
- The authors of this chapter prefer to place the patient in a supine position with the arm supported in an articulated shoulder positioner because this position facilitates conversion to an open procedure. Also, the supine position and the use of the articulated positioner allow the elbow to be placed in positions that facilitate access to multiple compartments and the use of intraoperative fluoroscopy.
- Preoperative evaluation and imaging is comparable to that of open surgical procedures.
- To protect the critical neurovascular structures, standard elbow arthroscopy principles should be followed during the process of entering the elbow and establishing a view.
- Entry into the joint typically is not difficult.
- Careful lavage is required to clear hematoma and visualize the fracture. A 3.5-mm shaver inserted through a second portal, with the blade directed toward the humerus and away from the important structures and capsule, will help débride the hematoma. The use of

 

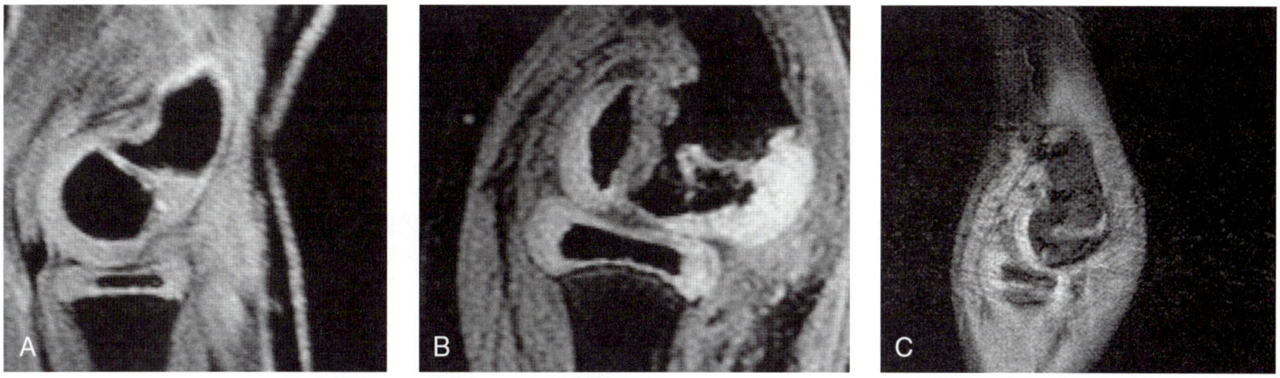

**Figure 4** Sagittal short tau inversion recovery (STIR) MRIs demonstrate a normal capitellum (**A**) and the preoperative appearance of a deformed lateral condyle resulting from osteonecrosis and fragmentation of the lateral condyle after fracture (**B**). **C,** Postoperative sagittal STIR MRI demonstrates the appearance of the elbow shown in panel B 6 months after epiphyseal recontouring. The final shape achieved is much closer to a circle (as opposed to the elliptical shape seen preoperatively). The patient regained functional range of motion, but the physeal bar re-formed.

**Table 1** Results of Arthroscopic Reduction and Internal Fixation of Elbow Fracture[a]

| Authors (Year) | No. of Patients | Procedure or Approach | Mean Patient Age in Years (Range) | Mean Follow-up in Months (Range) | Results |
|---|---|---|---|---|---|
| Adams et al (2007) | 6 | Coronoid | 37 (12-46) | 31.8 (NR) | Flexion/extension of 9°-133°<br>Pronation/supination, 87°/79°<br>Mayo Elbow Performance score, 100 (5 patients; unavailable for 1 patient)<br>Complications: heterotopic ossification and ulnar neuropathy |
| Michels et al (2007) | 14 | Radial head | 37.5 (19-57) | 66 (12-132) | Avg Mayo Elbow Performance score, 97.6<br>79% excellent and 21% good |
| Hausman et al (2007) | 6 | Pediatric lateral condyle | 4 (1.75-5.75) | 8 (5.3-11) | Full active ROM<br>1 patient had signs of osteonecrosis |
| Kuriyama et al (2010) | 2 | Capitellum | Patient 1: 42<br>Patient 2: 34 | Patient 1: 20<br>Patient 2: 17 | Patient 1: Normal active ROM<br>Patient 2: Active flexion/extension of 5°-125°, 90° supination, 85° pronation, and signs of osteonecrosis |

NR = not reported, ROM = range of motion.
[a] All studies are level IV evidence.

a tourniquet and a careful, methodical process of débridement also are helpful.

- Low inflow pressures (<30 mm Hg) should be used. The elbow rapidly distends at a critical level between 30 and 35 mm Hg. Below that threshold, minimal swelling occurs, even with extended working times. The use of low inflow pressures also facilitates conversion to an open approach, if necessary.
- Arthroscopic fracture fixation is easier when performed at least 48 hours after fracture to avoid the persistent oozing of blood from the fracture. During this delay, hematoma seals the fracture surfaces, allowing low inflow pressures of 25 to 30 mm Hg to be used.

## Instruments/Equipment/Implants Required

- Useful implants and instruments include small, cannulated screws; a suture retriever; fiber resin–reinforced suture; a Freer elevator with a hole drilled in the blade; a small rake or double skin hook with the tines filed and shortened for grabbing and reducing fractures; and a selection of arthroscopic suture-passing instruments.

- The use of separate trocars and cannulas is helpful because entering the joint with a trocar alone provides improved tactile feedback by eliminating the extra drag of the cannula on the tissues.

## Procedures

### PEDIATRIC LATERAL CONDYLE FRACTURE

- A proximal anteromedial portal is established with the use of a semiblunt trocar.
- Initial lavage is performed.
- The proximal anterolateral portal is established with an inside-out technique. Alternatively, if adequate visualization is obtained by lavage alone, this portal may be established from the outside.
- A 3.5-mm shaver is used for further lavage to improve visualization. In small children, typically those younger than 4 or 5 years, the use of a wrist arthroscope and a 2.9-mm shaver may be preferred. (This procedure has been performed in children as young as 2 years.) In patients older than 5 years, adult-sized instruments are typically used.
- The fracture surface is identified, and the fixation pins (minimum size, 0.062-in) are provisionally placed (**Figure 5**). Pins can also be placed from the outside in. At least one pin should penetrate the secondary ossification center.
- To minimize the number of passes, the arthroscope may be advanced to the bone of the secondary ossification center, the camera withdrawn, and the fixation pin drilled through the remaining cannula, which is held against the bone of the ossification center.
- The pin is extracted from the leading end as it exits the lateral side of the elbow.

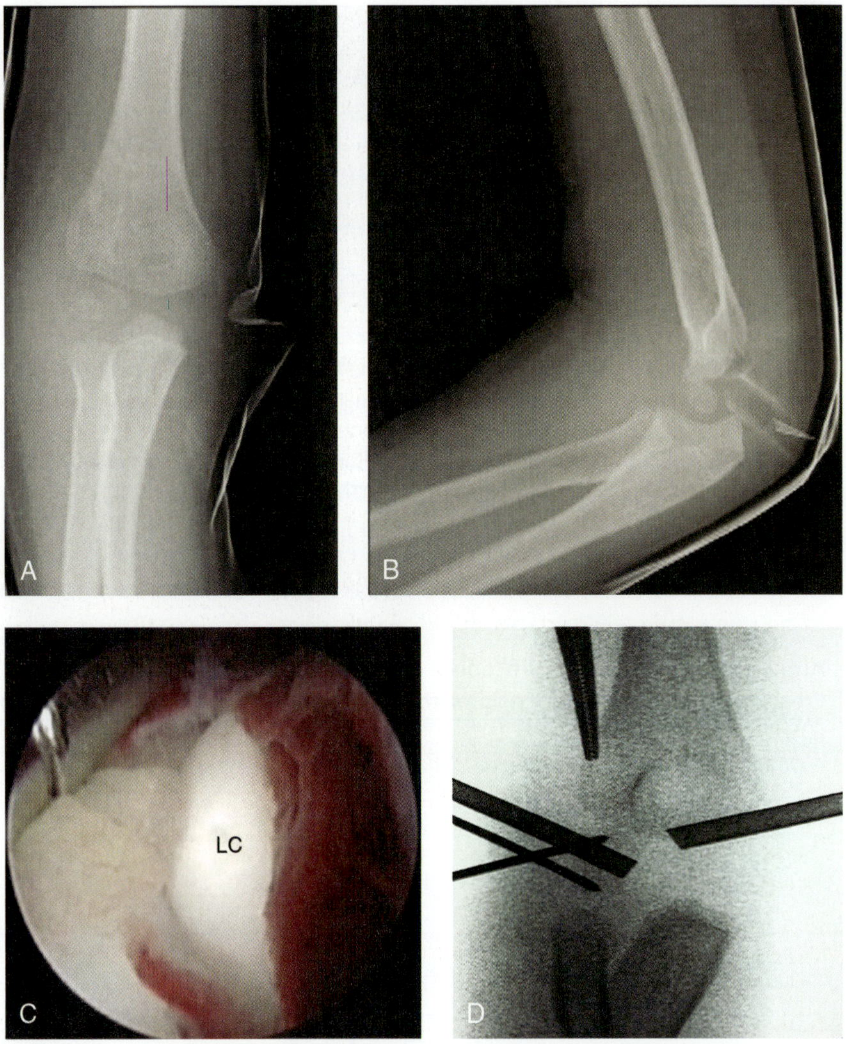


**Figure 5** AP (**A**) and lateral (**B**) radiographs demonstrate a displaced lateral condyle in a 4-year-old patient. **C,** Arthroscopic view from the medial portal demonstrates the lateral condyle fragment. The surgeon is preparing to advance the medial cannula to the fracture site for pin placement in the lateral condyle (LC). **D,** AP fluoroscopic image demonstrates provisional fixation with two previously positioned Kirschner wires.

- The arthroscope is replaced in the anteromedial portal to view the tip of the pin at the surface of the bone.
- The pin is used as a joystick to manipulate the condylar fragment, and the accuracy of the reduction is assessed.
- Two or three pins are inserted to fix the fracture.
- A transverse transcondylar pin adds considerable rotational stability. If possible, one of the pins should be directed transversely into the trochlea.
- In patients with marked displacement or rotation of the fracture, adequate reduction may not be possible. In these patients, standard open reduction or the use of a small incision to assist with reduction may be needed.

### CAPITELLUM AND TROCHLEA FRACTURES

- A proximal anteromedial portal is established.
- Hematoma is evacuated as described previously.

 

- Capitellum fractures frequently partially reduce on elbow extension and displace on elbow flexion. A trocar introduced in the proximal anterolateral portal can help push the articular fragment distally. The trocar or a Freer elevator is inserted in the radiocapitellar joint and used in shoehorn fashion to help the radial head glide proximally over the capitellum. When the elbow is flexed, the radial head helps maintain the reduction (**Figure 6, A** and **B**).
- The fracture is inspected from a transtricipital or distal posterolateral portal.
- A shaver inserted in the posterior radiocapitellar soft-spot portal is used to débride loose fragments. This step is important because of the high incidence of comminution or plastic deformation of the posterior wall of the lateral condyle, which can impede an anatomic reduction.
- As the arthroscope is advanced down the lateral gutter into the anterior compartment, the lateral trochlea is visualized and the reduction assessed.
- Frequently, the fragment will be found to be rotated, with the lateral trochlear ridge proximal. In this situation, a Freer elevator or small skin hook can be used to pull the trochlea distally to de-rotate the fragment.
- After accurate reduction is confirmed, guidewires are placed from posterior to anterior, entering through a small posterolateral incision over the flat surface of the posterior face of the lateral column.
- The guidewires are advanced until they are seen at the articular surface. The use of a 70° arthroscope, typically inserted through the posterior portal, may be helpful. Direct observation of the pin as it exits the capitellum assures optimal placement and correct length of cannulated screws (**Figure 6, C** and **D**). The longest screws possible should be used. Because of the spherical shape of the capitellum, undersizing or oversizing of screws may occur if screw lengths are estimated radiographically.
- To further increase the strength of fixation, a lateral-to-medial 2.5- or 2.7-mm transcondylar screw may be used.

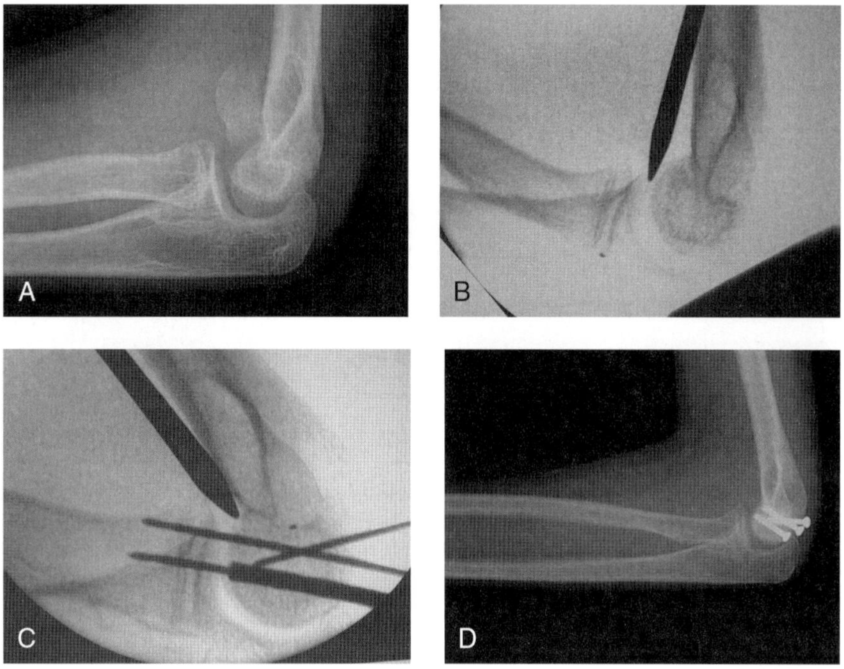


**Figure 6** **A,** Lateral radiograph of the elbow from a 14-year-old boy demonstrates a double-hump sign, indicating an anterior coronal shearing fracture extending to the lateral trochlear ridge. **B,** Lateral fluoroscopic image demonstrates arthroscopically assisted fracture reduction. **C,** Lateral fluoroscopic image demonstrates arthroscopically assisted reduction and percutaneous fixation of the fracture. **D,** Lateral radiograph demonstrates final fixation at 1 month postoperatively.

## UNICONDYLAR FRACTURES OF THE DISTAL HUMERUS

- Placement of the patient in a supine position and use of a shoulder positioner facilitate this procedure by applying longitudinal traction to the elbow.
- Visualization and reduction are similar to that described previously for the capitellum fracture. However, a thicker (3-mm) Steinmann pin may be needed to manipulate the comparatively larger fragment with attached muscle origins (**Figure 7, A**).
- After the reduction is confirmed arthroscopically and radiographically, the fracture is temporarily fixed with transcondylar Kirschner wires or pins. A 3-mm Steinmann pin provides firm fixation for reduction and temporary stabilization (**Figure 7, B** and **C**).
- A medial or lateral midaxial incision is made for application of the plate. This dissection exposes the distal humerus, and no additional arthrotomy or musculotendinous dissection is required.
- In the reduction of a lateral column fracture, care must be taken to protect the ulnar nerve by not advancing the pin too far medially.
- In the reduction of a medial column fracture, the incision should be

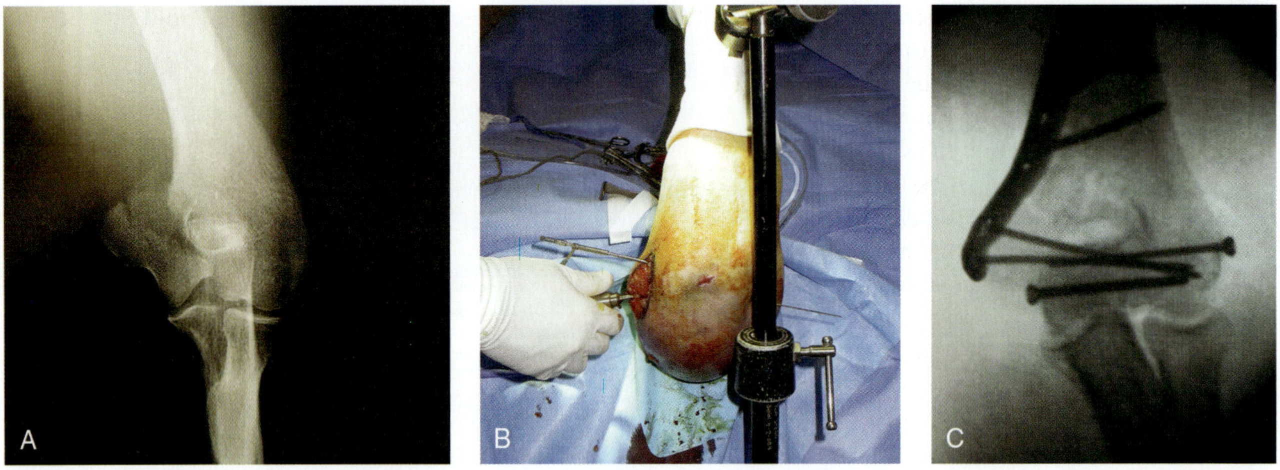


**Figure 7** **A,** AP radiograph of an elbow demonstrates a medial condyle fracture with an intact lateral column. **B,** Intraoperative photograph shows a medial incision that was made to identify and protect the ulnar nerve. The muscle and capsule attachments are not dissected, and an arthrotomy is not needed. A Steinmann pin was inserted for manipulation, and the reduction was observed arthroscopically. After radiographic confirmation, the pin was advanced into the lateral column. **C,** AP fluoroscopic image demonstrates placement of a plate directly on the supracondylar ridge and the use of screws to achieve stable, strong fixation.

made before pin placement because of the proximity of the ulnar nerve, which should be identified and protected when the pin is inserted.

- After the pin is in place, arthroscopic and radiographic examinations are used to confirm adequate reduction.
- A precontoured plate is applied over the Kirschner wires or Steinmann pin in the correct position.
- The plate is provisionally fixed, and a second distal transcondylar screw is placed though the plate.
- The initial pin can be replaced with a transcondylar screw through the plate according to the O'Driscoll principles of distal humerus fracture fixation.
- The remaining proximal and distal screws are placed.

## CORONOID FRACTURES

- Standard anteromedial and anterolateral portals are used.
- Evacuating the hematoma with a 3.5-mm shaver will permit adequate visualization of the coronoid from the anterolateral portal.
- If considerable synovitis or hematoma is present, a limited anterior capsular débridement may be necessary to enable visualization of the fragment. The capsule should not be resected.
- Guidewires for cannulated screws are placed through the posterior, subcutaneous border of the proximal ulna into the bed of the coronoid fracture with the use of a mini C-arm for fluoroscopic guidance or a drill guide of the type used in anterior cruciate ligament repair.
- A small, modified skin hook is introduced through a cannula in the anteromedial portal to reduce and stabilize the coronoid fragment. With the reduction held in place, the guidewires are advanced into the coronoid fragment. The screws should angle 10° to 15° proximally to "trap" the coronoid and minimize the possibility of the trochlea pushing the fragment off the tip of the screw. When properly reduced, the coronoid should conform to the trochlea.
- If the fragment is too small to support two screws, one cannulated screw and a cerclage suture are used. The screw should be slightly undersized to avoid abrasion and breakage of the suture on the tip of the screw. A No. 2 fiber-reinforced suture is passed through the screw and retrieved with a suture shuttle technique along the medial or lateral side of the proximal ulna.
- To pass the suture laterally, a shuttle suture is introduced through an 18-gauge spinal needle inserted just proximal to the proximal radioulnar joint from the posterolateral surface of the elbow. The fixation suture and the shuttle are extracted through the lateral portal and shuttled to the posterior surface, where an arthroscopic sliding knot is used to cinch the coronoid fragment into place.

## POSTEROLATERAL ROTATORY INSTABILITY OF THE ELBOW

- In patients with acute injuries, an anchor is percutaneously placed under arthroscopic visualization just posterior and proximal to the origin of the LUCL at the lateral epicondyle. Arthroscopic suture-passing instruments are used to place a horizontal mattress suture through the ligament. The suture is tied through a small incision.

 

- In patients with chronic posterolateral instability, multiple sutures are placed in the lateral ulnohumeral ligament beginning at its most distal extent and progressing proximally. Sutures are placed in the lateral gutter and are retrieved with a retrograde suture retriever placed near the proximal attachment of the radial ulnohumeral ligament on the humerus. The sutures are pulled to evaluate tension and plication. After the tension and plication are deemed acceptable, the sutures are tied sequentially from distal to proximal, thereby plicating and tightening the posterolateral corner.
- To confirm adequate reconstruction, the elbow drive-through sign (the ability to move an arthroscope through the posterior central portal down the posterolateral gutter and straight across to the medial gutter) is tested. In a stable elbow, this maneuver is not possible.

#### RADIAL HEAD FRACTURES

- The radial head is viewed from the proximal anteromedial portal.
- A shaver is inserted through the proximal anterolateral portal.
- Reduction is accomplished with the use of a periosteal elevator or percutaneously placed Kirschner wires, which can be used as joysticks to maneuver the fracture fragments into position.
- After reduction is achieved, the cannulated screw guidewires can be passed into the radial diaphysis to allow placement of cannulated headless screws. Care must be taken to bury the threads beneath the articular surface to avoid impingement of the proximal radioulnar joint. The posterior radial head can be viewed through a soft-spot portal. The posterolateral working portal provides an optimal angle for screw entry.

#### PEDIATRIC SUPRACONDYLAR MALUNION

- Anteromedial and anterolateral portals are established slightly more distal than the typical portal positions to avoid anterior deflection by the apex of the deformity.
- The apex of the deformity is identified by dissecting with the shaver along the anterior cortex of the humerus, which is a relatively safe zone of dissection.
- The level of the intended osteotomy is confirmed radiographically.
- A barrel-shaped burr is used to cut a groove into the anterior cortex of the humerus. The requisite dimension of the anterior cut is calculated by using elementary trigonometry, and the cut is approximated by means of comparison with the known diameter of the burr.
- Kirschner wires or Steinmann pins are placed for fixation.
- The resection is continued past the midaxial line into the anterior surface of the posterior cortex.
- Gentle pressure applied with the surgeon's thumbs along the posterior cortex of the distal fragment will crack the posterior cortex, which is then flexed the desired amount.
- The pins are advanced to stabilize the osteotomy.
- Three previously placed 2-mm Kirschner wires or Steinmann pins, two lateral and one medial, are advanced under radiographic guidance, with care taken to avoid the ulnar nerve.
- The correction and alignment are confirmed radiographically.
- If varus alignment is observed, a biplanar osteotomy can be done by varying the cut across the anterior aspect of the elbow according to the preoperative calculations of the correction required.

#### EPIPHYSEAL RECONSTRUCTION

- A standard anteromedial portal is created.
- An anterolateral portal is created with a 25-gauge needle just superior to the capitellum.
- A 3.5-mm shaver is used to begin a thorough and meticulous débridement of the fibrous scar tissue at the site of the nonunion. Both surfaces must be cleaned and planed to ensure a broad surface of contact to optimize the potential for healing.
- Débridement of the posterior wall fragment exposes the bone of the physeal bar. This bone should be removed with aggressive use of a shaver or a burr until the white cartilage of the physeal plate is exposed. It is necessary to remove a substantial amount of tissue and bone.
- After the fracture surfaces are prepared, guidewires for cannulated screws are inserted from the posterior flat surface of the lateral condyle, as described previously for capitellum fractures.
- The anterior fragment is reduced, and the guidewires are advanced.
- After drilling is performed, cannulated screws are measured and inserted.

### Wound Closure

- The portal incisions are closed with absorbable sutures in the standard manner.

## Postoperative Regimen

Healing is prioritized over early range of motion. Usually, the small size of the fragment precludes aggressive, early exercises. The elbow is immobilized in a cast until the fracture has united, after which range-of-motion exercises are begun. However, the patients should be informed at the outset of treatment that a staged arthroscopic release may be necessary to restore motion, especially because motion was limited even before the first procedure.

## Limiting Adverse Events

The key steps in safe elbow arthroscopy are careful entry into the joint and establishment of an adequate working space to permit visualization and identification of the elbow anatomy. Because of the presence of hemarthrosis, the initial step is to perform gentle lavage in the joint using a small (3.5-mm) shaver with the blade directed toward the humerus to evacuate the blood. The clot is broken up with the shaver tip. Patience and persistence are required for this step, which can take 10 minutes to perform. If the surgical field cannot be cleared to permit a good view, the arthroscopy should be abandoned and a conventional, open approach used. Conversion to open surgery is easy if inflow pressures are kept below 30 mm Hg to avoid soft-tissue extravasation and swelling of the elbow. The technical steps used to reduce and repair the fracture are similar to those used in open surgery, and the same precautions apply.

## Bibliography


Abboud JA, Ricchetti ET, Tjoumakaris F, Ramsey ML: Elbow arthroscopy: Basic setup and portal placement. *J Am Acad Orthop Surg* 2006;14(5):312-318.

Adams JE, Merten SM, Steinmann SP: Arthroscopic-assisted treatment of coronoid fractures. *Arthroscopy* 2007;23(10):1060-1065.

Adams JE, Sanchez-Sotelo J, Kallina CF IV, Morrey BF, Steinmann SP: Fractures of the coronoid: Morphology based upon computer tomography scanning. *J Shoulder Elbow Surg* 2012;21(6):782-788.

Andrews JR, Carson WG: Arthroscopy of the elbow. *Arthroscopy* 1985;1(2):97-107.

Baker CL Jr, Jones GL: Arthroscopy of the elbow. *Am J Sports Med* 1999;27(2):251-264.

Bennett JM: Elbow arthroscopy: The basics. *J Hand Surg Am* 2013;38(1):164-167.

Broberg MA, Morrey BF: Results of treatment of fracture-dislocations of the elbow. *Clin Orthop Relat Res* 1987;(216):109-119.

Catterall A: Legg-Calvé-Perthes syndrome. *Clin Orthop Relat Res* 1981;(158):41-52.

Claessen FM, Louwerens JK, Doornberg JN, van Dijk CN, van den Bekerom MP, Eygendaal D: Hegemann's disease and fishtail deformity: Aetiopathogenesis, radiographic appearance and clinical outcome. *J Child Orthop* 2015;9(1):1-8.

Closkey RF, Goode JR, Kirschenbaum D, Cody RP: The role of the coronoid process in elbow stability: A biomechanical analysis of axial loading. *J Bone Joint Surg Am* 2000;82(12):1749-1753.

Dawson FA, Inostroza F: Arthroscopic reduction and percutaneous fixation of a radial neck fracture in a child. *Arthroscopy* 2004;20(suppl 2):90-93.

Dodson CC, Nho SJ, Williams RJ III, Altchek DW: Elbow arthroscopy. *J Am Acad Orthop Surg* 2008;16(10):574-585.

Doornberg JN, Ring D: Coronoid fracture patterns. *J Hand Surg Am* 2006;31(1):45-52.


 

Glotzbecker MP, Bae DS, Links AC, Waters PM: Fishtail deformity of the distal humerus: A report of 15 cases. *J Pediatr Orthop* 2013;33(6):592-597.

Guitton TG, Doornberg JN, Raaymakers EL, Ring D, Kloen P: Fractures of the capitellum and trochlea. *J Bone Joint Surg Am* 2009;91(2):390-397.

Hardy P, Menguy F, Guillot S: Arthroscopic treatment of capitellum fracture of the humerus. *Arthroscopy* 2002;18(4):422-426.

Hausman MR, Klug RA, Qureshi S, Goldstein R, Parsons BO: Arthroscopically assisted coronoid fracture fixation: A preliminary report. *Clin Orthop Relat Res* 2008;466(12):3147-3152.

Hausman MR, Qureshi S, Goldstein R, et al: Arthroscopically-assisted treatment of pediatric lateral humeral condyle fractures. *J Pediatr Orthop* 2007;27(7):739-742.

Holt MS, Savoie FH III, Field LD, Ramsey JR: Arthroscopic management of elbow trauma. *Hand Clin* 2004;20(4):485-495.

Hsu JW, Gould JL, Fonseca-Sabune H, Hausman MH: The emerging role of elbow arthroscopy in chronic use injuries and fracture care. *Hand Clin* 2009;25(3):305-321.

Kelly EW, Morrey BF, O'Driscoll SW: Complications of elbow arthroscopy. *J Bone Joint Surg Am* 2001;83(1):25-34.

Koehler SM, Sakamoto S, Abernathie BL, Hausman MR: Arthroscopic correction of a supracondylar malunion in a child. *Arthrosc Tech* 2015;4(3):e215-e221.

Kuriyama K, Kawanishi Y, Yamamoto K: Arthroscopic-assisted reduction and percutaneous fixation for coronal shear fractures of the distal humerus: Report of two cases. *J Hand Surg Am* 2010;35(9):1506-1509.

Labelle H, Bunnell WP, Duhaime M, Poitras B: Cubitus varus deformity following supracondylar fractures of the humerus in children. *J Pediatr Orthop* 1982;2(5):539-546.

Lynch GJ, Meyers JF, Whipple TL, Caspari RB: Neurovascular anatomy and elbow arthroscopy: Inherent risks. *Arthroscopy* 1986;2(3):191-197.

Métaizeau JP: Reduction and osteosynthesis of radial neck fractures in children by centromedullary pinning. *Injury* 2005;36(suppl 1):S75-S77.

Métaizeau JP, Prévot J, Schmitt M: Reduction and fixation of fractures of the neck of the radious be centro-medullary pinning: Original technic [French]. *Rev Chir Orthop Reparatrice Appar Mot* 1980;66(1):47-49.

Micheli LJ, Luke AC, Mintzer CM, Waters PM: Elbow arthroscopy in the pediatric and adolescent population. *Arthroscopy* 2001;17(7):694-699.

Michels F, Pouliart N, Handelberg F: Arthroscopic management of Mason type 2 radial head fractures. *Knee Surg Sports Traumatol Arthrosc* 2007;15(10):1244-1250.

Mitani M, Nabeshima Y, Ozaki A, et al: Arthroscopic reduction and percutaneous cannulated screw fixation of a capitellar fracture of the humerus: A case report. *J Shoulder Elbow Surg* 2009;18(2):e6-e9.

Morrey BF: Arthroscopy of the elbow. *Instr Course Lect* 1986;35:102-107.

Moskal MJ, Savoie FH III, Field LD: Elbow arthroscopy in trauma and reconstruction. *Orthop Clin North Am* 1999;30(1):163-177.

O'Driscoll SW: Optimizing stability in distal humeral fracture fixation. *J Shoulder Elbow Surg* 2005;14 (1 suppl S):S186-S194.

O'Driscoll SW, Bell DF, Morrey BF: Posterolateral rotatory instability of the elbow. *J Bone Joint Surg Am* 1991;73(3):440-446.

O'Driscoll SW, Morrey BF: Arthroscopy of the elbow: Diagnostic and therapeutic benefits and hazards. *J Bone Joint Surg Am* 1992;74(1):84-94.

Olsen SJ II, Fleisig GS, Dun S, Loftice J, Andrews JR: Risk factors for shoulder and elbow injuries in adolescent baseball pitchers. *Am J Sports Med* 2006;34(6):905-912.

Otsuka NY, Kasser JR: Supracondylar fractures of the humerus in children. *J Am Acad Orthop Surg* 1997;5(1):19-26.

Perez Carro L, Golano P, Vega J: Arthroscopic-assisted reduction and percutaneous external fixation of lateral condyle fractures of the humerus. *Arthroscopy* 2007;23(10):1131.e1 1131.e4.

Ring D, Jupiter JB, Gulotta L: Articular fractures of the distal part of the humerus. *J Bone Joint Surg Am* 2003;85(2):232-238.

Rolla PR, Surace MF, Bini A, Pilato G: Arthroscopic treatment of fractures of the radial head. *Arthroscopy* 2006;22(2): 233.e1-233.e6.

Savoie FH III, Nunley PD, Field LD: Arthroscopic management of the arthritic elbow: Indications, technique, and results. *J Shoulder Elbow Surg* 1999;8(3):214-219.

Savoie FH III, O'Brien MJ, Field LD, Gurley DJ: Arthroscopic and open radial ulnohumeral ligament reconstruction for posterolateral rotatory instability of the elbow. *Clin Sports Med* 2010;29(4):611-618.

Schneeberger AG, Sadowski MM, Jacob HA: Coronoid process and radial head as posterolateral rotatory stabilizers of the elbow. *J Bone Joint Surg Am* 2004;86(5):975-982.

Siparsky PN, Kocher MS: Current concepts in pediatric and adolescent arthroscopy. *Arthroscopy* 2009;25(12):1453-1469.

Smith JP III, Savoie FH III, Field LD: Posterolateral rotatory instability of the elbow. *Clin Sports Med* 2001;20(1):47-58.

Van Tongel A, Macdonald P, Van Riet R, Dubberley J: Elbow arthroscopy in acute injuries. *Knee Surg Sports Traumatol Arthrosc* 2012;20(12):2542-2548.

Vavken P, Müller AM, Camathias C: First 50 pediatric and adolescent elbow arthroscopies: Analysis of indications and complications. *J Pediatr Orthop* 2015; March 3 [Epub ahead of print].

 

SECTION 2
# Enthesopathy and Tendon Rupture

# Chapter 8

# Triceps Tendon Repair

*Joshua A. Baumfeld, MD*
*Eric T. Tolo, MD*

**Learning Objectives**

- Understand the indications for triceps tendon repair.
- Learn the current techniques for triceps tendon repair.
- Review and understand the current literature available for triceps tendon repair.

## Indications

Complete tears of the triceps tendon and those tears comprising greater than 50% of the tendon are considered for surgical repair (**Figure 1**). However, treatment must be individualized to each patient. Patients who are debilitated may benefit from nonsurgical treatment of complete tears because the lateral expansion and anconeus are often intact, allowing active, albeit weak, elbow extension (**Figure 2**). Partial tears comprising greater than 50% of the tendon are often managed surgically in young, healthy patients.

Partial tears comprising less than 50% of the tendon are often managed nonsurgically. However, active individuals may require surgical intervention if nonsurgical treatment is unsuccessful. Symptoms of partial tears include pain and weakness. Partial and complete tears of the triceps muscle belly are generally managed nonsurgically.

## Contraindications

Patients with severe medical comorbidities who are at risk for anesthetic or surgical complications should be treated nonsurgically. Patients with a history of infection or an active infection should not be treated surgically with allograft.

## Alternative Treatments

Nonsurgical management often consists of immobilization in a splint or cast for up to 4 weeks with the elbow at approximately 30° of flexion. Depending on the size of the tear, immediate rehabilitation of small partial-thickness tears

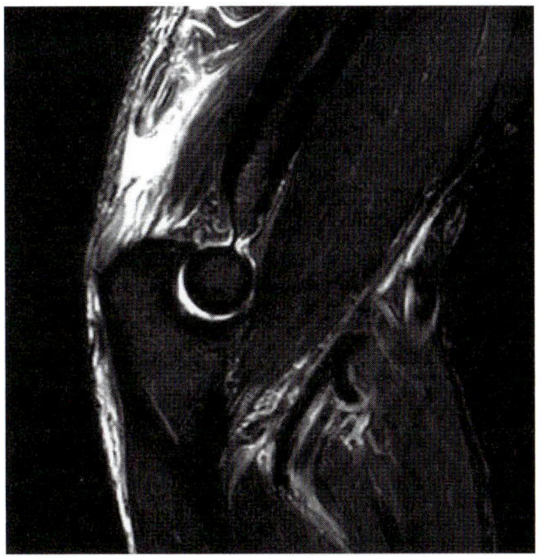

**Figure 1** Sagittal T2-weighted MRI of an elbow demonstrates a complete tear of the distal triceps tendon.

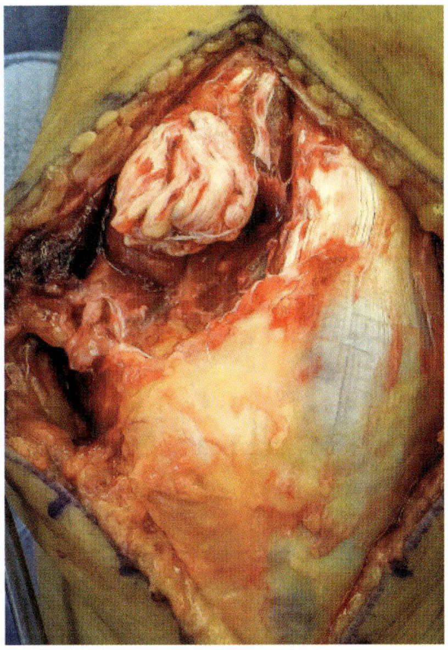

**Figure 2** Intraoperative photograph of an elbow shows a torn triceps tendon and an intact anconeus muscle.

*Dr. Tolo or an immediate family member serves as a board member, owner, officer, or committee member of the New England Orthopedic Society and the New England Shoulder and Elbow Society. Neither Dr. Baumfeld nor any immediate family member has received anything of value from or has stock or stock options held in a commercial company or institution related directly or indirectly to the subject of this chapter.*

**Table 1** Results of Triceps Tendon Repair[a]

| Authors (Year) | No. of Patients | Procedure or Approach | Mean Patient Age in Years | Mean Follow-up in Months (Range) | Success Rate (%) | Results |
|---|---|---|---|---|---|---|
| van Riet et al (2003) | 14 | Primary repair through trans-osseous cruciate drill holes | 50 | 93 | 100 | Avg ROM, 8°-138°<br>Peak strength averaged 92% of that of the unaffected extremity at >1 yr postoperatively |
| Mair et al (2004) | 19 (11 complete tears) | Primary suture repair | 29 | 34 | 95 | 18 patients returned to professional football |
| Sierra et al (2006) | 12 | Primary repair through trans-osseous drill holes using the Krackow or Bunnell suture technique (10 patients) or anconeus flap reconstruction (2 patients) | 50 | 16.8 (7-168) | 75 (full strength) | 9 patients had 5/5 strength, and 2 had 4/5 strength<br>Complications occurred in 3 patients |
| Bava et al (2012) | 5 | Single-row suture anchor repair | 46.8 | 32 (18-49) | 100 | Avg ASES score, 99.2 ± 1<br>Avg DASH score, 1.4 ± 3<br>Avg Mayo Elbow Performance Index, 95.8 ± 9 |
| Kokkalis et al (2013) | 11 | Double-row with Bunnell suture repair through crossed drill holes and proximal 2-3 anchors placed for medial row | 53 | 21 (12-40) | 82 (very satisfied) | VAS score improved from 8.5 to 2.4<br>Strength improved from 1.63/5 to 4.8/5<br>ROM was near normal in all patients, with an avg loss of 7° of extension |

ASES = American Shoulder and Elbow Surgeons elbow outcome; DASH = Disabilities of the Arm, Shoulder and Hand; ROM = range of motion; VAS = visual analog scale.
[a] All studies are level IV evidence.

may be attempted. The authors of this chapter prefer the use of either a hinged elbow brace that allows for locking and adjustment of the flexion position, or a removable thermoplastic splint set at approximately 30°. Active flexion is gradually increased as healing progresses.

## Results

Published results of the triceps tendon repair are summarized in **Table 1**. Because of the rarity of this injury, published results are limited. Some studies include heterogeneous patient populations treated with various repair techniques. Multiple techniques have yielded similar outcomes, with high rates of success and low rates of rerupture. Typically, the surgical techniques used consist of locked suturing of the triceps tendon and repair with crossed drill holes across the olecranon; the use of suture anchors in a single- or double-row configuration; a hybrid technique using a row of suture anchors as well as the passage of suture through the olecranon; the augmentation of a primary repair or attempted primary repair with an anconeus flap; or the use of either Achilles tendon allograft (with or without a bone block) or semitendinosus allograft or autograft (in patients with chronic tears in which the native tendon will not reach the olecranon).

## Techniques

### Setup/Exposure

- The patient is placed supine with the affected arm brought over and held at the chest.
- Alternatively, the patient is placed

 

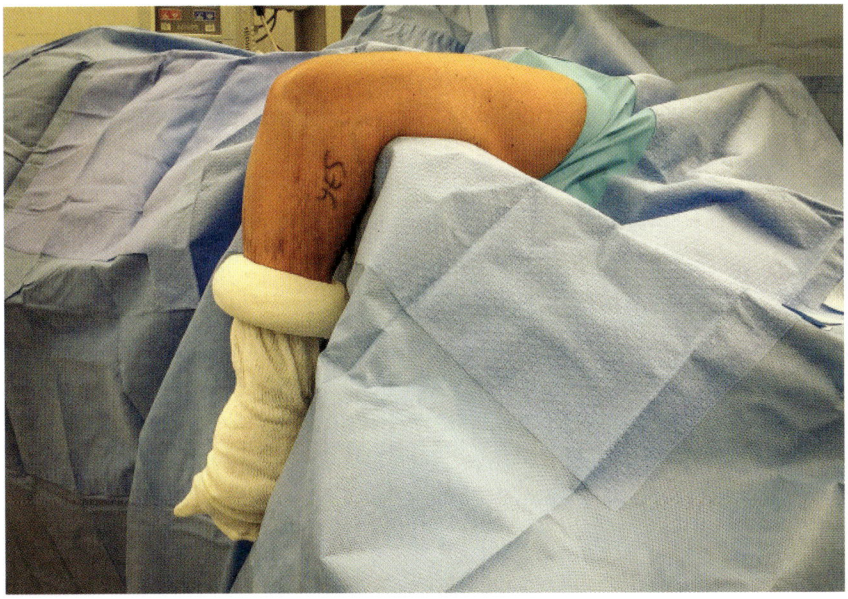

**Figure 3** Intraoperative photograph shows a patient placed in the lateral decubitus position, with the right elbow placed in an arm holder.

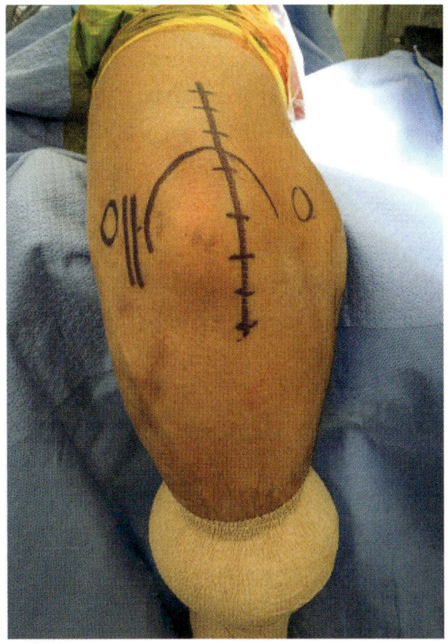

**Figure 4** Intraoperative photograph of an elbow shows the planned incision site for triceps tendon repair. The locations of the posterior midline incision (dashed line) and the ulnar nerve (parallel lines) are marked.

in the lateral decubitus position, and the affected arm is supported by a commercial arm holder (**Figure 3**).

- A posterior midline incision is made extending proximally to the musculotendinous junction of the triceps and distally approximately 3 cm from the olecranon tip (**Figure 4**). To perform an anconeus rotation flap reconstruction in the chronic setting, the posterior midline incision is lengthened distally to expose the anconeus.
- The ulnar nerve is identified medially (**Figure 5**).

## Instruments/Equipment/ Implants Required

- A No. 2 or No. 5 high-strength, braided, nonabsorbable suture is used.
- For direct repair through bone tunnels, a 2.0-mm drill with a Keith needle or straight suture passer is used.
- For repair with bone anchors, 3.5- to 5.0-mm anchors are used.
- A fluoroscopic C-arm may be useful for intraoperative imaging.

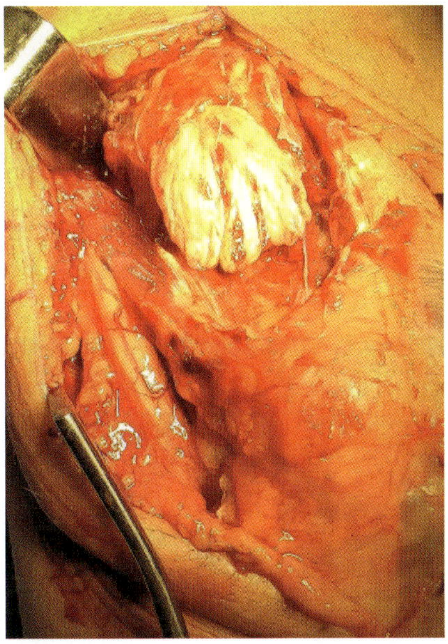

**Figure 5** Intraoperative photograph of an elbow shows the location of the ulnar nerve, which lies just medial to the torn triceps tendon.

## Procedure

- The degenerative tendon is débrided.
- In acute cases, a fleck of avulsed olecranon is commonly excised.
- In chronic cases, calcific changes in the tendon are commonly shelled out from the degenerative tendon (**Figure 6**).
- The olecranon is débrided before repair.
- The elbow is held in 40° 60° of flexion to determine the appropriate tension of the repair.

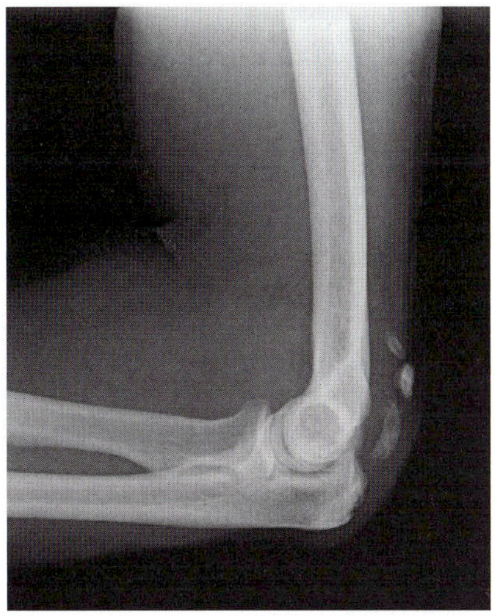

**Figure 6** Lateral radiograph of an elbow demonstrates a chronic triceps tendon tear with avulsion and calcifications.

- The goal of repair is to reattach healthy tendon to the original triceps footprint (**Figure 7**).
- In all repairs except the anconeus rotation flap reconstruction, the repaired triceps tendon should be sutured to the anconeus to augment the repair laterally. The common insertion has a mean width of 19 mm (range, 14 to 27 mm) and a mean thickness of 8 mm (range, 5 to 11 mm). The average distance from the posterior articular surface to the deepest insertion of the medial head is 16 mm (range, 12 to 20 mm), and the average length of the triceps bony footprint is 20.5 mm and the average width, 22.7 mm.

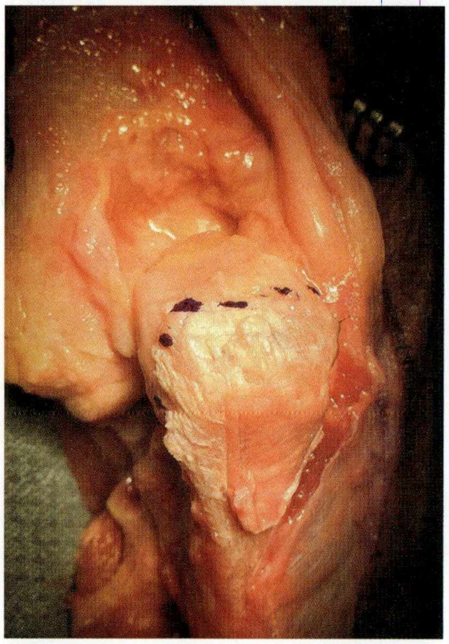

**Figure 7** Intraoperative photograph of an elbow shows the location of the triceps footprint, approximately 16 mm from the proximal tip of the articular surface.

**BONE TUNNEL TECHNIQUE**

- The suture is passed from distal to proximal in a locking fashion on the lateral and medial sides of the triceps tendon.
- The suture is tied proximally with the suture ends left free distally (**Figure 8, A**).
- Oblique drill holes are made in the olecranon to replicate the footprint.
- The free suture ends are passed through the drill holes using a Keith needle (**Figure 8, B**).
- To increase the surface area for repair, the sutures are passed with a free needle back into the distal extent of the triceps tendon (**Figure 8, C**).

**ANCHOR TECHNIQUE**

- Two bone anchors are placed into the medial and lateral olecranon.
- One free end of each suture from each anchor is placed in a locking fashion from distal to proximal. The suture strands from the same anchor that was placed in the tendon are then tied together proximally (**Figure 9, A**).
- The free suture ends from each anchor are then tensioned to deliver the triceps tendon to the olecranon, after which the suture ends are tied to one another (**Figure 9, B** and **C**).

**HYBRID BONE TUNNEL AND ANCHOR TECHNIQUE**

- Two bone anchors are placed into the medial and lateral olecranon.
- The sutures are passed and tied proximally and the free ends are tied as indicated previously, and the tendon is reapproximated to the olecranon.

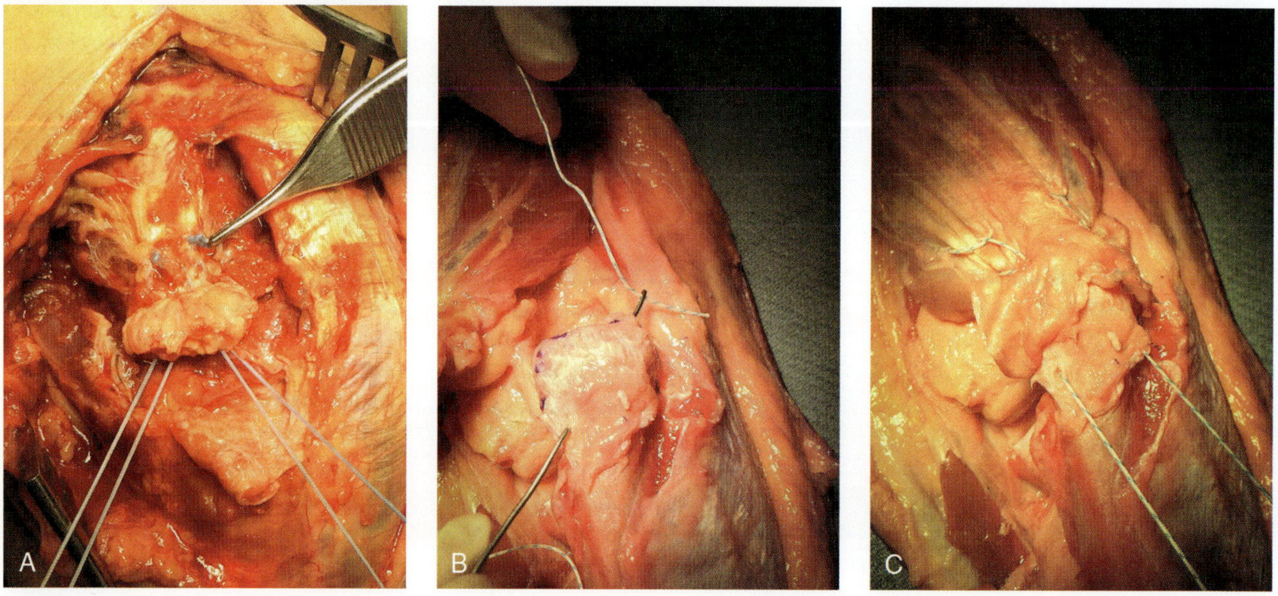


**Figure 8** Intraoperative photographs of an elbow show steps in the bone tunnel technique for triceps tendon repair. **A,** Locking sutures are used to grasp the tendon for a four-strand repair. **B,** Sutures are passed through bone tunnels in the olecranon. **C,** The triceps tendon is delivered to the bone and sutures are tied.

 

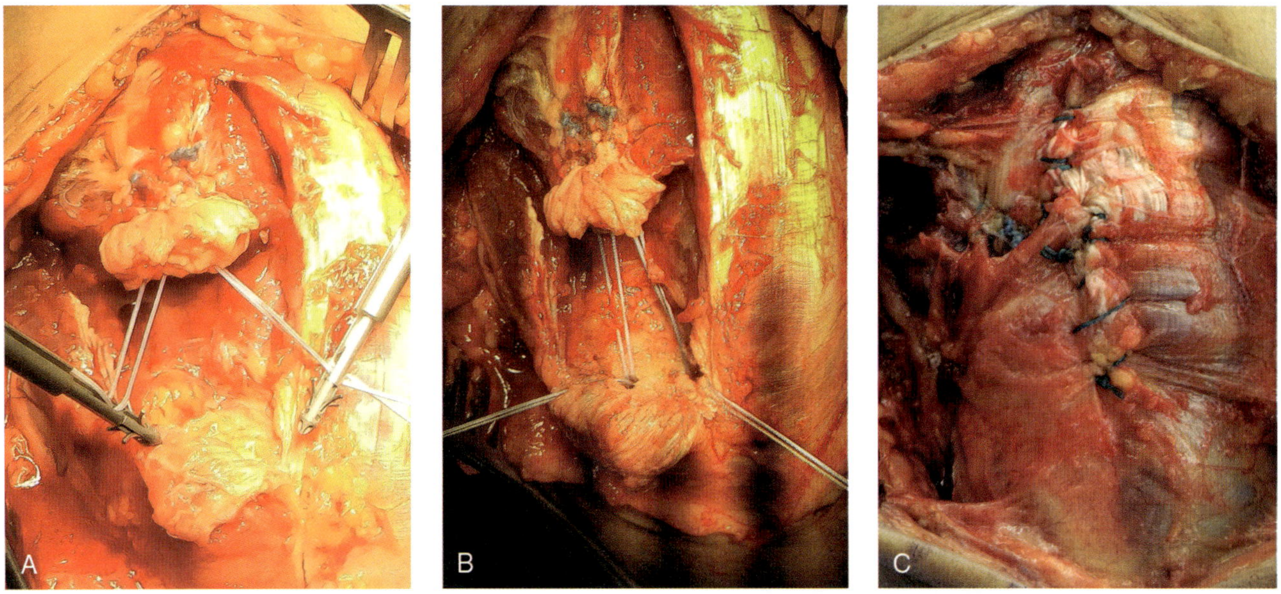

**Figure 9** Intraoperative photographs of an elbow show steps in the anchor technique for triceps tendon repair. **A,** The sutures are passed through two bone anchors. **B,** The anchors are placed into the olecranon at the triceps footprint. **C,** Appearance of the final repair with the lateral triceps tendon sutured to the intact anconeus.

- The free suture ends are passed with a free needle through the distal extent of the triceps tendon and then through transverse drill holes. The sutures are passed and tied.

#### ANCONEUS ROTATION FLAP RECONSTRUCTION

- The Kocher interval between the extensor carpi ulnaris muscle and the anconeus is used (**Figure 10, A**).
- The anconeus is mobilized from the ulnar and humeral attachments and is rotated over the proximal olecranon (**Figure 10, B**).
- The anconeus is repaired with drill holes and/or suture anchors.

#### ACHILLES TENDON ALLOGRAFT RECONSTRUCTION

- The remaining triceps tendon and muscle are mobilized.
- The allograft is secured distally at the olecranon. In the setting of bone deficiency, an Achilles allograft with attached calcaneal bone is affixed to the olecranon with a screw (**Figure 11**). In the setting of adequate bone stock, the allograft is secured to the triceps tendon using the bone tunnel repair, anchor repair, or hybrid repair technique as indicated previously.
- With the allograft expansion proximally, the tendon is wrapped around the musculotendinous junction of the triceps tendon and sutured in place with the elbow in 40° to 60° of flexion.

### Wound Closure

- Tension on the repair is assessed with the elbow in flexion.
- The wound is closed in a layered fashion.
- A posterior splint with side supports at 30° of flexion is placed.

## Postoperative Regimen

It is critical to protect the repair postoperatively. The patient must wear a splint for approximately 10 to 14 days postoperatively, with strict arm elevation for the first 72 hours. The initial splint is replaced with a static thermoplastic splint in 30° to 60° of flexion or a hinged elbow brace. Gentle passive, gravity-assisted extension and active flexion exercises are begun after the postoperative splint is removed; these exercises will limit stress on the repair. The goal with this rehabilitation protocol is to regain full range of motion by 6 to 8 weeks postoperatively. Resistance therapy is delayed until after tendon-bone healing has occurred, approximately 10 to 12 weeks postoperatively. The patient may not achieve full strength until 6 to 12 months postoperatively.

## Limiting Adverse Events

The ulnar nerve must be identified and protected during triceps tendon repair. Transposition of the ulnar nerve is rarely required. To minimize the risk of injury, the surgeon must take care when drilling across the olecranon and when using needle devices to pass suture adjacent to the ulnar nerve.

The surgeon should take care not to breach the articular surface (be aware of

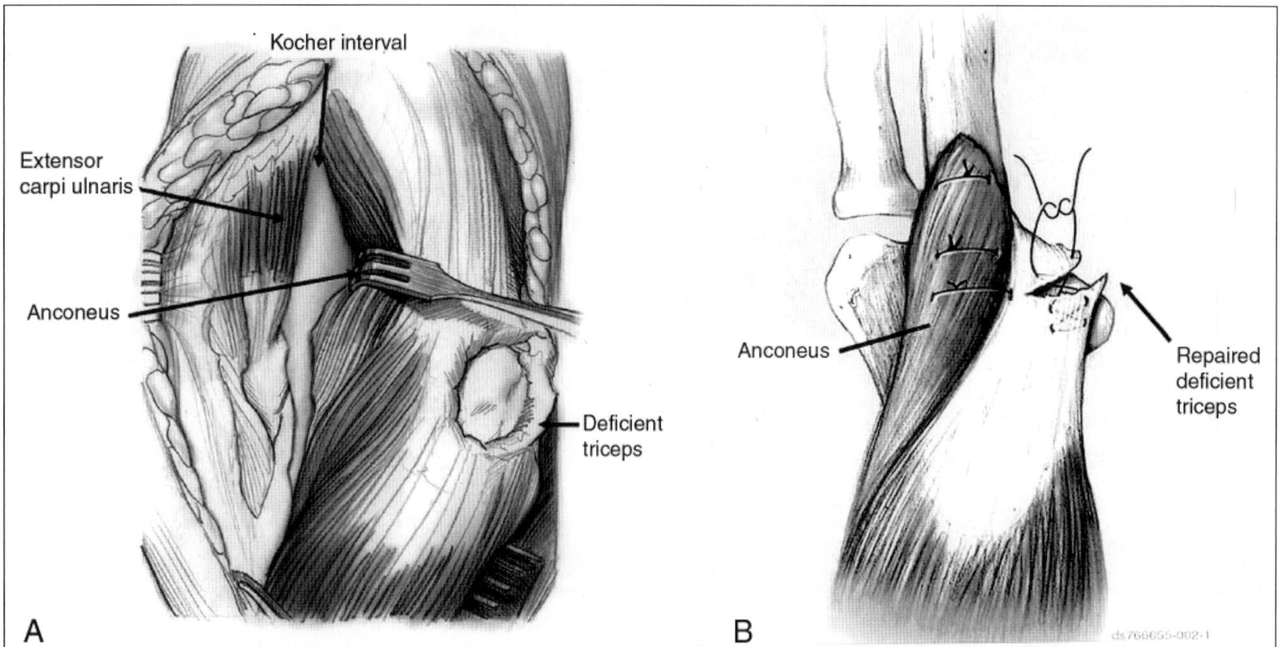


**Figure 10** Illustration of an elbow shows steps in anconeus rotation flap reconstruction for triceps tendon repair. **A,** The attachment of the anconeus to the lateral margin of the triceps allows the anconeus to serve as a reconstructive option for triceps deficiency. **B,** If the deficit in the triceps tendon is not too extensive, the anconeus may be mobilized and oriented over the tip of the olecranon. The tear or deficiency is repaired or reinforced with No. 5 nonabsorbable suture. (Reproduced with permission from the Mayo Foundation for Medical Education and Research, Rochester, MN.)

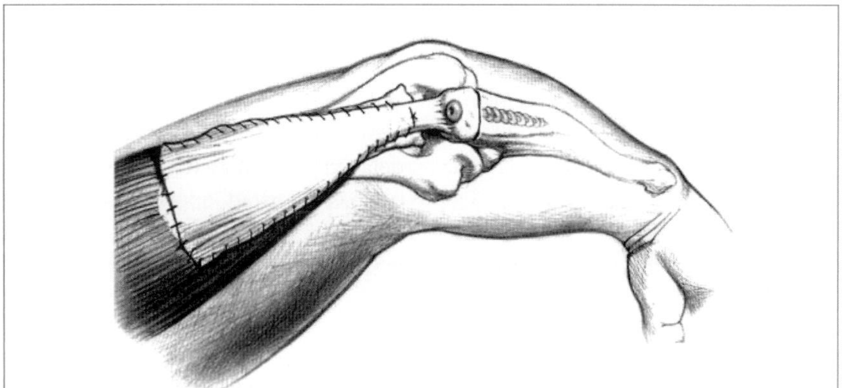

**Figure 11** Illustration of an elbow shows the final appearance of an Achilles tendon allograft reconstruction for triceps tendon repair. The proximal aspect of the graft is secured with multiple No. 1 interrupted and running sutures. (Reproduced with permission from the Mayo Foundation for Medical Education and Research, Rochester, MN.)

the position of the articular surface to avoid iatrogenic damage) when drilling holes and placing anchors into the olecranon. Anchors should be angled away from the articular surface. Intraoperative imaging is useful in confirming placement of surgical tools and anchoring devices.

Similar to the knee joint, the elbow is placed under high stresses, and meticulous wound closure is required to reduce the risk of dehiscence. The wound should be closed in a layered fashion, and the closure should provide enough resistance to allow early motion without the risk of wound dehiscence.

 

## Bibliography

Athwal GS, McGill RJ, Rispoli DM: Isolated avulsion of the medial head of the triceps tendon: An anatomic study and arthroscopic repair in 2 cases. *Arthroscopy* 2009;25(9):983-988.

Bava ED, Barber FA, Lund ER: Clinical outcome after suture anchor repair for complete traumatic rupture of the distal triceps tendon. *Arthroscopy* 2012;28(8):1058-1063.

Harris PC, Atkinson D, Moorehead JD: Bilateral partial rupture of triceps tendon: Case report and quantitative assessment of recovery. *Am J Sports Med* 2004;32(3):787-792.

Kokkalis ZT, Mavrogenis AF, Spyridonos S, Papagelopoulos PJ, Weiser RW, Sotereanos DG: Triceps brachii distal tendon reattachment with a double-row technique. *Orthopedics* 2013;36(2):110-116

Mair SD, Isbell WM, Gill TJ, Schlegel TF, Hawkins RJ: Triceps tendon ruptures in professional football players. *Am J Sports Med* 2004;32(2):431-434.

Sanchez-Sotelo J, Morrey BF: Surgical techniques for reconstruction of chronic insufficiency of the triceps: Rotation flap using anconeus and tendo achillis allograft. *J Bone Joint Surg Br* 2002;84(8):1116-1120.

Sierra RJ, Weiss NG, Shrader MW, Steinmann SP: Acute triceps ruptures: Case report and retrospective chart review. *J Shoulder Elbow Surg* 2006;15(1):130-134.

Strauch RJ: Biceps and triceps injuries of the elbow. *Orthop Clin North Am* 1999;30(1):95-107.

van Riet RP, Morrey BF, Ho E, O'Driscoll SW: Surgical treatment of distal triceps ruptures. *J Bone Joint Surg Am* 2003;85(10):1961-1967.

Yeh PC, Dodds SD, Smart LR, Mazzocca AD, Sethi PM: Distal triceps rupture. *J Am Acad Orthop Surg* 2010;18(1):31-40.

Yeh PC, Stephens KT, Solovyova O, et al: The distal triceps tendon footprint and a biomechanical analysis of 3 repair techniques. *Am J Sports Med* 2010;38(5):1025-1033.

# Chapter 9

# Distal Biceps Tendon Repair and Reconstruction

*Christopher C. Schmidt, MD*
*Claudius D. Jarrett, MD*

**Learning Objectives**

- Describe the distal biceps tendon and proximal radial anatomy and mechanics.
- Compare the reattachment sites and outcomes associated with either an anterior or posterior approach.
- Discuss the surgical options for the symptomatic chronic distal biceps tendon rupture.

## Indications

An improved understanding of the anatomy, mechanics, and surgical and nonsurgical management options has enhanced the ability to optimize function after complete avulsion of the distal biceps tendon. Distal biceps tendon rupture typically occurs in men between 20 and 50 years of age. Nonsurgical treatment results in diminished supination strength that is unsatisfying to some patients. Patient satisfaction is optimized with timely diagnosis, patient education, and shared decision-making. If surgical treatment is chosen, reattachment of the torn tendon to its native footprint is recommended.

Diagnosing a complete distal biceps tendon rupture is usually straightforward. Patients report a history of an eccentric contraction, a traumatic popping sensation, and pain. Physical examination often reveals ecchymosis, weak supination strength, and a positive hook test. The hook test is reported to be 100% sensitive and specific in detecting complete distal tears. The test is performed in 90° of elbow flexion and full isometric supination. The examiner should first test the uninjured arm, in which the biceps tendon is similar to a tight cord. The examiner hooks the tendon from the lateral side to avoid mistaking the lacertus fibrosus for an intact tendon. A negative result occurs when the biceps tendon is hooked without pain. If the cord cannot be hooked, complete rupture is diagnosed. The hook test helps to eliminate the diagnosis of myotendinous junction tears. Patients with myotendinous junction tears may report antecubital pain, ecchymosis, swelling, and/or weakness with elbow flexion and supination, but the tendon can be hooked; the test is negative for complete distal rupture. The reverse Popeye sign is commonly observed in patients with both a complete rupture and lacertus fibrosus tear. If the diagnosis remains unclear after the history and examination, elbow ultrasonography or MRI can be ordered.

The sharp pain after a complete rupture usually lessens with time, but some patients experience a chronic cramping sensation with activity and a loss of supination and flexion strength. The main indications for surgical treatment are to improve supination strength through a full arc of forearm rotation and limit fatigue pain. After a complete distal biceps tendon rupture, maximum supination strength decreases an average of 40% (range, 26% to 60%), and maximum flexion strength decreases an average of 20% (range, zero to 40%). Distal biceps tendon repair restores an average supination strength of 98% in pronation, 90% in neutral, and 74% in supination, as well as an average 95% flexion strength. Strong supination throughout the full arc of rotation helps in tasks such as loosening a tight bolt, swinging a bat or golf club, and stabilizing tools.

Studies of biceps deficiency demonstrate that patients often report fatigue with repetitive supination activities, compared with the uninjured side. This sensation of fatigue was initially

*Dr. Schmidt or an immediate family member serves as a paid consultant to or is an employee of Arthrex. Neither Dr. Jarrett nor any immediate family member has received anything of value from or has stock or stock options held in a commercial company or institution related directly or indirectly to the subject of this chapter.*

attributed to loss of endurance. However, recent research has attributed the fatigue to a lower initiating torque rather than a decrease in endurance of the remaining, intact musculotendinous units. That is, the torque generated by the remaining brachioradialis and supinator muscles does not change, but the absence of the biceps force lowers the starting torque that can be generated by the arm, which results in earlier fatigue during a given task. Furthermore, a patient with biceps deficiency has difficulty generating a supination torque in neutral-to-supinated positions without recruitment of the trunk muscles.

Surgical repair of a ruptured biceps tendon yields an average gain of 30% supination strength through a full arc of motion, an average increase in 15% flexion strength, a higher fatigue threshold, normal posture during end supination activities, and correction of the reverse Popeye deformity. However, some patients may prefer to avoid the risks, discomfort, and inconvenience of surgical treatment. To optimize outcomes, the surgeon should educate patients on the anticipated results, the functional implications of a biceps tendon deficiency, and the odds of potential surgical complications. After discussion of the risks and benefits of nonsurgical and surgical treatment, patients should choose the best option for their particular situation.

Chronicity of the injury should be addressed because an acute rupture (2 to 4 weeks after injury) is easier to repair and tends to have a lower complication rate because of preservation of the bicipital tunnel. Patients with a chronic rupture who are not satisfied with their comfort, strength, and/or perceived endurance may still be candidates for repair or reconstruction.

The goals of surgical management are to realign the tendon by externally rotating it 90°, reattach the tendon to the native footprint, and preserve the geometry of the radial tuberosity. The distal biceps tendon is approximately 4 cm long and is composed of distinct short and long heads. The tendon externally rotates 90° from its origin at the myotendinous junction to its insertion on the radial tuberosity (**Figure 1**). The short head is ulnar to the long head at its myotendinous junction, externally rotates in the bicipital tunnel, and inserts distal to the insertion of the long head on the footprint. The short head is a stronger elbow flexor because of its distal attachment. The long head generates a greater terminal supination torque because its attachment is more posterior than that of the short head. The biceps tendon inserts on the posterior aspect of the radial tuberosity and the center of the biceps footprint usually lies 6 to 7 mm anterior to the apex (**Figure 2**). The radial protuberance, which is part of the tuberosity anterior to the footprint of the tendon, functions as a mechanical cam to maximize supination torque throughout rotation (**Figure 2**).

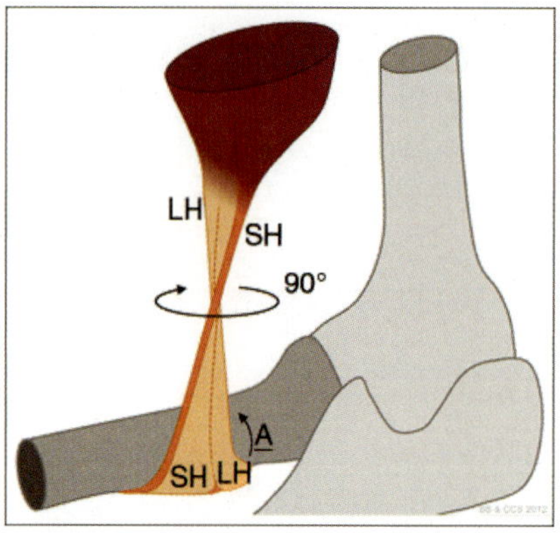


**Figure 1** Diagram shows the 90° external rotation of the biceps tendon as it approaches the tuberosity. The short head (SH) is on the ulnar side. With the rotation, the insertion of the short head is distal to that of the long head (LH). A = area of radius anterior to the insertion site. (Adapted with permission from Schmidt CC, Jarrett CD, Brown BT: The distal biceps tendon. *J Hand Surg Am* 2013;38[4]:811-821.)

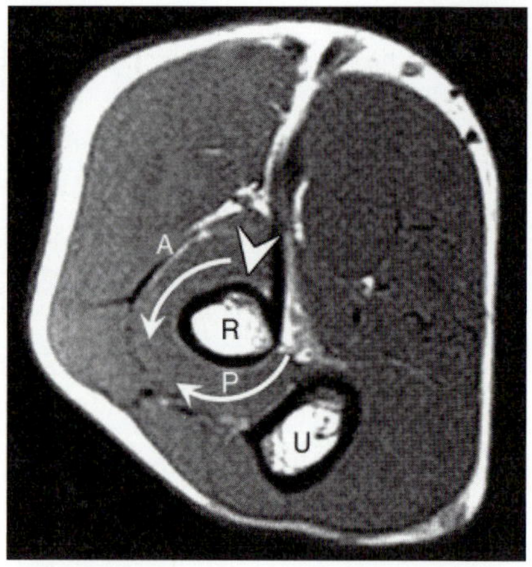


**Figure 2** Proton density axial MRI demonstrates the biceps tendon insertion site. The center of the tendon footprint inserts 6 to 7 mm anterior to the apex of the tuberosity (arrow). The protuberance (arrowhead), which is part of the tuberosity anterior to the biceps insertion, acts as a mechanical cam during supination. A = area of radius anterior to the insertion site, P = area of radius posterior to the insertion site, R = radius, U = ulna. (Adapted with permission from Schmidt CC, Diaz VA, Weir DM, Latona CR, Miller MC: Repaired distal biceps magnetic resonance imaging anatomy compared with outcome. *J Shoulder Elbow Surg* 2012;21[12]:1623-1631.)

Cadaver and clinical studies have demonstrated that reattaching the biceps tendon 6 mm anterior to its native footprint or 13 mm anterior to its apex results in losses in both the supination moment arm and strength from neutral to supinated positions (**Figure 3**). In two of six cadaver arms studied in 60° supination, an anterior repair converted the biceps tendon from a forearm supinator to a pronator. Additionally, reattaching the biceps tendon to a trough located in the tuberosity decreases the protuberance height and correspondingly reduces supination torque. The authors of this chapter suggest that reattaching the biceps tendon to its native footprint with preservation of the topographic anatomy of the radius should be the goal of surgical treatment. However, pathologic changes in the biceps tendon from chronic tendinopathy, rupture, and scarring can make restoring preinjury anatomy a challenge.

 

## Contraindications

Contraindications to surgical treatment include low functional demands, severe restrictions in elbow and forearm motion, active infection, and a compromised soft-tissue envelope.

## Alternative Treatments

Patients who undergo nonsurgical treatment can expect to lose approximately 40% of supination strength, experience decreased useful arc of rotation, lose 10% to 20% of flexion strength, and might experience fatigue pain. Many patients adapt well to the loss of supination strength without a substantial change in their lifestyle. For example, in one retrospective study of 16 patients treated nonsurgically, 6 patients reported supination weakness when performing activities such as turning a screwdriver, and 8 patients noted loss of strength when lifting heavy objects. However, the patients in the study had a mean score of 14 on the Disabilities of the Arm, Shoulder and Hand questionnaire (normative value, 10), and all 16 patients returned to their preinjury work.

## Results

### General Anatomic Considerations

Either an anterior approach (forearm in hypersupination) or a posterior extensor carpi ulnaris/supinator muscle–splitting approach (forearm in pronation) can be used to expose the radial tuberosity for repair (**Figure 4**). Recent cadaver and clinical studies have reported that an anterior approach together with the use of straight instruments often results in an anterior reattachment site that decreases the mechanical cam effect of the

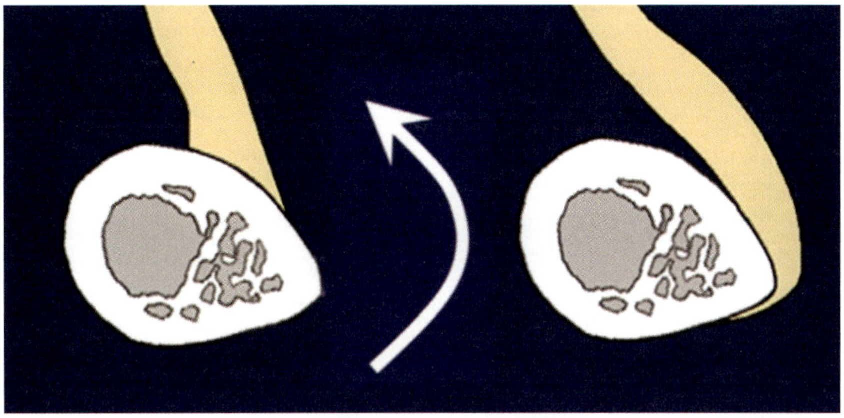

**Figure 3** Schematic of the native tendon (anatomic; right) and anterior (nonanatomic) repair (left). The center of the native tendon inserts 6 to 7 mm anterior to the apex. Anterior repair usually locates the tendon 6 mm anterior to the center of its footprint or 13 mm anterior to the apex. This nonanatomic reattachment site leads to loss of the supination cam (arrow) and can result in clinical weakness. (Adapted with permission from Schmidt CC, Jarrett CD, Brown BT: The distal biceps tendon. *J Hand Surg Am* 2013;38[4]:811-821.)

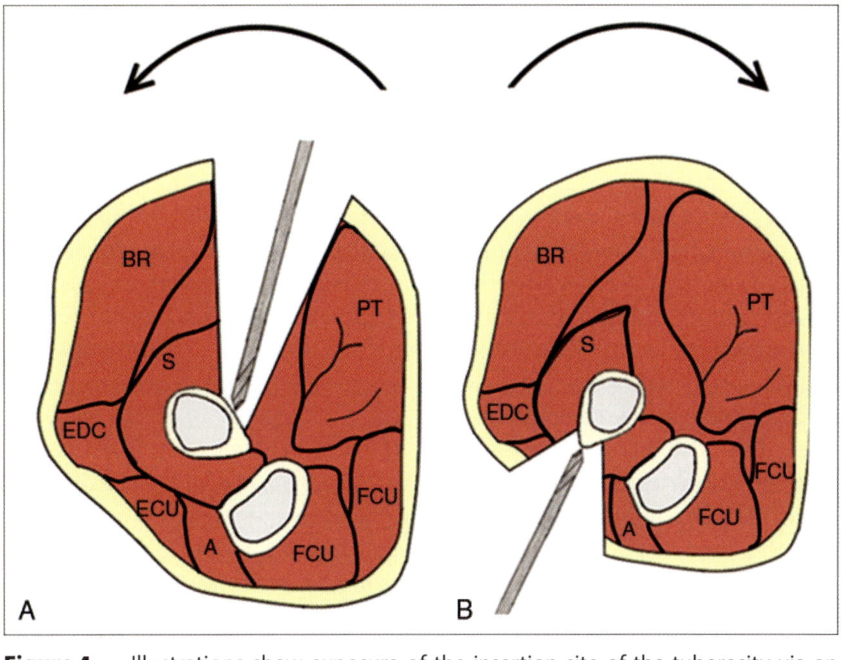


**Figure 4** Illustrations show exposure of the insertion site of the tuberosity via an anterior (Henry) approach with hypersupination (**A**) and via a posterior extensor carpi ulnaris muscle–splitting approach with maximum pronation (**B**). Arrows indicate direction of forearm motion. **A,** If an anterior approach and straight instruments are used, reattaching the biceps tendon to its native insertion site on the apex is difficult because of the bulky flexor pronator muscle mass and the pronated position of the tuberosity. **B,** A muscle-splitting approach and the use of straight instruments facilitate drilling at the apex of the tuberosity and allow reattachment of the tendon to its insertion site. A = anconeus muscle, BR = brachioradialis muscle, ECU = extensor carpi ulnaris muscle, EDC = extensor digitorum communis muscle, FCU = flexor carpi ulnaris muscle, PT = pronator teres muscle, S = supinator muscle. (Adapted with permission from Schmidt CC, Jarrett CD, Brown BT: The distal biceps tendon. *J Hand Surg Am* 2013;38[4]:811-821.)

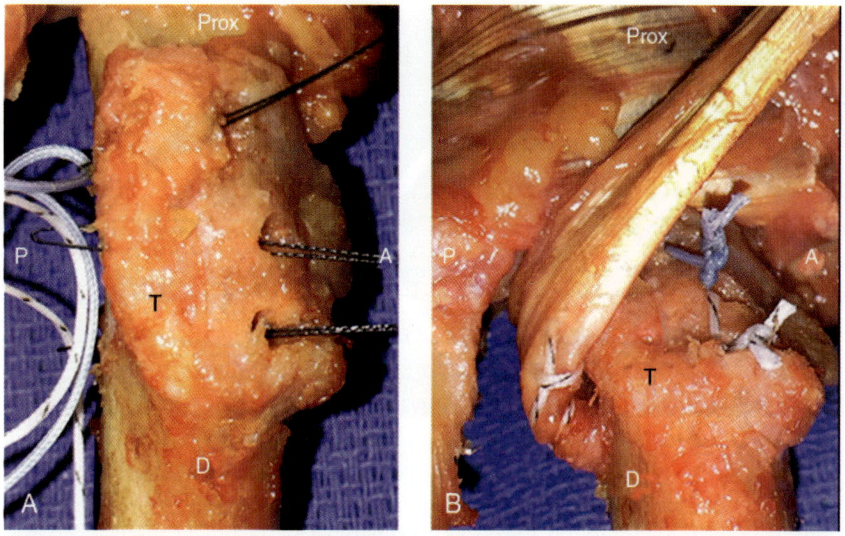


**Figure 5** Photographs of a cadaver model show reattachment of the biceps tendon posterior to the apex of the tuberosity using an anterior approach. **A,** Three drill holes are placed in the anterior tuberosity exiting just posterior to the apex of the tuberosity. A suture-shuttle device is used to pass the long head and short head sutures from posterior to anterior. **B,** The long head (solid stitch) and short head (striped stitch) are tied over bone bridges. The short head is distal to the long head. A = area of radius anterior to the insertion site, D = distal, P = posterior to the insertion site, Prox = proximal, T = apex of the radial tuberosity.

tuberosity (**Figures 2** and **3**). A solution to reestablish the supination cam is to drill posterior to the apex of the tuberosity and use suture shuttles to pull the tendon from front to back posteriorly around the apex. This method positions the tendon posterior to the protuberance and restores its native cam effect (**Figure 5**). A retrospective clinical study in which the tendon was repaired posterior to the apex of the tuberosity reported recovery of supination strength compared with the uninjured side throughout a full range of rotation. However, the authors of that study verified the repair location in only one patient (**Table 1**).

In contrast to an anterior approach, a posterior approach with the forearm in pronation provides the exposure needed to reliably reattach the torn tendon to its native footprint, approximately 6 to 7 mm anterior to its apex (**Figure 4**). The downside of the posterior approach is damage to the supinator muscle, which is partially split during the exposure. Supinator muscle injury is associated with loss of terminal supination strength, but the potential loss of strength is approximately three times less than that of a nonanatomic anterior insertion. In other words, an anatomic biceps reattachment is more important to return of full supination strength than iatrogenic supinator muscle injury.

## Acute Biceps Tendon Rupture

Overall outcomes of distal biceps tendon repair with either anterior or posterior approaches are good to excellent according to validated measures (**Tables 1** and **2**). However, only three published studies quantified the repair location, and only two studies measured isometric supination strength in pronation, neutral, and supination forearm positions. The studies in which an anterior approach was used reattached the tendon anterior to the native footprint and reported less supination strength in neutral (10%) and supinated (18% to 33%) positions, whereas supination strength in a pronated forearm position was maintained (**Table 1**). These findings may reflect the difficulty of reattaching the biceps tendon to the native insertion site using straight drill bits in the insertion of cortical buttons or suture anchors. The bulky flexor pronator muscle mass and the pronated position of the radial tuberosity hinder efforts to reattach the biceps tendon to the native insertion site (**Figure 4**). Mechanical cadaver model studies have shown that an anterior reattachment site results in a lesser supination moment arm and decreased torque in neutral and supinated forearm positions, but not in pronation. An explanation of this finding is that with the arm in the pronated position, the tendon remains wound around the bone and acts on the same point on the radial tuberosity regardless of the attachment site, whereas with the arm in the neutral or supinated position, the anteriorly reattached tendon prematurely unwinds and acts on a point on the radius anterior to the native attachment site (**Figure 6**). The anterior reattachment site does not restore the normal mechanical cam of the radial tuberosity and prevents the tendon from acting on the entire radial tuberosity. These clinical and cadaver model studies demonstrate that restoration of native force transmission to the bicipital tuberosity is critical for restoring supination strength through a full functional range of motion.

A clinical study using a posterior approach reported that anatomic reattachment sites were significantly correlated to the return of native supination strength ($P < 0.001$; **Table 2**). Compared with the anterior repair group, the posterior repair group demonstrated 14% greater supination strength in a supinated forearm position ($P < 0.027$). Previous outcome studies using a posterior approach reported an average drop in isometric supination strength in neutral forearm rotation of 9% but did not include verification of the reattachment site locations. Furthermore, two studies used a cortical trough in the repair,

 

**Table 1** Results of Anterior Repair of the Distal Biceps Tendon

| Authors (Year) | No. of Patients | Confirmation of Repair Site | Mean Patient Age in Years (Range) | Mean Follow-up in Months (Range) | Success Rate (%)[a] | Results | Level of Evidence |
|---|---|---|---|---|---|---|---|
| Grewal et al (2012) | 43 | No | 45.3 (38-53) | 24 | 96 | DASH score: 7.8 ± 12.9<br>Strength: 98% in neutral forearm position | I |
| Schmidt et al (2012) | 17 | Yes | 49 (33-67) | 27.9 (18-39) | 89 | DASH score: 7.7 (range, 0-49)<br>Strength: 100% with forearm in 60° of pronation, 90% with forearm in neutral position, 67% with forearm in 60° of supination | III |
| Tanner et al (2013) | 17 | In 1 patient | 54 (44-69) | 13 (6-25) | 93 | Strength: 91% in neutral forearm position[b] | IV |
| Hansen et al (2014) | 21 | Yes | 47.3 (35-66) | 44.2 (12-119) | 89 | DASH score: 10 ± 7<br>Strength: 85% with forearm in 10° of supination and 82% with forearm in 80° of supination[b] | IV |

DASH = Disabilities of the Arm, Shoulder and Hand.

[a] Success was defined as final DASH score <25, strength within 20% of the contralateral side, return to work, and no failure of repair.

[b] Isokinetic strength testing.

**Table 2** Results of Posterior Repair of the Distal Biceps Tendon

| Authors (Year) | No. of Patients | Confirmation of Repair Site | Mean Patient Age in Years (Range) | Mean Follow-up in Months (Range) | Success Rate (%)[a] | Results | Level of Evidence |
|---|---|---|---|---|---|---|---|
| Weinstein et al (2008) | 32 | No | 53 (39-79) | 42 | 100 | DASH score: 4 ± 7<br>Strength: 100% in neutral forearm position[b] | IV |
| Cil et al (2009) | 21 | No | 49 (35-67) | 57 (24-90) | 100 | DASH score: 3.6 ± 3.6<br>Strength: 91% in neutral forearm position | IV |
| Grewal et al (2012) | 40 | No | 45.3 (38-53) | 24 | 96 | DASH score: 5.5 ± 11.8<br>Strength: 92% in neutral forearm position | I |
| Schmidt et al (forthcoming) | 15 | Yes | 49.7 (36-68) | 17 (10-26) | 100 | DASH score: 4.0 ± 8.4<br>Strength: 92.2% in neutral forearm position, 81.3% in supinated forearm position | III |

DASH = Disabilities of the Arm, Shoulder and Hand.

[a] Success was defined as final DASH score <25, strength within 20% of the contralateral side, return to work, and no failure of repair.

[b] Isokinetic strength testing.

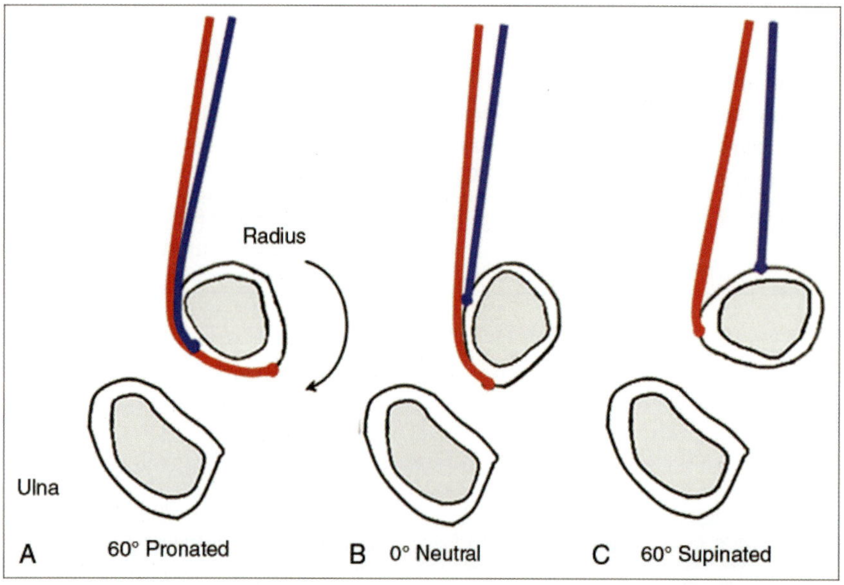


**Figure 6** Schematic diagrams depict the radius in relation to the ulna with the forearm in pronation (**A**), neutral (**B**), and supination (**C**). Red lines depict anatomic repair; blue lines depict anterior repair. Between neutral and supination, an anteriorly repaired tendon unwinds and can no longer generate torque (**B** and **C**). An anatomic repair remains wound around the radius between neutral and supination; thus, it maintains torque. Between pronation and neutral, both the anterior and anatomic repairs are wrapped around the radius and are capable of generating a moment arm. (Reproduced with permission from Schmidt CC, Weir DM, Wong AS, Howard M, Miller MC: The effect of biceps reattachment site. *J Shoulder Elbow Surg* 2010;19[8]:1157-1165.)

which has been shown to decrease the mechanical cam effect of the tuberosity and lead to supination weakness in a supinated forearm position. The authors of this chapter suspect that if the patients were tested in supination, they would experience a drop in torque comparable to that found in studies of the anterior approach. In contrast, the authors of a retrospective study reattached the tendon through a posterior approach with suture anchors without a cortical trough and reported no significant differences in isokinetic strength between repaired and uninjured arms. This finding supports the importance of preserving the radial geometry. The authors of a randomized prospective study reported no difference in supination strength in neutral position between anterior suture anchor and posterior trough repairs. The authors of this chapter suggest that the differences may be detectable only when measuring strength in different forearm positions. Most of the literature does not describe or verify reattachment locations, which seem to play an important role in determining postoperative supination strength and function.

## Chronic Biceps Tendon Rupture

Chronic biceps tendon ruptures are those that occur more than 4 weeks after injury. Primary repair of a chronic rupture is challenging because the muscle stiffens, the tendon shortens, and the bicipital tunnel becomes obliterated. However, primary repair using high elbow flexion angles (>60°) usually remains possible, thus avoiding the need for tendon graft reconstruction. Clinical outcomes and strength measurements of chronic reattachments seem comparable to those of acute repairs; however, rigorous strength testing has not been done (**Table 3**). An uninjured biceps tendon has an average length of 4 cm. Chronic ruptured tendons with as little as 1 cm of remaining tendon (enough to allow placement of four Krackow sutures) can be attached to the radius by flexing the elbow up to 100° without increasing the incidence of an elbow flexion contracture or the risk of repeat rupture (**Table 3**). Repairing the biceps tendon in high flexion requires either a posterior approach or an anterior approach with a pretied cortical button. Both techniques allow the tendon to be reduced to its footprint with elbow flexion, which eliminates the need to tie sutures in the restricted space of the antecubital fossa.

If the biceps musculotendinous junction and/or tendon are of poor quality, then tendon graft reconstruction is needed prior to repair. Graft materials including palmaris longus, flexor carpi radialis, fascia lata, semitendinosus, and Achilles tendon allograft have been reported. The authors of this chapter prefer to use Achilles tendon allograft because it eliminates donor site morbidity (**Table 3**).

**Video 9.1** Anatomic Distal Biceps Repair: Two Intramedullary Buttons or Modified Trough Technique and Chronic Distal Biceps Repair With Achilles Tendon Allograft. Christopher C. Schmidt, MD (12 min)

# Techniques

## Setup/Exposure

- Regional block with sedation is recommended to prevent violent rupture during awakening from general anesthesia.
- For both the anterior approach and the posterior approach, the patient is placed in the supine position.
- A tourniquet is placed high on the arm. If the patient has short arms and a chronic proximally retracted tendon, then a sterile tourniquet can be used.

 

**Table 3** Results of Repair of Chronic Rupture of the Distal Biceps Tendon[a]

| Authors (Year) | No. of Patients | Procedure or Approach | Mean Patient Age in Years (Range) | Mean Follow-up in Months (Range) | Success Rate (%)[b] | Results |
|---|---|---|---|---|---|---|
| Sanchez-Sotelo et al (2002) | 4 | Achilles allograft | 39 (31-43) | 34 (24-44) | 100 | Mean MEPS: 100<br>Strength: 4+ to 5 in neutral forearm position<br>Mean flexion/extension: 180°<br>Mean pronation/supination: 180° |
| Darlis and Sotereanos (2006) | 7 | Achilles allograft | 38 (30-52) | 29 (14-48) | 100 | Mean MEPS: 97<br>Mean strength: 87% in neutral forearm position[c]<br>Mean flexion/extension: 142°<br>Mean pronation/supination: 169° |
| Bosman et al (2012) | 5 | Primary repair | 47.2 (43-60) | 20.2 (12-28) | 100 | Mean MEPS: 100<br>Mean strength: 90% in neutral forearm position[c]<br>Mean flexion/extension: 169°<br>Mean pronation/supination: 171° |
| Morrey et al (2014) | 18 | Primary repair | 50 (38-67) | ≥12 | 100 | Mean MEPS: 100<br>Strength: 4+ to 5 in neutral forearm position<br>Mean flexion/extension: 135°<br>Mean pronation/supination: 160° |

MEPS = Mayo Elbow Performance Score.

[a] All studies are level IV evidence.

[b] Success was defined as final Disabilities of the Arm, Shoulder and Hand score <25; strength within 20% of the contralateral side; return to work; and no failure of repair.

[c] Isokinetic strength testing.

## Instruments/Equipment/ Implants Required

- The anterior repair requires a 2.5-mm drill bit, one to three suture shuttles, an 18-gauge spinal needle, a standard right-angle clamp, and two strong No. 2 sutures (one striped and one solid color) with needles on both ends.
- The posterior repair requires a long Kelly clamp, two strong No. 2 sutures (one striped and one solid color) with needles on both ends, two cortical buttons, and one 3.2-mm biceps drill pin.
- A posterior trough repair does not require the cortical buttons but does require a burr.
- Tendon reconstruction requires the same items as the posterior repair as well as Achilles tendon allograft.
- If cortical buttons are used during the repair, a mini C-arm is used to verify implant position.

## Procedure

### ANTERIOR APPROACH

- The patient is positioned supine with the arm abducted on an arm board.
- The patient's forearm should remain in maximum supination.
- An anterior incision starting distal to the antecubital fossa is made between the pronator teres and brachioradialis muscles (**Figure 4, A**).
- The basilic vein and the lateral antebrachial cutaneous nerve (LABCN) are identified and protected. The LABCN travels between the brachialis and biceps muscles. The nerve may be tethered farther medially than normal as a result of the pull from a retracted biceps.
- The torn biceps tendon is located and dissected free from scar tissue.
- A four-throw Krackow stitch is placed in the short head of the biceps tendon using a striped, strong No. 2 suture.
- A four-throw Krackow stitch is placed in the long head of the biceps with a solid-color, strong No. 2 suture.
- To facilitate visualization of the biceps tuberosity, an Army-Navy retractor is gently positioned around the brachioradialis to pull it radially.

- A second retractor placed underneath the pronator teres displaces the muscle ulnarly.
- The radial sensory nerve (RSN) lies under the brachioradialis, and the LABCN is just radial to the muscle, so care must be taken to allow periods of relaxation during retraction.
- The radial recurrent artery (leash of Henry) usually marks the position of the biceps tuberosity. The artery runs perpendicular to the long axis of the arm and must be ligated and divided to expose the tuberosity.
- To prepare the insertion site for reattachment of the tendon, any residual soft tissue remaining on the tuberosity is débrided to cortical bone. Postoperative MRI studies have clearly shown that the tendon reliably heals to cortical bone.
- Suture anchors or cortical buttons can be used to secure the tendon. However, the authors of this chapter prefer to route the tendon posterior to the apex and fasten it to bone with suture through drill tunnels.
- Three 2.5-mm drill holes are made along the anterior surface of the tuberosity from front to back, angling just posterior to the tuberosity. Drill holes exiting just posterior to the tuberosity facilitate retrieval of the suture shuttle devices (**Figure 5, A**). A 1.0-cm bone bridge should remain between each of the holes.
- An 18-gauge spinal needle is placed through one drill hole from front to back. A right-angle clamp is placed posterior to the tuberosity between the proximal radius and ulna to clamp the spinal needle. A suture shuttle is threaded through the spinal needle. The clamp is loosened, and the spinal needle is gently pulled anteriorly 5 mm to allow the suture shuttle device to rest in the clamp. The clamp is tightened, and the suture shuttle is pulled from the posterior side of the tuberosity.
- The preceding step is repeated two times, so that each of the three holes has a suture shuttle traveling from back to front (**Figure 5, A**).
- Care must be taken to ensure that the biceps tendon is externally rotated 90°, so that the short head (striped stitch) is distal to the long head (solid stitch; **Figure 5, B**).
- In preparation for suture shuttling, the outside limb of the short head (striped) suture is placed into the distal suture shuttle, the central limbs of the short head (striped) and long head (solid) sutures are placed into the central suture shuttle, and the outside limb of the long head (solid) suture is placed into the proximal suture shuttle (**Figure 5, A**).
- The tendon sutures are shuttled from back to front.
- The like sutures are tied together over the bone bridge to secure the biceps tendon around the apex onto the posterior border of the tuberosity in its correct orientation. In this way, the biceps tendon is repaired posterior to its footprint, which takes advantage of the native mechanical cam effect of the tuberosity and helps maintain a terminal supination force (**Figure 5, B**).

**POSTERIOR APPROACH**

- The design of the anterior incision depends on the location of the ruptured distal tendon.
- If the lacertus fibrosus is ruptured, the torn biceps usually is retracted proximally, folded into a ball, and surrounded by fluid and scar tissue. In this scenario, the ruptured tendon can be retrieved through an anterior 2-cm oblique incision just above the elbow flexion crease (**Figure 7**). Care should be taken to protect the LABCN, which may be attached to the tendon with scar tissue.

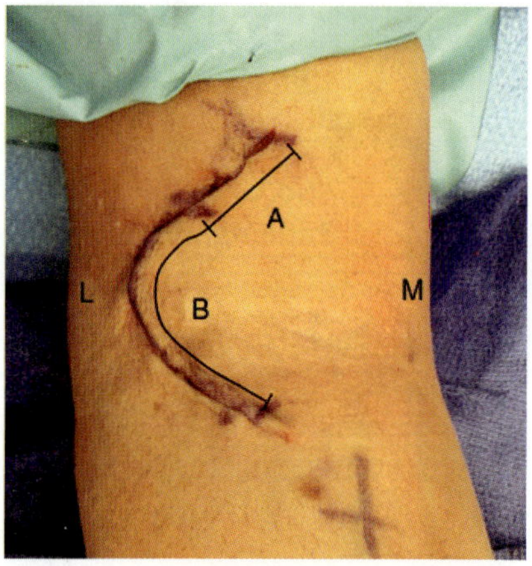


**Figure 7** Intraoperative photograph shows the position of the anterior incision used for finding and suturing the ruptured tendon during a muscle-splitting approach. If the lacertus fibrosus is ruptured, a 2-cm oblique incision (A) can be made above the elbow crease to locate the torn tendon. However, if the lacertus fibrosus is intact, the incision usually needs to be extended around the elbow flexion crease (B) because the ruptured tendon is located distally, usually connected by a pseudotendon to the tuberosity. L = lateral, M = medial.

- If the lacertus fibrosus is intact, the tendon usually is found to be tethered in the forearm and secured to the tuberosity by a thick pseudotendon. The distal end is usually encased in scar tissue and located in the proximal forearm between the pronator teres muscle and the brachioradialis muscle. An incision that curves around the elbow flexion crease laterally is often required to protect the neurovascular structures during tendon exposure and bicipital tunnel dissection (**Figure 7**). In chronic repairs, the path of the biceps to the radial tuberosity is often obscured by scar tissue, and the added incision length helps to avoid neurovascular injury. The lacertus fibrosus insertion into the biceps tendon is usually preserved, but it can be sacrificed if additional length is needed for the repair.

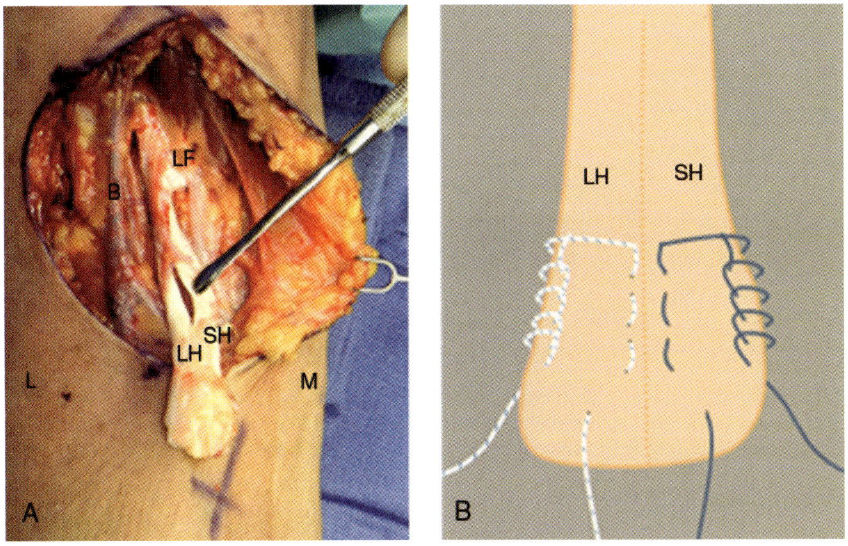


**Figure 8** **A,** Intraoperative photograph shows the short head (SH) and the long head (LH) of the biceps tendon. The short head is medial to the long head and connected to the lacertus fibrosus (LF). **B,** Schematic diagram shows the modified Krackow stitch. The outside limbs consist of four Krackow stitches. The inside limbs are running simple stitches, which will be the docking limbs. On each head, the running stitches exit in the center of the tendon. The Krackow stitches stop 5 to 10 mm from the tendon end and exit the tendon on the dorsal side. The stitch is design to compress the tendon to the footprint when the central docking limbs are pulled. L = lateral, M = medial.

- The scar is removed from the distal tendon end to expose native tendon.
- An effort is made to identify the short and long heads to ensure proper tendon alignment. If the heads cannot be identified, the medial portion is considered the short head and the lateral portion is considered the long head (**Figure 8, A**).
- A four-throw modified Krackow whipstitch is placed in each head, with the use of striped suture in the long head and solid suture in the short head (**Figure 8, B**).
- In each head, the outside limb of the stitch is locked, and the stitch ends 5 to 10 mm from the tendon end on the dorsal side. The central limb of the suture on each head is placed in a simple running pattern and finishes in the center of each head on the palmar side (**Figure 8, B**). When the tendon is externally rotated 90°, the palmar side will be adjacent to the footprint. The center limbs are passed through the cortical buttons and become the docking limbs (**Figure 8, B**). Two intramedullary cortical buttons have been shown to have similar time-zero mechanical failure strength as the native, uninjured tendon.
- The radial tuberosity is exposed posteriorly through a 3- to 4-cm incision starting 1.5 cm from the lateral epicondyle and 1.5 cm dorsal to the ulnar ridge.
- With the patient's forearm in pronation, the extensor carpi ulnaris muscle is split in line with its fibers (**Figure 4, B**). Forearm pronation positions the tuberosity in line with the incision and moves the posterior interosseous nerve anteriorly approximately 2 cm from the surgical field.
- The supinator muscle is incised directly over the tuberosity. The location of the tuberosity can be found by palpating the pronated forearm or using intraoperative C-arm imaging. The length of the supinator incision is limited to approximately 2 cm or the length of the tuberosity.
- The bicipitoradial bursa and tendon remnants are cleared from the tuberosity with a rongeur.
- A long Kelly clamp is placed from back to front in the bicipital tunnel.
- The tendon is passed from volar to dorsal along its native path. Forearm supination aids in tendon passage.
- Care is taken to externally rotate the tendon 90° so that the short head is repaired distal to the long head. The use of differently colored sutures is helpful in ensuring that the short and long heads are repaired in the proper orientation.
- The short and long heads are sutured to their respective footprint centroids (**Figure 9, A**). With the use of a 3.2-mm biceps drill pin, unicortical drill holes are made at the center of the footprint of each head (**Figure 9, B**). Care is taken to place the hole for the short head distal and the hole for the long head proximal/posterior on the footprint. The biceps drill pin is directed distally and angled 30° from the near cortex to aid in flipping the buttons against the near cortex. The docking limb of each suture is passed through the center holes of the cortical button and later will be pulled to compress the tendon against the cortex.
- The buttons for both the short head and the long head are placed in their respective drill holes (**Figure 10, A**). The buttons are flipped against the near cortex by pushing the button into the hole with the drill pin and pulling on the docking suture (**Figure 10, A**).
- After proper button location is confirmed, the docking stitches are pulled to compress their respective biceps heads against the footprint.

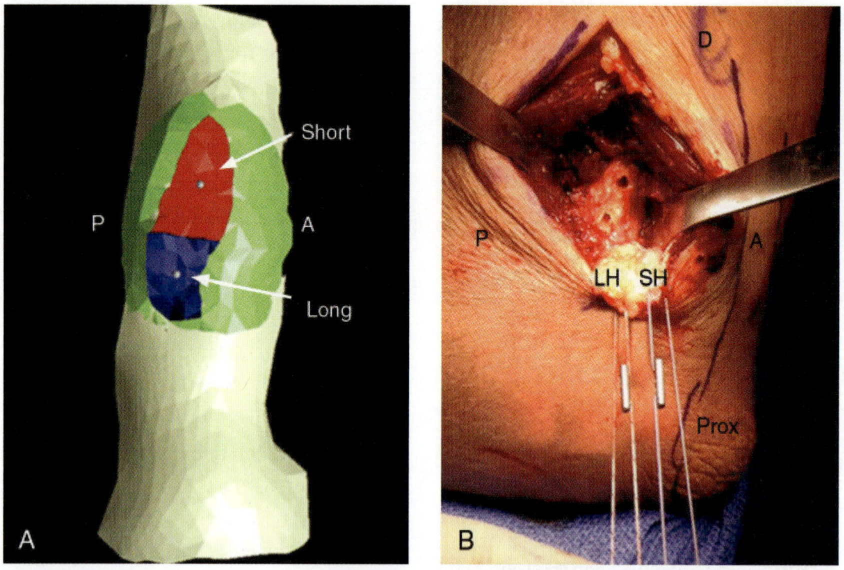


**Figure 9** **A,** A computer-generated model shows the centroids of the insertion sites of the short head and long head of the biceps tendon. **B,** Intraoperative photograph shows positioning of the drill holes for cortical buttons to replicate these centroids. The buttons are placed on the center limbs of each stitch. A = area of radius anterior to the insertion site, D = distal, LH = long head of the biceps tendon, P = posterior, Prox = proximal to the insertion site, SH = short head of the biceps tendon.

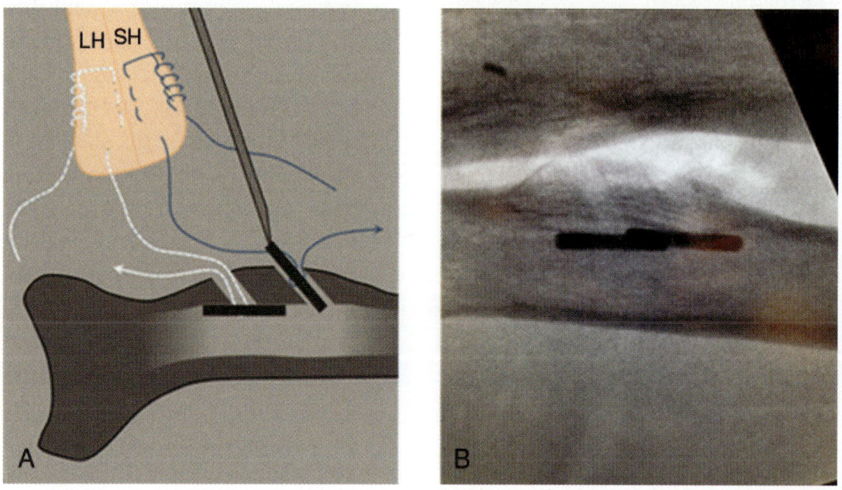


**Figure 10** **A,** Diagram shows placement of the cortical buttons for the short head of the biceps tendon (SH; solid stitch) and long head of the biceps tendon (LH; striped stitch) in their respective drill holes. The surgeon flips the buttons by pushing them into the canal with the back of the drill pin and simultaneously pulling on the docking suture. The tunnels for the buttons are drilled approximately 30° from the radial long axis. This position aids in flipping the button within the intramedullary canal. **B,** Intraoperative fluoroscopic image from a mini C-arm demonstrates the buttons correctly positioned flat against the near cortex before the knots are tied.

- Intraoperative fluoroscopy is used to confirm that both buttons are positioned parallel to and against the near intramedullary cortex (**Figure 10, B**).
- With the button acting as an intramedullary pulley, several knots are placed to complete the repair.
- An alternative to the cortical button technique is the trough repair, which is commonly used. The standard trough technique can be improved by placing the trough posterior to the apex of the tuberosity to take full advantage of the cam effect of the radial protuberance (**Figure 11, A**). To perform the trough repair, a socket measuring 7 mm wide by 10 mm long is burred posterior to the anatomic footprint (apex of the tuberosity), three holes are drilled 4 mm posterior to the socket, the sutures are passed through the three holes in a pattern similar to that described previously for the anterior repair, and the tendon is tied to bone (**Figure 11**).

**BICEPS RECONSTRUCTION**

- Biceps reconstruction is rarely needed because the tendon can usually be repaired in high flexion (>60°) with a posterior muscle-splitting approach using either the cortical button technique or the trough technique.
- However, if the biceps musculotendinous junction cannot be pulled or the tendon is of inadequate length or quality to hold four Krackow whipstitches, the muscle must be restored with an Achilles tendon allograft reconstruction.
- The exposure is similar to that used in the posterior approach but is extended both proximally and distally. The surgeon must remember to incise lateral to the elbow crease and that the distal limb is between the pronator teres and the brachioradialis muscles (**Figure 4, A**). The extended anterior exposure is needed to prevent injury to the LABCN and safely reestablish the bicipital tunnel.
- An Achilles tendon allograft is woven into the biceps remnant by cutting the allograft into three

 

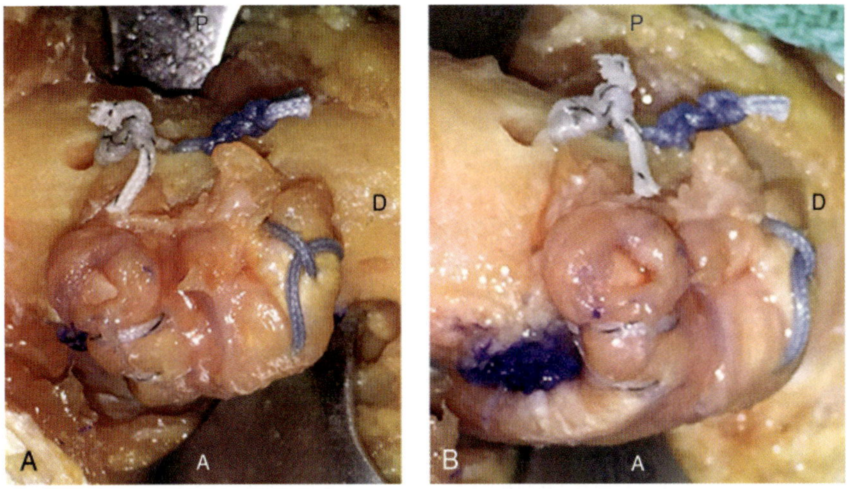


**Figure 11** Photographs of cadaver models show the trough repair technique. **A,** The trough is positioned posterior to the apex to preserve the radial protuberance (blue area). **B,** In the completed trough repair, the short head sutures are tied over the two distal holes and the long head sutures are tied over the two proximal holes. The tendon drapes over the protuberance of the tuberosity (blue area) to preserve its cam effect. A = area of radius anterior to the insertion site, D = distal, P = posterior.

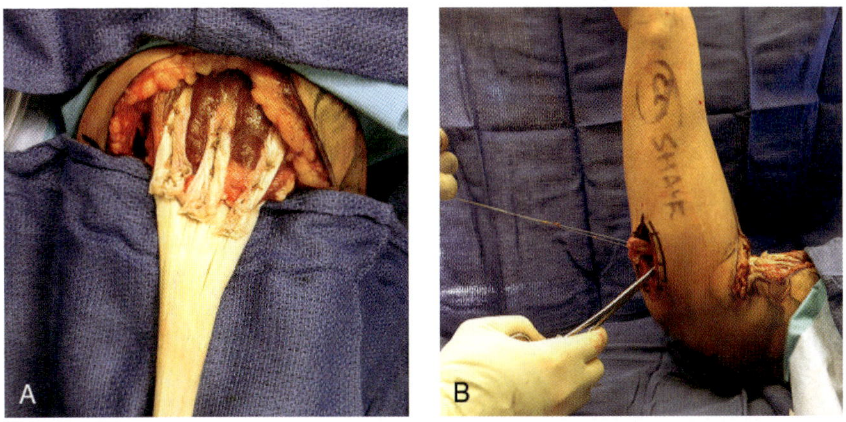


**Figure 12** Intraoperative photographs show an allograft reconstruction. **A,** The biceps musculotendinous junction is restored by dividing the allograft into three slips (tongues), passing them from posterior to anterior, suturing each slip together, and sandwiching the muscle between each slip. **B,** The muscle/graft construct is tensioned by flexing the elbow to 80°, pulling the tendon from front to back through the bicipital tunnel, and marking the intersection with the pronated radial tuberosity.

proximal tongues. Each tongue is passed through the biceps muscle from posterior to anterior and sutured to itself with absorbable No. 2 suture. The middle tongue is wrapped posterior to the remnant tendon (**Figure 12, A**).

- Multiple sutures are placed in a horizontal fashion between the anterior and posterior tongues, sandwiching the muscle between the tongues of the allograft.
- A posterior muscle-splitting approach is used to expose the tuberosity.
- Using a Kelly clamp, the graft is safely passed from front to back along the bicipital tunnel. If the bicipital tunnel is difficult to reestablish, the anterior interval between the pronator teres and the brachioradialis muscles should be developed to protect the neurovascular structures.
- To determine the length of the graft, the distal end of the graft is marked at its intersection with the tuberosity when the elbow is flexed to 80° and the forearm is pronated (**Figure 12, B**). The graft is then pulled back to the anterior incision and cut at the mark.
- Sutures are placed in the short and long heads of the biceps tendon, and the graft is passed from front to back a second time and affixed to the native footprint as described previously for the posterior approach.
- Care must be taken to ensure that the graft is externally rotated 90° to reconstruct the native anatomy.
- To complete the reconstruction, the graft is tensioned so that the arm rests in 80° of flexion. The authors of this chapter find that this high-flexion tension is needed to move the biceps muscle distally to an anatomic position that can correct the reverse Popeye sign.

### Wound Closure

- The extensor carpi ulnaris split is closed with a 2-0 absorbable stitch.
- All other skin incisions are closed with a subcutaneous 3-0 absorbable suture, followed by a 2-0 nonabsorbable stitch.

## Postoperative Regimen

Loss of elbow and forearm motion and rerupture are uncommon after repair or reconstruction of acute or chronic biceps rupture. The reattachment site is at the greatest risk of failure during the first 3 weeks postoperatively. For patients who undergo acute or chronic repair not requiring a high-flexion position (elbow flexed >60°), the elbow is immobilized in a supinated posterior splint for 2 weeks to allow the skin to heal and to prevent anterior healing of the biceps on the tuberosity. From 2 to 6 weeks, active and passive elbow and forearm range of motion is started with the goal of restoring full active motion. Patients are instructed not to pick up any object heavier than a one-half gallon of milk (<5 lb) and to avoid forceful supination. At 6 weeks, the restrictions are lifted, and gradual flexion and supination strengthening and endurance training commence.

High-flexion repairs and allograft reconstructions are protected for 2 weeks in a plaster splint and an additional 2 to 4 weeks in a custom-made plastic 90° elbow splint. The greatest risk during this period is early rerupture at the tuberosity and the myotendinous junction. Between 2 and 4 weeks postoperatively, patients are instructed to wear the splint at all times except when performing gentle elbow and forearm motion three times per day for 15 minutes each session. At 4 weeks, the splint becomes optional, and at 6 weeks it is discontinued. The goal of regaining full elbow and forearm motion in the first 6 weeks should have been discussed preoperatively with the patient. Strengthening and endurance exercises are gradually started after 10 weeks.

For all repairs, return to heavy labor occurs between 3 and 6 months, depending on patient motivation. Rerupture is uncommon during this period.

## Limiting Adverse Events

Commonly reported complications of biceps repair are posterior interosseous nerve palsy, LABCN and/or RSN paresthesia, heterotopic ossification, and rerupture. The rate of these complications ranges from 16% to 40%. Complications that may require revision surgery occur in approximately 6% of patients. Although an anterior reattachment site is not typically considered a complication, it can greatly affect postoperative function.

Posterior interosseous nerve palsy can occur with an anterior exposure of the tuberosity. The frequency of this complication is approximately 3%. The hypersupination required during an anterior repair brings the nerve in close proximity to the radial tuberosity. The use of a direct-pull retractor such as an Army-Navy retractor on the brachioradialis and lateral deep soft tissues can decrease the palsy rate. A levered retractor such as a Hohmann retractor should not be placed along the radial neck of the tuberosity. The posterior interosseous nerve also can be injured during placement of a guide pin for an extramedullary button. Directing the pin in a proximal/ulnar direction can mitigate this risk. Paresthesia of the LABCN and/or RSN also is more common with an anterior approach than with a posterior approach. In a prospective study comparing an anterior approach with a posterior muscle-splitting approach, LABCN palsy was seen in 40% of the anterior group compared with 7% of the muscle-splitting group ($P < 0.001$). The force and time of the brachioradialis retraction should be restricted to decrease the risk of nerve injury. Heterotopic ossification that limits forearm rotation occurs with equal frequency in the anterior and posterior muscle-splitting approaches. The previously discussed prospective study reported no clinically measurable loss of motion with either an anterior or posterior approach. The authors of this chapter recommend slow-release indomethacin at a dosage of 75 mg once per day for heterotopic ossification prophylaxis. All bone debris created during drilling or burring should be removed by means of irrigation. When a posterior muscle-splitting technique is used, the proximal ulna should not be exposed; the dissection plane should be through the extensor carpi ulnaris muscle, not the anconeus muscle. Rerupture is rare with modern fixation methods, occurring in approximately 2% of patients. If rerupture occurs, it generally occurs within the first 3 weeks after surgery. The failure rate of suture anchor fixation is higher than that of other fixation methods; however, this uncommon complication is typically accident-related or associated with patient noncompliance.

Surgical timing is a factor in the complication rate. The complication rate doubles when the repair is delayed for 2 to 4 weeks. During that time, the path of the biceps to the tuberosity becomes obliterated by scar tissue, which tends to increase the difficulty of surgical repair. Extra care must be taken to avoid excessive traction on the LABCN and the RSN during dissection of the tendon and reestablishment of the bicipital tunnel. Spreading with a curved Mayo scissors from the posterior exposure to the anterior exposure can help to open the tunnel. The repair should be scheduled in a timely manner before scarring increases the difficulty of repair.

## Acknowledgment

The authors thank Brandon T. Brown, MME, for his help in manuscript organization, figure creation, and video editing.

 

## Bibliography

Athwal GS, Steinmann SP, Rispoli DM: The distal biceps tendon: Footprint and relevant clinical anatomy. *J Hand Surg Am* 2007;32(8):1225-1229.

Baker BE, Bierwagen D: Rupture of the distal tendon of the biceps brachii: Operative versus non-operative treatment. *J Bone Joint Surg Am* 1985;67(3):414-417.

Bosman HA, Fincher M, Saw N: Anatomic direct repair of chronic distal biceps brachii tendon rupture without interposition graft. *J Shoulder Elbow Surg* 2012;21(10):1342-1347.

Cil A, Merten S, Steinmann SP: Immediate active range of motion after modified 2-incision repair in acute distal biceps tendon rupture. *Am J Sports Med* 2009;37(1):130-135.

Darlis NA, Sotereanos DG: Distal biceps tendon reconstruction in chronic ruptures. *J Shoulder Elbow Surg* 2006;15(5):614-619.

Eames MH, Bain GI, Fogg QA, van Riet RP: Distal biceps tendon anatomy: A cadaveric study. *J Bone Joint Surg Am* 2007;89(5):1044-1049.

Forthman CL, Zimmerman RM, Sullivan MJ, Gabel GT: Cross-sectional anatomy of the bicipital tuberosity and biceps brachii tendon insertion: Relevance to anatomic tendon repair. *J Shoulder Elbow Surg* 2008;17(3):522-526.

Freeman CR, McCormick KR, Mahoney D, Baratz M, Lubahn JD: Nonoperative treatment of distal biceps tendon ruptures compared with a historical control group. *J Bone Joint Surg Am* 2009;91(10):2329-2334.

Grewal R, Athwal GS, MacDermid JC, et al: Single versus double-incision technique for the repair of acute distal biceps tendon ruptures: A randomized clinical trial. *J Bone Joint Surg Am* 2012;94(13):1166-1174.

Hansen G, Smith A, Pollock JW, et al: Anatomic repair of the distal biceps tendon cannot be consistently performed through a classic single-incision suture anchor technique. *J Shoulder Elbow Surg* 2014;23(12):1898-1904.

Jarrett CD, Weir DM, Stuffmann ES, Jain S, Miller MC, Schmidt CC: Anatomic and biomechanical analysis of the short and long head components of the distal biceps tendon. *J Shoulder Elbow Surg* 2012;21(7):942-948.

Jobin CM, Kippe MA, Gardner TR, Levine WN, Ahmad CS: Distal biceps tendon repair: A cadaveric analysis of suture anchor and interference screw restoration of the anatomic footprint. *Am J Sports Med* 2009;37(11):2214-2221.

Morrey BF, Askew LJ, An KN, Dobyns JH: Rupture of the distal tendon of the biceps brachii: A biomechanical study. *J Bone Joint Surg Am* 1985;67(3):418-421.

Morrey ME, Abdel MP, Sanchez-Sotelo J, Morrey BF: Primary repair of retracted distal biceps tendon ruptures in extreme flexion. *J Shoulder Elbow Surg* 2014;23(5):679-685.

Nesterenko S, Domire ZJ, Morrey BF, Sanchez-Sotelo J: Elbow strength and endurance in patients with a ruptured distal biceps tendon. *J Shoulder Elbow Surg* 2010;19(2):184-189.

O'Driscoll SW, Goncalves LB, Dietz P: The hook test for distal biceps tendon avulsion. *Am J Sports Med* 2007;35(11):1865-1869

Prud'homme-Foster M, Louati H, Pollock JW, Papp S: Proper placement of the distal biceps tendon during repair improves supination strength: A biomechanical analysis. *J Shoulder Elbow Surg* 2015;24(4):527-532.

Sanchez-Sotelo J, Morrey BF, Adams RA, O'Driscoll SW: Reconstruction of chronic ruptures of the distal biceps tendon with use of an Achilles tendon allograft. *J Bone Joint Surg Am* 2002;84(6):999-1005.

Schmidt CC, Brown BT, Qvick LM, Stacowicz RZ, Latona CR, Miller MC: Factors that determine supination strength following distal biceps repair. *J Bone Joint Surg Am*, forthcoming.

Schmidt CC, Brown BT, Sawardeker PJ, DeGravelle M Jr, Miller MC: Factors affecting supination strength after a distal biceps rupture. *J Shoulder Elbow Surg* 2014;23(1):68-75.

Schmidt CC, Brown BT, Williams BG, et al: The importance of preserving the radial tuberosity during distal biceps repair. *J Bone Joint Surg Am* 2015;97(24):2014-2023.

Schmidt CC, Diaz VA, Weir DM, Latona CR, Miller MC: Repaired distal biceps magnetic resonance imaging anatomy compared with outcome. *J Shoulder Elbow Surg* 2012;21(12):1623-1631.

Schmidt CC, Jarrett CD, Brown BT: The distal biceps tendon. *J Hand Surg Am* 2013;38(4):811-821, quiz 821.

Schmidt CC, Weir DM, Wong AS, Howard M, Miller MC: The effect of biceps reattachment site. *J Shoulder Elbow Surg* 2010;19(8):1157-1165.

Tanner C, Johnson T, Muradov P, Husak L: Single incision power optimizing cost-effective (SPOC) distal biceps repair. *J Shoulder Elbow Surg* 2013;22(3):305-311.

Weinstein DM, Ciccone WJ II, Buckler MC, Balthrop PM, Busey TD, Elias JJ: Elbow function after repair of the distal biceps brachii tendon with a two-incision approach. *J Shoulder Elbow Surg* 2008;17(1 suppl):82S-86S.

## Video Reference

Schmidt CC: Video. *Anatomic Distal Biceps Repair: Two Intramedullary Buttons or Modified Trough Technique and Chronic Distal Biceps Repair With Achilles Tendon Allograft.* Pittsburgh, PA, 2016.

 

# Chapter 10

# Distal Biceps Tendinopathy

*Joideep Phadnis, MBChB, MRCS, FRCS (Tr & Orth)*

*Gregory I. Bain, MBBS, FRACS, FAOrthA, PhD*

**Learning Objectives**

- Identify the anatomy and pathoanatomy of distal biceps tendinopathy and partial tears.
- Understand the diagnosis and classification of distal biceps tendinopathy and partial tears.
- Articulate the principles of management of distal biceps tendinopathy and partial tears.

## Indications

Tendinopathy and partial tears of the distal biceps tendon are uncommon and often overlooked. In patients who have tendinopathy, outcomes of nonsurgical treatment are good. In patients who have a substantial partial tear, outcomes of surgical repair are typically good. Endoscopy facilitates a dynamic visual assessment of the biceps tendon and footprint. Footprint repair restores the anatomic attachment site and likely will restore the normal mechanics and strength of the distal biceps tendon.

### Anatomy

The biceps brachii is the primary supinator and an important flexor of the elbow. It arises from and inserts as two distinct heads. In the upper arm, the short head runs ulnar to the long head with a variable amount of interdigitation between the two muscle bellies. At the musculotendinous junction, the lacertus fibrosus arises as a layered structure predominantly from the long head to completely encircle the proximal forearm flexor muscles and attach onto the medial and lateral aspect of the anterior ulna. Beyond the lacertus fibrosus, the short head attaches more distally on the radial tuberosity, although the size of the tuberosity footprint and the exact location of each head on the tuberosity can vary. The short head is the dominant flexor of the elbow but also contributes a supination force when the forearm is in a neutral or pronated position. Because of the variation in size and orientation of the tuberosity relative to the coronal plane, some people may be more susceptible than others to impingement of the distal biceps against the ulna, particularly during rotation.

The distal biceps tendon receives its blood supply from the brachial artery proximally and the recurrent radial artery distally. The existence of a hypovascular zone approximately 2 cm in size close to the tendon insertion may further predispose this region to pathology.

The bicipitoradial bursa is a teardrop-shaped structure that lies between the biceps and the brachialis proximally and encircles the entire distal tendon. Because the bicipitoradial bursa adheres to the ulnar aspect of the tendon, effusions within the bursa accumulate on the radial aspect of the tendon and can result in substantial fluid collection proximally if the bursa is inflamed.

### Pathology

Biceps tendinopathy is a disease of the tendon, whereas enthesopathy is a disease of the tendon insertion. The two pathologies often coexist and manifest as a painful clinical condition. The intensity of symptoms and magnitude of disability vary. Histopathology reveals no evidence of inflammation. Instead, the tendon demonstrates mucoid degeneration, disorganization of collagen bundles, chondroid metaplasia, and increased production of matrix metalloproteinases as well as expression of multiple growth factors. The tendinopathy can be classified into four grades

*Dr. Bain or an immediate family member serves as a board member, owner, officer, or committee member of the Shoulder and Elbow Society of Australia, the Australian Hand Surgery Society, and the International Society for Sport Traumatology of the Hand. Neither Dr. Phadnis nor any immediate family member has received anything of value from or has stock or stock options held in a commercial company or institution related directly or indirectly to the subject of this chapter.*

**Table 1** Classification of Distal Biceps Pathology

| Grade | Injury | Clinical Findings | Hook Test Grade | MRI Findings | Recommended Management |
|---|---|---|---|---|---|
| 0 | Tendinopathy, bursitis | Atraumatic, tender, swollen<br>Often occurs in older women with comorbidities | N | Bursitis, fluid, tendinopathy | Nonsurgical management, bursectomy, biopsy |
| 1A | Low-grade partial defect (<50%) | Pain and weakness against resistance | N, A1 | Bursitis, effusion, footprint irregularity | Débridement |
| 1B | Isolated head rupture | Weakness against resistance | A1 | Isolated head avulsion | Repair of isolated head rupture |
| 1C | High-grade partial defect (>50%) | Pain and weakness against resistance | A1 | Incomplete footprint detachment | Detachment and reattachment of tendon |
| 2 | Complete tendon rupture, lacertus fibrosus intact | Tendon medialized by intact lacertus fibrosus<br>Marked weakness of supination | A2 | Complete footprint detachment<br>Tendon within sheath | Offer of repair |
| 3 | Complete tendon and lacertus fibrosus rupture with retraction | Retracted muscle<br>Marked weakness of supination | A3 | Complete footprint detachment<br>Retracted tendon and muscle | Offer of repair |
| 4A | Chronic rupture | Tendon medialized by intact lacertus fibrosus<br>Marked weakness of supination | A1, A2 | Complete footprint detachment and contracted tendon within sheath (A2)<br>A pseudotendon may bridge the native tendon to the footprint (A1) | Offer of repair |
| 4B | Chronic retracted rupture | Retracted muscle<br>Marked weakness | A3 | Complete footprint detachment<br>Retracted tendon within fibrous cocoon | Offer of repair in flexion or with tendon graft |

A = abnormal, N = normal.

ranging from no tear (grade 0) to partial tears of more than half of the tendon (grade 1C). Additional grades have been defined to classify complete tendon ruptures (**Table 1**). This framework can provide a useful guide for clinical diagnosis, imaging options, and patient-specific treatment.

## Clinical Presentation

Patients with biceps tendinopathy report a deep-seated anterior ache in the elbow that worsens with specific activities. Patients often associate a specific event with the onset of their symptoms. Although a traumatic injury in the setting of long-standing pathophysiology is possible, the pathology is more likely to be the result of a long-standing problem that is newly symptomatic. The potential for misinterpretation in this regard is important because patients who are in pain may choose more invasive treatments if they perceive themselves to be damaged and in need of repair—a perception that is rare among patients who perceive their pain to be the result of the gradual changes associated with tendinopathy and enthesopathy.

Although distal biceps rupture is unusual in women, tendinopathy may be less uncommon. Women who have biceps tendinopathy tend to be older than men with the same condition, and women may have predisposing metabolic conditions such as diabetes, renal disease, and hypothyroidism.

Pain from tendinopathy may be the result of bicipitoradial bursitis, impingement of a hypertrophic radial tuberosity, or partial tearing of the tendon insertion. Exudate associated with the bursitis may produce a bicipitoradial effusion that can extend into the antecubital fossa and has even been reported to cause neurovascular compression.

## Physical Examination

Deep-seated pain in the anterior elbow is commonly reported. Fullness of the antecubital fossa is sometimes present

 

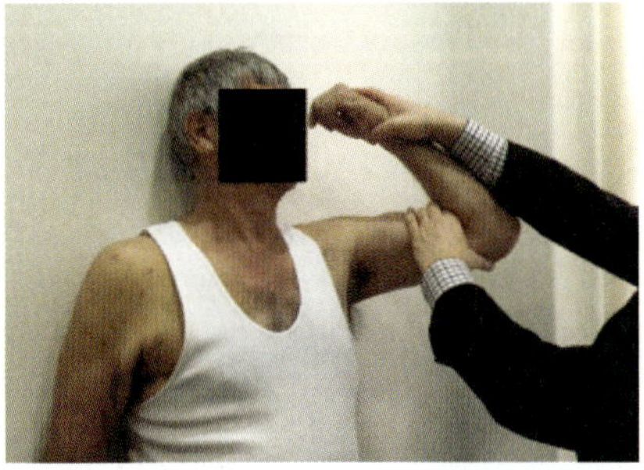

**Figure 1** Clinical photograph shows testing of flexion and supination power. With the patient's shoulder and elbow flexed, the examiner palpates the biceps tendon to assess for pain and weakness.

**Table 2** Interpretation of Hook Test Results

| Finding | Grade | Features of Tendon |
|---|---|---|
| Normal | N | Taut, unyielding, and symmetric with contralateral arm |
| Abnormal | A1 | Taut but yielding and asymmetric with contralateral arm |
| Abnormal | A2 | Lax and asymmetric |
| Abnormal | A3 | Absent cord |

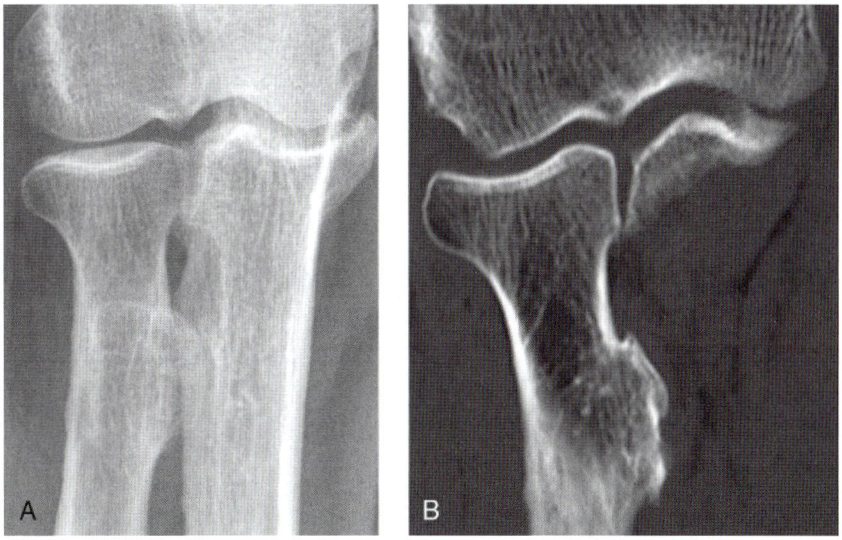


**Figure 2** AP radiograph (**A**) and coronal CT scan (**B**) of the elbow from a patient with tendinopathy and a partial-thickness defect of the distal biceps. The hypertrophic radial tuberosity may be predisposed to impingement against the ulna during pronation of the forearm.

as a result of fluid collection related to the bicipitoradial bursa.

Supination against resistance may elicit pain, and the patient may experience tenderness on palpation of the tendon insertion. Forearm rotation occasionally elicits reproducible pain and crepitus because of impingement of a prominent radial tuberosity and hypertrophic bursa against the proximal ulna.

The hook test is used for the diagnosis of complete distal biceps rupture (**Table 2**). Patients with distal biceps tendinopathy have a negative hook test result, but the biceps tendon yields and is markedly tender during the test.

Supination strength testing usually is performed at 90° of flexion and full forearm supination. The authors of this chapter also test both flexion and supination strength with the patient's arm in full elbow flexion, forearm supination, and 90° of shoulder flexion. This position places the biceps musculotendinous unit at its shortest length, making it more difficult for the muscle to generate force and resulting in more pronounced pain and weakness than is revealed when the test is performed in the standard manner (**Figure 1**).

## Imaging

Whereas acute complete distal biceps rupture is diagnosed by history and examination, tendinopathy is difficult to diagnose definitively without imaging. Radiographic imaging may show an unusually large radial tuberosity (**Figure 2**) or calcific spiculation in the tendon close to its insertion. Ultrasonography is best performed by a radiologist who is experienced in musculoskeletal ultrasonography. Ultrasonography is relatively inexpensive and readily available and is an option for patients who are unable to undergo MRI. It also allows dynamic assessment of tuberosity impingement. Historically, the effectiveness of ultrasonography of the distal biceps tendon has been limited by tendon anisotropy and the difficulty of imaging the tendon insertion. More recently, a pronator window technique has been described to overcome these problems. This technique uses the flexor-pronator musculature as an acoustic window. It is performed with the elbow at 90° of flexion and the forearm fully supinated. The transducer is placed parallel to the biceps tendon over the flexor-pronator mass to facilitate visualization of the tendon and its insertion coursing deep to the brachial artery.

The use of MRI with the arm in the flexion, abduction, and supination position provides the best assessment of the biceps tendon pathology and footprint because the entire length of the tendon and the footprint is seen on one image. Tendinopathy is associated with an effusion, altered intratendinous signal intensity, bursitis, and sometimes a peritendinous ganglion (**Figure 3**). Although partial tears can be observed on MRI, the sensitivity of MRI in the diagnosis of a partial

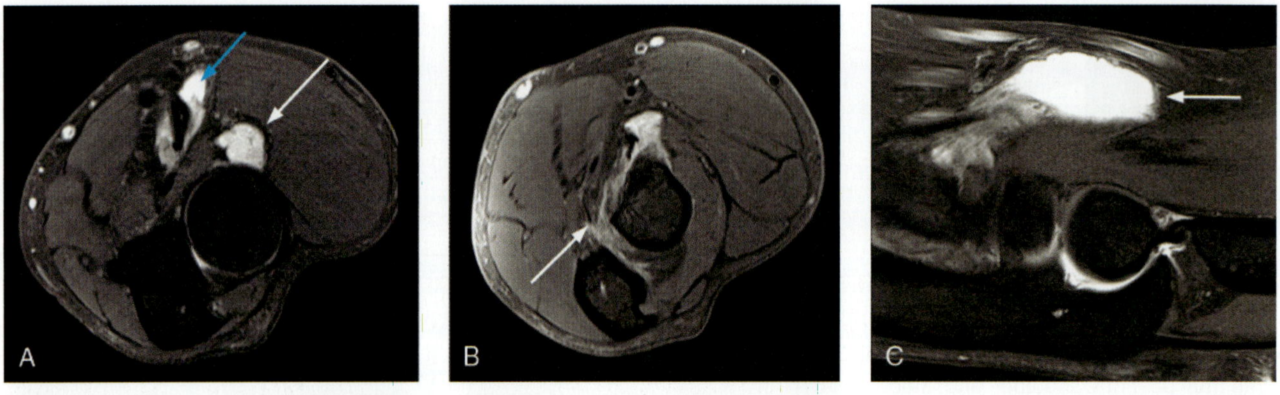


**Figure 3** MRIs of an elbow. **A,** Axial T2-weighted MRI demonstrates effusion around the biceps tendon (blue arrow) and within the bicipitoradial bursa (white arrow). **B,** Axial T2-weighted MRI demonstrates extensive partial-thickness defects at the biceps insertion (arrow). **C,** Sagittal T2-weighted MRI demonstrates the full extent of proximal fluid collection related to the biceps tendinopathy (arrow).

biceps tear is substantially lower than that of a complete tear (59% versus 100%), and quantification of tear size is challenging. Therefore, if the clinical presentation is typical, tendinopathy may be diagnosed in the presence of a normal MRI.

### Diagnostic Endoscopy

Although MRI and ultrasonography reliably identify tendinopathy, they may not provide an accurate measurement of distal biceps tendon defects. Accurate measurement is important because large defects of the tendon footprint may cause mechanical symptoms and weakness that may be improved by reconstructive procedures. The patient's symptoms and examination findings must be considered together with the imaging findings because radiologic changes do not necessarily correlate with symptoms. In patients with appropriate symptoms and clinical findings, endoscopic assessment can be used as a diagnostic tool to assess and quantify the pathoanatomy, including the integrity and quality of the tendon, the degree of footprint coverage, and the tension of the tendon. Any existing bursitis, synovitis, or partial tendon tears can be managed with débridement or endoscopically assisted tendon detachment and reattachment.

## Contraindications

The authors of this chapter consider surgical treatment in patients who are unsatisfied with their symptoms after 6 months of nonsurgical treatment. Surgical treatment is more readily offered to patients with weakness and a relatively recent onset of symptoms associated with an apparent injury than to patients with an insidious onset of symptoms or an underlying metabolic condition. Even if the patient has an apparent history of injury, the condition is usually chronic and latent. Ultimately, the choice to pursue surgical management of tendinopathy depends on patient and surgeon preference. The role of the surgeon is not to prescribe treatment but to educate and inform the patient that surgical treatment is not always required or necessary.

## Alternative Treatments

Although many other tendinopathies, such as tendinopathy of the extensor carpi radialis brevis, are known to be self-limiting, the natural history of distal biceps tendinopathy is not fully understood. Physical therapy can include heat, massage, ultrasonography, and an eccentric training program, but the effect of these treatment modalities compared with that of placebo treatment or no treatment is unknown.

The authors of this chapter suggest that a patient with a history of an acute injury in a previously pain-free elbow is more likely to have a partial tear, whereas a patient with an insidious onset of symptoms and/or underlying metabolic comorbidities is more likely to have tendinopathy without a substantial partial tear. In the experience of the authors of this chapter, patients with a partial tear are less likely than patients with only tendinopathy to be satisfied with nonsurgical treatment. Therefore, the authors typically offer surgical treatment to patients with a partial tear, usually after a trial of nonsurgical treatment of up to 6 months. Patients with tendinopathy are initially referred to a physical therapist. Activity modification often decreases symptoms; however, rest has not been proved to modify the course of the disease, and patients may remain active if they prefer. Oral NSAIDs and corticosteroid injections are occasionally used for temporary pain relief to facilitate eccentric exercises. However, corticosteroid injections are catabolic. They weaken the tendon and may accelerate tendon degeneration, increase the risk of development of fissures or defects, and predispose the tendon to a complete rupture. The authors of this chapter do not use platelet-rich plasma because they have found that this treatment is often uncomfortable for the patient and the current literature does not show a clear benefit compared with other nonsurgical modalities.

## Results

Treatment of biceps tendinopathy is debated and is based on a few retrospective case series. The general consensus is that tendinopathy can usually be managed nonsurgically. The authors of this chapter think that more extensive partial tears (>50% tendon involvement) are better managed surgically, although this figure is not evidence based. Published case series generally report good results of tendon detachment, débridement, and reattachment for the management of distal biceps tendinopathy (**Table 3**).

Several small case series have reported the outcome of surgical treatment of patients with tendinopathy and partial tears of the distal biceps. The authors of one series recommended detaching and reattaching the tendon rather than performing an in situ repair because one patient in the series had an inferior outcome after in situ repair. Several authors subsequently reported good results of detachment and suture anchor reattachment of the tendon.

No controlled studies of injection for the management of biceps tendinopathy have been published. Ultrasonographically guided corticosteroid injection for biceps tendinopathy without partial tears was associated with resolution of symptoms in 16 of 22 patients (73%) at a mean of 23 months after injection. In one study, the use of platelet-rich plasma with dry needling for the management of distal biceps tendinopathy resulted in improvement in six patients, but repeat injection was performed in two patients.

**Video 10.1** Anatomic Distal Biceps Tendon Repair. Joideep Phadnis, MBChB, MRCS, FRCS (Tr & Orth) (5 min)

## Techniques

Distal biceps endoscopy has both diagnostic and therapeutic purposes. In patients with partial biceps tendon tears, it allows a thorough assessment of the integrity and footprint of the tendon. In the experience of the authors of this chapter, the partial tear typically occurs in the distal short head of the biceps tendon. The bicipitoradial bursa and the frayed tendon edges can be débrided, or the tendon can be detached and reattached using an endoscopically assisted footprint repair technique (**Figure 4**).

The authors of this chapter suggest that reattaching the biceps tendon to its native footprint on the most ulnar aspect of the radial tuberosity is likely to be beneficial. Performing this reattachment through a single-incision technique is not possible because the forearm cannot be supinated enough to allow safe drilling or suture anchor placement through a single anterior incision. A double-incision technique with the use of suture anchors to restore the footprint is available but has been associated with radioulnar synostosis.

The authors of this chapter suggest, on the basis of a cadaver model, that the single-incision footprint technique better restores the native moment arm of the biceps and provides superior restoration of supination torque. Although the technique can be performed with endoscopic assistance or as an open procedure, the use of endoscopy facilitates decision making in the presence of a partial tear and provides superior visualization during the repair.

### Setup/Exposure

- The patient is positioned supine, with the arm placed on an arm table.
- General anesthesia is administered.
- The entire arm is prepped and draped.
- A sterile tourniquet is applied to the arm.
- The surgeon sits in the area of the patient's axilla, with the assistant on the side of the patient opposite the surgeon and the nurse at the end of the arm table.
- The viewing screen and nonsterile arthroscopic equipment are placed on the opposite side of the patient.

### Instruments/Equipment/Implants Required

#### DISTAL BICEPS ENDOSCOPY

- A 4.0-mm, 30° arthroscope is used.
- A hood attachment for the arthroscope is preferred but not essential.
- Nylon tape is required.
- A 4.0-mm full-radius resector without teeth is necessary.
- A bipolar cautery device is required.

#### FOOTPRINT REPAIR

- A cortical button is used.
- A 2.5-mm drill is required.
- A wide-bore epidural needle is necessary.
- Two No. 2 braided nonabsorbable composite sutures are used.
- Two different-colored No. 1 monofilament sutures are needed.

### Procedure

#### ESTABLISHMENT OF PORTALS

- A 2.5-cm longitudinal incision is made 2 cm distal to the anterior elbow crease. This incision serves as the portal for the arthroscope and instruments.
- A posterior accessory portal can be established with an inside-out technique by passing a switching stick between the radius and ulna to exit in the posterior forearm. This portal is used for preparation of the tuberosity.

**Table 3** Results of Management of Distal Biceps Tendinopathy and Partial Defects

| Authors (Year) | No. of Patients | Procedure or Approach | Mean Patient Age in Years (Range) | Mean Follow-up in Months (Range) | Success Rate (%)[a] | Results | Level of Evidence |
|---|---|---|---|---|---|---|---|
| Bourne and Morrey (1991) | 3 | Transosseous repair (2 release and repair, 1 in situ repair) | 49 (38-58) | 16 (12-24) | 66 | Good flexion strength, suboptimal supination strength<br>In situ repair was inferior<br>No complications | IV |
| Dürr et al (2000) | 4 | 3 nonsurgical, 1 surgical (transosseous repair) | 59 (40-82) | 6.5 (1-12) | 100 | No complications | IV |
| Vardakas et al (2001) | 7 | Suture anchor repair | 52 (38-58) | 9.5 (7-14) | 100 | No complications | IV |
| Kelly et al (2003) | 8 | Transosseous release and repair | 50 (36-60) | NA | 100 | No complications | IV |
| Dellaero and Mallon (2006) | 7 | Suture anchor release and repair | 42.7 (22-60) | 30.6 (25-39) | 100 | 2 patients had LABCN palsy | IV |
| Frazier et al (2010) | 17 | Suture anchor repair or transosseous repair | 48 (14-70) | 32 (12-96) | 90 | 2 patients had LABCN palsy<br>1 patient had asymptomatic heterotopic ossification<br>1 patient had rerupture (treated with suture repair) | IV |
| Maree et al (2011) | 20 | Corticosteroid injection (22 elbows) | 46 (16-72) | 23 (8-60) | 73 | 16 of 22 elbows had full recovery<br>No complications | IV |
| Ruch et al (2014) | 15 | Suture anchor repair | 55 (38-75) | NA | NA | 14 patients had disruption of lateral fibers<br>1 patient had a single head tear (short head)<br>5 patients had intratendinous ganglions<br>Complications: transient LABCN palsy in 8 patients, posterior interosseous nerve palsy in 3 patients | III |

LABCN = lateral antebrachial cutaneous nerve, NA = not available.

[a] Success defined by authors based on improvement in patient symptoms after treatment. Heterogeneous methods of patient assessment were used.

 

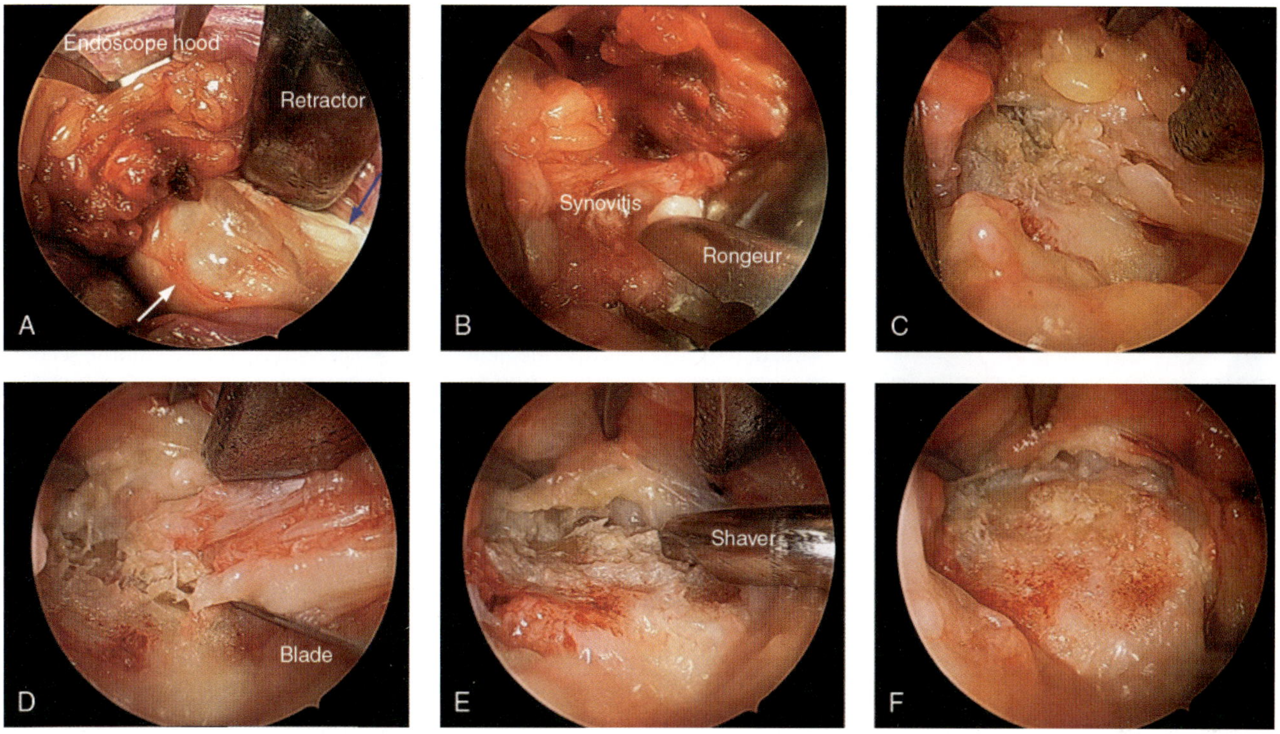


**Figure 4** Endoscopic images of an elbow show treatment of a partial defect of the distal biceps tendon. **A,** A fluid-filled bicipitoradial bursa (white arrow) is present on the radial aspect of the distal biceps tendon (blue arrow). **B,** The bursa is entered with the endoscope, and extensive synovitis is débrided. **C,** The bursa is resected. Note the tears on the undersurface of the tendon, the uncovered footprint, and the discolored, amorphous appearance of the diseased tissue. **D,** A blade is used to release the fissured tendon from the tuberosity. **E,** The tuberosity is prepared using a shaver. **F,** The tuberosity has been prepared for reattachment of the tendon. Note the punctate bleeding without removal of all cortical bone.

**DIAGNOSTIC PROCEDURE**

- The distal biceps tendon and its bicipitoradial bursa are identified by blunt dissection through the viewing portal.
- The bicipitoradial bursa is incised on its radial aspect to allow introduction of the hooded scope.
- A dry endoscopic technique facilitates clear identification of tissue planes and avoids fluid extravasation into the soft tissues. Occasional fogging of the lens is addressed by wiping with an alcohol swab.
- Alternatively, to remove fogging, blood, or bone debris from the lens, the lens can be wiped on the fat in the soft tissues. This method works in a similar manner to the use of glycine.
- Diagnostic endoscopy including assessment of the bursa, proximal radius, and distal biceps tendon is performed. The tendon is inspected dynamically through forearm rotation.
- The integrity of the footprint is tested with the use of traction on a nylon tape passed around the tendon and a hook probe at the axilla where the tendon inserts onto the tuberosity.
- The frayed, laminated, or partially torn tendon is débrided.
- The bursitis is débrided.
- To avoid the risk of inadvertent injury to adjacent structures, débridement is performed with handheld instruments or with a full-radius resector (without teeth) with the suction turned off. The aperture must be in full view whenever the resector is active.
- The small veins are the structure at greatest risk during débridement and must be avoided, especially on the ulnar side of the tendon near its attachment.
- If a substantial tear of one head is observed, the authors of this chapter release both heads so that advancement of the torn head onto the footprint does not result in the other head becoming abnormally tight.
- To release the tendon, curved scissors are placed into the axilla between the tendon attachment and the radial tuberosity. The tendon is released under endoscopic visualization.

**FOOTPRINT REPAIR**

- The footprint repair can be performed open or with endoscopic assistance (**Figures 4** and **5**). The

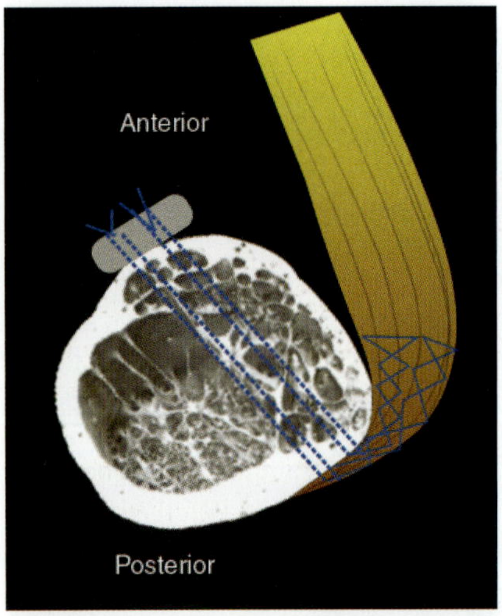


**Figure 5** Schematic diagram depicts the single-incision distal biceps footprint repair technique. The biceps tendon is wrapped around the radial tuberosity in its anatomic location and secured over the anterior radius with transosseous sutures tied over a cortical button.

technique is the same. Endoscopy facilitates improved diagnosis and visualization of the pathoanatomy of the distal biceps.

- After the tendon is released from its native footprint, the detached tendon stump is retrieved from the wound and débrided back to normal tendon.
- Two locking Krackow stitches of No. 2 braided nonabsorbable composite suture are placed in the tendon with a minimum of three throws along the tendon length, resulting in four suture strands exiting near the tip of the tendon. The sutures should exit on the superior surface of the tendon so that when the tendon is positioned on the tuberosity, the sutures will act as a tension band holding the tendon onto the débrided footprint and will not interpose between the tendon and the bone healing surface.
- The hooded endoscope is reinserted.
- Supplementary right-angle retractors are placed to aid visualization.
- Any remaining bursa is resected to allow clear visualization of the tuberosity.
- The tuberosity is débrided until punctate bleeding is visible, without decorticating the tuberosity. A shaver, rongeur, or curet can be used for this step.
- Alternatively, if the tuberosity is considerably prominent, an arthroscopic burr can be used for débridement. Because this débridement is performed in the depth of the bursa, the authors of this chapter have the assistant slowly add saline while the surgeon continues to work with the burr on low-pressure suction to keep the bone cool and remove the debris.
- Because the posterior aspect of the tuberosity (the true biceps footprint) can be difficult to débride through the anterior portal, a second working portal can be established by passing a switching stick between the ulna and radius to exit posteriorly.
- The shaver can be passed into the wound through the posterior portal to débride the back side of the tuberosity.
- Two oblique 2.5-mm drill holes are created from the anterior aspect of the radius. These holes should exit just behind the dorsal ulnar edge of the tuberosity.
- The patient's arm is pronated 40° from the fully supinated position.
- The drill is positioned on the anterolateral radius and aimed obliquely toward the posterior tuberosity.
- This position re-creates the footprint and ensures that the cortical button will not impinge on the repaired biceps tendon.
- A wide-bore epidural needle is loaded with a No. 1 looped monofilament suture such that a 1- to 2-cm loop of suture protrudes from the tip.
- The needle and its loop are passed through the first drill hole. A curved clip is preplaced to grasp the needle and the monofilament loop.
- After the needle is grasped, it is withdrawn, leaving the suture in the clip.
- The clip is withdrawn, and the suture loop is used to advance the sutures from the tendon.
- Visualization with the endoscope facilitates identification of the loop.
- The step is repeated for the second drill hole with a differently colored suture.
- The previously prepared biceps tendon is oriented so that when the suture is shuttled, the short head will be distal and the long head proximal.
- The sutures are shuttled through the drill holes. Both sutures from the radial Krackow stitch are placed into the distal drill hole, and both sutures from the ulnar Krackow stitch are placed into the proximal drill hole.
- The braided nonabsorbable suture strands are passed through the holes in the cortical button.
- With the patient's forearm in supination, traction is placed on the distal sutures to fully reduce the tendon onto the footprint. This step allows the proximal sutures to be easily tied.
- The distal sutures are tied.

### Wound Closure

- The tourniquet is released, and hemostasis is achieved.
- The wound is closed in standard fashion.

## Postoperative Regimen

Postoperatively, a light dressing is applied over the incision. A sling is provided for comfort only. Range-of-motion exercises are begun immediately postoperatively. After the wound has healed, a light sport-specific rehabilitation program is begun. Lifting is limited to the weight of a cup of tea for the first 6 weeks postoperatively. Heavy lifting is avoided for at least 3 months.

## Limiting Adverse Events

For distal biceps endoscopy, the elbow should be positioned in slight flexion with a bump under the forearm. This position reduces the anterior soft-tissue tension and allows easier access for the endoscope. A dry endoscopic technique and a hooded scope help avoid excessive swelling and provide optimal clarity of view. The hood is used as a retractor to increase the working space. To protect the neurovascular structures on the medial aspect of the biceps, the bursa should be entered on its radial aspect. Because partial tears are most frequently seen on the undersurface of the tendon at its attachment to the tuberosity, the surgeon should perform a dynamic assessment of the tendon while viewing the tendon footprint. To ensure safe tissue débridement, a full-radius resector without teeth and with minimal suction should be used. Intermittent fluid irrigation and low suction is used to maintain a clear view and a dry working space. Small vessels that can cause bleeding and obscure visualization should be retracted. A transverse vessel usually crosses the field at the distal aspect of the incision.

For footprint repair, the incision should be made 3 to 4 cm distal to the transverse elbow crease. This incision avoids vessels from the leash of Henry and lies directly over the radial tuberosity. The tendon and tuberosity should be prepared thoroughly to promote healing. While making the drill holes, the surgeon should reduce the supination on the forearm slightly. This technique helps the surgeon start the drill holes more radially on the anterior aspect of the radius, allows the drill holes to exit just behind the tuberosity, and ensures that the anterior cortical button does not impinge against the tendon after the tendon is reattached. Suture retrieval from the posteromedial aspect of the tuberosity is a difficult part of the procedure. Preplacing a curved clip for suture retrieval and ensuring that the monofilament loop is outside the tip of the needle facilitates this step. The surgeon must ensure that the whipstitched suture limbs exit on the ulnar surface of the tendon. This technique creates a tension-band effect and minimizes interposition of suture material between the tendon and bone. The sutures in the short head (medial two limbs) should be shuttled through the distal drill hole to re-create the normal 90° external rotation of the distal biceps and place the tendon on the tuberosity in the correct orientation. To maintain reduction of the tendon to the footprint when tying the sutures over the cortical button, the surgeon should maintain tension on the distal sutures while tying the proximal sutures first.

## Bibliography

Barker SL, Bell SN, Connell D, Coghlan JA: Ultrasound-guided platelet-rich plasma injection for distal biceps tendinopathy. *Shoulder & Elbow* 2015;7(2):110-114.

Bourne MH, Morrey BF: Partial rupture of the distal biceps tendon. *Clin Orthop Relat Res* 1991;(271):143-148.

Dellaero DT, Mallon WJ: Surgical treatment of partial biceps tendon ruptures at the elbow. *J Shoulder Elbow Surg* 2006;15(2):215-217.

Dürr HR, Stäbler A, Pfahler M, Matzko M, Refior HJ: Partial rupture of the distal biceps tendon. *Clin Orthop Relat Res* 2000;(374):195-200.

Eames MH, Bain GI, Fogg QA, van Riet RP: Distal biceps tendon anatomy: A cadaveric study. *J Bone Joint Surg Am* 2007;89(5):1044-1049.

Festa A, Mulieri PJ, Newman JS, Spitz DJ, Leslie BM: Effectiveness of magnetic resonance imaging in detecting partial and complete distal biceps tendon rupture. *J Hand Surg Am* 2010;35(1):77-83.

Forthman CL, Zimmerman RM, Sullivan MJ, Gabel GT: Cross-sectional anatomy of the bicipital tuberosity and biceps brachii tendon insertion: Relevance to anatomic tendon repair. *J Shoulder Elbow Surg* 2008;17(3):522-526.

Frazier MS, Boardman MJ, Westland M, Imbriglia JE: Surgical treatment of partial distal biceps tendon ruptures. *J Hand Surg Am* 2010;35(7):1111-1114.

Jarrett CD, Weir DM, Stuffmann ES, Jain S, Miller MC, Schmidt CC: Anatomic and biomechanical analysis of the short and long head components of the distal biceps tendon. *J Shoulder Elbow Surg* 2012;21(7):942-948.

Jockel CR, Mulieri PJ, Belsky MR, Leslie BM: Distal biceps tendon tears in women. *J Shoulder Elbow Surg* 2010;19(5):645-650.

Kelly EW, Steinmann S, O'Driscoll SW: Surgical treatment of partial distal biceps tendon ruptures through a single posterior incision. *J Shoulder Elbow Surg* 2003;12(5):456-461.

Maffulli N, Khan KM, Puddu G: Overuse tendon conditions: Time to change a confusing terminology. *Arthroscopy* 1998;14(8):840-843.

Maree MN, Vrettos BC, Roche SJ, Osch GV: Distal biceps tendinopathy: Conservative treatment. *Shoulder & Elbow* 2011;3(2):104-108.

O'Driscoll SW, Goncalves LB, Dietz P: The hook test for distal biceps tendon avulsion. *Am J Sports Med* 2007;35(11):1865-1869.

Phadnis J, Bain G: Endoscopic-assisted distal biceps footprint repair. *Tech Hand Up Extrem Surg* 2015;19(2):55-59.

Prud'homme-Foster M, Louati H, Pollock JW, Papp S: Proper placement of the distal biceps tendon during repair improves supination strength: A biomechanical analysis. *J Shoulder Elbow Surg* 2015;24(4):527-532.

Ruch DS, Watters TS, Wartinbee DA, Richard MJ, Leversedge FJ, Mithani SK: Anatomic findings and complications after surgical treatment of chronic, partial distal biceps tendon tears: A case cohort comparison study. *J Hand Surg Am* 2014;39(8):1572-1577.

Seiler JG III, Parker LM, Chamberland PD, Sherbourne GM, Carpenter WA: The distal biceps tendon: Two potential mechanisms involved in its rupture. Arterial supply and mechanical impingement. *J Shoulder Elbow Surg* 1995;4(3):149-156.

Smith J, Finnoff JT, O'Driscoll SW, Lai JK: Sonographic evaluation of the distal biceps tendon using a medial approach: The pronator window. *J Ultrasound Med* 2010;29(5):861-865.

Vardakas DG, Musgrave DS, Varitimidis SE, Goebel F, Sotereanos DG: Partial rupture of the distal biceps tendon. *J Shoulder Elbow Surg* 2001;10(4):377-379.

## Video Reference

Phadnis J: Video. *Anatomic Distal Biceps Tendon Repair.* Worthington, United Kingdom, 2016.

 

# Chapter 11
# Lateral and Medial Epicondylitis

*Jennifer Moriatis Wolf, MD*

**Learning Objectives**

- Describe the evidence and recommendations for steroid and blood-based injections.
- Describe indications for surgery for lateral and medial epicondylitis.

## Indications

Lateral epicondylitis and medial epicondylitis are enthesopathies occurring at the extensor carpi radialis brevis (ECRB) origin and the medial flexor-pronator origin, respectively. Despite the suffix *-itis*, they are not inflammatory. Lateral epicondylitis occurs approximately six times more frequently than medial epicondylitis. Onset of both conditions typically occurs in middle age. Some researchers theorize that these conditions are the result of overuse and microscopic tearing of the tendon origin, but these theories have not been proved.

Management of lateral and medial epicondylitis is primarily nonsurgical. Evidence suggests that epicondylitis resolves on its own over an extended period. In a randomized controlled trial comparing physical therapy with steroid injection in 185 patients, success rates at 1 year were 91% in the physical therapy cohort, 69% in the steroid cohort, and 83% in a control group. The results of this study can be used to help educate patients about the available treatment options. Nonsurgical treatment can also include physical therapy, the use of which is supported in high-level studies. Extracorporeal shock wave therapy and ultrasonography have been shown to be equivalent to placebo treatment in randomized trials. Corticosteroid injections, long the mainstay of treatment, have been shown to be effective for short-term pain relief (≤6 weeks) but to have minimal effect thereafter.

Other nonsurgical options include injection of blood-based products such as autologous whole blood or platelet-rich plasma (PRP), injection of botulinum toxin, and proliferation therapy using hypertonic glucose or saline injections. Autologous blood injections were originally described in a study published in 2003. The authors of the study noted resolution of pain and improved function in 28 patients with chronic tennis elbow who received one or two injections of whole blood mixed with lidocaine (**Figure 1**). Injection of PRP, which is obtained through centrifugation of whole blood to isolate the platelet-enriched serum, has been attempted because PRP is thought to have a higher concentration of growth factors than does whole blood. Comparative studies have shown positive results from both whole blood injection and PRP injection, but superiority of one over the other has not been shown. Some researchers support injection of botulinum toxin because of the theory that temporarily paralyzing the muscle will allow the tendon origin to heal; however, analysis of surgical specimens has not revealed evidence of damage that needs to heal. A multicenter randomized controlled trial comparing botulinum toxin injection with steroid injection and placebo injection with 18-week follow-up demonstrated superiority of botulinum toxin injection on the basis of clinical pain scores; however, it is important to recognize that one or more authors reported industry support for this study. A more recent meta-analysis of randomized trials of botulinum toxin showed a moderate effect of botulinum toxin for pain relief but no difference in grip compared with placebo. However, this treatment has not been widely adopted, likely because of its cost and the complication of grip weakness described in several studies. In a randomized controlled trial comparing dextrose injections with dextrose–morrhuate sodium injections or observation without injection in 32 patients, improved Patient-Rated Tennis Elbow Evaluation scores were

*Dr. Wolf or an immediate family member serves as a board member, owner, officer, or committee member of the American Foundation for Surgery of the Hand, the American Society for Surgery of the Hand, and the Ruth Jackson Orthopaedic Society.*

noted at 16 weeks in the two injection groups compared with the observation group.

Surgical treatment should be reserved for patients in whom nonsurgical treatment has failed to achieve satisfactory results. In one study, researchers reported a 90% response rate with improvement in pain in select patients with a minimum of 6 months of previous failed nonsurgical treatment. Surgical management of lateral epicondylitis can include percutaneous or open release of the ECRB origin or open or arthroscopic débridement of pathologic tissue at the ECRB origin (**Figure 2**) with or without reattachment of the ECRB origin. Data on the surgical management of medial epicondylitis are limited. The authors of one study recommended débridement of the nidus of pathologic tissue in the medial conjoint tendon and attention to potential concomitant ulnar neuropathy (**Figure 3**).

## Contraindications

Because evidence supports the time-limited nature of epicondylitis, nonsurgical treatment should be attempted before surgical treatment is considered. Additionally, if the patient's symptoms are consistent with radial tunnel syndrome (compression of the posterior interosseous nerve in the proximal forearm), surgical treatment at the lateral epicondyle will not address this issue. In fact, many patients with so-called recalcitrant epicondylitis actually have radial tunnel syndrome. Caution is necessary when undertaking surgical treatment in patients with severe skin atrophy resulting from multiple corticosteroid injections. The local tissue may be hyperesthetic, and a surgical incision often worsens this problem.

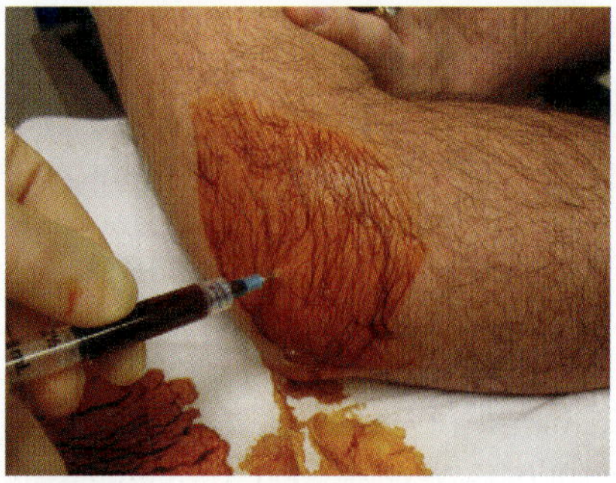

**Figure 1** Clinical photograph of an elbow shows an autologous blood injection at the extensor origin administered under sterile conditions.

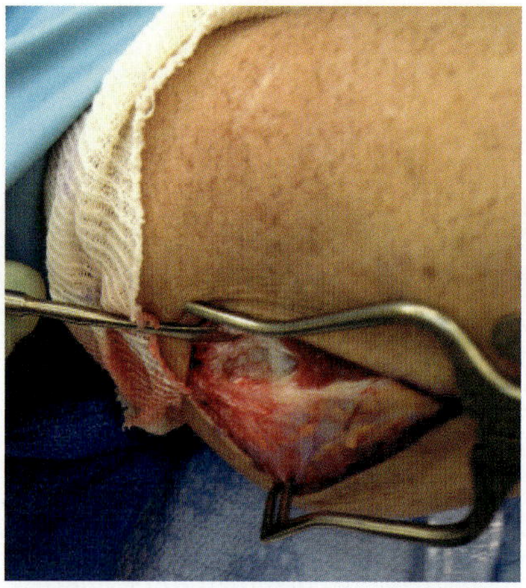

**Figure 2** Intraoperative photograph of an elbow shows open débridement of the lateral epicondyle.

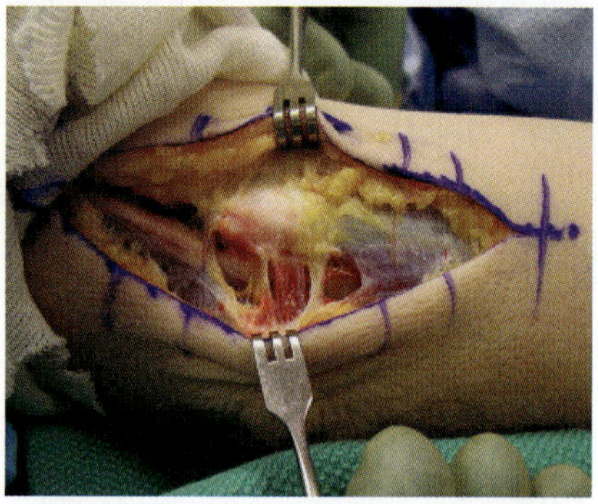

**Figure 3** Intraoperative photograph shows exposure of the medial side of the elbow flexor-pronator mass and the ulnar nerve during surgical treatment of medial epicondylitis.

**Table 1** Results of Nonsurgical and Surgical Management of Lateral and Medial Epicondylitis

| Authors (Year) | Number of Patients | Procedure or Approach | Mean Patient Age in Years (Range) |
|---|---|---|---|
| Dunn et al (2008) | 83 | Open Nirschl débridement | 46 (23-70) |
| Thanasas et al (2011) | 28 | Injection of PRP or injection of autologous blood | PRP group, 35.9 (34-55)<br>Autologous blood group, 36.6 (29-52) |
| Coombes et al (2013) | 165 | Corticosteroid injection or physical therapy | 49.7 (NA) |
| Solheim et al (2013) | 295 | Open or arthroscopic tendon release | 46 (NA) |

NA = not available; PRP = platelet-rich plasma; quickDASH = quick Disabilities of the Arm, Shoulder and Hand.

 

## Alternative Treatments

As noted previously, nonsurgical management of lateral and medial epicondylitis includes physical therapy, injections, and observation. Newer alternative treatments include percutaneous radiofrequency ablation and percutaneous microresection, both of which are performed under ultrasonographic guidance. Evidence for these procedures is limited. Radiofrequency ablation was reported retrospectively in 34 patients with tennis elbow; patients experienced a 78% reduction in pain, and Mayo Elbow Performance Index scores had improved at 6 months. A retrospective study of ultrasonographically guided microresection, performed under sterile conditions through a small stab incision at the elbow, showed positive results at 1 year in 19 of 20 patients, with relief of pain and improved function measured by visual analog scale and Disabilities of the Arm, Shoulder and Hand scores.

## Results

Results from select studies on nonsurgical and surgical management of lateral and medial epicondylitis are summarized in **Table 1**. Level I studies of nonsurgical treatment show similar outcomes for observation compared with therapy and steroid injection, and similar improvement with various blood-based injections. Good results have been reported in surgical studies; however, these studies are retrospective in nature.

## Techniques

### Open Débridement of the Lateral Epicondyle

#### SETUP/EXPOSURE

- The patient is positioned supine, with the extremity placed on an arm table.
- A tourniquet is placed high on the arm.
- An oblique incision approximately 4 to 5 cm in length is marked, centered at the lateral epicondyle (**Figure 4, A**).
- The incision is deepened through the skin and subcutaneous tissues, exposing the fascia over the lateral ECRB origin (**Figure 4, B**).
- The fascia is opened in the interval between the extensor carpi radialis longus and the extensor carpi ulnaris, exposing the deeper ECRB.
- The origin of the ECRB is opened in its midpoint longitudinally, exposing the edge of the lateral epicondyle and the tissue at the origin of the muscle. It is not necessary to open the joint (**Figure 4, C**).

#### INSTRUMENTS/EQUIPMENT/IMPLANTS REQUIRED

- Rongeurs are used.
- Osteotomes are required.

#### PROCEDURE

- Tissue that appears frayed, friable, or gray is removed.
- The lateral epicondyle is abraded with a rongeur or an osteotome to produce a bleeding edge.
- The author of this chapter also cuts the branches of the posterior cutaneous nerve of the forearm that innervate the area.

#### WOUND CLOSURE

- The fascia of the extensor carpi radialis longus and the extensor carpi ulnaris are closed over the lateral epicondyle with absorbable sutures.
- The skin is closed with a running subcuticular absorbable suture.

**Table 1** Results of Nonsurgical and Surgical Management of Lateral and Medial Epicondylitis (*continued*)

| Mean Follow-up in Years (Range) | Success Rate (%) | Results | Level of Evidence |
|---|---|---|---|
| 12.6 (10-14) | 84 | Improved American Shoulder and Elbow Surgeons and Nirschl scores | IV |
| 0.5 | Autologous blood, 41.6<br>PRP, 67.5 | Improved pain visual analog scale and Liverpool Elbow scores | I |
| 1 | Steroid injection, 83<br>Placebo injection, 96<br>Physical therapy, 91<br>No physical therapy, 88 | Success measured by patient-rated global rating of change | I (2 × 2 factorial trial) |
| 4.2 (NA) | Open, 67<br>Arthroscopic, 78 | Success rates based on improved quickDASH score | III |

NA = not available; PRP = platelet-rich plasma; quickDASH = quick Disabilities of the Arm, Shoulder and Hand.

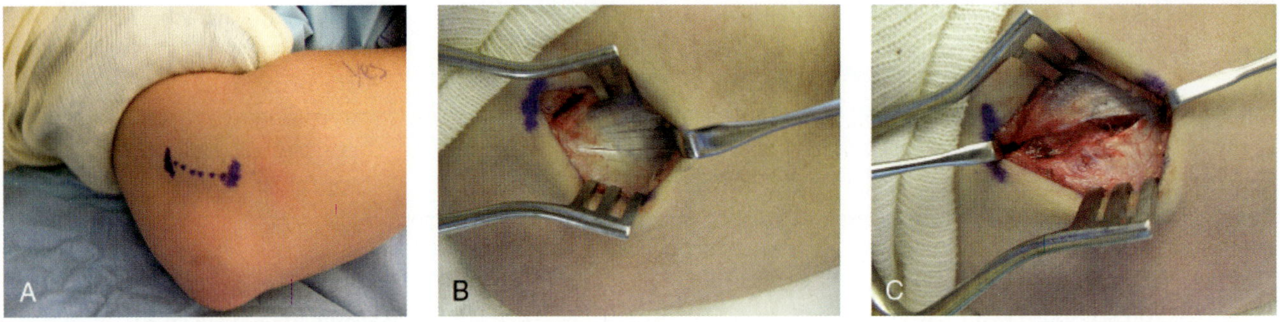


**Figure 4** Intraoperative photographs of an elbow show steps in open débridement of the lateral epicondyle. **A,** An oblique incision marked over the lateral epicondyle. **B,** The opening of the skin and subcutaneous tissue to expose the extensor origin. **C,** Exposure of the origin of the extensor carpi radialis brevis through the interval between the extensor carpi radialis longus and the extensor carpi ulnaris.

## Débridement of the Medial Epicondyle

### SETUP/EXPOSURE

- The patient is positioned supine, with the extremity placed on an arm table.
- A tourniquet is placed high on the arm.
- In patients with concomitant ulnar nerve compression or neuritis, a curved incision can be marked below the medial epicondyle to allow exposure of the ulnar nerve.
- The skin and subcutaneous tissues are incised, exposing the fascia over the flexor-pronator origin on the medial epicondyle.
- The ulnar nerve is identified posterior to the epicondyle (**Figure 5**).

### PROCEDURE

- The flexor-pronator origin is opened within its anterior half, typically at the interval between the pronator and the flexor carpi radialis.
- The nidus of pathologic tissue is débrided. This is characterized as thickened fibrous bands adjacent to the medial epicondylar origin.

### WOUND CLOSURE

- Wound closure is similar to that described previously for lateral epicondylar débridement.
- The fascia are closed over the epicondyle with absorbable sutures.
- The skin is closed with a running subcuticular absorbable suture.

## Postoperative Regimen

After either of the procedures described in this chapter, a bulky sterile dressing is placed over the incision site, and a long arm splint that includes the wrist is applied to keep the elbow in 90° of flexion. The splint is removed 10 days postoperatively, and a physical therapist instructs the patient in active motion and stretching of the elbow and wrist. Strengthening of the arm is initiated 2 months postoperatively.

## Limiting Adverse Events

Overuse of corticosteroid injections should be avoided because it can result in skin atrophy and destabilization of the supporting ligaments of the elbow. Surgical complications in the management of lateral epicondylitis include injury to the lateral ulnar collateral ligament, which is best avoided by taking care not to dissect too far inferiorly at the lateral epicondyle, and neuroma formation, which can be avoided with careful sectioning and removal of the branches of the posterior cutaneous nerve in this area. Skin hypersensitivity is a potential complication of primary or revision surgical procedures performed through atrophied skin. Anconeus transposition has been described as an option for coverage and padding. The authors of one study reported improved outcomes in patients with lateral epicondylitis who were treated with elbow débridement combined with anconeus transfer in comparison with patients treated with débridement alone. Complications of medial epicondylar débridement include injury to the medial antebrachial cutaneous nerve branches crossing the area. Such injury is avoided by careful dissection and preservation of these nerve twigs.

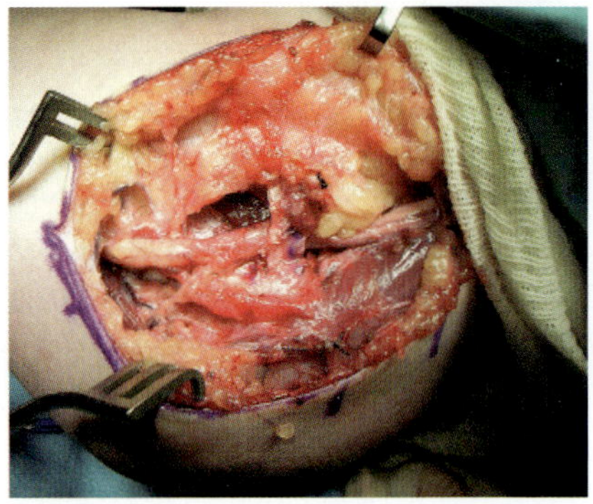

**Figure 5** Intraoperative photograph of an elbow shows exposure of the ulnar nerve and the flexor-pronator mass in preparation for débridement of the medial epicondyle.

 

## Bibliography

Brinks A, Koes BW, Volkers AC, Verhaar JA, Bierma-Zeinstra SM: Adverse effects of extra-articular corticosteroid injections: A systematic review. *BMC Musculoskelet Disord* 2010;11:206.

Chanlalit C, Limsricharoen W: Posterolateral rotatory instability from multiple steroids injections for tennis elbow: A case report. *J Med Assoc Thai* 2013;96(suppl 1):S104-S107.

Cohen MS, Romeo AA: Open and arthroscopic management of lateral epicondylitis in the athlete. *Hand Clin* 2009;25(3):331-338.

Coombes BK, Bisset L, Brooks P, Khan A, Vicenzino B: Effect of corticosteroid injection, physiotherapy, or both on clinical outcomes in patients with unilateral lateral epicondylalgia: A randomized controlled trial. *JAMA* 2013;309(5):461-469.

Dellon AL, Kim J, Ducic I: Painful neuroma of the posterior cutaneous nerve of the forearm after surgery for lateral humeral epicondylitis. *J Hand Surg Am* 2004;29(3):387-390.

Di Stefano V, Nixon JE: Skin and fat atrophy complications of local steroid injection. *Pa Med* 1974;77(1):38.

Dunn JH, Kim JJ, Davis L, Nirschl RP: Ten- to 14-year follow-up of the Nirschl surgical technique for lateral epicondylitis. *Am J Sports Med* 2008;36(2):261-266.

Edwards SG, Calandruccio JH: Autologous blood injections for refractory lateral epicondylitis. *J Hand Surg Am* 2003;28(2):272-278.

Gabel GT, Morrey BF: Medial epicondylitis, in Morrey BF, ed: *The Elbow and Its Disorders*. Philadelphia, PA, Saunders, 2000, pp 537-542.

Gabel GT, Morrey BF: Operative treatment of medical epicondylitis: Influence of concomitant ulnar neuropathy at the elbow. *J Bone Joint Surg Am* 1995;77(7):1065-1069.

Gonzalez MH, Lotfi P, Bendre A, Mandelbroyt Y, Lieska N: The ulnar nerve at the elbow and its local branching: An anatomic study. *J Hand Surg Br* 2001;26(2):142-144.

Haker E, Lundeberg T: Pulsed ultrasound treatment in lateral epicondylalgia. *Scand J Rehabil Med* 1991;23(3):115-118.

Kalichman L, Bannuru RR, Severin M, Harvey W: Injection of botulinum toxin for treatment of chronic lateral epicondylitis: Systematic review and meta-analysis. *Semin Arthritis Rheum* 2011;40(6):532-538.

Koh JS, Mohan PC, Howe TS, et al: Fasciotomy and surgical tenotomy for recalcitrant lateral elbow tendinopathy: Early clinical experience with a novel device for minimally invasive percutaneous microresection. *Am J Sports Med* 2013;41(3):636-644.

Lin CL, Lee JS, Su WR, Kuo LC, Tai TW, Jou IM: Clinical and ultrasonographic results of ultrasonographically guided percutaneous radiofrequency lesioning in the treatment of recalcitrant lateral epicondylitis. *Am J Sports Med* 2011;39(11):2429-2435.

Martinez-Silvestrini JA, Newcomer KL, Gay RE, Schaefer MP, Kortebein P, Arendt KW: Chronic lateral epicondylitis: Comparative effectiveness of a home exercise program including stretching alone versus stretching supplemented with eccentric or concentric strengthening. *J Hand Ther* 2005;18(4):411-419, quiz 420.

Mishra A, Pavelko T: Treatment of chronic elbow tendinosis with buffered platelet-rich plasma. *Am J Sports Med* 2006;34(11):1774-1778.

Placzek R, Drescher W, Deuretzbacher G, Hempfing A, Meiss AL: Treatment of chronic radial epicondylitis with botulinum toxin A: A double-blind, placebo-controlled, randomized multicenter study. *J Bone Joint Surg Am* 2007;89(2):255-260.

Rabago D, Lee KS, Ryan M, et al: Hypertonic dextrose and morrhuate sodium injections (prolotherapy) for lateral epicondylosis (tennis elbow): Results of a single-blind, pilot-level, randomized controlled trial. *Am J Phys Med Rehabil* 2013;92(7):587-596.

Raeissadat SA, Rayegani SM, Hassanabadi H, Rahimi R, Sedighipour L, Rostami K: Is platelet-rich plasma superior to whole blood in the management of chronic tennis elbow: One year randomized clinical trial. *BMC Sports Sci Med Rehabil* 2014;6:12.

Regan W, Wold LE, Coonrad R, Morrey BF: Microscopic histopathology of chronic refractory lateral epicondylitis. *Am J Sports Med* 1992;20(6):746-749.

Rose NE, Forman SK, Dellon AL: Denervation of the lateral humeral epicondyle for treatment of chronic lateral epicondylitis. *J Hand Surg Am* 2013;38(2):344-349.

Ruch DS, Orr SB, Richard MJ, Leversedge FJ, Mithani SK, Laino DK: A comparison of débridement with and without anconeus muscle flap for treatment of refractory lateral epicondylitis. *J Shoulder Elbow Surg* 2015;24(2):236-241.

Sayegh ET, Strauch RJ: Does nonsurgical treatment improve longitudinal outcomes of lateral epicondylitis over no treatment? A meta-analysis. *Clin Orthop Relat Res* 2015;473(3):1093-1107.

Shiri R, Viikari-Juntura E, Varonen H, Heliövaara M: Prevalence and determinants of lateral and medial epicondylitis: A population study. *Am J Epidemiol* 2006;164(11):1065-1074.

Smidt N, Assendelft WJ, Arola H, et al: Effectiveness of physiotherapy for lateral epicondylitis: A systematic review. *Ann Med* 2003;35(1):51-62.

Smidt N, Assendelft WJ, van der Windt DA, Hay EM, Buchbinder R, Bouter LM: Corticosteroid injections for lateral epicondylitis: A systematic review. *Pain* 2002;96(1-2):23-40.

Smidt N, van der Windt DA, Assendelft WJ, Devillé WL, Korthals-de Bos IB, Bouter LM: Corticosteroid injections, physiotherapy, or a wait-and-see policy for lateral epicondylitis: A randomised controlled trial. *Lancet* 2002;359(9307):657-662.

Solheim E, Hegna J, Øyen J: Arthroscopic versus open tennis elbow release: 3- to 6-year results of a case-control series of 305 elbows. *Arthroscopy* 2013;29(5):854-859.

Staples MP, Forbes A, Ptasznik R, Gordon J, Buchbinder R: A randomized controlled trial of extracorporeal shock wave therapy for lateral epicondylitis (tennis elbow). *J Rheumatol* 2008;35(10):2038-2046.

Szabo RM: Steroid injection for lateral epicondylitis. *J Hand Surg Am* 2009;34(2):326-330.

 

Thanasas C, Papadimitriou G, Charalambidis C, Paraskevopoulos I, Papanikolaou A: Platelet-rich plasma versus autologous whole blood for the treatment of chronic lateral elbow epicondylitis: A randomized controlled clinical trial. *Am J Sports Med* 2011;39(10):2130-2134.

Thornton SJ, Rogers JR, Prickett WD, Dunn WR, Allen AA, Hannafin JA: Treatment of recalcitrant lateral epicondylitis with suture anchor repair. *Am J Sports Med* 2005;33(10):1558-1564.

# Chapter 12

# Management of Medial Collateral Ligament Insufficiency of the Elbow

*Michael J. Carroll, MD, FRCSC*

*Kenneth J. Faber, MD, MHPE, FRCSC*

**Learning Objectives**

- Understand medial elbow anatomy relevant to medial collateral ligament insufficiency.
- Understand how to evaluate a patient who has medial collateral ligament insufficiency.
- Understand the indications and contraindications for medial collateral ligament reconstruction.
- Understand the medial collateral ligament reconstruction technique preferred by the authors of this chapter.
- Understand the outcomes of surgical management for medial collateral ligament insufficiency.

## Indications

Medial collateral ligament (MCL) reconstruction of the elbow was first described by Jobe in the mid 1980s. Currently, several technical modifications of the Jobe technique (modified Jobe technique, docking technique) are commonly used. Many patients are successfully treated nonsurgically, and one of the key factors in patient care is patient selection. Current areas of interest include the epidemiology of MCL reconstruction and outcome optimization.

The elbow is an inherently stable joint because of its conforming articular geometry. The joint capsule as well as the collateral ligaments provide additional static stability, and the surrounding muscles provide dynamic stabilizing forces. The MCL complex consists of the anterior, posterior, and transverse bundles. The anterior bundle, which is the primary restraint against valgus instability, originates on the anteroinferior margin of the medial epicondyle and inserts on the sublime tubercle of the ulna. Valgus stability is enhanced by the dynamic contribution of the flexor-pronator mass.

Valgus instability is the result of acute MCL rupture such as elbow dislocation or chronic attenuation (usually the result of repetitive valgus torque). A throwing athlete may recall a sudden pop, describe localized pain, or report a loss of throwing velocity or accuracy. In a throwing athlete, a sudden pop is likely acute deterioration of a chronic attenuation. Relevant physical examination findings include focal tenderness at the origin, at the insertion, or along the course of the MCL.

Several physical examination maneuvers, including the valgus stress test, the moving valgus stress test, and the milking maneuver, may be used in the evaluation of a patient with valgus instability. The valgus stress test is performed with the patient's shoulder abducted and maximally externally rotated, which anchors the arm by fixing the shoulder in place, and the elbow positioned in 25° to 30° of flexion, which unlocks the olecranon from its fossa and relaxes the anterior capsule. The examiner applies a valgus stress to the elbow while placing a finger on the medial ulnohumeral joint to assess the amount of opening. The degree of opening is compared with that of the unaffected elbow, taking the patient's natural laxity into consideration.

The moving valgus stress test was first described in 2005. This test is 100% sensitive and 75% specific for pain related to MCL pathology. The moving valgus stress test is performed with the patient's shoulder placed in 90° of abduction. Beginning with the elbow in full flexion, the examiner places one

*Dr. Faber or an immediate family member has received royalties from and serves as a paid consultant to Exactech. Neither Dr. Carroll nor any immediate family member has received anything of value from or has stock or stock options held in a commercial company or institution related directly or indirectly to the subject of this chapter.*

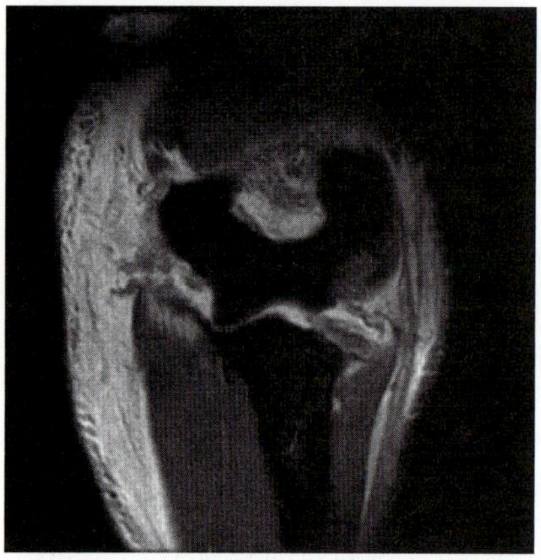

**Figure 1** Coronal fast inversion recovery MRI of an elbow demonstrates medial collateral ligament disruption as well as concomitant injury to the flexor-pronator mass and bony injury to the capitellum.

hand at the patient's elbow and the other at the patient's wrist and generates sufficient valgus torque to bring the patient's shoulder into maximal external rotation. The valgus torque is maintained as the examiner quickly moves the patient's elbow from maximal flexion to 30° of extension. Reproduction of activity-related medial elbow pain between 70° and 120° indicates a positive test.

Standard AP, lateral, and oblique radiographs of the elbow are obtained to evaluate for MCL-specific features such as an avulsion fracture of the medial epicondyle, a sublime tubercle fracture, posteromedial olecranon osteophytes, intrasubstance calcification of the MCL, or asymmetry of the articular surfaces. Imaging also should be examined for signs of arthritis and loose bodies. Valgus stress radiographs of the affected elbow may be obtained and compared with those of the contralateral elbow to determine the amount of joint-space widening; however, the utility of comparative valgus stress radiographs is limited because side-to-side differences in joint-space widening exist in asymptomatic athletes, and there is no universally agreed-upon threshold value that is diagnostic of an MCL tear. Currently, MRI with or without contrast is considered the preferred imaging modality for evaluation of MCL pathology (**Figure 1**).

The decision to undergo MCL reconstruction is individualized and based on several factors, including the acuity of the injury, the amount of dysfunction, athletic or functional demands, the ability to modify activity or occupation, and the acceptance and understanding of the rehabilitation protocol. Many patients, including recreational and competitive athletes, can be treated nonsurgically with activity modification, such as avoiding a particular sport or switching to a playing position that lessens valgus moment about the elbow, or with rehabilitation programs that focus on forearm strengthening, core muscle strengthening, upper extremity flexibility training, and additional coaching to improve throwing mechanics. MCL reconstruction is considered in patients who are dissatisfied with their level of medial elbow pain and their athletic performance after nonsurgical management; accept the risks, discomforts, and inconveniences of surgery; and are prepared to undergo a lengthy rehabilitation protocol.

## Contraindications

MCL reconstruction is contraindicated in patients who have asymptomatic or incomplete MCL tears and in those who will be unable to comply with a rigorous rehabilitation protocol. Although no guidelines exist, diffuse, advanced degenerative changes involving the articular surface also are considered a contraindication to reconstruction.

## Alternative Treatments

Nonsurgical management is the first line of treatment for almost all patients who have medial-sided elbow pain caused by MCL insufficiency. Young patients who have MCL insufficiency should be counseled on the likelihood of a pitching career. Although a return to a high school or collegiate competitive sport is possible after MCL reconstruction, one study reported that no pitcher who underwent MCL reconstruction during high school or college progressed to the major leagues. Palliative treatments include rest, NSAIDs, and cryotherapy. A progressive elbow range of motion and flexor-pronator strengthening protocol is initiated as symptoms improve. In most patients, ligament reconstruction with a tendon graft is preferred rather than MCL repair; however, one study reported favorable outcomes after primary MCL repair in young athletes. In that study, of the patients treated with MCL repair after at least 3 months of unsuccessful nonsurgical management, 69% experienced acute onset of symptoms, and 31% could not recall a particular inciting event and were classified as having gradual onset of symptoms. The role of elbow arthroscopy in conjunction with MCL reconstruction is controversial. Elbow arthroscopy may be useful in patients who have associated intra-articular pathology such as posteromedial ulnohumeral osteophytes, chondral lesions, or loose bodies.

## Results

High-level evidence on the outcomes of patients who underwent surgical treatment for MCL insufficiency is lacking. Based on retrospective studies of throwing athletes, MCL reconstruction typically improves function and allows a large percentage of competitive athletes to return to sport at their preinjury level (**Table 1**). Several modifications to the Jobe or docking techniques have been introduced; however, comparative data on the relative advantages and

 

**Table 1** Results of Medial Collateral Ligament (MCL) Reconstruction[a]

| Authors (Year) | No. of Patients | Procedure or Approach | Mean Patient Age in Years (Range) | Mean Follow-up in Months (Range) | Success Rate | Results |
|---|---|---|---|---|---|---|
| Jobe et al (1986) | 16 | Jobe technique, primarily with palmaris longus autograft | 17.4 (20-31) | 51 (24-117) | 62% of patients returned to their preoperative level of sport | 12.5% of patients had ulnar nerve symptoms<br>6% of patients had superficial infection |
| Conway et al (1992) | 56 | Jobe technique, primarily with palmaris longus autograft | 23.7 (15-24) | 75.6 (24-180) | Conway-Jobe rating scale score: 64% excellent, 14% good | 21% of patients had ulnar nerve symptoms<br><2% of patients had hematoma |
| Dodson et al (2006) | 100 | Docking technique, primarily with palmaris longus autograft | 22 (16-43) | 36 (24-60) | Conway-Jobe rating scale score: 90% excellent, 7% good | 2% of patients had ulnar nerve symptoms<br>1% of patients had elbow stiffness |
| Cain et al (2010) | 743 | Modified Jobe technique, primarily with palmaris longus autograft | 21.5 (14-59) | 38.4 (24-130) | 83% of patients returned to previous level of sport or higher | 16% of patients had ulnar nerve symptoms<br>4% of patients had graft site superficial infection<br><1% of patients had medial epicondyle fracture<br><1% of patients had MCL failure |
| Savoie et al (2013) | 116 | Jobe technique or docking technique, with or without an interference screw | 20.4 (14-32) | 39 (24-72) | Conway-Jobe rating scale score: 80% excellent, 13% good | 3% of patients had ulnar nerve symptoms<br><1% of patients had hematoma, medial epicondyle fracture, stitch abscess, or flexor-pronator complex tear |

[a] All studies are level IV evidence.

disadvantages of each technique are insufficient. A recent systematic review reported that ulnar nerve neurapraxia was the most common complication after MCL reconstruction, with a lower incidence of ulnar nerve neurapraxia reported in patients who underwent MCL reconstruction with the use of the modified docking technique. Regardless of the technique used for MCL reconstruction, the rate of revision reconstruction procedures is low. The authors of this chapter prefer to use a double-strand docking technique with an ipsilateral palmaris longus tendon autograft.

**Video 12.1** Hybrid Technique for Reconstruction of the Medial Collateral Ligament of the Elbow. J. Michael Bennett, MD; Thomas L. Mehlhoff, MD; Rodney K. Baker (6 min)

# Technique

## Setup/Exposure

- The patient is examined preoperatively to determine the presence of a palmaris longus tendon. To do this, the patient is asked to flex his or her wrist against resistance with the small finger and thumb tightly apposed. If the ipsilateral palmaris longus tendon is absent, the palmaris longus tendon from the contralateral forearm is used for the graft. If both palmaris longus tendons are absent, the ipsilateral gracilis tendon can be harvested.
- The graft selected determines the type of anesthesia used. If a palmaris longus tendon is used, the procedure is performed under a combination of regional anesthesia and sedation. If a gracilis tendon is used, the procedure is performed under general anesthesia.
- The patient is positioned supine

with a small bump placed beneath the contralateral scapula.

- The shoulder is abducted, the arm is externally rotated, and the surgical limb is prepped free and placed on a hand table.
- If performing concomitant elbow arthroscopy or harvesting the contralateral palmaris longus or gracilis tendon, the standard surgical setup requires modifications.

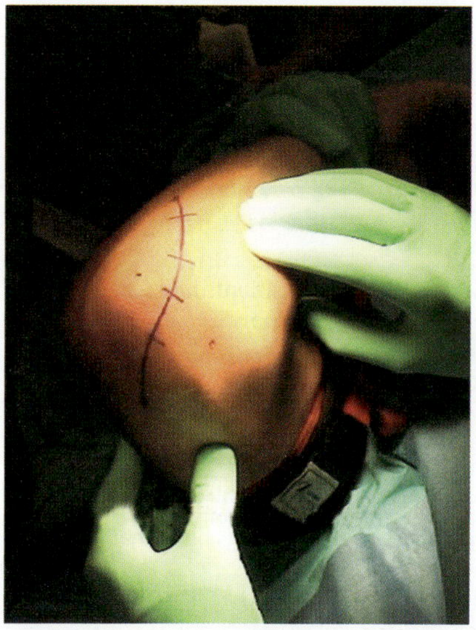

**Figure 2** Intraoperative photograph of an elbow shows superficial surgical exposure via a medial approach. A gently curving posterior skin incision facilitates access to the medial side of the elbow and minimizes risk of injury to the cutaneous nerves.

- A curvilinear posterior skin incision is made on the medial elbow (**Figure 2**). The incision is taken directly down to the fascia, allowing a full-thickness flap to be raised. The medial antebrachial cutaneous nerve is typically identified just superficial to the fascial layer, coursing anterior to the medial epicondyle. Care is taken to ensure that the medial antebrachial cutaneous nerve remains within the skin flap to minimize the risk of iatrogenic injury.
- The ulnar nerve is identified proximally and traced distally. An in situ release of the ulnar nerve is performed as it passes through the cubital tunnel. The overlying fascia is released distally as the ulnar nerve passes between the two heads of the flexor carpi ulnaris (FCU).

## Instruments/Equipment/ Implants Required

- A sterile tourniquet is required.
- Bipolar cautery is used.
- Small, blunt retractors are necessary.
- Heavy absorbable and nonabsorbable braided suture are used.
- A suture-retrieving device is necessary.
- A 3.5-mm and a 2-mm drill bit are used.
- A small, round-tipped burr is necessary.
- A cortical button may be necessary.

## Procedure

- The palmaris longus tendon is harvested before exposing the medial side of the elbow. The subcutaneous course of the palmaris longus tendon is identified, and a single 5-mm transverse incision is made directly over the palmaris longus tendon, slightly proximal to the wrist crease. Care is taken to expose and confirm the palmaris longus tendon, clearly differentiating it from the median nerve.
- The palmaris longus tendon is released distally and captured with a heavy, nonabsorbable suture (**Figure 3, A**). A closed tendon stripper is used to harvest the graft (**Figure 3, B**). The eventual posterior limb of the palmaris longus tendon also is captured with a heavy, nonabsorbable suture using a running, locking technique. The graft is placed in a moist sponge and then placed on the back table.
- The fascia overlying the FCU is incised to expose the anterior bundle of the MCL. A blunt elevator is used to separate the muscle in line with its fibers and deepen it to the level of the capsule. The MCL

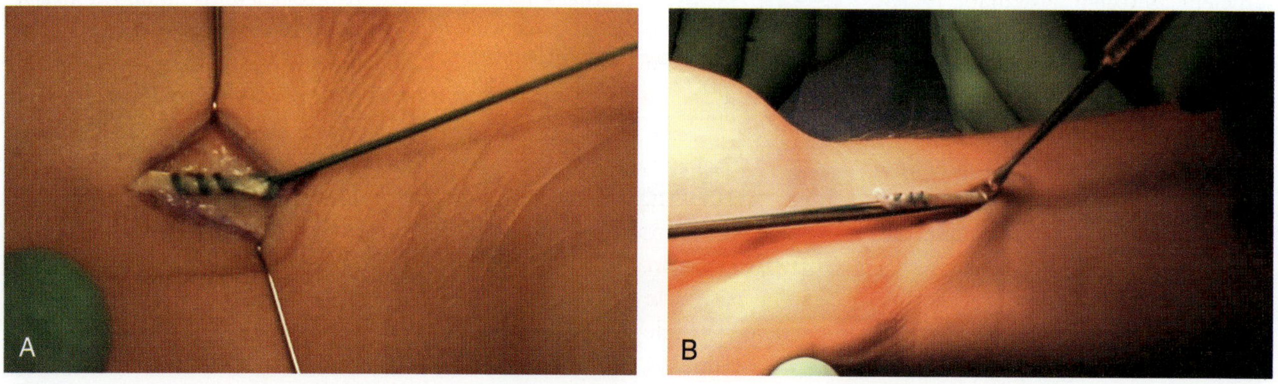

**Figure 3** Intraoperative photographs of a wrist show harvest of palmaris longus tendon graft. **A,** The palmaris longus tendon is captured with the use of a heavy, nonabsorbable suture. **B,** Tension is applied to the palmaris longus tendon graft while the tendon stripper is placed and gently advanced.

 

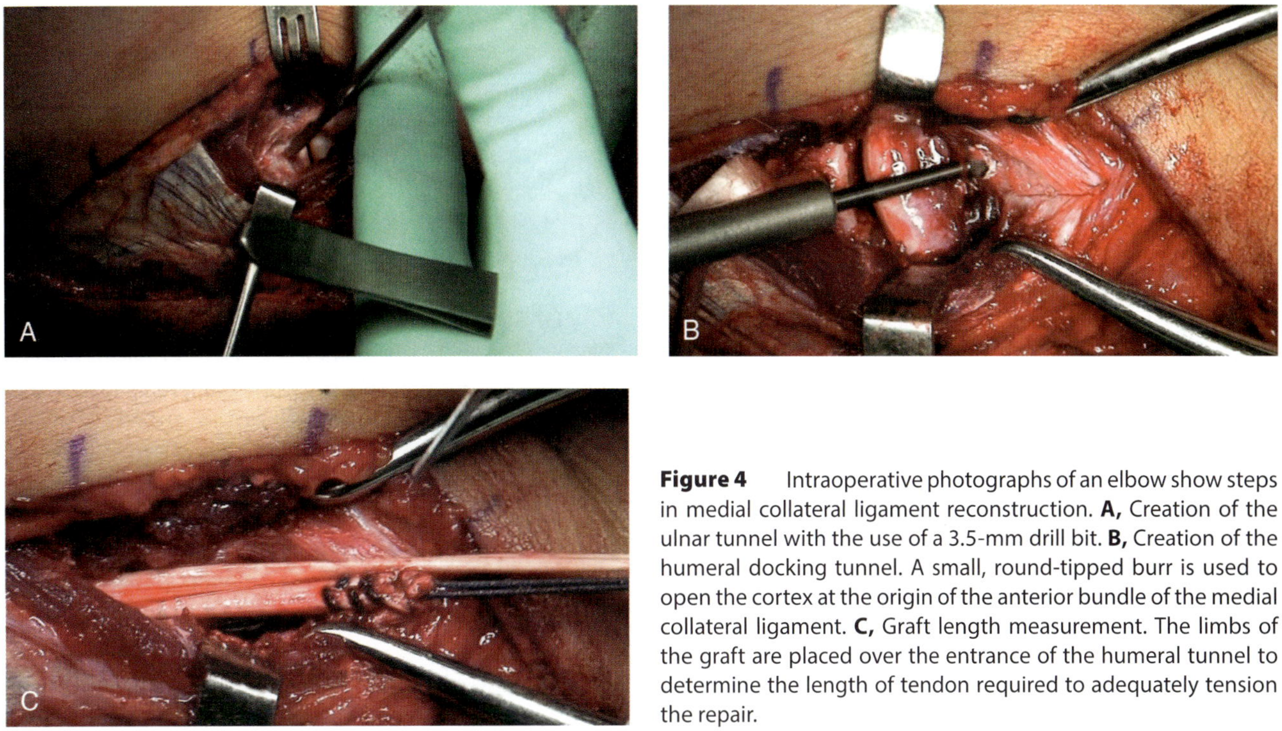

**Figure 4** Intraoperative photographs of an elbow show steps in medial collateral ligament reconstruction. **A,** Creation of the ulnar tunnel with the use of a 3.5-mm drill bit. **B,** Creation of the humeral docking tunnel. A small, round-tipped burr is used to open the cortex at the origin of the anterior bundle of the medial collateral ligament. **C,** Graft length measurement. The limbs of the graft are placed over the entrance of the humeral tunnel to determine the length of tendon required to adequately tension the repair.

is exposed along its length from the medial epicondyle to approximately 5 cm distal to the sublime tubercle of the ulna.

- The MCL is visualized and the nature of the tear is examined.
- To facilitate placement of the humeral tunnels, a small sleeve of soft tissue is sharply elevated off the anterior one-half of the medial epicondyle.
- The ulnar tunnel is created using a 3.5-mm drill bit (**Figure 4, A**). Blunt retractors are inserted to protect the ulnar nerve, and two converging drill holes are created just distal to the anterior and posterior margins of the sublime tubercle. The holes are spaced 1 cm apart to prevent fracture of the bridging cortical bone. A curved curet or sharp reduction clamp is used to connect the drill holes. A suture-passing device is used to deliver the shuttling sutures, followed by the graft, through the tunnel.
- The larger humeral tunnel, which accepts both limbs of the tendon graft, is created using a small burr at the origin of the anterior bundle of the MCL, which can be visualized directly and typically lies at the anterior-inferior margin of the medial epicondyle. The burr tip is advanced 10 to 20 mm on a trajectory anterior to the intermuscular septum, with care taken to remain unicortical (**Figure 4, B**). A 2-mm drill bit is used to create two holes in the cortex, such that a Y-shaped tunnel is fashioned.
- With the forearm positioned in supination and a slight varus stress applied to the elbow, the graft is positioned over the entrance of the larger humeral tunnel. The length of tendon required to adequately tension the graft within the humeral tunnel is measured and marked using a sterile skin marker (**Figure 4, C**). A similar length of tendon is then captured with a heavy running, locked nonabsorbable suture, and excess tendon is excised.
- The sutures of the anterior limb of the graft are shuttled through the larger humeral tunnel and retrieved through the smaller humeral tunnel.
- The posterior limb of the graft, which was captured earlier with a running, locking suture, is shuttled into the larger humeral tunnel, and the suture limbs are retrieved through the smaller humeral tunnel.
- Repairable portions of the native ligament and capsule are closed over the graft using a nonabsorbable braided suture.
- The graft is tensioned, and the suture limbs are tied over the bone bridge. If required, the bone bridge is reinforced by tying the sutures over a cortical button.

## Wound Closure

- Before wound closure, the tourniquet is deflated, and hemostasis is achieved using bipolar cautery.
- A standard three-layer closure

is performed. The FCU fascia is repaired with interrupted No. 1 absorbable braided suture. A 4-0 absorbable braided suture is used to close the subcutaneous skin layer. The skin is closed with simple stitches using a 3-0 nonabsorbable monofilament suture.

## Postoperative Regimen

A posterior splint is applied with the elbow flexed to 90° and the forearm fully supinated. At 10 to 14 days postoperatively, the splint is replaced with a varus-valgus restraining brace, and short-arc active elbow flexion-extension exercises are initiated with the forearm maintained in full supination. Forearm rotation is performed only with the elbow flexed beyond 90°. At 6 to 8 weeks postoperatively, the brace is discontinued, and full, unrestricted range of motion is encouraged. Strengthening begins at 12 weeks postoperatively. Gradual return to sport is permitted at 4 to 6 months postoperatively, provided motion and strength have been reestablished.

## Limiting Adverse Events

The most common complication after MCL reconstruction is ulnar nerve neurapraxia. Although the ulnar nerve does not require routine anterior transposition, it does require proximal and distal exposure for adequate visualization and protection. To minimize the risk of a traction-related ulnar nerve neurapraxia, the ulnar nerve is tagged with a light drain, which is tied rather than secured with a clamp. The ulnar nerve should be mobilized and transposed if its position precludes adequate exposure of the MCL or intended placement of the humeral tunnels. Ulnar nerve irritation may result from adjacent knot placement. To avoid ulnar nerve irritation, the knots should be placed on the medial supracondylar ridge or anterior to the intermuscular septum.

Fracture through the humeral or ulnar bone tunnels can be avoided by ensuring that they are adequately spaced. If a fracture is encountered, the graft can be stabilized using a suspensory cortical button or tied over a post. Clinical instability may persist postoperatively if the graft is improperly tensioned. Failure attributed to the viscoelastic properties of the tendon, such as creep, can be minimized by placing the graft in a tensioning device on a back table during exposure of the elbow or by cycling and pretensioning the graft before it is docked in the humeral tunnel.

## Bibliography


Armstrong AD, Dunning CE, Faber KJ, Duck TR, Johnson JA, King GJ: Rehabilitation of the medial collateral ligament-deficient elbow: An in vitro biomechanical study. *J Hand Surg Am* 2000;25(6):1051-1057.

Cain EL Jr, Andrews JR, Dugas JR, et al: Outcome of ulnar collateral ligament reconstruction of the elbow in 1281 athletes: Results in 743 athletes with minimum 2-year follow-up. *Am J Sports Med* 2010;38(12):2426-2434.

Conway JE, Jobe FW, Glousman RE, Pink M: Medial instability of the elbow in throwing athletes: Treatment by repair or reconstruction of the ulnar collateral ligament. *J Bone Joint Surg Am* 1992;74(1):67-83.

Dodson CC, Thomas A, Dines JS, Nho SJ, Williams RJ III, Altchek DW: Medial ulnar collateral ligament reconstruction of the elbow in throwing athletes. *Am J Sports Med* 2006;34(12):1926-1932.

Dugas JR, Ostrander RV, Cain EL, Kingsley D, Andrews JR: Anatomy of the anterior bundle of the ulnar collateral ligament. *J Shoulder Elbow Surg* 2007;16(5):657-660.

Ellenbecker TS, Mattalino AJ, Elam EA, Caplinger RA: Medial elbow joint laxity in professional baseball pitchers: A bilateral comparison using stress radiography. *Am J Sports Med* 1998;26(3):420-424.

Jobe FW, Stark H, Lombardo SJ: Reconstruction of the ulnar collateral ligament in athletes. *J Bone Joint Surg Am* 1986;68(8):1158-1163.


 

Morrey BF, Tanaka S, An KN: Valgus stability of the elbow: A definition of primary and secondary constraints. *Clin Orthop Relat Res* 1991;(265):187-195.

O'Driscoll SW, Lawton RL, Smith AM: The "moving valgus stress test" for medial collateral ligament tears of the elbow. *Am J Sports Med* 2005;33(2):231-239.

Savoie FH III, Morgan C, Yaste J, Hurt J, Field L: Medial ulnar collateral ligament reconstruction using hamstring allograft in overhead throwing athletes. *J Bone Joint Surg Am* 2013;95(12):1062-1066.

Savoie FH III, Trenhaile SW, Roberts J, Field LD, Ramsey JR: Primary repair of ulnar collateral ligament injuries of the elbow in young athletes: A case series of injuries to the proximal and distal ends of the ligament. *Am J Sports Med* 2008;36(6):1066-1072.

Watson JN, McQueen P, Hutchinson MR: A systematic review of ulnar collateral ligament reconstruction techniques. *Am J Sports Med* 2014;42(10):2510-2516.

## Video Reference

Bennett JM, Mehlhoff TL, Baker RK: Video excerpt. *Hybrid Technique for Reconstruction of the Medial Collateral Ligament of the Elbow.* Houston, TX, Fonden Orthopedic Group, 2010.

# Chapter 13

# Lateral Collateral Reconstruction With Free Tendon Graft to Manage Lateral Collateral Ligament Insufficiency

*H. Mike Kim, MD*

*April D. Armstrong, BSc(PT), MD, MSc, FRCSC*

**Learning Objectives**

- Understand the underlying pathology of posterolateral rotatory instability (PLRI) of the elbow.
- Understand the clinical presentation and diagnosis of PLRI.
- Understand the indications and contraindications of lateral collateral ligament (LCL) reconstruction using a free graft.
- Learn the docking technique for LCL reconstruction using autologous gracilis graft and understand the overall clinical results of LCL reconstruction.

## Indications

Acute elbow dislocation involves various degrees of capsular ligament detachment. In most cases, the capsular ligaments are avulsed from the humeral attachment, which typically starts from the lateral aspect of the elbow and propagates medially. Therefore, the lateral collateral ligament (LCL) is almost always disrupted in acute elbow dislocation, but disruption of the medial collateral ligament (MCL) varies depending on the injury severity. In the absence of an associated fracture such as a simple elbow dislocation, closed reduction followed by a short period of immobilization usually is sufficient to achieve a stable elbow joint with no substantial sequelae. In patients with such injury, the capsular ligaments typically are avulsed from their humeral attachments and heal, provided the elbow is protected from further stresses. In the presence of concomitant fracture, such as complex elbow dislocation, surgery typically is required to address the fractures and ligamentous disruptions after initial closed reduction of the dislocation.

Recurrent subluxation of the elbow joint, that is, posterolateral rotatory instability (PLRI), is uncommon. PLRI typically results not from insufficiency of the LCL complex in general, but from insufficiency of the LCL in particular. PLRI after elbow dislocation most commonly occurs in adolescence. Other conditions associated with PLRI include iatrogenic injury to the LCL during débridement to manage lateral epicondylitis; connective tissue disorders such as Ehlers-Danlos syndrome; and long-standing cubitus varus deformity, such as malunion of a supracondylar fracture sustained in childhood. Additionally, PLRI can be a sequela of steroid injection to manage lateral epicondylitis.

In PLRI, the elbow rotates away from the distal humerus on the lateral side, resulting in posterolateral subluxation of the radiocapitellar joint on elbow extension, forearm supination, and valgus stress. Patients with PLRI may present with nonspecific, vague pain on the lateral elbow that is often accompanied by locking, catching, or clicking, particularly on extension and weight bearing. Patients may also describe a feeling of instability; however, frank dislocation in acute or recurrent elbow dislocations is uncommon. Clinical examination of patients with PLRI can be equivocal, with few obvious signs of the condition.

The pivot shift test can be used to evaluate for PLRI. To perform the pivot shift test, the patient is positioned supine with the arm placed over the head to lock and stabilize the shoulder in

*Dr. Armstrong or an immediate family member is a member of a speakers' bureau or has made paid presentations on behalf of and serves as a paid and unpaid consultant to Zimmer and serves as a board member, owner, officer, or committee member of the American Orthopaedic Association. Neither Dr. Kim nor any immediate family member has received anything of value from or has stock or stock options held in a commercial company or institution related directly or indirectly to the subject of this chapter.*

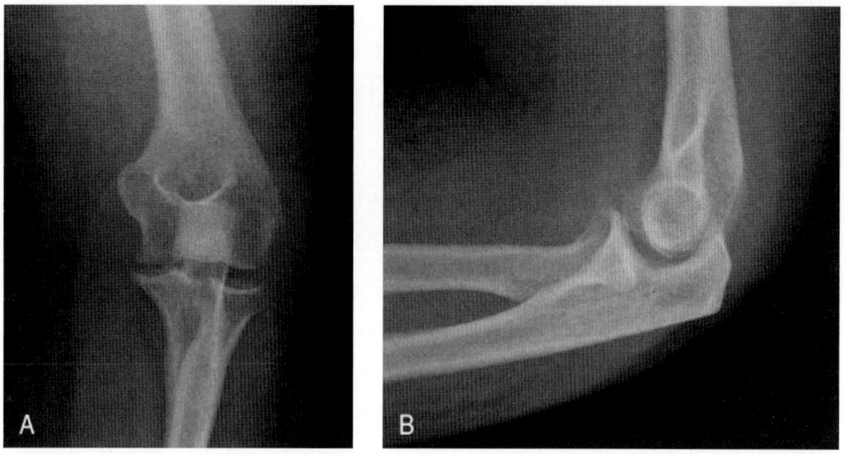


**Figure 1** Plain radiographs obtained 3 weeks after closed reduction of traumatic posterolateral dislocation in the left elbow of a 51-year-old patient. **A,** AP radiograph demonstrates increased radiocapitellar joint space, with slight medial translation of the ulna relative to the trochlea. **B,** Lateral radiograph demonstrates a slight increase in the ulnohumeral distance (drop sign) and posterior subluxation of the radial head relative to the capitellum.

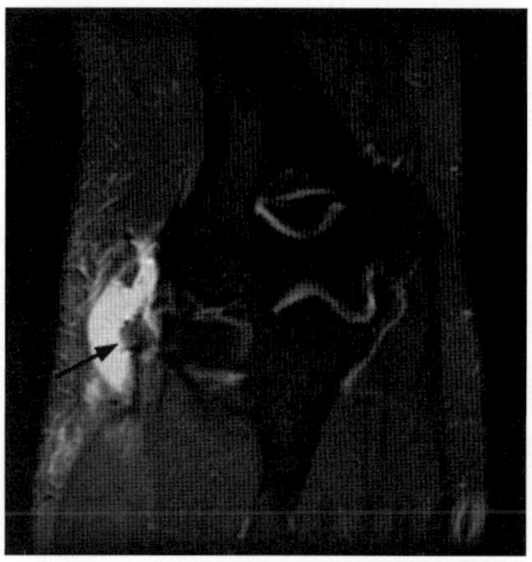

**Figure 2** MRI of the right elbow of a 45-year-old patient who presented with symptoms of posterolateral rotatory instability after open débridement to manage lateral epicondylitis. The lateral collateral ligament complex and extensor tendons (arrow) are detached from the lateral epicondyle, and the resulting fluid-filled subcutaneous cyst is visible.

external rotation, and with the forearm in supination and the elbow in extension. Valgus stress and axial load are applied to the elbow by the examiner. In the setting of PLRI, the radiocapitellar joint subluxates in this position. As the examiner slowly flexes the elbow while maintaining valgus stress, supination, and axial loading, the radiocapitellar joint reduces with a visible or palpable clunk. Dimpling of the skin may appear prior to joint reduction. In the awake patient, signs of a positive test are apprehension, dimpling of the skin, or clear subluxation. In the patient who is under anesthesia, the test is positive if a palpable or visible clunk is noted. This test is not always diagnostic, however, regardless whether the patient is awake or under anesthesia.

Four other tests are known to be useful in diagnosing PLRI: the posterolateral drawer test, the floor push-up test, the chair push-up test, and the tabletop relocation test. To perform the posterolateral drawer test, the examiner places the patient's elbow in 90° of flexion and then applies a posteriorly directed force to the lateral aspect of the proximal forearm to subluxate the joint. The test is positive if the patient exhibits apprehension or elbow subluxation occurs. In the floor push-up test, the patient pushes up from a prone position with the forearms in maximum supination and pronation. The test is positive if apprehension occurs as the elbow is extended from a flexed position with the forearm in supination, but not with the forearm in pronation. For the chair push-up test, the patient sits on a chair with armrests with the elbows flexed 90°, the forearm in supination, and the shoulders in slight abduction and is asked to rise by pushing himself or herself up from the armrest using only upper extremity force. If the patient is reluctant to extend the elbow fully as he or she rises from the chair because of apprehension or instability, the test is considered positive. For the tabletop relocation test, the patient presses up on a table using the affected arm, with the forearm in supination. To relieve patient apprehension on elbow extension, the examiner can push on the radial head to prevent subluxation.

In the acute setting, associated fractures can be seen radiographically. A slight increase in the ulnohumeral distance (that is, drop sign) and posterior subluxation of the radial head relative to the capitellum can be seen on the lateral view (**Figure 1**). The usefulness of MRI in the diagnosis of LCL insufficiency is controversial, especially in cases of chronic laxity with no anatomic disruption. However, MRI should be used to evaluate the integrity of the LCL and extensor muscles in the setting of a high index of suspicion for PLRI (**Figure 2**). In the acute setting, three-dimensional CT can be helpful in evaluating associated osseous injuries and intra-articular osteochondral fragments.

LCL reconstruction rather than repair is indicated in most patients who exhibit chronic insufficiency and in whom good-quality ligamentous tissue amenable for repair or imbrication is lacking. Little is known about the natural history of LCL insufficiency. LCL reconstruction may not be successful in elderly and physically inactive patients because of the low healing potential of graft tendons and the presence of osteopenia. Thus, surgery is optional in these patient groups.

 

## Contraindications

LCL reconstruction alone should not be performed in the setting of concomitant osseous abnormalities that contribute to the instability, such as cubitus varus deformity of the distal humerus or deficiency of the radial head or coronoid process. LCL reconstruction using bone tunnels is contraindicated in skeletally immature patients because the tunnels would cross the growth plate of the distal humerus. In patients with acute elbow fracture or dislocation, however, direct repair of the ligament complex is indicated. In the setting of advanced elbow arthritis, LCL reconstruction can be considered to prevent recurrent dislocation; however, the prognosis is guarded because of the persistence of arthritic symptoms even after successful reconstruction.

## Alternative Treatments

Currently, direct repair or reconstruction of the LCL is the most effective treatment for patients with substantial symptoms. Braces and physical therapy are of little use to these patients.

## Results

Several studies have been done on direct repair and reconstruction of LCL using various grafts and fixation techniques (**Table 1**). Currently, LCL reconstruction using tendon graft seems to provide a higher success rate than ligament repair, with better stability and function. Mild extension deficit, which is not uncommon after reconstruction, is a generally accepted outcome because the most unstable position is full extension. The authors of this chapter describe LCL reconstruction using autologous gracilis tendon graft and performed using the docking technique.

## Technique

### Setup/Exposure

- The patient is positioned supine, and an arm board is used.
- A combination of regional and general anesthesia is used.
- The method of prepping and draping used varies depending on the graft selected. Graft choices include the palmaris longus tendon, semitendinosus tendon, plantaris tendon, triceps tendon or fascia, split Achilles tendon, fascia lata, fourth toe extensor tendon, and various allografts; however, the authors of this chapter prefer to use autologous gracilis tendon graft from the ipsilateral leg. The ipsilateral leg is preferred because it is more convenient to approach from the same side as the surgical side.
- After the ipsilateral extremities are prepped and draped, sterile tourniquets are applied to the proximal arm and thigh.
- If the diagnosis has been confirmed, graft harvest is performed first.
- A linear skin incision measuring 4 cm long is made at the anteromedial aspect of the proximal tibia over the insertion of the pes anserinus.
- The sartorius fascia is sharply opened and reflected along its proximal margin to expose the underlying insertion of the gracilis tendon.
- The gracilis tendon is detached from its tibial insertion as distally as possible, taking care to preserve the underlying MCL. The saphenous nerve is typically located superficial to the sartorius tendon at the level of the knee joint, and overzealous deep dissection should be avoided.
- A No. 2 braided nonabsorbable suture is applied to the distal end of the tendon in a locking fashion.
- Any existing accessory insertions of the gracilis are released to avoid premature amputation of the tendon during harvest.
- A tendon stripper is used to detach the tendon at the proximal musculotendinous junction.
- The residual muscle is scraped off the proximal end of the tendon.
- The tendon is kept in moistened gauze on the back table.
- A skin incision is made over the lateral aspect of the elbow starting 2 to 3 cm proximal to the lateral epicondyle.
- The incision is extended distally and diagonally toward the subcutaneous border of the proximal ulnar shaft. A narrow stripe of fat often exists in the interval between the extensor carpi ulnaris (ECU) and the anconeus muscles. This stripe is helpful in locating the Kocher interval (**Figure 3, A**).
- The fascia over the Kocher interval is opened with a scalpel.
- The anconeus muscle is elevated from the underlying LCL starting at the distal part of the Kocher interval. Starting the elevation in this manner is preferred because it affords the clearest distinction of the anconeus muscle from the underlying LCL, especially in cases of chronic insufficiency, in which the LCL is often attenuated or defective proximally.
- The anconeus muscle is retracted posteriorly to expose the supinator crest of the proximal ulna (**Figure 3, B**).
- The ECU is sharply detached from the underlying LCL and retracted anteriorly.
- The lateral epicondyle and part of the supracondylar ridge are cleared of soft tissue. Part of the extensor muscle origin and triceps must be elevated from the distal humerus to obtain sufficient exposure of the bone for drilling and suture passing later in the procedure.

**Table 1** Results of Direct Repair and Reconstruction of the Lateral Collateral Ligament[a]

| Author(s) (Year) | No. of Patients | Procedure or Approach (No. of Patients) | Mean Patient Age in Years (Range) | Mean Follow-up in Months (Range) | Success Rate (%) | Results |
|---|---|---|---|---|---|---|
| O'Driscoll et al (1991) | 5 | Direct repair (2), LCL repair with augmentation with palmaris longus graft (2), LCL repair with augmentation with triceps fascia graft (1) | 12 (5-40) | 20 (15-30) | 100 | Stability was achieved in 4 patients, and 1 patient died of an unrelated cause |
| Nestor et al (1992) | 11 | Direct repair (3), LCL reconstruction using palmaris longus graft (bone tunnels) alone (5) or combined with synthetic ligamentous augmentation device (2), LCL reconstruction with triceps graft (1) | 28 (9-46) | 42 (24-68) | 73 | Excellent results were achieved with direct repair<br>Subjective instability was reported in 3 patients treated with reconstruction, 1 poor result with failure occurred at 3 mo postoperatively (after LCL reconstruction using palmaris longus graft and synthetic augmentation device), and 1 failure occurred at 3 mo postoperatively |
| Lee and Teo (2003) | 10 | Direct repair (4), LCL reconstruction with palmaris longus or semitendinosus graft (bone tunnels) (6) | 34 (20-50) | 24.1 (7-52) | 100 | Results were excellent in 3 patients treated with LCL reconstruction, good in 5, and fair in 2 (one after direct repair and one after LCL reconstruction) |
| Eygendaal (2004) | 12 | LCL reconstruction with triceps tendon graft (interference screw) | 35 (19-65) | 23 (17-28) | 92 | Stability was achieved in 11 patients, and 1 patient had a positive pivot shift test<br>Function was excellent in 9 patients, good in 2, and moderate in 1 |
| Sanchez-Sotelo et al (2005) | 44 | Direct repair (12), LCL reconstruction with palmaris longus, triceps fascia, Achilles tendon, plantaris, or semitendinosus graft (bone tunnels) (32) | 35 (9-80) | 72 (12-180) | 89 | Stability was achieved in 39 patients<br>Function was excellent in 19 patients, good in 13, fair in 7, and poor in 5 |
| Jones et al (2012) | 8 | LCL reconstruction with palmaris longus graft (bone tunnels, docking technique) | 39.8 (17-57) | 85.2 (62.4-112.8) | 100 | Stability was achieved in 6 patients, and 2 patients reported occasional instability<br>Function was excellent in 4 patients and good in 4<br>All patients were satisfied with their results |
| Lin et al (2012) | 14 | LCL reconstruction with palmaris longus or gracilis graft (bone tunnels) | 31.6 (18-60) | 49 (24-72) | 93 | Stability was achieved in 13 patients; the 1 case of instability was corrected with MCL reconstruction<br>Function was excellent in 10 patients, good in 3, and fair in 1 |

LCL = lateral collateral ligament, MCL = medial collateral ligament.
[a] All studies are level IV evidence.

 

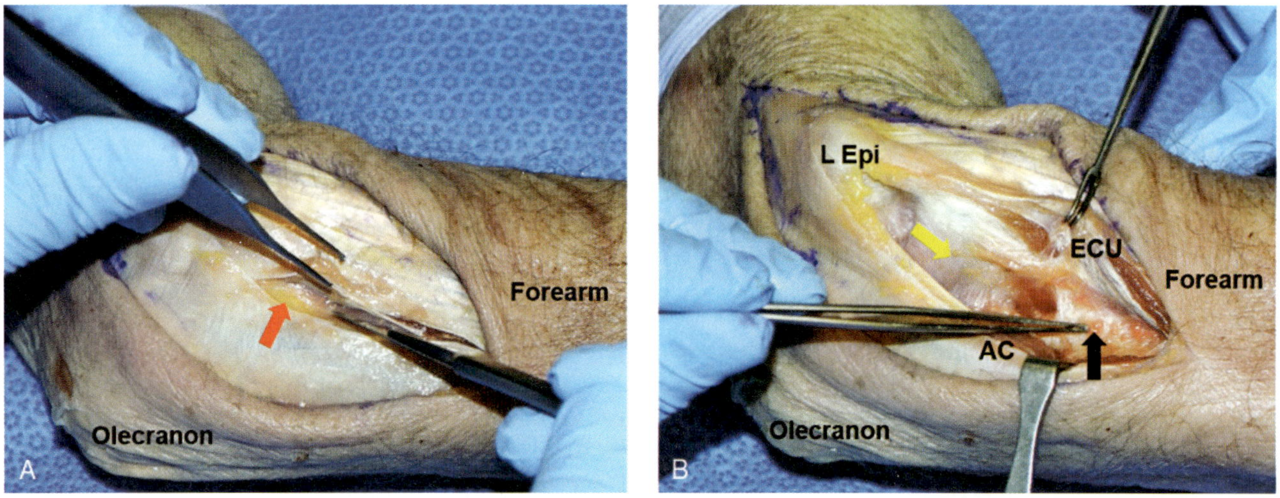


**Figure 3** **A,** Intraoperative photograph of the skin incision made along the Kocher interval. The narrow stripe of fat (red arrow) marks the interval between the extensor carpi ulnaris and anconeus. **B,** Intraoperative photograph shows the anconeus (AC) elevated from the underlying lateral collateral ligament (yellow arrow) and retracted posteriorly to expose the supinator crest (black arrow) of the proximal ulna. The extensor carpi ulnaris (ECU) has been detached from the underlying lateral collateral ligament and retracted anteriorly. L Epi = lateral epicondyle.

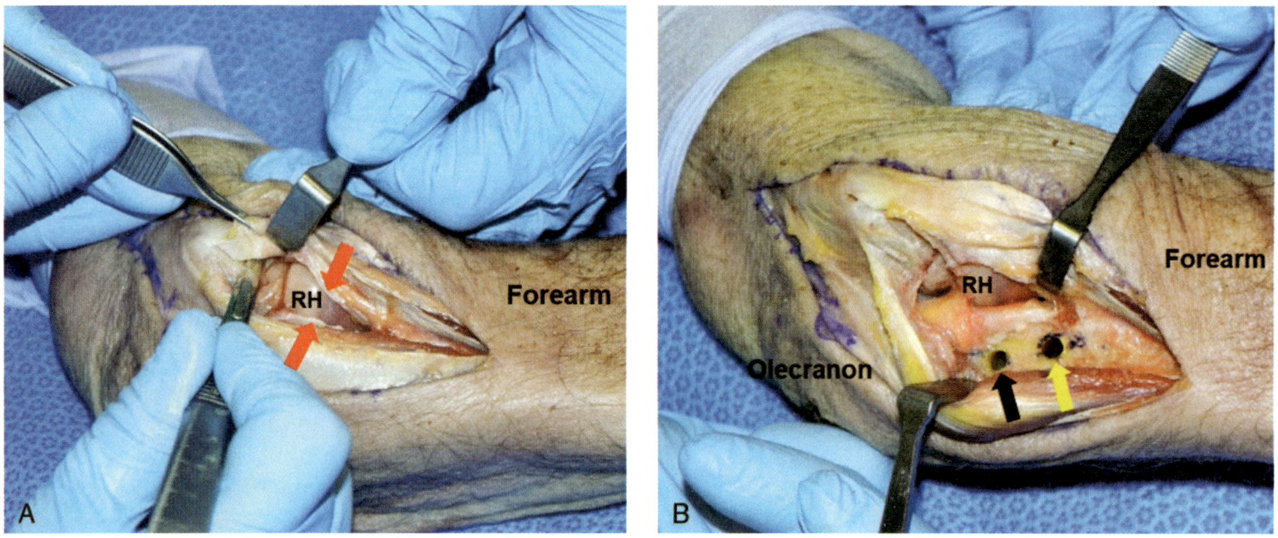


**Figure 4** **A,** Intraoperative photograph shows the longitudinal incision made along the remaining lateral collateral ligament tissue (red arrows) to allow inspection of the joint for intra-articular pathology. **B,** Intraoperative photograph shows the bone tunnel made on the ulna at the proximal end of the supinator crest or at the level of the radial neck (yellow arrow), using a 4-mm round burr. A second bone tunnel (black arrow) was made using the same burr 1.5 cm proximal to the first tunnel near the base of the annular ligament. The tunnels are angled toward each other so that they converge within the ulna. Sufficient bony bridge between the two tunnels was retained. RH = radial head.

## Instruments/Equipment/ Implants Required

- A 4-mm round burr is needed to create the humeral docking and ulnar bone tunnels.
- A 1.5-mm side-cutting burr or 2-mm drill bit is needed to create suture-passing tunnels at the lateral epicondyle.
- Small curved curets are used.
- A suture passer is required, such as a Hewson suture passer.
- No. 2 braided nonabsorbable sutures are used.
- Instruments for tendon harvest are required, such as a tendon stripper.

## Procedure

- After the LCL has been fully exposed, a longitudinal incision is

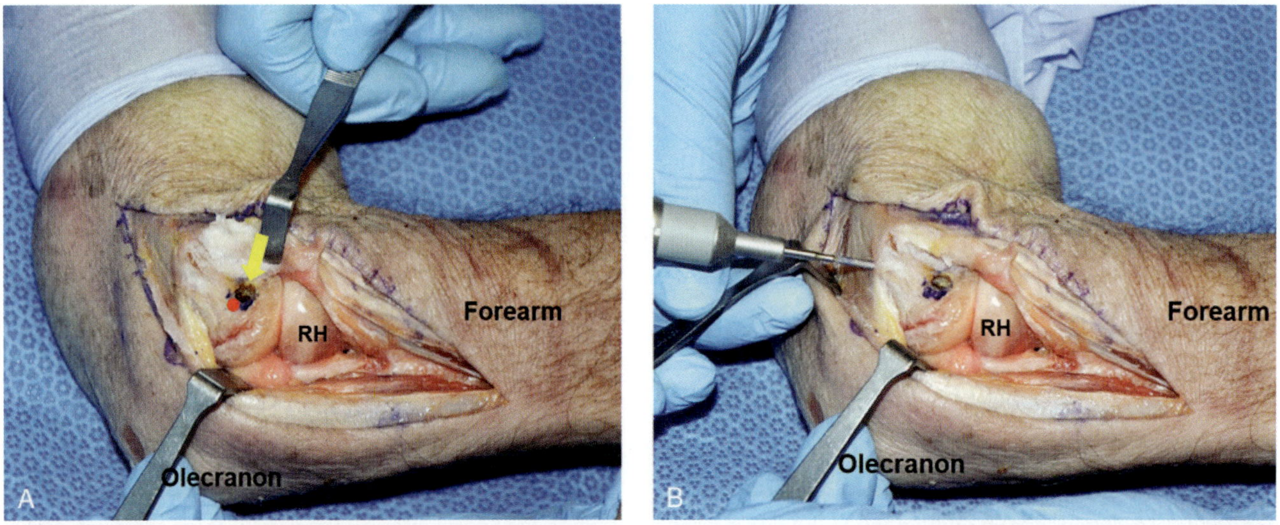


**Figure 5** Intraoperative photographs show steps in the creation of a docking tunnel in the distal humerus. **A,** A 4-mm round burr was used to create a 15-mm-deep bone tunnel at the isometric point of the lateral epicondyle (yellow arrow). For comparison, a red dot marks the anatomic isometric point, which is located at the center of rotation of the capitellum near the tip of the lateral epicondyle. **B,** The two suture-passing tunnels over the anterior and posterior sides of the superior aspect of the lateral epicondyle were created with a 2-mm side-cutting burr. The tunnels were directed toward the docking tunnel, and a bony bridge was left between them. RH = radial head.

made along the remaining LCL tissue.

- The elbow joint is inspected for intra-articular pathology (**Figure 4, A**).
- A 4-mm round burr is used to create a bone tunnel on the ulna, either at the proximal end of the supinator crest or at the level of the radial neck.
- A second bone tunnel is made 1 to 2 cm proximal to the first tunnel near the base of the annular ligament (**Figure 4, B**).
- The two tunnels should be directed toward each other so that they converge within the ulna.
- It is important to obtain a bony bridge at least 1 cm wide between the two tunnels to avoid inadvertent fracture of the bridge.
- Sequentially sized, curved curets are used to connect the two tunnels, taking care not to violate the bony bridge.
- Using the same 4-mm round burr as described previously, a 15-mm-deep bone tunnel is made at the isometric point of the lateral epicondyle. The anatomic isometric point is located at the center of rotation of the capitellum near the tip of the lateral epicondyle. However, to ensure that the graft is taut in extension at the point at which the elbow becomes unstable, the tunnel should be made slightly anterior and proximal to the true anatomic isometric point (**Figure 5, A**).
- Using a 2-mm side-cutting burr or drill bit, two additional bone tunnels are made over the anterior and posterior sides of the superior aspect of the lateral epicondyle. These two tunnels are directed toward the docking tunnel, taking care to retain a bony bridge measuring at least 1 cm wide (**Figure 5, B**).
- A small hemostat is placed in the docking hole to aid in confirming the point at which the suture-passing tunnels connect during drilling.
- A No. 2 suture is attached to one end of the graft tendon, and a suture retriever is used to pass the graft tendon through the ulnar tunnels in a distal-to-proximal direction (**Figure 6, A**).
- Graft passage can be facilitated by trimming the leading end of the graft tendon and applying mineral oil to the tendon.
- The longitudinal incision made in the remaining LCL tissue is closed with a 2-0 absorbable suture using a running Krackow stitch (**Figure 6, B**). The two suture limbs are left intact to be passed through the docking and suture-passing tunnels later in the procedure.
- Using a suture retriever, the two suture limbs from the graft and one suture limb from the LCL closure are shuttled through the docking tunnel and the posterior suture-passing tunnel (**Figure 7, A**). The graft is pulled and docked in the tunnel. While maintaining tension on the graft suture through the tunnel, the length of the tendon that will lie in the 15-mm-deep docking tunnel is estimated and marked with a pen on the other

 

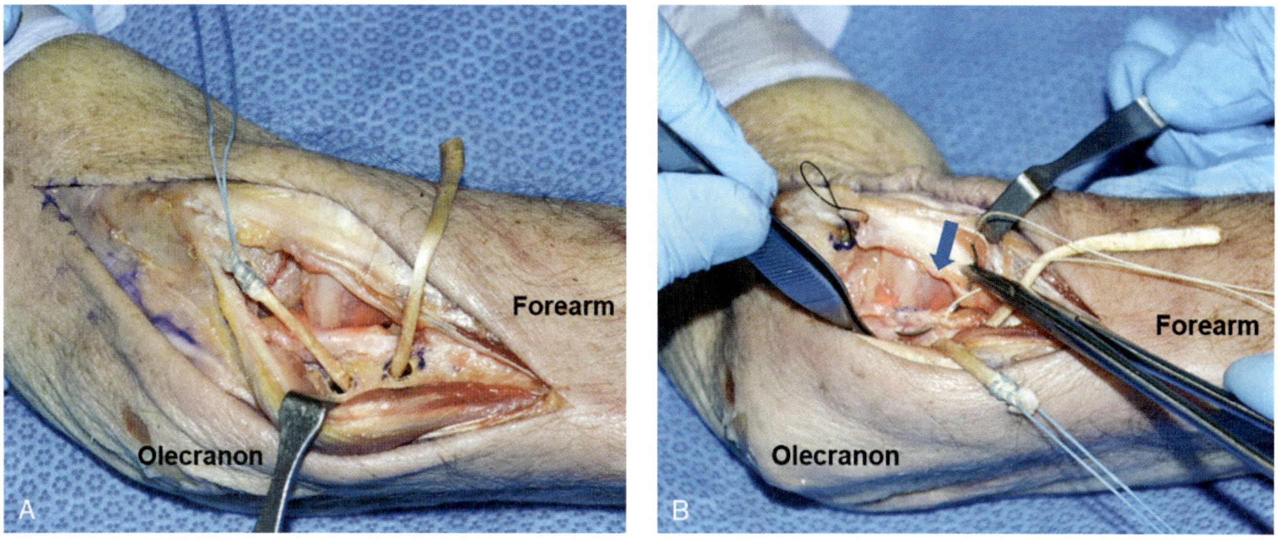


**Figure 6** **A,** Intraoperative photograph shows passage of graft tendon through the ulnar tunnels in a distal-to-proximal direction. **B,** Intraoperative photograph shows placement of a 2-0 absorbable suture using a running Krackow stitch to close the longitudinal incision made in the remaining lateral collateral ligament tissue (arrow).

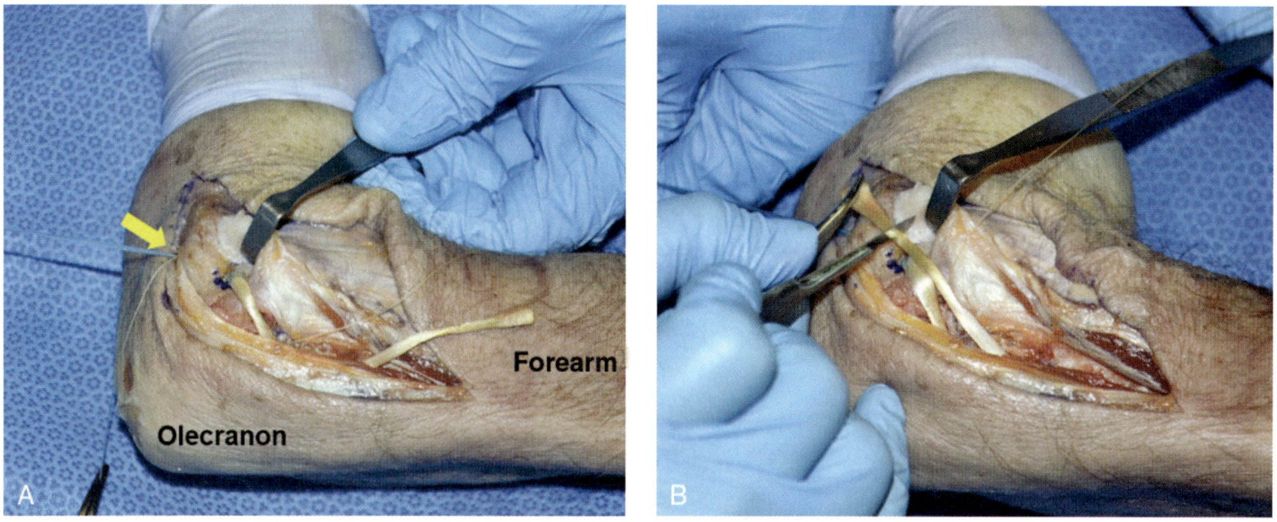


**Figure 7** **A,** Intraoperative photograph shows the appearance of the two suture limbs from the graft and one suture limb from the lateral collateral ligament closure after they were passed through the docking tunnel and the posterior suture-passing tunnel (arrow) and after the graft was pulled and docked in the tunnel. **B,** After marking the estimated length of the tendon that will lie in the docking tunnel, the remaining portion of the tendon is cut off using a scalpel.

limb of the graft tendon. To ensure proper graft tension, the tendon is cut 1 to 2 mm shorter than the estimated length. The remaining portion of the tendon is removed (**Figure 7, B**).

- A No. 2 nonabsorbable suture is applied to the tendon end using a running Krackow stitch.
- Using a suture retriever, the new No. 2 suture limbs and the other suture limb from the LCL closure are shuttled through the docking and anterior suture-passing tunnels.
- Next, both limbs of the graft tendon are docked in the tunnel (**Figure 8, A**). The remaining LCL tissue should lie beneath the graft tendon limbs so that it is interposed between the graft and radial head.
- The 2-0 absorbable sutures from the LCL are tied over the bone bridge.
- Then, with the elbow in 90° of flexion, full pronation, and slight valgus, the No. 2 sutures from the graft are tied. Graft tension is checked

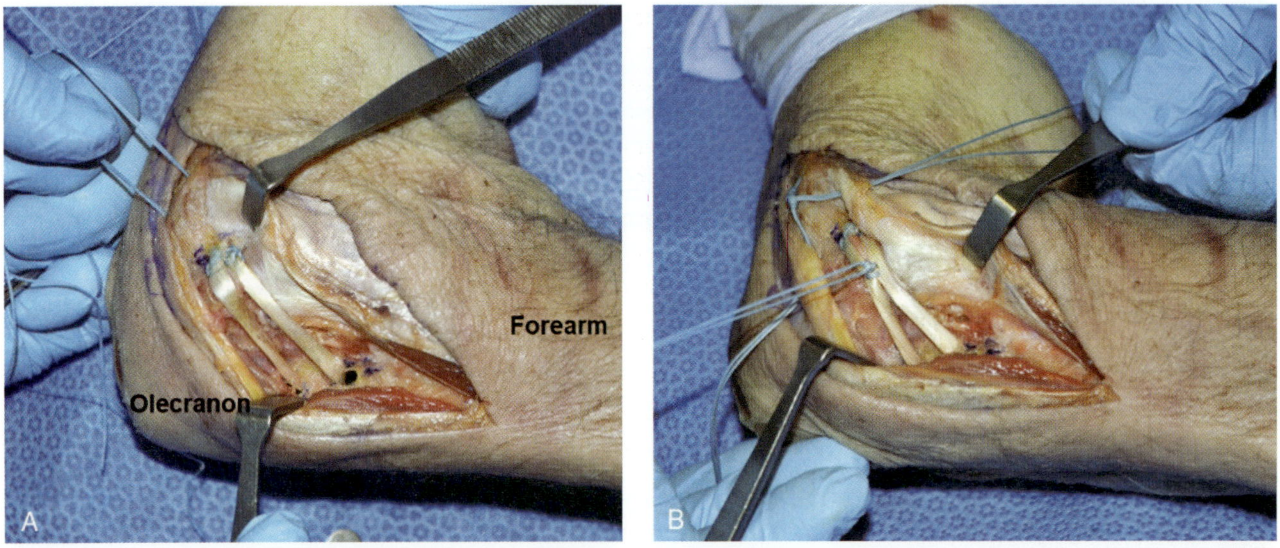


**Figure 8** **A,** Intraoperative photograph shows the appearance of both limbs of the graft tendon after they were pulled into the docking tunnel. **B,** Intraoperative photograph shows the graft tendon limbs sutured to each other with nonabsorbable suture as well as the remaining suture limbs from the graft left for later use in closing the proximal portion of the extensor muscles and fascia.

throughout elbow range of motion (ROM), paying special attention to the graft tension with the elbow in extension.

- If additional tension is needed, a few throws of a nonabsorbable suture can be applied to suture the graft tendon limbs to each other (**Figure 8, B**).
- The remaining suture tails from the graft can be used to close the proximal portion of the extensor muscles and fascia.

### Wound Closure

- The tourniquet is deflated, and meticulous hemostasis is performed.
- After the wound is irrigated, the anconeus muscle and ECU fascia are closed with No. 2 nonabsorbable sutures, the subcutaneous tissue is closed with 2-0 absorbable sutures, and the skin is closed with 3-0 nylon sutures.
- A compressive dressing is applied, followed by a posterior splint with the elbow in 90° of flexion and the forearm fully pronated.

## Postoperative Regimen

The elbow is immobilized in the initial posterior splint for 1 week, with the elbow in 90° of flexion and the forearm in pronation. After that first week, a static elbow brace is applied with the elbow held in 90° of flexion and the forearm in full pronation. Active and active-assisted ROM exercises of the elbow with the forearm in pronation are begun 1 week postoperatively. The exercises should be performed four to six times per day with the brace off. The elbow should be in the brace at all other times to avoid placing inadvertent varus stress on the elbow. Elbow extension is limited to 30° initially and then is gradually increased until full extension is achieved 4 weeks postoperatively. Flexion is not limited postoperatively. Full active forearm rotation into pronation and supination with the elbow in 90° of flexion is begun 1 week postoperatively. Supination in elbow extension is not allowed until 6 weeks postoperatively. Use of the brace is discontinued 6 to 8 weeks postoperatively, at which time full, active ROM of the elbow is allowed. Resistance exercises remain prohibited, however. Strengthening exercises are begun approximately 12 weeks after full elbow motion has been achieved. Unrestricted return to previous activities is allowed approximately 6 to 9 months postoperatively.

## Limiting Adverse Events

Reported complications of LCL reconstruction with free tendon graft include intraoperative fracture of the ulnar bone tunnels, delayed laxity, donor-site morbidity, decreased ROM, and persistent pain. Meticulous surgical technique and clear patient instructions on postoperative care and rehabilitation are required to minimize the risk of complications and optimize outcomes.

To avoid fracture of the bone bridge, the two ulnar tunnels should be made at least 1 cm apart. Additionally, overzealous handing of the bony bridge should be avoided when using the curved curets to connect the two tunnels. When using a commercial guide, it is important to ensure that the guide does not move after the first tunnel is made.

Accurate placement of the humeral docking tunnel is a critical step in the procedure. To ensure that the graft is taut on elbow extension, the tunnel should be made slightly anterior and proximal to the true isometric point so that the graft is positioned at the center of the isometric point on elbow extension.

It is important to reapproximate the remaining LCL tissue and place it underneath the graft tendon to avoid direct contact between the graft tendon and the radial head. To ensure proper tension on the graft, the elbow should be concentrically reduced while it is kept in full pronation, 90° of flexion, and slight valgus when the graft sutures are tied over the bony bridge.

The need to avoid varus stress in the early postoperative period must be emphasized to the patient. Additionally, it is important to stress the need to wear the elbow brace at all times except when performing the exercises and the need to maintain the elbow at the side during the exercises. In the first 6 weeks postoperatively, forearm supination is allowed only with the elbow in 90° of flexion.

## Bibliography


Arvind CH, Hargreaves DG: Tabletop relocation test: A new clinical test for posterolateral rotatory instability of the elbow. *J Shoulder Elbow Surg* 2006;15(6):707-708.

Coonrad RW, Roush TF, Major NM, Basamania CJ: The drop sign, a radiographic warning sign of elbow instability. *J Shoulder Elbow Surg* 2005;14(3):312-317.

Eygendaal D: Ligamentous reconstruction around the elbow using triceps tendon. *Acta Orthop Scand* 2004;75(5):516-523.

Jones KJ, Dodson CC, Osbahr DC, et al: The docking technique for lateral ulnar collateral ligament reconstruction: Surgical technique and clinical outcomes. *J Shoulder Elbow Surg* 2012;21(3):389-395.

Lee BP, Teo LH: Surgical reconstruction for posterolateral rotatory instability of the elbow. *J Shoulder Elbow Surg* 2003;12(5):476-479.

Lin KY, Shen PH, Lee CH, Pan RY, Lin LC, Shen HC: Functional outcomes of surgical reconstruction for posterolateral rotatory instability of the elbow. *Injury* 2012;43(10):1657-1661.

Magee T: Accuracy of 3-T MR arthrography versus conventional 3-T MRI of elbow tendons and ligaments compared with surgery. *AJR Am J Roentgenol* 2015;204(1):W70-W75.

Nestor BJ, O'Driscoll SW, Morrey BF: Ligamentous reconstruction for posterolateral rotatory instability of the elbow. *J Bone Joint Surg Am* 1992;74(8):1235-1241.

O'Driscoll SW: Reconstruction of the lateral collateral ligament, in Yamaguchi K, King GJW, McKee MD, O'Driscoll SWM, eds: *Advanced Reconstruction Elbow.* Rosemont, IL, American Academy of Orthopaedic Surgeons, 2007, pp 159-165.

O'Driscoll SW, Bell DF, Morrey BF: Posterolateral rotatory instability of the elbow. *J Bone Joint Surg Am* 1991;73(3):440-446.

O'Driscoll SW, Jupiter JB, King GJ, Hotchkiss RN, Morrey BF: The unstable elbow. *Instr Course Lect* 2001;50:89-102.

O'Driscoll SW, Spinner RJ, McKee MD, et al: Tardy posterolateral rotatory instability of the elbow due to cubitus varus. *J Bone Joint Surg Am* 2001;83(9):1358-1369.

Potter HG, Weiland AJ, Schatz JA, Paletta GA, Hotchkiss RN: Posterolateral rotatory instability of the elbow: Usefulness of MR imaging in diagnosis. *Radiology* 1997;204(1):185-189.

Regan W, Lapner PC: Prospective evaluation of two diagnostic apprehension signs for posterolateral instability of the elbow. *J Shoulder Elbow Surg* 2006;15(3):344-346.

Sanchez-Sotelo J, Morrey BF, O'Driscoll SW: Ligamentous repair and reconstruction for posterolateral rotatory instability of the elbow. *J Bone Joint Surg Br* 2005;87(1):54-61.

Terada N, Yamada H, Toyama Y: The appearance of the lateral ulnar collateral ligament on magnetic resonance imaging. *J Shoulder Elbow Surg* 2004;13(2):214-216.

 

# SECTION 3
# *Elbow Arthroplasty*

# Chapter 14

# Osteochondral Graft Reconstruction for Osteochondritis Dissecans of the Capitellum

*Donald S. Bae, MD*

**Learning Objectives**

- Understand the indications for osteochondral autologous transplantation in the management of osteochondritis dissecans of the capitellum.
- Understand the technique of an anconeus-splitting approach to the capitellum for single-plug transplantation.
- Recognize common pitfalls and complications associated with osteochondral autologous transplantation in the adolescent elbow.

## Indications

Osteochondritis dissecans (OCD) of the elbow is thought to be caused by repetitive microtrauma to the vulnerable chondroepiphysis of the capitellum, resulting in subchondral bone necrosis, articular cartilage failure, and, ultimately, loose-body formation. OCD is most commonly seen in early adolescent patients and typically manifests as lateral elbow pain, loss of elbow motion, and mechanical symptoms of locking and catching. Numerous classification schemes have been proposed for OCD, and they all categorize these lesions as either stable or unstable (**Table 1**). In addition, OCD lesions may be categorized as contained or uncontained based on the presence or absence of intact surrounding articular cartilage and preservation of the bony lateral column of the distal humerus.

Surgical treatment is typically recommended for patients with symptomatic, unstable OCD lesions. Loose body removal, chondroplasty, internal fixation, and/or marrow stimulation (such as by means of drilling or microfracture) have all been proposed; however, healing and return to sport rates of only 40% to 80% have been reported with these techniques. In efforts to improve healing rates and maximize functional outcomes, osteochondral autologous transplantation (OAT) has been proposed as an alternative surgical option, with the theoretical advantages of replacing the diseased subchondral bone and overlying articular surface with viable bone and hyaline cartilage, respectively. Initial reports of OAT in the knee have shown very favorable early to midterm results.

Although osteochondral graft reconstruction is suitable for managing all unstable OCD lesions, OAT may be particularly well suited for patients with deep or uncontained lesions and patients who have experienced failure of prior OCD surgery.

## Contraindications

Rest and activity modification are the current treatment standards for stable OCD lesions, with healing expected in 50% to 90% of patients, particularly in younger patients with early-stage OCD. Although no absolute contraindications exist for the use of osteochondral grafting for unstable lesions, a few considerations are worth mentioning. In skeletally immature patients with considerable growth remaining, the short distance between the articular surface and the distal humeral physis may preclude osteochondral grafting. Stable, press-fit stabilization of the OAT plug requires a minimum depth of grafting that might result in physeal disruption. Furthermore, OAT is more challenging in patients with limited elbow flexion because access to the capitellum with an anconeus-splitting approach is precluded by extension contracture of the elbow. Extensive capitellar involvement may be managed with a mosaicplasty

*Dr. Bae or an immediate family member has stock or stock options held in Cempra, Johnson & Johnson, Kythera Biopharmaceuticals, and Vivus and serves as a board member, owner, officer, or committee member of the American Academy of Orthopaedic Surgeons, the American Society for Surgery of the Hand, and the Pediatric Orthopaedic Society of North America.*

**Table 1** International Cartilage Repair Society Classification of Osteochondritis Dissecans

| Grade | Stability | Features |
|---|---|---|
| I | Stable | Cartilage intact, softened, but continuous |
| II | Stable | Partial discontinuity |
| III | Unstable | Complete discontinuity, in situ |
| IV | Unstable | Complete discontinuity, intra-articular loose body |

technique, although the ability to restore a smooth congruous articular surface is limited and the requisite placement of convergent OAT grafts may compromise stability.

## Alternative Treatments

Unstable in situ OCD lesions also may be managed with internal fixation. Bone plugs, headless variable-pitch compression screws, bioabsorbable tacks, and pull-out wires have been proposed, with the best results seen in younger patients with lesions that are less than 8 mm deep.

For grade IV lesions with intra-articular loose bodies, alternatives to OAT include loose body removal, chondroplasty, and microfracture or marrow stimulation. With these techniques, efforts are made to provide a more congruous radiocapitellar articulation by stimulating fibrocartilage formation in the OCD lesion.

## Results

Multiple published studies demonstrate that osteochondral grafting for OCD lesions results in pain relief, healing, and return to competitive sport in greater than 85% to 90% of patients with unstable lesions (**Table 2**). In studies of adolescent patients, high rates of pain relief and return to participation in baseball were reported after osteochondral grafting that involved the mosaicplasty technique with donor grafts from the knee. Similarly, good to excellent healing and functional improvement were noted in an older patient cohort treated with mosaicplasty.

Successful OCD reconstruction also has been achieved using osteochondral grafts harvested from the articular rib head. One study noted complete pain relief in a small number of adolescent patients treated with costal osteochondral grafting, with most patients returning to baseball. Another study reported 100% pain relief and return to sport in a larger cohort of patients treated with OAT using a single plug from the fifth or sixth rib head. Most patients in the study were adolescents, but one patient was middle-aged. High rates of pain relief and return to sports were reported in a series of adolescents with advanced OCD lesions who were treated with osteochondral autograft harvested from the rib head and augmented with bone graft and/or internal fixation.

## Techniques

Many osteochondral grafting techniques exist, but the author of this chapter prefers to perform an elbow arthroscopy first, followed by single-plug OAT with an anconeus-splitting approach. Donor osteochondral grafts are harvested from the lateral femoral condyle through a limited lateral parapatellar arthrotomy.

### Setup/Exposure

- The patient is placed in the supine position.
- Nonsterile tourniquets are placed on the upper brachium and the upper thigh of the ipsilateral lower limb.
- A small hand table or an arm board may be placed in line with the upper extremity to support the limb during OAT (**Figure 1**).
- The upper and lower extremities are prepped and draped in the usual sterile fashion.
- Although numerous commercially available arm holders are available, the author of this chapter prefers to use finger traps placed on the index and long fingers with 3 to 5 lb of counterweight. This allows suspension of the upper extremity, thereby facilitating circumferential access to the elbow and stabilization of the elbow at the desired degree of flexion-extension (**Figure 2**).

### Instruments/Equipment/Implants Required

- For elbow arthroscopy in children and adolescents, 2.7- or 2.9-mm 30° arthroscopes and arthroscopic shavers are used.
- Arthroscopic graspers of varying sizes should be available to facilitate loose-body removal, if necessary.
- In addition to standard surgical instruments for soft-tissue dissection, small Gelpi retractors are particularly helpful during capitellar exposure.
- Donor and recipient cylindrical Osteochondral Autograft Transfer System (OATS, Arthrex) chisels are used; 6-, 8-, and 10-mm–diameter chisels should be available.
- Intraoperative fluoroscopy is not needed for OATS reconstruction of the capitellum.

 

**Table 2** Results of Osteochondral Grafting to Manage Osteochondritis Dissecans[a]

| Authors (Year) | Number of Patients | Procedure or Approach | Mean Patient Age in Years (Range) | Mean Follow-up in Months (Range) | Success Rate (%) | Results |
|---|---|---|---|---|---|---|
| Iwasaki et al (2006) | 8 | Mosaicplasty from knee | 14 (11-16) | 24 (14-42) | 87.5 (pain relief) | 7 patients were pain free, and 6 patients returned to baseball<br>The mean Timmerman and Andrews score improved from 140 to 183 |
| Yamamoto et al (2006) | 18 | Mosaicplasty from knee | 13.6 (10-16) | 41.7 (25-63) | 94 (pain relief) | 17 patients had decreased pain, and 16 patients returned to throwing<br>The mean Timmerman and Andrews score improved from 150.8 to 180.6 |
| Iwasaki et al (2009) | 19 | Mosaicplasty from knee | 14.2 (11-19) | 45.1 (24-87) | 94 (pain free) | 18 patients were pain free, and 17 patients returned to playing baseball<br>The mean Timmerman and Andrews score improved from 131 to 191 |
| Mihara et al (2010) | 7 | Osteochondral graft from rib | 13.3 (11-15) | 37.4 (24-92) | 100 (return to sport) | 6 patients returned to baseball<br>The mean Timmerman and Andrews score improved from 141.4 to 185 |
| Ovesen et al (2011) | 10 | Mosaicplasty from knee | 18 (13-27) | 30 (10-60) | 89 (pain free) | 8 patients were pain free<br>The mean MEPS improved from 71 to 93.5 |
| Shimada et al (2012) | 26 | Single plug from rib | 16 (12-43) | 36 (24-51) | 100 | All patients had improved pain and returned to ADLs and sport participation<br>The mean Timmerman and Andrews score improved from 111 to 180<br>5 patients had secondary surgery |
| Maruyama et al (2014) | 33 | Mosaicplasty from knee | 13.6 (11-17) | 28.4 (12-76) | 91 (pain free) | 30 patients were pain free and 31 returned to baseball<br>The mean Timmerman and Andrews score improved from 143 to 190 |
| Nishinaka et al (2014) | 22 | Single plug from rib, with or without internal fixation | 13.9 (12-16) | 27 (12-77) | 100 | All patients had improved pain and returned to sports<br>The mean Timmerman and Andrews score improved from 121.5 to 169.2<br>4 patients required secondary surgery |

ADLs = activities of daily living, MEPS = Mayo Elbow Performance Score.

[a] All studies are level IV evidence.

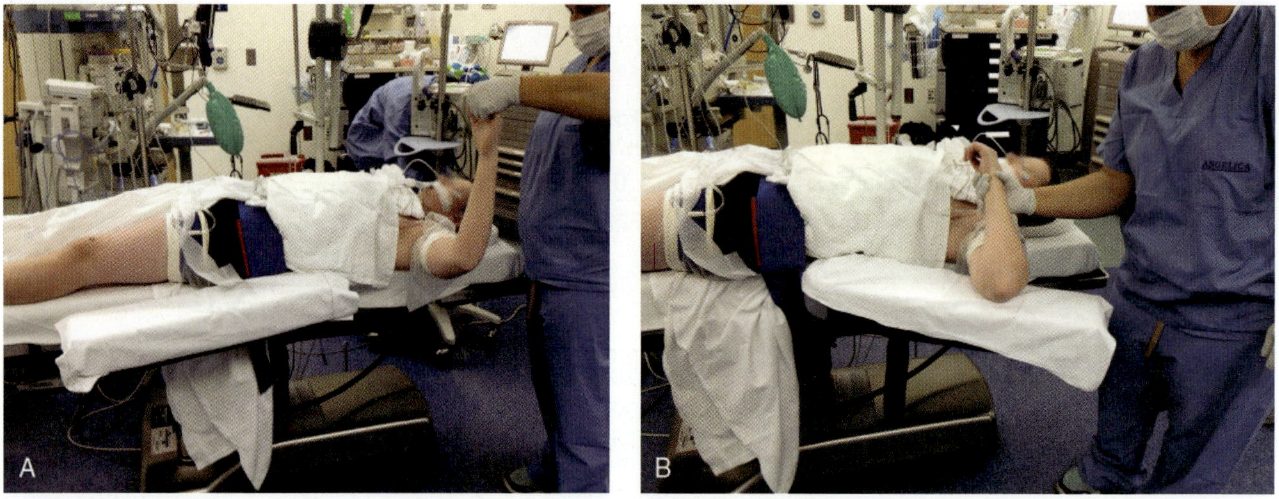

**Figure 1** Preoperative photographs show supine patient positioning for osteochondral autologous transplantation. **A,** The surgeon holds the upper limb in preparation for placement on an arm board. **B,** The appearance of the upper extremity placed in a hyperflexed position on an arm board. (Copyright Children's Orthopaedic Surgery Foundation, Boston, MA.)

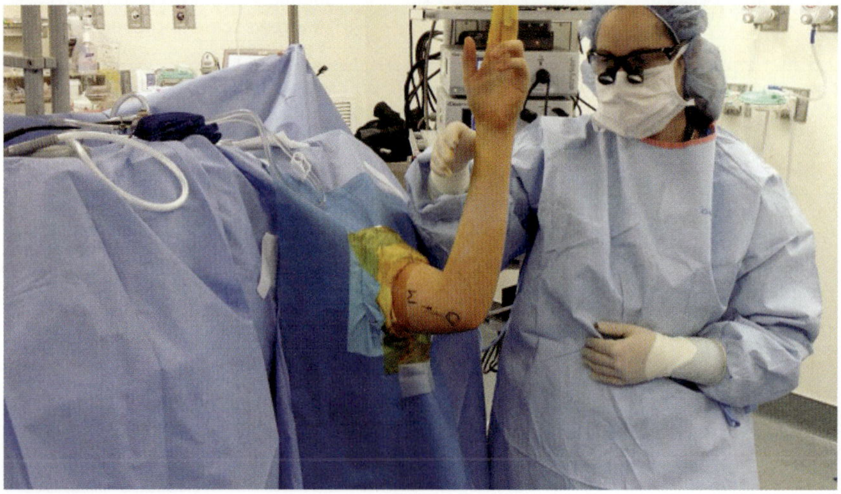

**Figure 2** Preoperative photograph shows the use of finger traps and a balanced counterweight of 4 lb to facilitate stable suspension of the limb and circumferential access during elbow arthroscopy. (Copyright Children's Orthopaedic Surgery Foundation, Boston, MA.)

## Procedure

- The patient's elbow is suspended in 90° flexion, and the elbow joint is insufflated with 10 to 20 mL of sterile saline introduced through a direct lateral (soft-spot) portal.
- A proximal anteromedial viewing portal (Poehling portal) is established.
- A 3- to 4-mm incision is created 2 to 3 cm proximal to the medial epicondyle, just anterior to the palpable medial intermuscular septum.
- The arthroscope is introduced and directed toward the radial head, taking care to maintain contact with the anterior humerus to avoid neurovascular injury.
- An initial arthroscopic survey is performed, and loose bodies in the anterior compartment are identified.
- The removal of any loose bodies may be performed through a standard anterolateral working portal, which is created just superior to the radiocapitellar articulation (**Figure 3**).
- The elbow is extended to enable evaluation of the OCD lesion and facilitate limited débridement of the synovitis.
- The arthroscope and the cannula are removed, the finger trap suspension is undone, and the arm is placed on a hand table or an arm board.
- The limb is exsanguinated with an elastic Esmarch bandage, and an upper-extremity tourniquet is inflated to 250 mm Hg.
- The elbow is hyperflexed, and a longitudinal incision is created over the palpable capitellum between the lateral epicondyle and lateral border of the olecranon (**Figure 4, A**).
- Dissection is performed through the subcutaneous tissues, and the fascia overlying the anconeus is incised in line with the skin incision (**Figure 4, B**).
- The anconeus muscle fibers are split and retracted to reveal the joint capsule.
- The capsule is incised, and a small Gelpi retractor is placed to

 

facilitate exposure of the capitellum (**Figure 5**).

- The typical grade IV OCD lesion is carefully examined, and the margins of intact articular cartilage and the quality of the underlying subchondral bone are noted. Commercially available sizers should be available to quantify the diameter of the lesion, which typically measures 8 to 10 mm.
- The chisel appropriate for the recipient site is placed in the region overlying the OCD lesion. It is imperative that the chisel is oriented perpendicular to the articular surface.
- The chisel is impacted to a depth of 10 to 15 mm, and the abnormal bone from the OCD lesion is removed. The depth of the recipient site is carefully measured, and confirmation is made that no cortical breach has occurred. This completes preparation of the recipient site (**Figure 6**).
- Attention is then turned to the knee.
- After the limb is exsanguinated with an Esmarch bandage and the tourniquet on the proximal thigh is inflated to 250 mm Hg, a small lateral parapatellar incision is created just superior to the palpable joint line (**Figure 7, A**).
- Dissection is performed through the subcutaneous tissues and the deep fascia.
- A lateral parapatellar arthrotomy is created, leaving a cuff of tissue on the patella to facilitate subsequent closure.
- With the knee in full extension, the patella is gently retracted medially, and the non–weight-bearing anterior surface of the lateral condyle is visualized. The ideal location for donor graft harvest is above the sulcus terminalis but below the distal femoral physis (**Figure 7, B**).
- The chisel appropriate for the donor

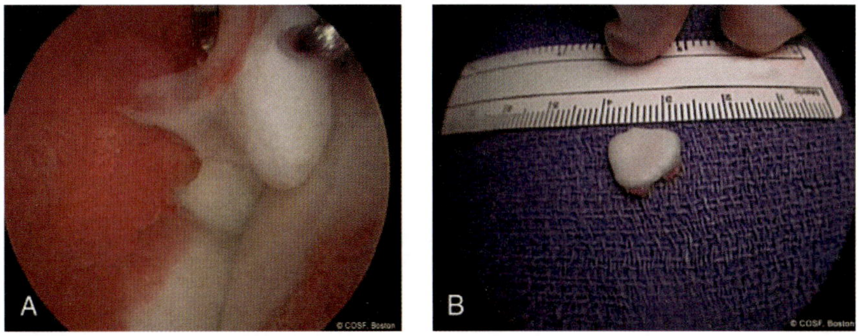


**Figure 3** **A,** Arthroscopic image obtained from a proximal anteromedial viewing portal in a right elbow demonstrates removal of an osteochondral loose body through an anterolateral working portal. **B,** Appearance and size of the osteochondral loose body after excision. (Copyright Children's Orthopaedic Surgery Foundation, Boston, MA.)

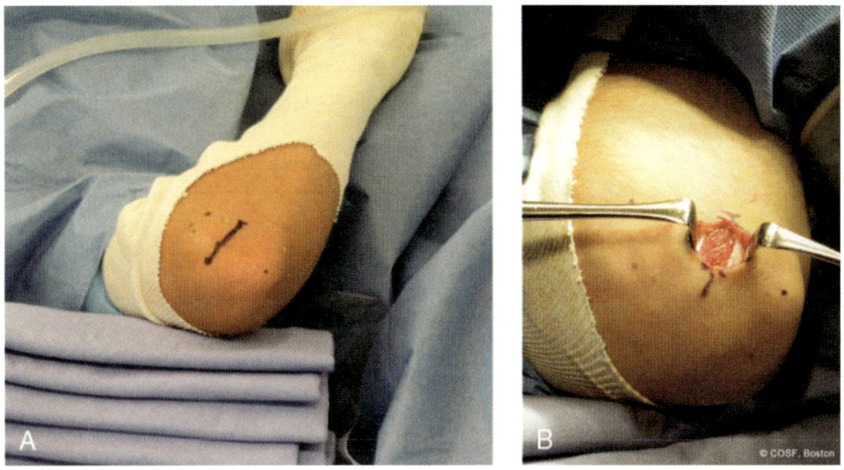


**Figure 4** Intraoperative photographs of a patient undergoing osteochondral grafting to manage osteochondritis dissecans. **A,** The planned surgical incision overlying the capitellum is marked on the right elbow, which is in hyperflexion. **B,** The fascia of the anconeus is split in line with the skin incision. (Copyright Children's Orthopaedic Surgery Foundation, Boston, MA.)

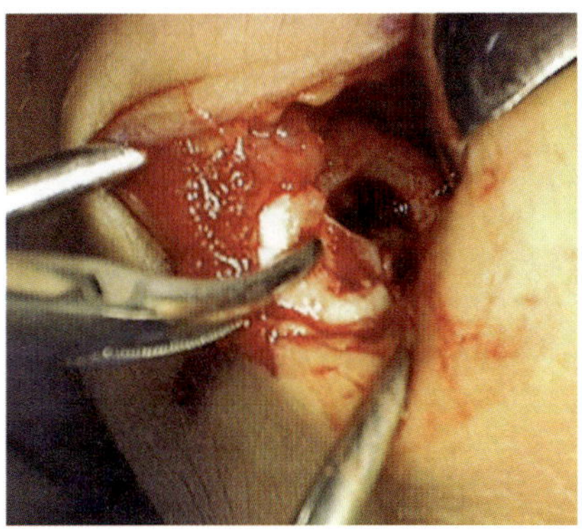

**Figure 5** Intraoperative photograph shows removal of an unstable osteochondritis dissecans lesion with an anconeus-splitting approach. (Copyright Children's Orthopaedic Surgery Foundation, Boston, MA.)

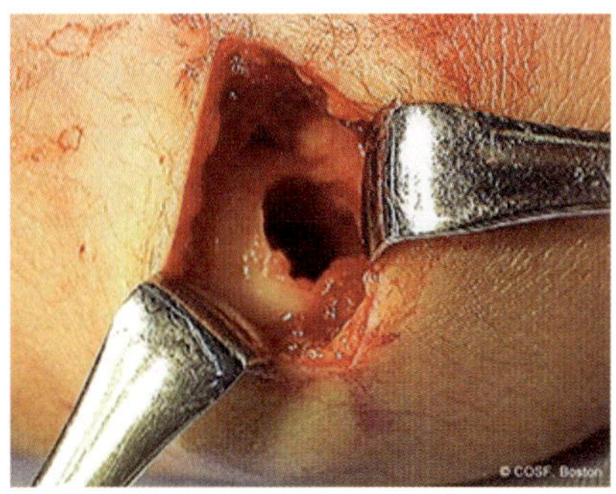

**Figure 6** Intraoperative photograph shows preparation of the recipient site in osteochondral autologous transplantation in a right elbow. (Copyright Children's Orthopaedic Surgery Foundation, Boston, MA.)

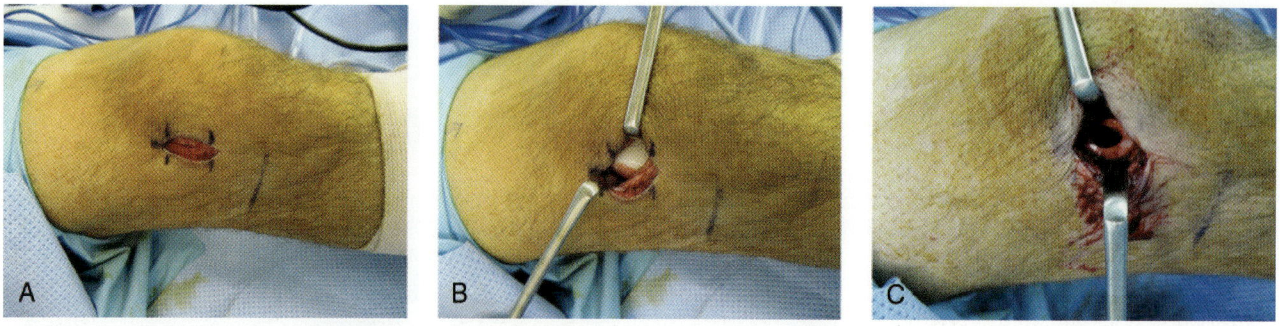


**Figure 7** Intraoperative photographs show harvest of a donor osteochondral plug from a patient's knee. **A,** Appearance of a small lateral parapatellar incision. **B,** Arthrotomy has been performed, and the patella has been gently retracted medially to allow visualization and access to the non–weight-bearing surface of the lateral femoral condyle. **C,** Appearance of the donor site after plug harvest. (Copyright Children's Orthopaedic Surgery Foundation, Boston, MA.)

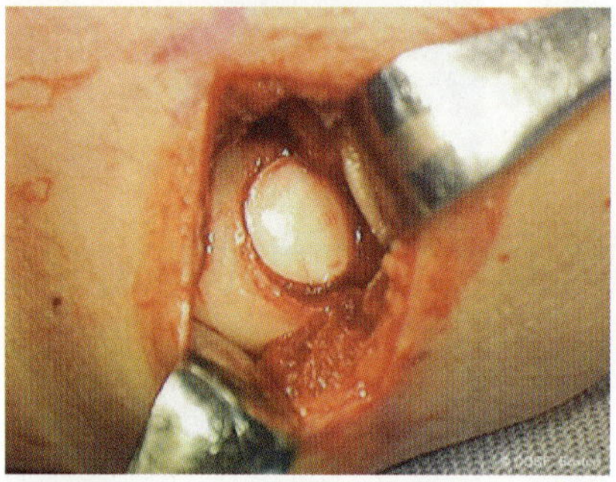

**Figure 8** Photograph of the final intraoperative appearance of the capitellar reconstruction after graft placement by means of osteochondral autologous transplantation. (Copyright Children's Orthopaedic Surgery Foundation, Boston, MA.)

site is placed on the lateral condyle, taking great care to orient the chisel orthogonal to the articular surface.

- The donor site chisel is impacted to a depth 1 to 2 mm greater than the measured recipient site defect.
- The chisel is withdrawn, and the osteochondral plug harvest is completed (**Figure 7, C**).
- The donor site chisel—with the osteochondral plug within—is moved to a separate table in the operating room, where the end of the osteochondral plug is delivered from the chisel. The donor plug is sized to a depth of 0.5 to 1 mm shorter than the recipient site, and any excess bone is removed.
- The bony end of the plug is flattened by using a No. 15 blade or a fine rongeur.
- The donor osteochondral graft is gently placed into the recipient site in the elbow. The orientation of the graft must be preserved during delivery to facilitate press fitting and avoid inadvertent fracture of the graft. To minimize trauma to the hyaline cartilage cells, overzealous impaction with a mallet must be avoided.
- The graft is seated either flush with the adjacent cartilage surface or slightly countersunk in relation to it (**Figure 8**).
- The elbow is taken through a full range of motion (ROM) and evaluated for crepitus and plug instability.

### Wound Closure

- The elbow wound is copiously irrigated with sterile saline solution.
- The capsule is reapproximated with 2-0 polyglactin suture.
- The anconeus fascia and subcutaneous tissues are closed with absorbable 3-0 and 4-0 polyglactin sutures, and the skin is closed with a 4-0 poliglecaprone suture.
- Arthroscopy portals are similarly closed with poliglecaprone or other absorbable monofilament sutures.
- The knee parapatellar arthrotomy is similarly closed with 2-0 or 0 polyglactin suture.
- The deep fascia of the knee is closed in layers with 2-0 and 3-0 polyglactin suture, and the skin is reapproximated with poliglecaprone subcuticular suture.
- Bulky sterile bandages are applied to the elbow and the knee, followed by application of a bivalve long arm cast and a knee immobilizer.

## Postoperative Regimen

Although osteochondral grafts are inherently stable and many surgeons initiate immediate elbow ROM after surgery, the author of this chapter prefers to immobilize the limb in a long arm cast for 2 weeks postoperatively. After the cast is removed and the wounds are inspected, gentle ROM is initiated, with the goal of achieving full elbow flexion-extension by the 6th postoperative week. At 6 weeks after surgery, physical therapy is initiated to restore any remaining limitations in elbow ROM and begin gradual strengthening.

Sport-specific activities are typically restricted for 6 months postoperatively, although many athletes are able to return to sport earlier. Criteria for return

 

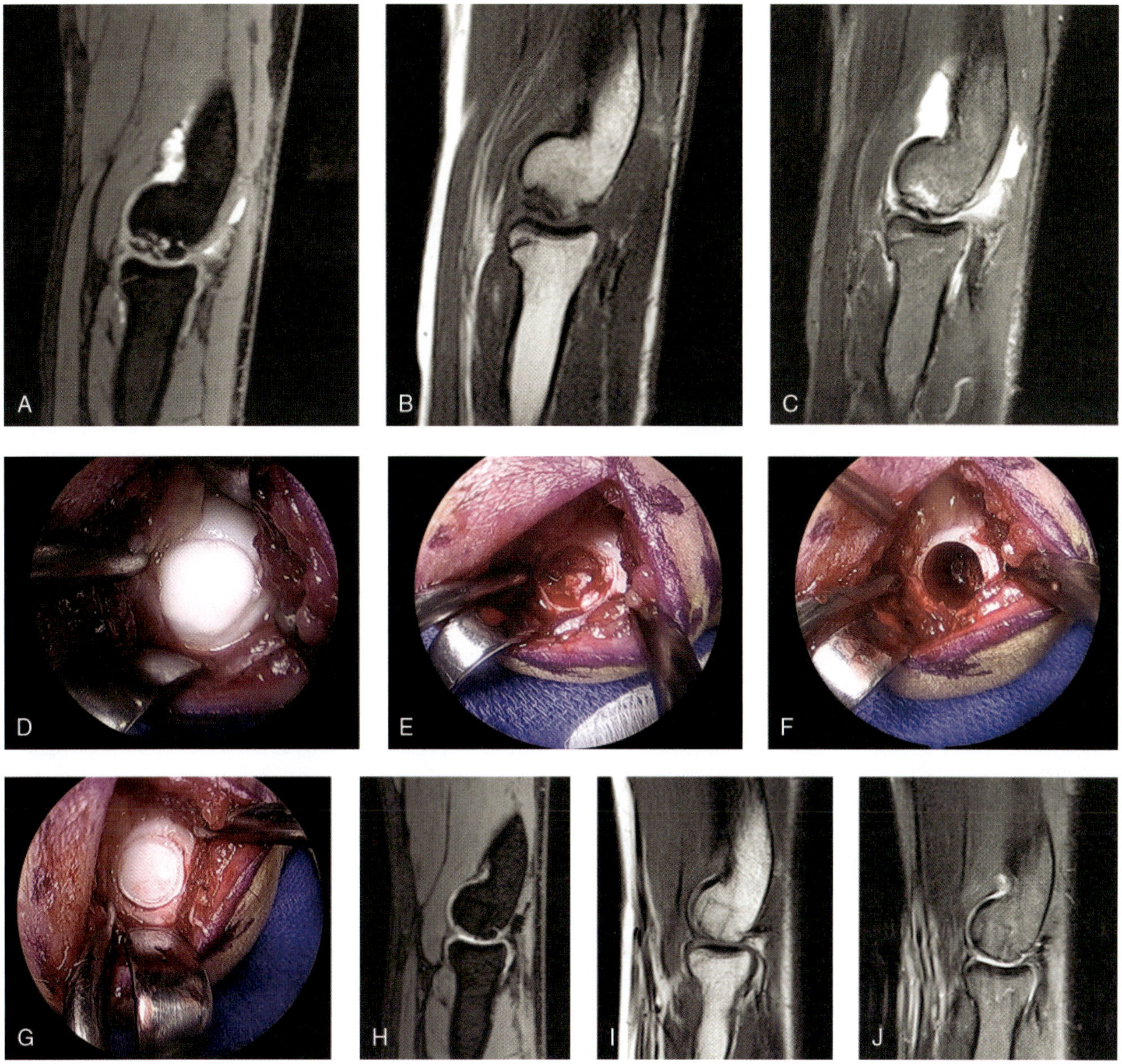


**Figure 9** MRIs from a 16-year-old female gymnast who underwent osteochondral autologous transplantation. Preoperative double-echo steady state (DESS) (**A**), T1-weighted (**B**), and short tau inversion recovery (STIR) (**C**) MRIs demonstrate an unstable osteochondritis dissecans lesion with subchondral bone involvement. **D,** Appearance of a large, unstable, in situ fragment noted intraoperatively. **E,** Appearance of the osteocartilaginous defect after loose-body removal. **F,** Intraoperative appearance after preparation of the graft recipient site. **G,** Intraoperative appearance of the restored articular contour after graft placement. Excellent articular congruity and bony healing is demonstrated on DESS (**H**), T1-weighted (**I**), and STIR (**J**) MRIs obtained 6 months postoperatively. (Copyright Children's Orthopaedic Surgery Foundation, Boston, MA.)

to high-risk activities, such as baseball pitching, gymnastics, and wrestling, include resolution of pain and tenderness, full restoration of elbow motion, elbow strength greater than or equal to 90% that of the contralateral elbow, and radiographic evidence of healing (**Figure 9**). With regard to the knee, weight bearing as tolerated is allowed immediately after surgery. A knee immobilizer is offered for comfort, particularly in patients with temporary gait abnormalities caused by quadriceps inhibition or pain.

## Limiting Adverse Events

Patient selection is important to limit adverse events. Osteochondral graft reconstruction with an anconeus-splitting approach is challenging in patients with obesity and those with limited elbow flexion; in both cases, the radial head cannot be fully flexed away from the capitellum. A posterolateral approach may be considered in these patients. Furthermore, OAT may not be the appropriate primary reconstruction option in very young patients, in whom osteochondral graft placement might lead to disturbance of the lateral distal humeral physis.

Careful surgical technique when preparing the recipient site and harvesting and placing the graft material is important to limit adverse events. When the elbow is in hyperflexion, the capsule is closely apposed to the capitellum, and a capsulotomy must be performed gently to avoid injury to the capitellar articular cartilage. Furthermore, distal extension of the surgical approach is limited by the annular ligament. As soon as the radial head is visualized, the capsular incision is ceased to avoid disruption of the annular ligament. It is critically important that the recipient site chisel is impacted precisely along the desired trajectory, orthogonal to the cartilage surface, with the limb firmly stabilized. Eccentric blows with a mallet on the chisel may lead to suboptimal preparation of the recipient site, leading to difficulties in extracting the recipient bone as well as the loss of press-fit stability during graft placement.

Although a surgeon may be tempted to harvest osteochondral donor plugs very superiorly on the lateral femoral condyle, locating and protecting the distal femoral physis is important in skeletally immature patients. Donor graft harvest may be safely performed superior to the sulcus terminalis, above the weight-bearing portion of the distal femur. Harvesting with the knee in terminal extension facilitates appropriate donor site selection.

For press-fit stability, the diameter of the donor osteochondral plug should be slightly greater than the diameter of the recipient site. To achieve such stability, particularly in athletic adolescents with more dense bone, every effort must be made to match the trajectory of the donor graft with that of the recipient site during delivery. Furthermore, slightly undersizing the donor graft length by 0.5 to 1 mm minimizes the risk of graft prominence. Undersizing is important because a prominent graft may result in early failure. Although sharp excision of any prominent cartilage from a graft placed too proud may be tempting, doing so removes the important superficial fibers of the hyaline cartilage surface.

## Bibliography


Andrews JR, Carson WG: Arthroscopy of the elbow. *Arthroscopy* 1985;1(2):97-107.

Baumgarten TE, Andrews JR, Satterwhite YE: The arthroscopic classification and treatment of osteochondritis dissecans of the capitellum. *Am J Sports Med* 1998;26(4):520-523.

Brittberg M, Winalski CS: Evaluation of cartilage injuries and repair. *J Bone Joint Surg Am* 2003;85(suppl 2):58-69.

Byrd JW, Jones KS: Arthroscopic surgery for isolated capitellar osteochondritis dissecans in adolescent baseball players: Minimum three-year follow-up. *Am J Sports Med* 2002;30(4):474-478.

Gudas R, Gudaitė A, Pocius A, et al: Ten-year follow-up of a prospective, randomized clinical study of mosaic osteochondral autologous transplantation versus microfracture for the treatment of osteochondral defects in the knee joint of athletes. *Am J Sports Med* 2012;40(11):2499-2508.

Gudas R, Simonaityte R, Čekanauskas E, Tamošiūnas R: A prospective, randomized clinical study of osteochondral autologous transplantation versus microfracture for the treatment of osteochondritis dissecans in the knee joint in children. *J Pediatr Orthop* 2009;29(7):741-748.

Harada M, Ogino T, Takahara M, Ishigaki D, Kashiwa H, Kanauchi Y: Fragment fixation with a bone graft and dynamic staples for osteochondritis dissecans of the humeral capitellum. *J Shoulder Elbow Surg* 2002;11(4):368-372.


 

Hennrikus WP, Miller PE, Micheli LJ, Waters PM, Bae DS: Internal fixation of unstable in situ osteochondritis dissecans lesions of the capitellum. *J Pediatr Orthop* 2015;35(5):467-473.

Iwasaki N, Kato H, Ishikawa J, Masuko T, Funakoshi T, Minami A: Autologous osteochondral mosaicplasty for osteochondritis dissecans of the elbow in teenage athletes. *J Bone Joint Surg Am* 2009;91(10):2359-2366.

Iwasaki N, Kato H, Ishikawa J, Saitoh S, Minami A: Autologous osteochondral mosaicplasty for capitellar osteochondritis dissecans in teenaged patients. *Am J Sports Med* 2006;34(8):1233-1239.

Kobayashi K, Burton KJ, Rodner C, Smith B, Caputo AE: Lateral compression injuries in the pediatric elbow: Panner's disease and osteochondritis dissecans of the capitellum. *J Am Acad Orthop Surg* 2004;12(4):246-254.

Maruyama M, Takahara M, Harada M, Satake H, Takagi M: Outcomes of an open autologous osteochondral plug graft for capitellar osteochondritis dissecans: Time to return to sports. *Am J Sports Med* 2014;42(9):2122-2127.

Matsuura T, Kashiwaguchi S, Iwase T, Takeda Y, Yasui N: Conservative treatment for osteochondrosis of the humeral capitellum. *Am J Sports Med* 2008;36(5):868-872.

Mihara K, Suzuki K, Makiuchi D, Nishinaka N, Yamaguchi K, Tsutsui H: Surgical treatment for osteochondritis dissecans of the humeral capitellum. *J Shoulder Elbow Surg* 2010;19(1):31-37.

Mihara K, Tsutsui H, Nishinaka N, Yamaguchi K: Nonoperative treatment for osteochondritis dissecans of the capitellum. *Am J Sports Med* 2009;37(2):298-304.

Miyamoto W, Yamamoto S, Kii R, Uchio Y: Oblique osteochondral plugs transplantation technique for osteochondritis dissecans of the elbow joint. *Knee Surg Sports Traumatol Arthrosc* 2009;17(2):204-208.

Nishinaka N, Tsutsui H, Yamaguchi K, Uehara T, Nagai S, Atsumi T: Costal osteochondral autograft for reconstruction of advanced-stage osteochondritis dissecans of the capitellum. *J Shoulder Elbow Surg* 2014;23(12):1888-1897.

Nobuta S, Ogawa K, Sato K, Nakagawa T, Hatori M, Itoi E: Clinical outcome of fragment fixation for osteochondritis dissecans of the elbow. *Ups J Med Sci* 2008;113(2):201-208.

Oka Y, Ohta K, Fukuda H: Bone-peg grafting for osteochondritis dissecans of the elbow. *Int Orthop* 1999;23(1):53-57.

Ovesen J, Olsen BS, Johannsen HV: The clinical outcomes of mosaicplasty in the treatment of osteochondritis dissecans of the distal humeral capitellum of young athletes. *J Shoulder Elbow Surg* 2011;20(5):813-818.

Poehling GG, Whipple TL, Sisco L, Goldman B: Elbow arthroscopy: A new technique. *Arthroscopy* 1989;5(3):222-224.

Ruchelsman DE, Hall MP, Youm T: Osteochondritis dissecans of the capitellum: Current concepts. *J Am Acad Orthop Surg* 2010;18(9):557-567.

Shi LL, Bae DS, Kocher MS, Micheli LJ, Waters PM: Contained versus uncontained lesions in juvenile elbow osteochondritis dissecans. *J Pediatr Orthop* 2012;32(3):221-225.

Shimada K, Tanaka H, Matsumoto T, et al: Cylindrical costal osteochondral autograft for reconstruction of large defects of the capitellum due to osteochondritis dissecans. *J Bone Joint Surg Am* 2012;94(11):992-1002.

Takahara M, Mura N, Sasaki J, Harada M, Ogino T: Classification, treatment, and outcome of osteochondritis dissecans of the humeral capitellum. *J Bone Joint Surg Am* 2007;89(6):1205-1214.

Takeda H, Watarai K, Matsushita T, Saito T, Terashima Y: A surgical treatment for unstable osteochondritis dissecans lesions of the humeral capitellum in adolescent baseball players. *Am J Sports Med* 2002;30(5):713-717.

Yamamoto Y, Ishibashi Y, Tsuda E, Sato H, Toh S: Osteochondral autograft transplantation for osteochondritis dissecans of the elbow in juvenile baseball players: Minimum 2-year follow-up. *Am J Sports Med* 2006;34(5):714-720.

Zlotolow DA, Bae DS: Osteochondral autograft transplantation in the elbow. *J Hand Surg Am* 2014;39(2):368-372.

 

# Chapter 15

# Distal Humeral Hemiarthroplasty

*Jeffery S. Hughes, MBBS, FRACS*

**Learning Objectives**

- Understand the indications for distal humeral hemiarthroplasty.
- Identify patients who are most likely to benefit from distal humeral hemiarthroplasty.

## Introduction

Although developments in open reduction and internal fixation (ORIF) and total elbow arthroplasty (TEA) have advanced the management of distal humeral fracture, there are clinical situations in which neither technique is optimal. Distal humeral hemiarthroplasty (DHH) offers patients who have extensive joint comminution or entire articular surface involvement in whom ORIF cannot provide reliable outcomes or patients who have physical demands that exceed those allowed after TEA with an alternative for a stable functional elbow.

DHH was first reported in 1947. Recently, the use of DHH as a potential surgical treatment of distal humerus disorders has increased. As understanding of the anatomy and biomechanics of the elbow as well as the availability of anatomic prostheses have improved, the advantages of DHH compared with other treatments currently used to manage complex fractures of the distal humerus or pathology that destroys large segments of the distal humeral articular joint surface have been recognized.

Early studies on DHH reported the use of a small number of implants for a variety of pathologies, including trauma, inflammatory arthritis, and tumor management. Early prostheses were custom-made or nonanatomic (capitellocondylar, Kudo [Biomet]) or had anatomic components (Stevens-Street).

DHH is an alternative to ORIF, interposition arthroplasty, and TEA that should be considered for the management of complex elbow pathology, depending on a patient's activity level and infirmity. The decision to perform DHH is based on the general advantages of the procedure compared with ORIF and TEA as well as patient-specific lifestyle factors and functional status. DHH eliminates the risks of nonunion, malunion, loss of fixation, and stiffness associated with ORIF and the risk of polyethylene wear associated with TEA. In addition, DHH is not subject to a lifetime 6.6-lb (3-kg) weight-bearing restriction and has a lower incidence of component loosening compared with TEA, which makes it a more suitable choice for healthy, high-demand patients.

*Dr. Hughes or an immediate family member has received royalties from, is a member of a speakers' bureau or has made paid presentations on behalf of, and serves as a paid consultant to Zimmer Biomet.*

## Indications

The indications for DHH continue to evolve as clinical data from longitudinal studies offer direction with regard to the results that can be achieved with DHH and the patients in whom DHH can be used appropriately. Trauma and its sequelae account for most articular surface problems of the distal humerus. Complex fractures of the capitellum and trochlea are particularly difficult. DHH offers several potential advantages to healthy, active patients who have high activity demands after linked TEA.

The selection of ORIF, bone grafting, DHH, TEA, or radiocapitellar arthroplasty depends on load-bearing articular column involvement (**Figure 1**) as well as patient age and activity level. Currently, the indications for DHH include acute trauma, such as comminuted bicolumnar intra-articular fractures in which ORIF will not result in sufficient stability to allow for early range of motion (ROM), unreconstructible capitellar and trochlear fractures, and coronal shear fractures of the capitellum and lateral trochlea with low transverse fracture of the epicondyles; salvage of failed internal fixation; unreconstructible malunion or nonunion of the distal humerus; osteonecrosis of the trochlea with collapse of the subchondral bone; and tumors of

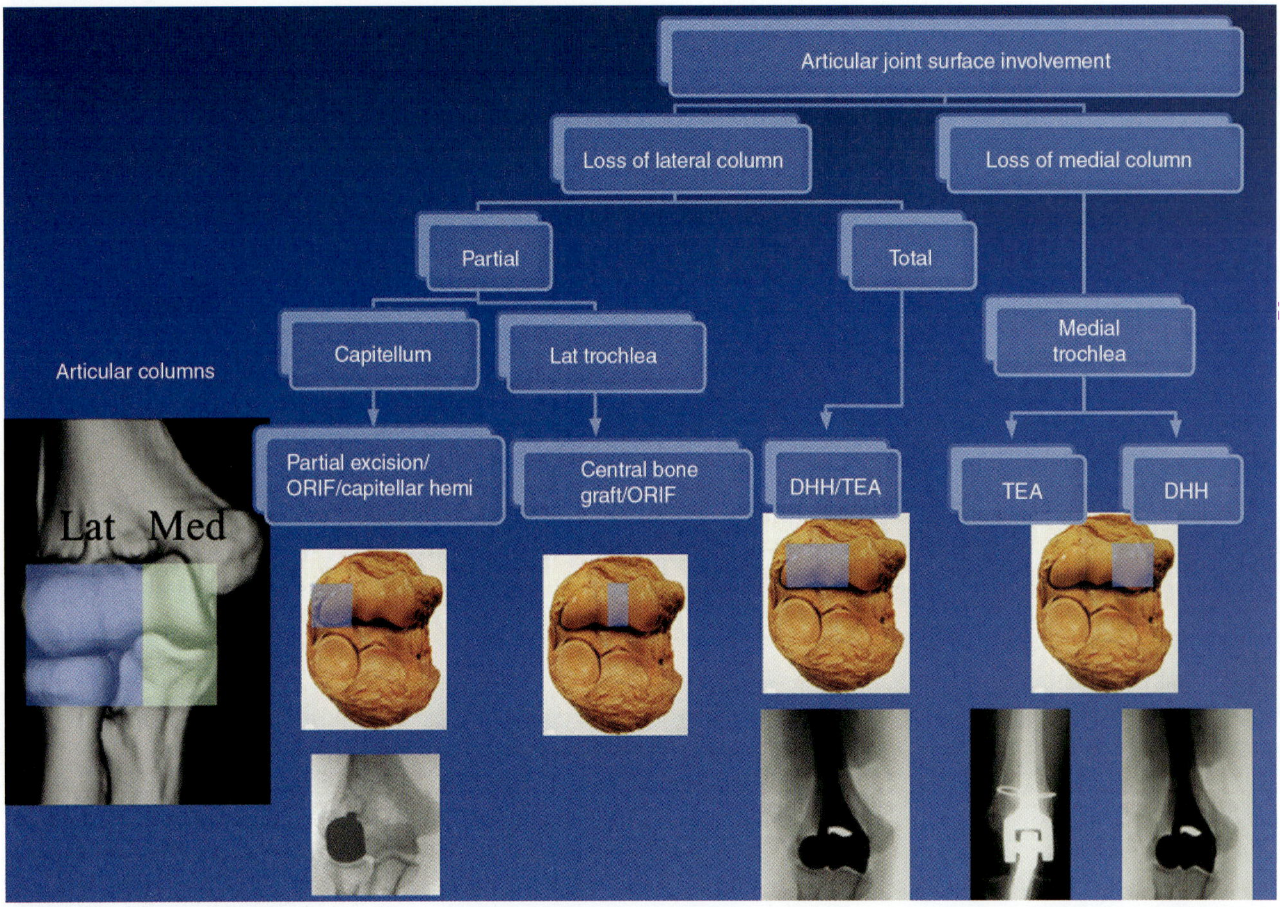


**Figure 1** Treatment algorithm for unreconstructible distal humerus fracture. The involvement of the distal articular joint surface is determined based on loss of the articular surface of the medial column (Med) or the lateral column (Lat). The lateral column includes the capitellum and lateral trochlea, and the medial column includes the medial trochlea. The articular segment or segments that are lost determine the treatment option. DHH = distal humeral hemiarthroplasty, Hemi = hemiarthroplasty, ORIF = open reduction and internal fixation, TEA = total elbow arthroplasty.

the trochlea in which resection allows for preservation of the epicondyles and collateral ligaments.

In early studies, patients who had rheumatoid arthritis reported stiff, painful joints after DHH; however, this may not be the case for all patients. DHH may be of value in younger patients experiencing burnout or in low-demand patients being treated with disease-modifying antirheumatic drugs who have an eburnated but congruent joint. In the experience of the author of this chapter, the use of DHH for the management of primary osteoarthritis is unpredictable with regard to pain relief and ROM.

The condyles, coronoid process, and radial head must be intact or repairable to ensure elbow stability. The metaphyseal condyles and columns must be intact or repairable to ensure prosthesis stability. The medial collateral ligament and the lateral collateral ligament must be intact or repairable. Preoperative imaging should include AP and lateral radiographs of the elbow. Because it is often unclear whether a fracture is reconstructible or will require DHH, CT also should be considered to aid in the evaluation of articular column involvement. If reconstruction is not achievable, a radiograph of the contralateral elbow can aid in accurate templating (**Figure 2**). Prosthesis sizing is based on the direct correlation between the AP dimensions of the normal articular surface and the radii of the capitellum and trochlea. In addition, simultaneous alignment of the longitudinal axis of the radial neck with the center of the capitellum and of the prosthetic trochlea with the trochlea or sigmoid fossa should be confirmed on an AP radiograph.

Advances in the understanding of elbow anatomy and biomechanics have helped determine the correct shape and size of joint surfaces as well as the landmarks for appropriate implantation that will ensure good stability and function. A near-anatomic DHH spool was designed in 1974. Experience with the mechanism of humeral component loosening that was associated with TEA dictated that DHH implants be stemmed and, preferably, have an anterior flange that resists joint reactive forces. The only TEA system currently available that allows for DHH is the Latitude EV Total Elbow Prosthesis (Tornier; **Figure 3**). This prosthesis has three stem sizes (each with an anterior flange) and six modular anatomic spools. Although reconstruction of the epicondyles is preferred, a central axis hole allows for suture fixation of collateral ligament repair if necessary. The Latitude EV Total Elbow Prosthesis theoretically allows for conversion to a semiconstrained TEA; however, the practicality of this conversion has yet to be demonstrated. In the experience of the author of this chapter, the only loose stems observed have been in prostheses with nonflanged alternatives (such as the Sorbie-Questor prosthesis [Wright Medical Technology]). Chondral wear is characteristic of all joint hemiarthroplasties. Biomechanical studies on the Latitude EV Total Elbow Prosthesis and its contact stresses provide insight into the mode of wear as well as how current prostheses should be implanted and potentially modified in the future.

## Contraindications

Absolute contraindications to DHH include overt local or distant foci of infection; inadequate neurovascular status; insufficient bony support; poor soft-tissue coverage; and unstable fracture of the radial head, the coronoid, or both. In addition, a nonanatomic sigmoid fossa as a result of developmental humeral insufficiency (such as fishtail deformity) results in poor congruency with a DHH; therefore, TEA may be a more suitable procedure. Relative contraindications to DHH include articular cartilage damage of the radial head and sigmoid fossa as a result of chronic fracture arthrofibrosis or inflammatory arthropathy.

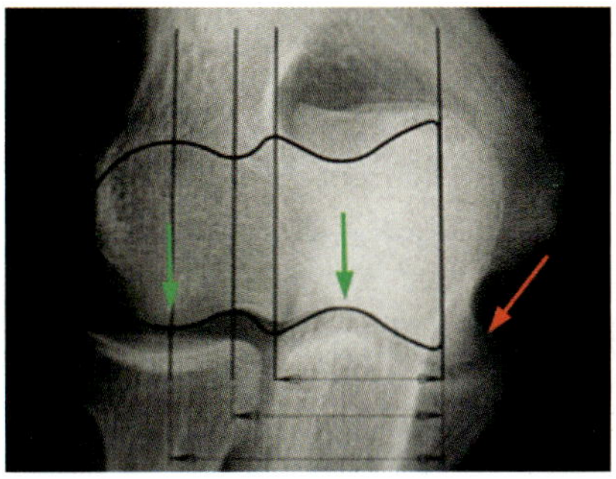

**Figure 2** AP radiograph of an elbow demonstrates preoperative templating, which helps ensure correct anatomic component selection. When the prosthetic trochlea matches the anterior coronoid, the center of the radial head aligns with the capitellum (green arrows). The currently available prosthetic spools do not articulate anatomically with the anteromedial facet of the sigmoid fossa, which may result in medial notching (red arrow). (Adapted from Hughes JS, Parsons M: Distal humeral hemiarthroplasty, in Yamaguchi K, King GJ, McKee MD, O'Driscoll SW, eds: *Advanced Reconstruction: Elbow.* Rosemont, IL, American Academy of Orthopaedic Surgeons, 2007, pp 219-228.)

## Alternative Treatments

Nonsurgical management of displaced intra-articular distal humerus fractures, including cast immobilization and acceptance of displacement of the bony fragments and early mobilization, may be considered in infirm or low-demand patients.

The goals of surgery for displaced intra-articular distal humerus fractures include anatomic restoration of the joint surface and rigid fixation that allows for early ROM. ORIF remains the preferred method of surgical treatment because successful ORIF restores the native articulation of the elbow joint. If fixation is tenuous, a period of immobilization is prescribed to allow for incipient union. Most patients who undergo a period of immobilization regain good elbow motion; however, contracture release is recommended for patients in whom good elbow motion cannot be regained. Studies have reported a substantial rate of unsatisfactory outcomes and a high complication rate in patients who undergo ORIF for the management of comminuted intra-articular fractures, which indicates the difficulty in achieving the goals of surgical management in patients with complex fractures.

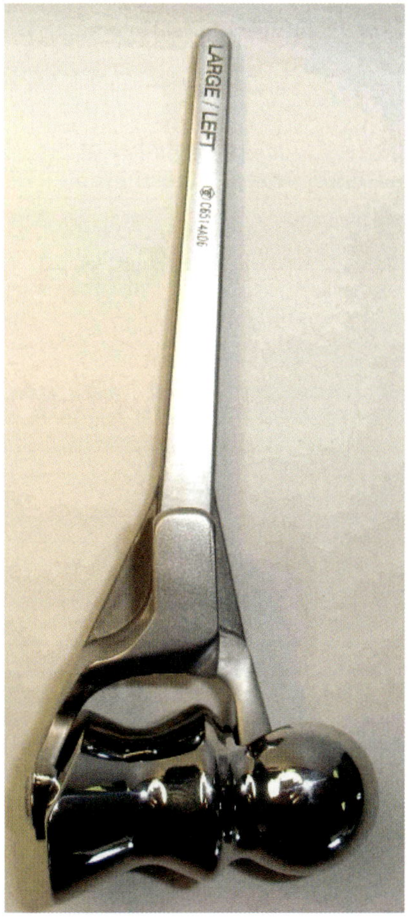


**Figure 3** Clinical photograph shows the Latitude EV Total Elbow Prosthesis (Tornier). The prosthesis has an anatomic spool and an anterior flange, which, if grafted, helps prevent stem loosening. (Reproduced from Hughes JS, Parsons M: Distal humeral hemiarthroplasty, in Yamaguchi K, King GJ, McKee MD, O'Driscoll SW, eds: *Advanced Reconstruction: Elbow.* Rosemont, IL, American Academy of Orthopaedic Surgeons, 2007, pp 219-228.)

**Table 1** Results of Distal Humeral Hemiarthroplasty (DHH)

| Authors (Year) | Number of Prostheses | Prosthesis | Mean Patient Age in Years (Range) | Mean Follow-up in Months (Range) | Results |
|---|---|---|---|---|---|
| Mellen and Phalen (1947) | 4 | Acrylic custom | 22.5 (19-28) | (9-18) | Good pain relief<br>Follow-up time noted for only 3 patients |
| Street and Stevens (1974) | 10 | Anatomic metal spool | NA (16-64) | NA (12-84) | 4 of 5 elbows with posttraumatic lesions were pain free<br>Poor ROM in the 3 elbows with rheumatoid arthritis<br>The other 2 elbows were managed for ankylosis secondary to hemophilia |
| Shifrin and Johnson (1990) | 1 | Custom | 19 | 252 | Good pain relief and ROM |
| Swoboda and Scott (1999) | 7 | Capitellocondylar | 38 (20-50) | NA (25-109) | 1 prosthesis was removed due to infection<br>4 patients were pain free and 2 experienced minimal pain<br>Mean 27° increase in flexion arc |
| Parsons et al (2005) | 8 | Sorbie-Questor (Wright Medical Technology) | 61 (46-83) | 24 (NA) | Mean ASES score, 80<br>Mean extension, 22°<br>Mean flexion, 126°<br>Patients with acute fractures had better outcomes compared with those with chronic fractures |
| Adolfsson and Hammer (2006) | 4 | Kudo (Biomet) | 80 (79-89) | 10 (3-14) | MEPS: 3 excellent outcomes and 1 good outcome<br>Mean extension, 20°<br>Mean flexion, 126° |
| Burkhart et al (2011) | 10 | Latitude Total Elbow Prosthesis (Tornier) | 75.2 (NA) | 12.1 (NA) | MEPS: 9 good to excellent outcomes and 1 fair outcome<br>Mean extension, 17.5°<br>Mean flexion, 124.5° |
| Adolfsson and Nestorson (2012) | 8 | Kudo | 79 (71-89) | 48 (30-72) | Mean MEPS, 89<br>Mean extension, 31°<br>Mean flexion, 126° |
| Argintar et al (2012) | 10 | Latitude Total Elbow Prosthesis | 73.4 (56-77) | 12 (NA) | Mean MEPS, 77.2<br>Mean DASH score, 35.1<br>Mean extension, 22°<br>Mean flexion, 121° |

ASES = American Shoulder and Elbow Surgeons; DASH = Disabilities of the Arm, Shoulder and Hand; EQ-5D = EuroQol EQ-5D Health Questionnaire; MEPS = Mayo Elbow Performance Score; NA = not available; ROM = range of motion.

TEA has gained acceptance as a primary treatment for comminuted intra-articular distal humerus fractures in infirm, low-demand, elderly patients who have osteoporotic bone. However, the application of TEA in healthy, active patients increases the risk of early prosthesis failure.

## Results

The longest follow-up of DHH with a custom prosthesis is 20 years; the results of that study included good pain relief and functional ROM. The literature on DHH is limited to a few small case series (**Table 1**). One study involved 10 elbows that were managed with distal humeral anatomic spools without stems. Poor ROM and unstable implants were reported in five elbows with rheumatoid arthritis. Four of five elbows with posttraumatic lesions were pain free and had good functional ROM. A study on the use of capitellocondylar humeral

 

**Table 1** Results of Distal Humeral Hemiarthroplasty (DHH) (*continued*)

| Authors (Year) | Number of Prostheses | Prosthesis | Mean Patient Age in Years (Range) | Mean Follow-up in Months (Range) | Results |
|---|---|---|---|---|---|
| Smith and Hughes (2013) | 26 | Sorbie-Questor or Latitude Total Elbow Prosthesis | 60 (29-85) | 80 (25-133) | 17 patients were available for follow-up<br>Mean ASES scores: pain, 9.9; function, 25; satisfaction, 9.1<br>Mean MEPS, 90<br>Mean QuickDASH score, 19<br>Mean EQ-5D index, 0.84<br>Mean EQ-5D visual analog score, 80<br>Mean extension, 17°<br>Mean flexion, 133°<br>Chondral erosion associated with time since DHH |
| Hohman et al (2014) | 8 | Latitude Total Elbow Prosthesis | 64 (33-75) | 36 (26-60) | Mean MEPS, 80<br>Mean DASH score, 31<br>Mean extension, 19°<br>Mean flexion, 120° |

ASES = American Shoulder and Elbow Surgeons; DASH = Disabilities of the Arm, Shoulder and Hand; EQ-5D = EuroQol EQ-5D Health Questionnaire; MEPS = Mayo Elbow Performance Score; NA = not available; ROM = range of motion.

prostheses (nonanatomic) in patients who had rheumatoid arthritis reported variable results. A study on the use of the Sorbie-Questor prosthesis in four patients with acute trauma and four patients with chronic trauma reported a mean ROM from 22° to 126° and improved pain levels in all patients. Overall, pain relief was better after treatment in the acute period compared with treatment of chronic trauma.

Loss of articular cartilage in the sigmoid fossa and over the radial head may lead to incomplete pain relief, reduced function, and uncertain longevity. This is reflected in the experience of the author of this chapter, who reported that American Shoulder and Elbow Surgeons (ASES) elbow scores were better in patients treated acutely compared with patients who underwent delayed or salvage procedures.

In a 2013 study on the medium- and long-term outcomes of 26 patients who underwent DHH for the management of intra-articular distal humerus fractures and their sequelae, 4 patients died and 4 patients were revised to TEA. Of the four revisions, two were performed to address periprosthetic fractures and two to address primary component loosening (all in prostheses that did not have an anterior flange). Other complications included ulnar neuropathy in four patients, severe stiffness in one patient, and wound necrosis in one patient. Seventeen of the 26 patients were assessed at mean follow-up of 80 months. Postoperatively, the patients demonstrated a good functional arc and reported good function, good patient satisfaction, and very little pain. There was no evidence of instability postoperatively. Radiologic evidence of ulnar wear was observed in 13 patients and may have been at least partially related to prosthetic design. Worse wear was associated with a higher ASES elbow pain score, a lower ASES elbow satisfaction score, and a lower EuroQol EQ-5D Health Questionnaire visual analog scale score for quality of life. The degree of wear correlated with time after surgery but not with patient age at the time of surgery. A systematic review of 116 patients reported good or excellent results in 67% of the patients with fracture indications and 58% of the patients with nonfracture indications. Complications occurred in 27% of the patients with fracture indications and 32% of the patients with nonfracture indications.

## Techniques

### Setup/Exposure

- Timing of DHH in relation to acute trauma does not seem to be crucial given that DHH is undertaken within 7 to 10 days after injury. It may be more appropriate to transfer the patient to a center that has staff who are expert in managing elbow trauma and performing elbow arthroplasty and other fracture management techniques.
- In rare patients, soft-tissue constraints indicate that an immediate DHH is not appropriate; these patients may be treated with stabilization with an external fixator and delayed DHH (**Figure 4**).

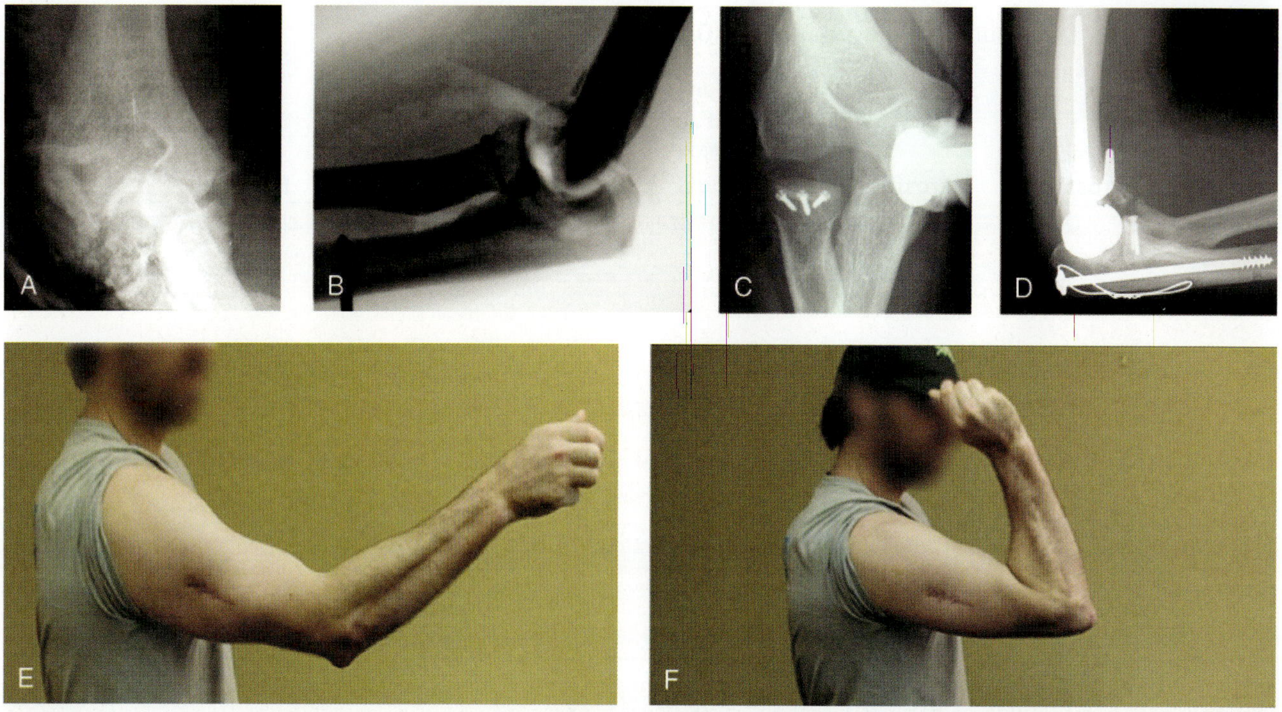


**Figure 4** Images of the elbow from a 26-year-old man who underwent stabilization with an external fixator and distal humeral hemiarthroplasty (DHH). **A,** AP radiograph demonstrates compound traumatic loss of the trochlea and capitellum, radial head fracture, and 10 cm of segmental radial nerve loss. Lateral (**B**) and AP (**C**) radiographs demonstrate immediate débridement and reduction out to length with an external fixator as well as open reduction and internal fixation of the radial head. **D,** Lateral radiograph demonstrates implantation of a Latitude EV Total Elbow Prosthesis (Tornier) via an olecranon osteotomy to preserve the collateral ligaments, which took place 3 months after skin coverage and healing of the radial head (lateral bony column). At 6 months postoperatively, the patient underwent tendon transfers to address the radial nerve deficit. **E** and **F,** Postoperative photographs show a functional arc of 30° to 120° with some restriction of forearm rotation as a result of heterotopic ossification of the radial neck.

- Often, only after a fracture is exposed can it be deemed irreparable. Thus, both ORIF implants and DHH prostheses should be available for patients who have severely comminuted fractures (**Figure 5, A**).
- The patient is placed in the lateral decubitus position, and the patient's arm is secured on an arm support (**Figure 5, B**).
- A tourniquet is applied as proximal as possible. This allows for free use of the image intensifier intraoperatively and adequate clearance for elbow flexion to 120°, which facilitates insertion of the component.
- The administration of parenteral antibiotics is routine; however, the author of this chapter also administers intravenous regional antibiotics in the surgical arm after exsanguination. The author of this chapter routinely administers prophylactic intravenous regional antibiotics; 1 g of cefazolin in 50 mL of sterile saline is suitable for most patients. If an alternative antibiotic is required, it must have no tissue toxicity. For example, vancomycin is not appropriate for DHH.
- Deep flaps are developed via a posterior incision to allow access to the epicondyles.
- A chevron osteotomy provides exposure for ORIF (if achievable) or DHH.
- The ulnar nerve is released and, usually, is transposed, especially if there is a fracture that involves the articular columns (**Figure 5, C**). This exposure preserves the collateral ligaments, which facilitates early mobilization (**Figure 5, D**).
- Triceps-on approaches are advantageous because they maintain the extensor mechanism; however, they result in reduced visualization of the articulation and make it difficult to balance the joint, which may increase the risk of instability.

## Instruments/Equipment/ Implants Required

- An external fixator is used.
- ORIF implants should be available.
- DHH prostheses should be available.
- A tourniquet is used.
- An image intensifier is used.
- Parenteral and regional antibiotics are administered.

 

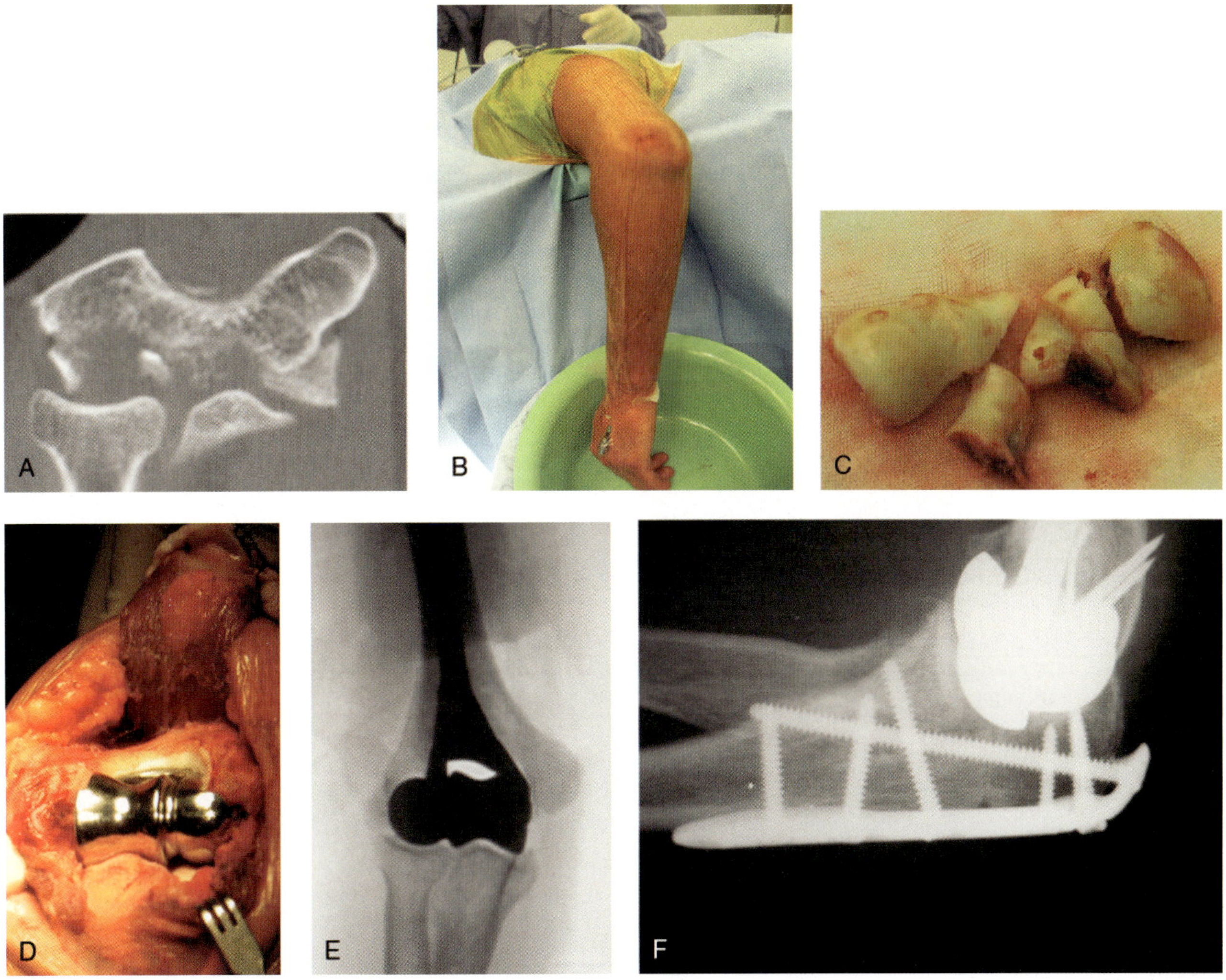


**Figure 5** Images from a 62-year-old woman who underwent distal humeral hemiarthroplasty after a fall. **A,** Preoperative CT scan of the elbow demonstrates a comminuted distal humerus fracture. **B,** Intraoperative photograph shows the patient placed in the lateral decubitus position with her arm supported to allow elbow flexion to 120°. **C,** Photograph shows a comminuted fracture of the distal articular joint that involved all of the lateral column and most of the medial column. **D,** Intraoperative photograph of the elbow shows that an olecranon osteotomy provides adequate exposure for insertion of the humeral component, leaves the collateral ligaments intact, and allows for intraoperative templating of the anatomic spools, which helps ensure selection of an appropriately sized spool. The axis of rotation of the component is aligned with a line that extends from the anteroinferior aspect of the medial epicondyle to the lateral epicondyle. **E,** AP radiograph demonstrates an implanted Latitude EV Total Elbow Prosthesis (Tornier) with accurate restoration of the joint axis and good joint congruency. **F,** Lateral radiograph demonstrates fixation of the olecranon osteotomy with an olecranon plate and cancellous bone graft. (Reproduced from Hughes JS, Parsons M: Distal humeral hemiarthroplasty, in Yamaguchi K, King GJ, McKee MD, O'Driscoll SW, eds: *Advanced Reconstruction: Elbow*. Rosemont, IL, American Academy of Orthopaedic Surgeons, 2007, pp 219-228.)

## Procedure

### ACUTE PATHOLOGY

- The triceps is reflected, and the articular segment is wrapped in saline-soaked gauze to protect the articular cartilage.
- The fracture is assessed, and if DHH is planned, the humerus is broached in preparation for stem insertion.
- If ORIF of a supracondylar column is required, a trial component or broach is left in situ to preserve the intramedullary canal for the prosthesis.
- Freehand bone cuts often are necessary to allow for appropriate placement of the prosthesis.
- Reconstruction of the bony columns and the collateral ligament origins is required when performing a DHH.
- Care is taken to maintain the joint axis. Periarticular plate systems may aid in maintaining the joint axis; however, the complexity of DHH increases substantially with each additional column reconstruction.

**Table 2** Complications of Distal Humeral Hemiarthroplasty

| Complication | Cause | Solution |
|---|---|---|
| Intraoperative flexion contracture | Oversized spool<br>Prosthetic axis distal to ligament axis<br>Capsular contracture | Check the preoperative template<br>Place the trial spool directly onto the radial head and coronoid<br>Insert the implant deeper<br>Release the anterior capsule |
| Joint translocation | Undertensioned collateral ligament repair<br>Overtensioned collateral ligament repair | Reassess ligament repair |
| Rotatory instability | Component malrotation<br>Incomplete restoration of columnar length<br>Failed LCL repair | Perform radiographic EUA<br>Address identifiable causes |
| Radiocapitellar mismatch | Incorrect spool size<br>PLRI | Revise the spool<br>Assess for instability |
| Olecranon osteotomy nonunion | Inadequate fixation<br>Inadequate biology | Ensure accurate reduction<br>Ensure rigid ORIF<br>Bone graft all osteotomies |
| Ulnar neuritis | Traumatic neurapraxia<br>Increased neural tension<br>Ulnar instability | Assess for neurolysis<br>Assess for transposition<br>Check depth of implant insertion and ulnar transposition |
| Painful joint | Overstuffed joint<br>Arthrolysis<br>Sepsis (*Staphylococcus epidermidis* or *Propionibacterium acnes*)<br>Loose prosthesis<br>Nonunion (condyle/osteotomy) | Downsize the spool<br>Revise to TEA<br>Obtain serology/aspirate/perform staged TEA<br>Obtain serology/aspirate/perform TEA<br>Obtain serology/perform ORIF with or without bone graft |
| Stiff elbow | Overstuffed joint<br>Arthrofibrosis<br>Heterotopic ossification | Downsize spool<br>Assess whether position of joint axis needs to be revised<br>Perform surgical release of the contracture at 6 months postoperatively |

EUA = examination under anesthesia, LCL = lateral collateral ligament, ORIF = open reduction and internal fixation, PLRI = posterolateral rotatory instability, TEA = total elbow arthroplasty.

As with comminuted supracondylar humerus fractures, some shortening may aid in obtaining stable fixation.

- The correct depth and rotation of implant insertion is determined by aligning the axis of the component with the origins of the medial collateral ligament (anteroinferior border of the medial epicondyle) and the humeral insertion points of the lateral collateral ligament (center of the lateral epicondyle).
- Varus-valgus alignment is determined by centering the prosthetic stem in the humeral canal with the aforementioned alignments correct. The correct depth, rotation, and valgus-varus orientation can be accurately restored in this manner.
- Preoperative templating helps determine implant selection. The Latitude EV Total Elbow Prosthesis does not allow for using large stems with small spools; therefore, a best fit is most likely determined by spool selection.
- Spool selection is verified intraoperatively by positioning the spool on the anterior sigmoid fossa and radial head, confirming that the center of the radial head aligns with the center of the capitellum and that there is good trochlear congruency (**Figure 5, E**).
- With the trial implant in situ, the elbow is moved through full elbow flexion and extension to ensure that the joint is not overstuffed as a result of an oversized spool or too-distal placement of the joint axis. If the joint demonstrates any tendency toward instability or translocation, the prosthesis is likely misaligned relative to the ligament attachments. The prosthesis is realigned accordingly, and the tracking of the articulation is rechecked (**Table 2**). A cement restrictor and antibiotic-impregnated cement are used to cement the component.

 

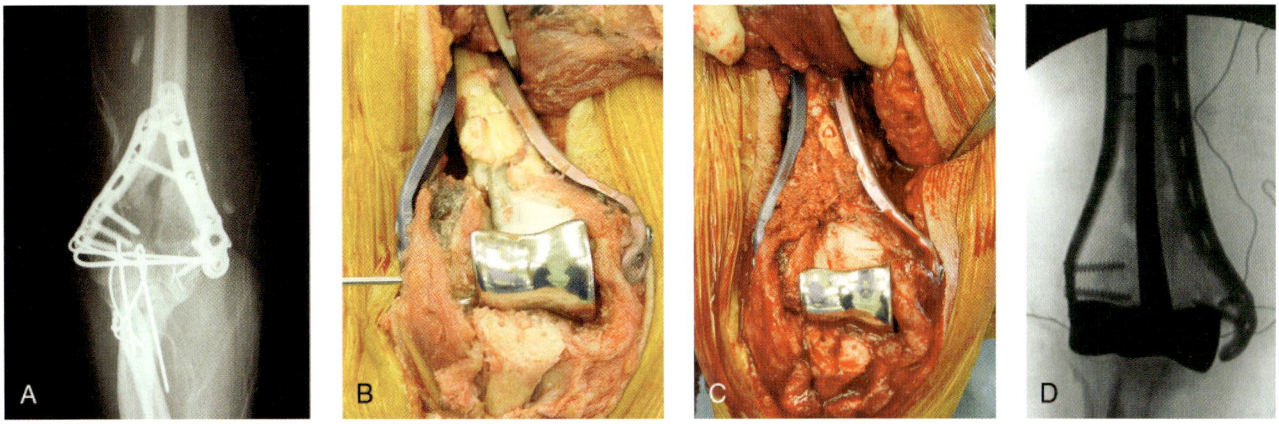


**Figure 6** Images of an elbow with distal humerus nonunion that was managed with distal humeral hemiarthroplasty. **A,** AP radiograph demonstrates an established nonunion of the distal humerus with complete loss of the articular surface of the lateral column. Intraoperative photographs (**B** and **C**) and fluoroscopic image (**D**) show column reconstruction with periarticular plates and autologous bone graft. (Panels B, C, and D reproduced from Hughes JS, Parsons M: Distal humeral hemiarthroplasty, in Yamaguchi K, King GJ, McKee MD, O'Driscoll SW, eds: *Advanced Reconstruction: Elbow*. Rosemont, IL, American Academy of Orthopaedic Surgeons, 2007, pp 219-228.)

- Occasionally, the anterior flange bone graft may be too thick, which can displace the axis of rotation too anteriorly. If this occurs, the bone graft should be reduced in size or placed after the stem is in situ and the cement has cured.
- The olecranon osteotomy is fixed with a strong tension-band wire construct or an olecranon plate, which is buried at the time that the extensor and flexor muscles are repaired. The medial and lateral aspects of the osteotomy are always grafted with cancellous bone to minimize the risk of osteotomy nonunion (**Figure 5, F**).
- Fixation and tracking of the DHH is assessed with the image intensifier before closure to ensure joint stability and that no screws enter the articulation. Full ROM also should be present.
- The ulnar nerve is inspected to confirm that it is stable and is not compressed when the arm is flexed. If the ulnar nerve is compromised, it is transposed.

#### NONACUTE PATHOLOGY

- DHH can be used to salvage malunion, nonunion (**Figure 6**), or tumor of the distal humerus in patients in whom major segments of the distal humeral articular surface cannot be preserved.
- To manage nonunion, a thorough surgical débridement is performed, and tissue is sent for culture and histopathology. If clinical parameters and surgical findings suggest infection, there is a low threshold to débride the wound, insert an antibiotic spacer, and wait for extended culture results.
- The principles of column reconstruction, joint axis restoration, and accurate component placement are the same as those for patients who have acute fractures.
- A shortening osteotomy and autologous bone grafting may be required.
- The use of a prosthesis with an anterior flange that is bone grafted is important to ensure long-term stem fixation, especially if complex column reconstructions are undertaken, because they may compromise metaphyseal fixation of the stem.
- Currently, no long-stem prosthetic options are available.

### Wound Closure

- The tourniquet is released and hemostasis is obtained.
- More recently, the author of this chapter has begun using vacuum dressings to minimize wound swelling and discharge.

## Postoperative Regimen

After adequate fixation is achieved, a protocol of elevation, ice application, compression, and passive ROM from 20° to 100° with the use of a self-guided program of flexion/extension stretches or a continuous passive motion machine is begun. Occasionally, if ORIF is inadequate to allow early ROM the elbow is immobilized for 1 month postoperatively before active, self-assisted stretching exercises are begun. Nighttime extension static splinting is used for patients who are at risk for flexion contracture. Active strengthening exercises are begun 4 to 6 weeks postoperatively, at which time union of the osteotomy should be progressing. Patients are advised to limit heavy or repetitive loads on the elbow and to avoid high-impact activities.

## Limiting Adverse Events

The most common adverse events after DHH are implant-related irritation, ulnar neuropathy, and elbow laxity. Less common early complications include fracture, inordinate pain or stiffness, infection, heterotopic ossification, implant loosening, weakness, posterolateral rotatory instability, and wound breakdown. Late complications include painful chondral wear, arthrosis of the sigmoid fossa or radial head, and implant loosening. Elbow instability, joint stiffness, and implant loosening may be related to surgical technique (**Table 2**). Loosening of the humeral stem is uncommon, especially in prostheses with an anterior flange that is bone grafted; however, periprosthetic fracture may be a precursor to implant loosening. Ulnar neuropathy has been identified as a complication in some patients; therefore, ulnar nerve transposition is currently performed more frequently than it was in the past.

Most revision surgeries are related to the removal of bothersome plates, screws, and wires; ulnar neuropathy; and stiffness, including heterotopic ossification. A medial trochlear osteophyte that seems to be caused by edge loading of the anatomic spool on the sigmoid fossa has developed in some patients. The implications of medial trochlear osteophytes are unclear.

## Acknowledgment

The author wishes to acknowledge John E. Farey, MBBS, who assisted in the writing and preparation of this chapter.

## Bibliography

Adolfsson L, Hammer R: Elbow hemiarthroplasty for acute reconstruction of intraarticular distal humerus fractures: A preliminary report involving 4 patients. *Acta Orthop* 2006;77(5):785-787.

Adolfsson L, Nestorson J: The Kudo humeral component as primary hemiarthroplasty in distal humeral fractures. *J Shoulder Elbow Surg* 2012;21(4):451-455.

Argintar E, Berry M, Narvy SJ, Kramer J, Omid R, Itamura JM: Hemiarthroplasty for the treatment of distal humerus fractures: Short-term clinical results. *Orthopedics* 2012;35(12):1042-1045.

Barr JS, Eaton RG: Elbow reconstruction with a new prosthesis to replace the distal end of the humerus: A case report. *J Bone Joint Surg Am* 1965;47(7):1408-1413.

Beckett KS, McConnell P, Lagopoulos M, Newman RJ: Variations in the normal anatomy of the collateral ligaments of the human elbow joint. *J Anat* 2000;197(pt 3):507-511.

Burkhart KJ, Nijs S, Mattyasovszky SG, et al: Distal humerus hemiarthroplasty of the elbow for comminuted distal humeral fractures in the elderly patient. *J Trauma* 2011;71(3):635-642.

Cobb TK, Morrey BF: Total elbow arthroplasty as primary treatment for distal humeral fractures in elderly patients. *J Bone Joint Surg Am* 1997;79(6):826-832.

Dunn J, Kusnezov N, Pirela-Cruz M: Distal humeral hemiarthroplasty: Indications, results, and complications. A systematic review. *Hand (N Y)* 2014;9(4):406-412.

Frankle MA, Herscovici D Jr, DiPasquale TG, Vasey MB, Sanders RW: A comparison of open reduction and internal fixation and primary total elbow arthroplasty in the treatment of intraarticular distal humerus fractures in women older than age 65. *J Orthop Trauma* 2003;17(7):473-480.

 

Gambirasio R, Riand N, Stern R, Hoffmeyer P: Total elbow replacement for complex fractures of the distal humerus: An option for the elderly patient. *J Bone Joint Surg Br* 2001;83(7):974-978.

Gramstad GD, King GJ, O'Driscoll SW, Yamaguchi K: Elbow arthroplasty using a convertible implant. *Tech Hand Up Extrem Surg* 2005;9(3):153-163.

Hohman DW, Nodzo SR, Qvick LM, Duquin TR, Paterson PP: Hemiarthroplasty of the distal humerus for acute and chronic complex intra-articular injuries. *J Shoulder Elbow Surg* 2014;23(2):265-272.

Lapner M, Willing R, Johnson JA, King GJ: The effect of distal humeral hemiarthroplasty on articular contact of the elbow. *Clin Biomech (Bristol, Avon)* 2014;29(5):537-544.

Macausland WR: Replacement of the lower end of the humerus with a prosthesis: A report of four cases. *West J Surg Obstet Gynecol* 1954;62(11):557-566.

Mellen RH, Phalen GS: Arthroplasty of the elbow by replacement of the distal portion of the humerus with an acrylic prosthesis. *J Bone Joint Surg Am* 1947;29(2):348-353.

Miller BS, Harper WP, Hughes JS, Sonnabend DH, Walsh WR: Regional antibiotic prophylaxis in elbow surgery. *J Shoulder Elbow Surg* 2004;13(1):57-59.

Parsons M, O'Brien RJ, Hughes JS: Elbow hemiarthroplasty for acute and salvage reconstruction of intra-articular distal humerus fractures. *Techniques in Shoulder & Elbow Surgery* 2005;6(2):87-97.

Ray PS, Kakarlapudi K, Rajsekhar C, Bhamra MS: Total elbow arthroplasty as primary treatment for distal humeral fractures in elderly patients. *Injury* 2000;31(9):687-692.

Shifrin PG, Johnson DP: Elbow hemiarthroplasty with 20-year follow-up study: A case report and literature review. *Clin Orthop Relat Res* 1990;(254):128-133.

Smith GC, Hughes JS: Unreconstructable acute distal humeral fractures and their sequelae treated with distal humeral hemiarthroplasty: A two-year to eleven-year follow-up. *J Shoulder Elbow Surg* 2013;22(12):1710-1723.

Street DM, Stevens PS: A humeral replacement prosthesis for the elbow: Results in ten elbows. *J Bone Joint Surg Am* 1974;56(6):1147-1158.

Swoboda B, Scott RD: Humeral hemiarthroplasty of the elbow joint in young patients with rheumatoid arthritis: A report on 7 arthroplasties. *J Arthroplasty* 1999;14(5):553-559.

Venable CS: An elbow and an elbow prosthesis: Case of complete loss of the lower third of the humerus. *Am J Surg* 1952;83(3):271-275.

# Chapter 16

# Radiocapitellar Prosthetic Arthroplasty

*Reid W. Draeger, MD*

**Learning Objectives**

- Learn appropriate indications and contraindications for radiocapitellar prosthetic arthroplasty.
- Become familiar with outcomes of radiocapitellar prosthetic arthroplasty from the limited number of published case studies.
- Learn the surgical steps necessary to perform radiocapitellar prosthetic arthroplasty, noting in particular certain key steps that help limit adverse events.

## Indications

Radiocapitellar prosthetic arthroplasty, although uncommonly performed, is an option for the management of isolated radiocapitellar degeneration in patients in whom radial head excision would be inadequate or would leave a too-unstable joint. In patients with an incompetent lateral collateral ligament (LCL) complex or chronic Essex-Lopresti lesions, radiocapitellar prosthetic arthroplasty helps to re-create normal elbow kinematics; however, the arthroplasty must be coupled with LCL repair or reconstruction, or with interosseous membrane reconstruction. Although radial head excision may be sufficient to manage isolated radiocapitellar degenerative arthritis and posttraumatic arthritis of the radiocapitellar joint, radiocapitellar prosthetic arthroplasty may be an alternative treatment option. Additionally, radiocapitellar prosthetic arthroplasty may be performed to manage lateral elbow joint damage in an elbow with an intact LCL complex or torn LCL complex that is reparable or reconstructible, if other management options fail. Malunited or nonunited capitellar fractures (especially those extending into the lateral trochlea) may be managed with radiocapitellar prosthetic arthroplasty if capitellar fracture fragment excision alone is insufficient.

## Contraindications

Radiocapitellar prosthetic arthroplasty is contraindicated in patients who have derangement of the elbow joint that extends out of the radiocapitellar joint into the ulnohumeral joint. In addition, radiocapitellar prosthetic arthroplasty is contraindicated in patients who have an active infection. The lateral elbow ligaments must be either intact, reparable, or reconstructible for the radiocapitellar prosthesis to be sufficiently stabilized after placement. Radiocapitellar prosthetic arthroplasty also is contraindicated in patients in whom the radial shaft and radial head are malaligned with the capitellum because the radial head component is unlikely to articulate correctly with the capitellar component.

## Alternative Treatments

Nonsurgical management for radiocapitellar prosthetic arthroplasty is sufficient for many patients and includes activity modification, therapy to maximize function, and adaptation. Alternative surgical treatments to radiocapitellar prosthetic arthroplasty include open or arthroscopic débridement, synovectomy, anconeus interposition arthroplasty, radial head excision, and capitellar excision. Careful review of a patient's physical examination and radiographs may help facilitate proper patient selection for radiocapitellar prosthetic arthroplasty. Pain at extreme elbow flexion and extension may indicate impinging osteophytes, which may be more effectively managed with the use of open or arthroscopic débridement rather than radiocapitellar prosthetic arthroplasty. Pain at rest may indicate synovitis, which may be more effectively managed with the use of synovectomy rather than radiocapitellar prosthetic arthroplasty. Pain throughout the arc of motion indicates damage to the articular surface. Patients

*Dr. Draeger or an immediate family member has stock or stock options held in GlaxoSmithKline.*

in whom damage to the articular surface is limited to the radiocapitellar joint may be effectively treated with radial head excision, capitellar excision, anconeus interposition arthroplasty, or radiocapitellar prosthetic arthroplasty. Both the radial head and capitellum contribute to elbow stability; therefore, they should be resected only in patients who have intact medial and lateral ulnar collateral ligaments. Radiocapitellar prosthetic arthroplasty and anconeus interposition arthroplasty should be considered if ligamentous instability in patients who have advanced radiocapitellar arthritis precludes radial head or capitellar excision. Anconeus interposition arthroplasty may offer some advantages over radiocapitellar prosthetic arthroplasty because it preserves native bone stock; however, radiocapitellar prosthetic arthroplasty has been reported to restore normal elbow kinematics, especially in patients who have an intact or repaired medial ulnar collateral ligament.

## Results

The few available studies on the outcomes of radiocapitellar prosthetic arthroplasty are case series that range from 3 to 43 patients and report general rather than short-term outcomes (the longest mean follow-up reported is just more than 7 years postoperatively; **Table 1**). Some patients underwent only capitellar resurfacing arthroplasty, and other patients underwent radiocapitellar prosthetic arthroplasty. Most patients who underwent radiocapitellar prosthetic arthroplasty had substantial improvements in Mayo Elbow Performance Scores, with most patients scoring excellent or good results. Few patients underwent revision surgery during the short evaluation periods. Higher-quality evidence is necessary to further validate radiocapitellar prosthetic arthroplasty as a reliable and favorable procedure; however, such evidence is difficult to obtain because radiocapitellar prosthetic arthroplasty is so rarely indicated.

**Video 16.1** Radiocapitellar Arthroplasty of the Elbow: Surgical Technique. Matthias Vanhees, MD; Frederik Verstreken, MD; Roger P. van Riet, MD, PhD (12 min)

## Techniques

### Setup/Exposure

- General anesthesia is typically used for radiocapitellar prosthetic arthroplasty because there may be patient discomfort with the use of a tourniquet if the patient is placed in the semilateral position with a beanbag placed under the ipsilateral shoulder.
- The patient is placed in either the semilateral or supine position.
- Semilateral positioning of the patient on a beanbag should allow the surgical extremity to rest across the chest without an assistant holding it in place. The shoulder should be positioned such that it is easily abducted for intraoperative fluoroscopic imaging.
- With the patient placed supine, use of a hand table may help in positioning the surgical extremity but may interfere with fluoroscopic imaging. Thus, use of a hand table is at the surgeon's discretion.
- A sterile tourniquet is placed high in the axilla and inflated.
- A 10-cm longitudinal incision centered over the lateral epicondyle is made between the tip of the olecranon and the lateral epicondyle (**Figure 1, A**).
- Using a scalpel, full-thickness skin flaps are sharply elevated off the deep fascia to expose the extensor musculature origin at the lateral epicondyle.
- The anterior and posterior margins of the radial head are palpated, and a longitudinal incision that extends from the lateral epicondyle to a point no farther than 2 cm distal to the radiocapitellar joint is made through the fascia to expose the radiocapitellar joint (**Figure 1, B**). This incision should be made with the patient's forearm in full pronation to distance the incision from the posterior interosseous nerve and should be made well anterior to the LCL complex, which is anterior to the Kocher interval between the anconeus and extensor carpi ulnaris muscles. The Kocher interval exposes the radiocapitellar joint too posteriorly and violates the LCL complex.
- Wide exposure is necessary to place both the capitellar and radial head components. A lateral epicondyle osteotomy allows for wide exposure of the entire radiocapitellar joint and avoids iatrogenic damage to the LCL complex. The lateral epicondyle osteotomy can be easily secured at the end of the procedure with the use of headless compression screws.

### Instruments/Equipment/Implants Required

- There are two implants currently available for radiocapitellar prosthetic arthroplasty: the UNI-Elbow Radio Capitellum System (Stryker; **Figure 2, A** and **B**) and the Lateral Resurfacing Elbow (Biomet; **Figure 2, C**). The technique discussed in this chapter pertains to the UNI-Elbow Radio Capitellum System because it is the only implant currently cleared by the FDA for radiocapitellar prosthetic arthroplasty in the United States.
- Cement is necessary for the capitellar component and should be available.

 

**Table 1** Results of Radiocapitellar Prosthetic Arthroplasty[a]

| Author(s) (Year) | No. of Patients | Procedure or Approach | Mean Patient Age in Years (Range) | Mean Follow-up in Months (Range) | Success Rate (%) | Results |
|---|---|---|---|---|---|---|
| Pooley (2007) | 43 (44 elbows) | 22 hemi-LRE arthroplasty (capitellar resurfacing only); 22 total LRE arthroplasty (capitellar resurfacing and radial head arthroplasty) | 52 (40-75) | 9 (9-18) | 95 | Results only reported for 10 patients<br>MEPS: 6 excellent results, 3 good results, and 1 fair result<br>2 patients had complications necessitating revision surgery: 1 deep infection leading to removal of components, 1 triceps muscle dehiscence requiring repair |
| Heijink et al (2008) | 3 | Custom radiocapitellar hemiarthroplasty (Stryker) with metallic capitellar resurfacing component and metal-backed polyethylene radial head prosthesis | 43 (37-50) | 87 (25-173) | 100 | MEPS: 2 excellent results and 1 good result<br>No further revision surgery procedures |
| Giannicola et al (2012) | 24[b] | 17 total LRE arthroplasty; 3 hemi-LRE arthroplasty (capitellum only) | 55 (31-73) | 23 (6-47) | 80 | 19 patients had good to excellent results, with significant improvement of MEPS, modified ASES scores, QuickDASH scores, and arc of motion ($P = 0.001$ for each measure)<br>16 patients were satisfied with their outcome, and 4 patients were unsatisfied with their outcome (3 with recurrent elbow stiffness and 1 with worsening of ulnar neuropathy)<br>3 patients underwent revision surgery (1 open elbow arthrolysis with HO excision, 1 soft-tissue release with HO excision, and 1 débridement with ulnar nerve neurolysis)<br>1 patient with Parkinson disease had a chronically dislocated prosthesis but refused further treatment |
| Heijink et al (2014) | 6 | UNI-Elbow Radio Capitellum arthroplasty (Stryker) | 52 (40-69) | 50 (30-64) | 100 | All patients had substantial improvement in MEPS (3 excellent results and 3 good results)<br>No implant failures<br>All patients were satisfied with their outcome at final follow-up |

ASES = American Shoulder and Elbow Surgeons elbow assessment; HO = heterotopic ossification; LRE = Lateral Resurfacing Elbow (Biomet); MEPS = Mayo Elbow Performance Score; QuickDASH = Quick Disabilities of the Arm, Shoulder and Hand.

[a] All studies are level IV evidence.

[b] 20 patients were available for follow-up.

 

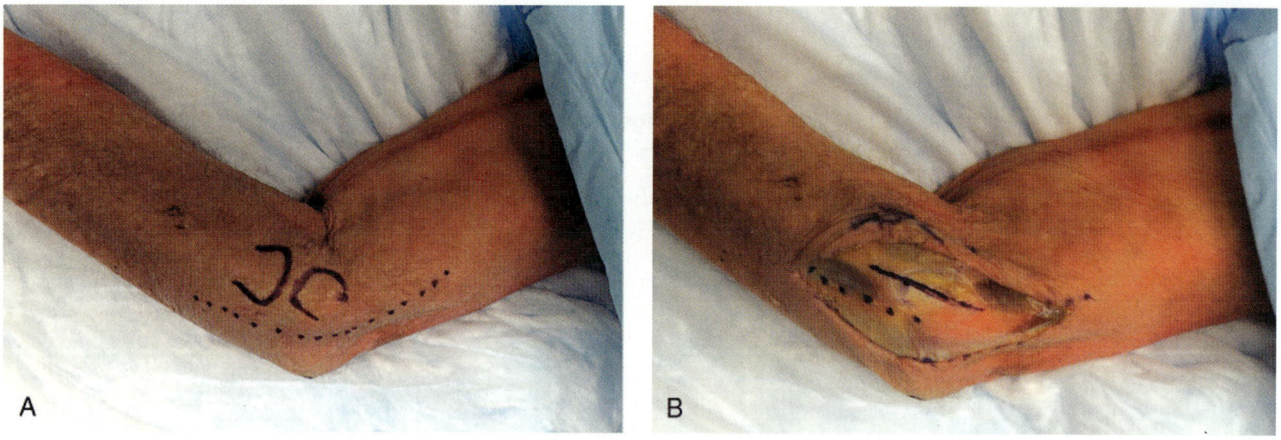


**Figure 1** Clinical photographs of the elbow of a cadaver model show the proposed incisions for radiocapitellar prosthetic arthroplasty. **A,** The lateral incision is a Kocher-type skin incision with proximal extension along the lateral column of the distal humerus. The radial head and capitellum are marked. **B,** The fascial incision, which is used to approach the radiocapitellar joint, is made by palpating the anterior and posterior margins of the radial head and making a longitudinal incision that bisects these points and is centered over the radiocapitellar articulation. The exposure of Kaplan (solid line) splits the extensors longitudinally. The more posterior Kocher interval between the anconeus and extensor carpi ulnaris (dotted line) is not selected because it affords less access to the anterior radiocapitellar joint and violates the lateral collateral ligament complex.

- Standard fluoroscopy is useful for multiple steps of the procedure, including establishing the center of rotation of the distal humerus and verifying placement of the prosthesis.
- Standard instruments for elbow procedures, including large rake retractors, self-retaining retractors, and narrow Richardson retractors to help with exposure, are helpful for radiocapitellar prosthetic arthroplasty.
- A microsagittal saw and sharp, narrow osteotomes should be available for the lateral epicondyle osteotomy.
- Small headless compression screws should be available for fixation of the lateral epicondyle osteotomy.

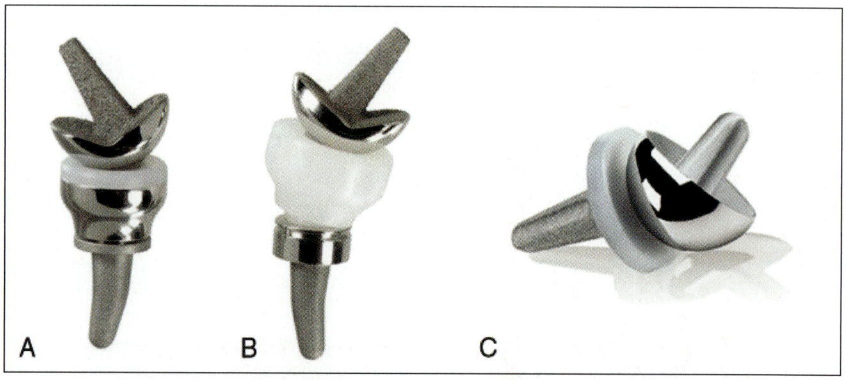


**Figure 2** Photographs show available implants for radiocapitellar prosthetic arthroplasty. **A** and **B,** The UNI-Elbow Radio Capitellum System (Stryker) is the only implant currently cleared for radiocapitellar prosthetic arthroplasty in the United States. **C,** The Lateral Resurfacing Elbow (Biomet) is available for radiocapitellar prosthetic arthroplasty outside of the United States. (Panels A and B copyright Stryker Corporation, Kalamazoo, MI, and panel C reproduced with permission from Zimmer Biomet, Warsaw, IN.)

## Procedure

- The radiocapitellar joint is entered via a more anterolateral elbow (Kaplan) exposure, which splits the extensor musculature and exposes the radial head to the neck.
- Proximal dissection is carried up the lateral column, which allows for visualization of the anterior joint.
- To gain full access to both the posterior and anterior aspects of the radiocapitellar joint, a lateral epicondyle osteotomy is performed with a microsagittal saw and completed with an osteotome. The site of the lateral epicondyle osteotomy is illustrated in **Figure 3, A**.
- A transverse, axial counter-cut is made just proximal to the lateral epicondyle. The osteotomy is performed distally in a longitudinal direction with the use of a longitudinal saw cut in the coronal plane; this axial counter-cut is made just medial to the prominence of the lateral epicondyle but does not violate the articular cartilage of the capitellum and proceeds in an anterior-to-posterior fashion. The counter-cut prevents fracture or propagation of the osteotomy site proximally.
- To complete the osteotomy, the longitudinal saw cut can be taken

 

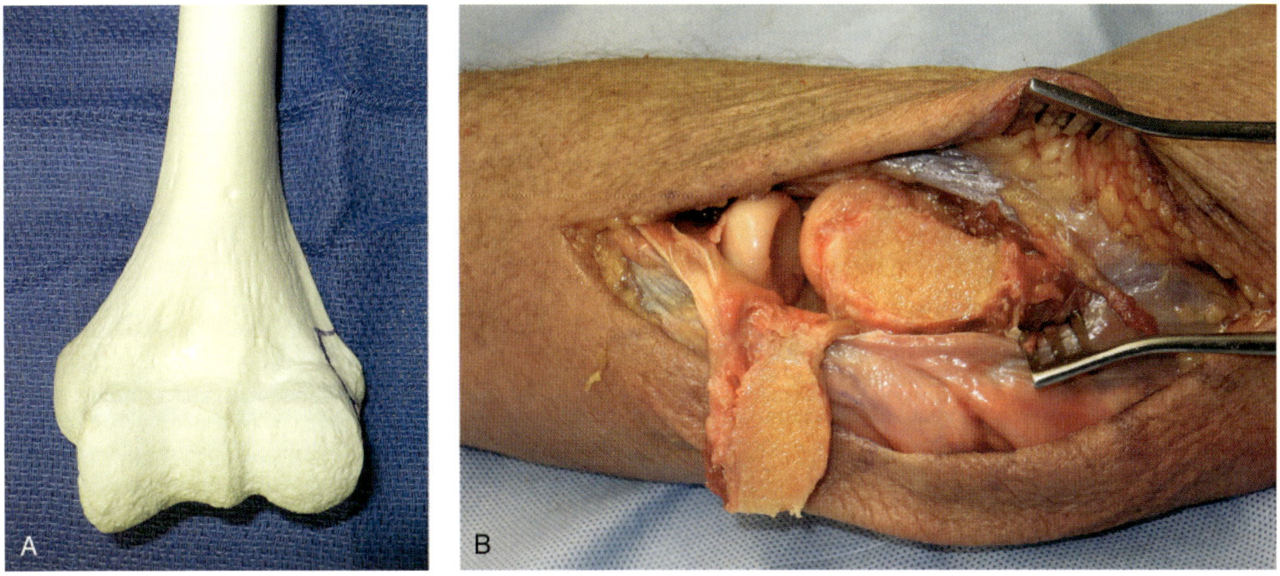


**Figure 3** **A,** Photograph of the distal humerus of a bone model shows the site for a lateral epicondyle osteotomy. **B,** Intraoperative photograph of the elbow of a cadaver model shows a lateral epicondyle osteotomy, which results in wide exposure of both the anterior and posterior aspects of the radiocapitellar joint.

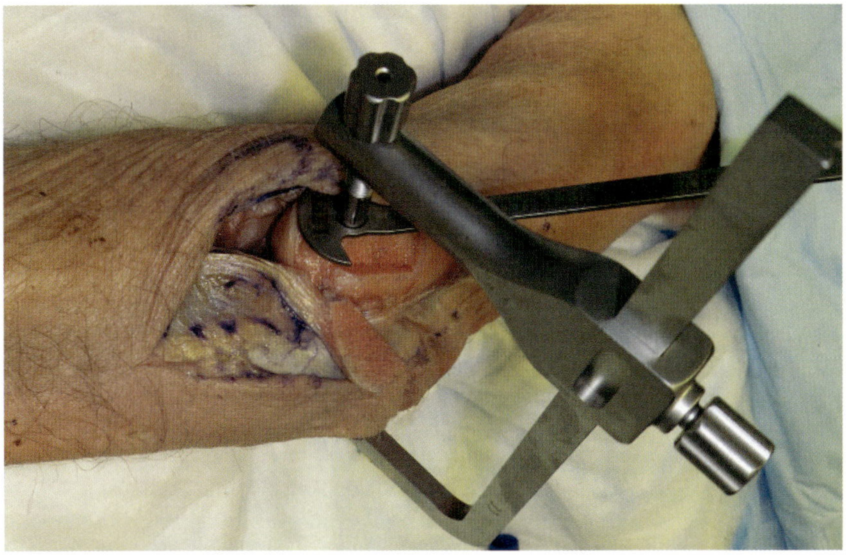

**Figure 4** Intraoperative photograph of the elbow of a cadaver model shows correct placement of a capitellar centering guide. The drill guide is tightened in place after the capitellar centering guide is situated in the correct position and a guidewire has been driven through the lateral aspect of the capitellum at its center of rotation but not through the medial cortex of the distal humerus.

straight posteriorly until it exits the lateral distal humerus, or a posterior longitudinal counter-cut can be made in the coronal plane posterior to the origin of the LCL complex (**Figure 3, B**).

- Alternatively, the LCL can be taken down from its origin at the lateral epicondyle and repaired later through bone tunnels or with the use of suture anchors. A lateral epicondyle osteotomy may help provide more reliable tensioning and better healing of the repaired LCL.
- The center of rotation of the capitellum is established by placing a Kirschner wire (K-wire) through the capitellum, which can be done with the aid of a capitellar centering guide (**Figure 4**). The medial targeting arm of the capitellar centering guide is placed over the medial epicondyle, and the lateral part of the capitellar centering guide is placed on the lateral aspect of the capitellum and positioned to mirror its curvature. The geometry of the nondiseased capitellum must be taken into consideration when placing the capitellar centering guide because advanced degenerative changes can substantially distort the geometry of the capitellum.
- A K-wire is placed through the capitellar centering guide. Placement of the K-wire in the center of rotation of the distal humerus is confirmed via multiplanar fluoroscopic imaging.

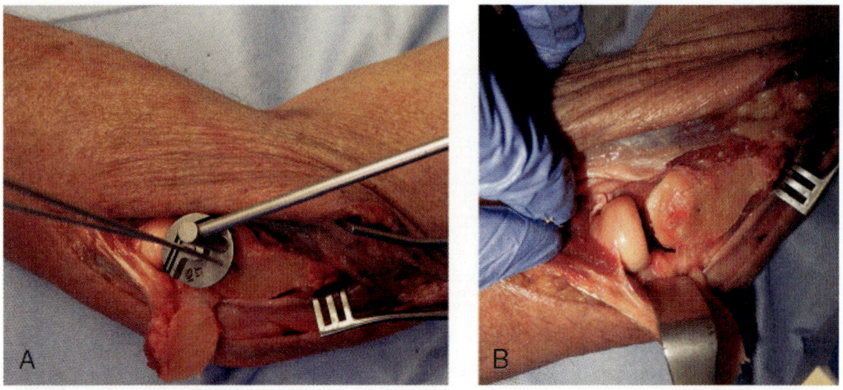


**Figure 5** Intraoperative photographs of the elbow of a cadaver model show capitellar resection. **A,** A capitellar cutting guide is placed over the center-of-rotation guidewire and oriented so that the handle of the capitellar cutting guide is in line with the humeral shaft. The capitellar cutting guide is secured with an additional oblique Kirschner wire before the cuts are made. **B,** Only a small amount of subchondral bone has been removed with the cuts, which creates a chevron-shaped cut surface on the capitellum.

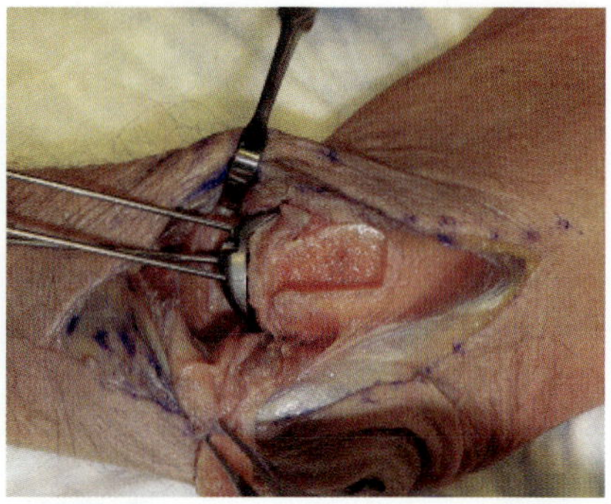

**Figure 6** Intraoperative photograph of the elbow of a cadaver model shows placement of a capitellar trial, which is secured with two oblique guidewires and one central guidewire that is directed up the intramedullary canal of the humerus to guide reaming and broaching for the stem of the implant.

- Alternatively, the guidewire may be placed freehand with the use of fluoroscopic imaging or an anterior cruciate ligament (ACL) targeting guide. If an ACL targeting guide is used, the surgeon should be mindful of the ulnar nerve during placement of the medial anchor point of the ACL targeting guide.
- To place the appropriate cuts for the implant, a capitellar cutting guide is placed over the guidewire, and the handle of the capitellar cutting guide is aligned with the humeral shaft (**Figure 5, A**).
- Capitellar cutting guides are available in multiple sizes. The surgeon should select the one that most closely matches the patient's capitellum.
- Although each capitellar cutting guide has two cutting surfaces, the distal cutting surface affords sufficient bone removal for capitellar implant placement in most patients.
- The anterior joint capsule is retracted, and a sagittal counter-cut is made at the medial aspect of the capitellum with the use of a microsagittal saw to prevent propagation of the distal capitellar cuts into the trochlea.

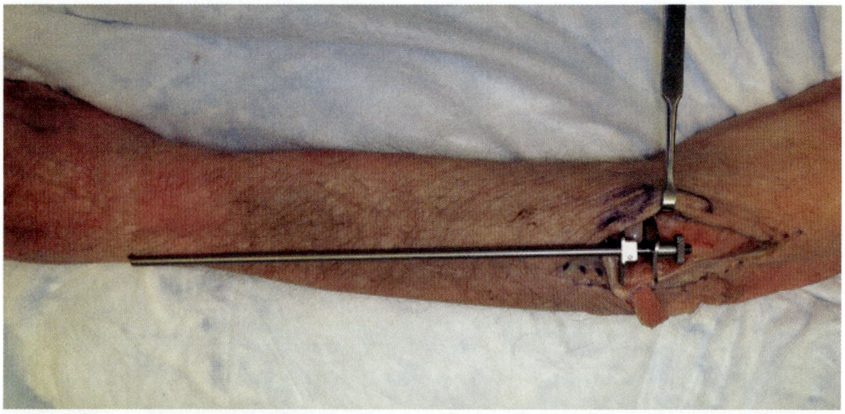

**Figure 7** Intraoperative photograph of the forearm of a cadaver model shows correct placement of a radial head cutting guide. The radial head cutting guide is placed in the radiocapitellar joint, and the guide rod is pointed toward the ulnar styloid.

- The distal capitellar cuts are made from lateral to medial in the chosen slots, terminating at the medial capitellar counter-cut (**Figure 5, B**).
- The cut capitellar bone is excised, and an appropriately sized capitellar trial implant is placed. At the time of final implant placement, cement will act as a grout to fill in any gaps at the cut surface. If the cut surface is oblique and the trial toggles, freehand freshening of the cuts may be necessary.
- The capitellar trial is secured with up to three diverging K-wires. The medial-most, central guidewire is directed up the axis of the distal humerus (**Figure 6**).
- All the K-wires except the medial-most central K-wire are removed, and the capitellar trial is extracted by sliding it over the central guidewire. Fluoroscopic imaging of the guidewire can help ensure its central location in the capitellum and that sufficient bone stock is present both anteriorly and posteriorly.
- A cannulated drill is used over the central guidewire to ream a hole for the stem of the capitellar prosthesis.

 

The drill should be inserted to, but not through, the posterior cortex of the humerus.

- A cannulated rasp is oriented with the outrigger pointed directly lateral and aligned with the point of the chevron capitellar cut. Fluoroscopic imaging can confirm the presence of anterior and posterior bone stock about the rasp.
- The radius is prepared for radial head arthroplasty before placement of the final capitellar implant.
- A radial head cutting guide is placed into the radiocapitellar joint and positioned with the proximal paddle flush with the radial head. The guide rod is aligned with the ulnar styloid to identify the axis of rotation of the forearm and to guide the radial neck cut, which is made perpendicular to the axis of rotation of the forearm to allow for proper mating of the radial head and capitellar arthroplasty components (**Figure 7**).
- The cut is made along the distal aspect of the collar of the radial head cutting guide.
- Radial head resection allows for additional exposure and working room about the capitellum; therefore, it can be performed before the capitellum is addressed.
- The resected radial head is measured to determine sizing for the implant. The implant is sized based on the diameter of the concave surface of the radial head.
- If the concave surface of the resected radial head measures between two implant sizes, the surgeon should select the smaller radial head implant to avoid overstuffing the joint.
- The radial neck is broached with successively larger broaches.
- The surgeon should begin with the smallest broach and upsize the broach until it fits snugly in the radial canal.

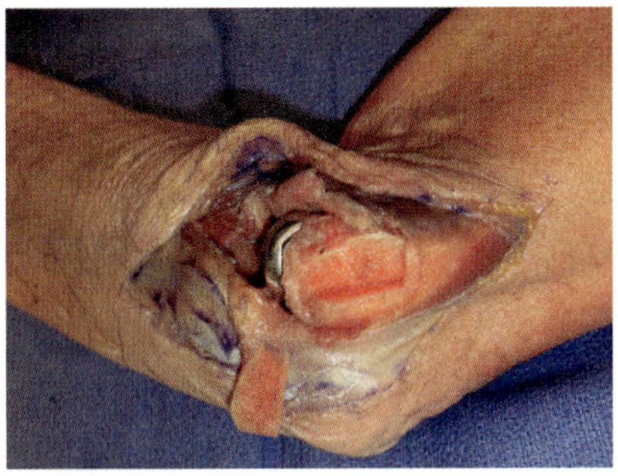

**Figure 8** Intraoperative photograph of the elbow of a cadaver model shows final placement of a capitellar implant. No cement was used in this example; however, the use of cement on the baseplate (not the stem) of the capitellar prosthesis is recommended for additional fixation.

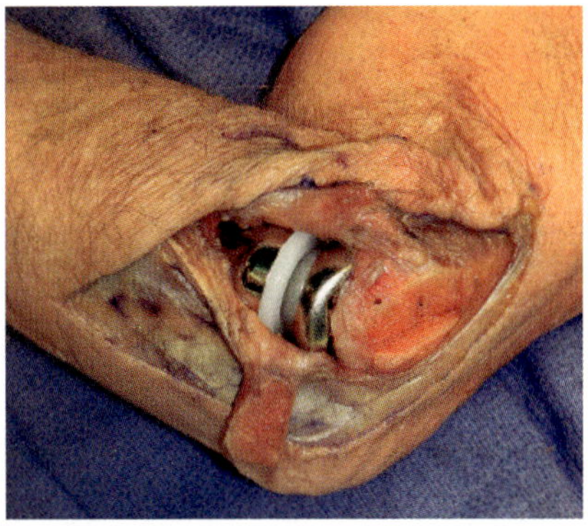

**Figure 9** Intraoperative photograph of the elbow of a cadaver model shows final placement of radial head and capitellar prostheses. Stability of the prostheses is evaluated with the elbow in pronation, supination, flexion, and extension.

- The appropriate-size capitellar component is selected.
- Cement is mixed and placed on the baseplate of the prosthesis. Often, cement is not needed in the intramedullary canal along the stem unless poor bone stock is encountered.
- The capitellar implant is placed in the hole that was broached for the stem and impacted into place with an impactor (**Figure 8**).
- Excess cement is removed from around the capitellar prosthesis, and the cement is allowed to harden.
- A trial stem that is one size smaller than that for which was broached is selected and assembled to a trial radial head. This trial component is inserted into the radial neck, and the articulation is tested with the final capitellar component to confirm adequate articulation of the components in elbow flexion, extension, pronation, and supination.
- A nonabrasive barrier such as a sponge should be placed between the metallic radial head trial and the metallic capitellar implant to prevent scratching.
- Fluoroscopic images can be obtained during trialing of the radial head component to evaluate the ulnohumeral articulation, ensure that the joint space appears symmetric both medially and laterally, and ensure that the selected radial head implant does not overstuff the joint.
- The use of cement for the radial head prosthesis is at the discretion of the surgeon. The radial head prosthesis described in this chapter is designed for press-fit applications, and cement is rarely needed to secure the prosthesis.
- An appropriately sized radial head implant designed for use with a capitellar implant (polyethylene articulation on a cobalt-chrome baseplate and stem) is selected, assembled on the back table, and impacted into the canal (**Figure 9**).
- The radiocapitellar joint is reduced, and joint stability is assessed in flexion, extension, pronation, and supination.

## Wound Closure

- The lateral epicondyle osteotomy is carefully rotated back into alignment and held in a reduced position with the use of two K-wires, which provides substantial provisional stability to the arthroplasty. The joint is taken through a range of

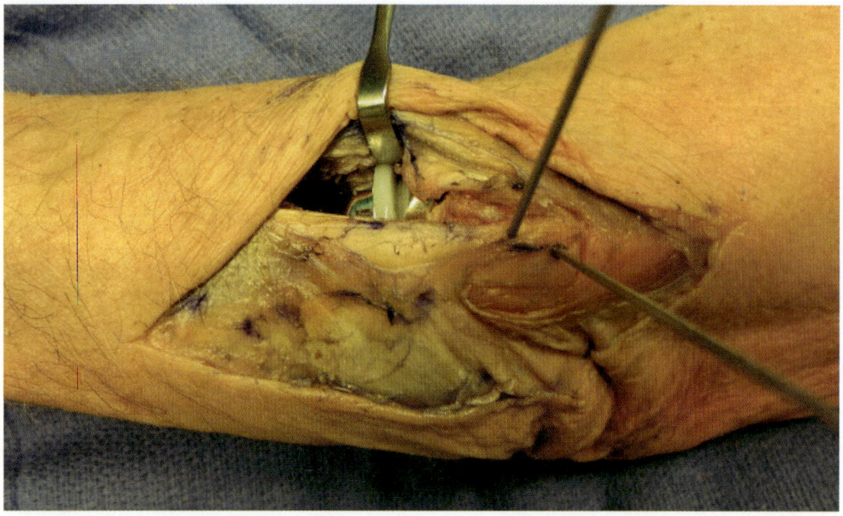

**Figure 10** Intraoperative photograph of the elbow of a cadaver model shows provisional fixation of a lateral epicondyle osteotomy with the use of two Kirschner wires. This fixation reattaches the lateral collateral ligament complex at the appropriate tension and location and provides substantial stability to the radiocapitellar joint.

motion with the osteotomy provisionally fixed to ensure stability in flexion, extension, pronation, and supination (**Figure 10**).

- The lateral epicondyle osteotomy can be fixed in multiple ways, including with cannulated headless compression screws, noncannulated screws, or cerclage wire. Headless compression screws can be placed over the guidewires that are used for provisional fixation of the osteotomy and can be advanced until they are not prominent laterally, which minimizes hardware irritation.
- The tourniquet is released, and meticulous hemostasis is attained with the use of electrocautery. The use of a drain is dictated by the amount of hemorrhage in the surgical field. If in doubt, the surgeon should use a drain because hematoma, seroma, and hemarthrosis formation can greatly contribute to stiffness at the elbow joint.
- The split in the extensor fascia is closed with the use of absorbable suture. The deep dermal layer is closed with the use of absorbable suture. The skin is closed with the use of nonabsorbable monofilament suture.

## Postoperative Regimen

A postoperative supraclavicular block with a nerve catheter may help control postoperative pain. The author of this chapter prefers to assess the patient's postoperative neurovascular status before supraclavicular block placement. The author of this chapter prefers to splint the elbow in extension for 48 to 72 hours postoperatively to help prevent a flexion contracture. A compressive sleeve and strict elevation helps lessen postoperative edema and, consequently, limits postoperative stiffness. The elbow splint is removed 48 to 72 hours postoperatively, at which time early active and active therapist-assisted range of motion is initiated under the guidance of an occupational therapist. Flexion and extension in full pronation help minimize stress on the LCL. Pronation and supination with the elbow held in 90° of flexion also are encouraged to help minimize stress on the LCL. A resting thermoplastic splint that holds the elbow in a comfortable resting position is fabricated and worn at night and between active and active-assisted range-of-motion exercises, which are performed multiple times per day. Elbow motion with the shoulder abducted should be avoided in the early postoperative period because it places obligate varus stress on the elbow and LCL.

## Limiting Adverse Events

To avoid damage to the lateral ulnar collateral ligament, the surgeon should enter the radiocapitellar joint via a more anterior (Kaplan) exposure, which splits the extensor musculature and adequately exposes the radiocapitellar joint for the lateral epicondyle osteotomy. Damage to the lateral ulnar collateral ligament that is not addressed during radiocapitellar prosthetic arthroplasty can lead to instability and failure. The surgeon should split the extensor musculature to a point no further than 2 cm distal to the radiocapitellar joint. This incision should be made with the patient's forearm in full pronation to minimize risk to the posterior interosseous nerve.

A lateral epicondyle osteotomy helps ensure wide exposure of the entire radiocapitellar joint and allows for reliable reattachment of the lateral ulnar collateral ligament at the end of the procedure. Radial head resection allows for additional exposure of the radiocapitellar joint, which facilitates instrumentation of the capitellum.

Accurate determination of the center of rotation of the capitellum is critical to ensure proper placement of the capitellar cuts and ultimate capitellar prosthesis placement. A capitellar centering guide or other targeting guide should be used to accurately locate the center of rotation of the capitellum. The center of rotation of the capitellum should be confirmed with the use of multiplanar fluoroscopic imaging because deformity can make the use of guides less reliable.

The surgeon should make a sagittal counter-cut at the medial border of the capitellum with either a microsagittal saw or osteotome to help prevent propagation of the capitellar cuts into the trochlea. The posterior cortex of the humerus should not be violated with either the cannulated drill or the capitellar broaches during preparation of the humerus for the capitellar implant.

Trialing of the radial head with the final capitellar component is important and allows for adjustment of the radial head prosthesis so that it maintains appropriate articulation with the ulnohumeral joint. If gapping at the ulnohumeral joint is noticed during radial head trialing, the radial head component should be further recessed and additional radial neck resection may be necessary. Gapping noted at the radiocapitellar joint during trialing may indicate that the capitellar component is recessed and the radial head component should be placed proud.

## Bibliography


Baghdadi YM, Morrey BF, Sanchez-Sotelo J: Anconeus interposition arthroplasty: Mid- to long-term results. *Clin Orthop Relat Res* 2014;472(7):2151-2161.

Giannicola G, Angeloni R, Mantovani A, et al: Open debridement and radiocapitellar replacement in primary and post-traumatic arthritis of the elbow: A multicenter study. *J Shoulder Elbow Surg* 2012;21(4):456-463.

Giannicola G, Sacchetti FM, Antonietti G, Piccioli A, Postacchini R, Cinotti G: Radial head, radiocapitellar and total elbow arthroplasties: A review of recent literature. *Injury* 2014;45(2):428-436.

Heijink A, Morrey BF, Cooney WP III: Radiocapitellar hemiarthroplasty for radiocapitellar arthritis: A report of three cases. *J Shoulder Elbow Surg* 2008;17(2):e12-e15.

Heijink A, Morrey BF, Eygendaal D: Radiocapitellar prosthetic arthroplasty: A report of 6 cases and review of the literature. *J Shoulder Elbow Surg* 2014;23(6):843-849.

Kelly EW, Bryce R, Coghlan J, Bell S: Arthroscopic debridement without radial head excision of the osteoarthritic elbow. *Arthroscopy* 2007;23(2):151-156.

McLaughlin RE II, Savoie FH III, Field LD, Ramsey JR: Arthroscopic treatment of the arthritic elbow due to primary radiocapitellar arthritis. *Arthroscopy* 2006;22(1):63-69.

Morrey BF, Schneeberger AG: Anconeus arthroplasty: A new technique for reconstruction of the radiocapitellar and/or proximal radioulnar joint. *J Bone Joint Surg Am* 2002;84(11):1960-1969.

Pooley J: Unicompartmental elbow replacement: Development of a lateral replacement elbow (LRE) arthroplasty. *Techniques in Shoulder & Elbow Surgery* 2007;8(4):204-212.

Sabo MT, Shannon H, De Luce S, et al: Elbow kinematics after radiocapitellar arthroplasty. *J Hand Surg Am* 2012;37(5):1024-1032.


## Video Reference


Vanhees M, Verstreken F, van Riet RP: Video. *Radiocapitellar Arthroplasty of the Elbow: Surgical Technique*. Antwerp, Belgium, 2015.

# Chapter 17

# Unlinked Total Elbow Arthroplasty

*Jonah Hebert-Davies, MD, FRCSC*
*Graham J.W. King, MD, MSc, FRCSC*
*Shawn William O'Driscoll, MD, PhD*
*Ken Yamaguchi, MD, MBA*

**Learning Objectives**

- Understand native elbow stability and problems with standard elbow arthroplasty.
- Understand the history and reasons for previous failures with unlinked total elbow implants.
- Review surgical techniques to perform an unlinked total elbow arthroplasty.

## Indications

Historically, total elbow arthroplasty (TEA) was used to manage elbow degeneration in patients with low physical demands and who had rheumatoid arthritis. The advent of linked TEA expanded the indications for TEA to include patients who require posttraumatic reconstruction. As the indications for TEA expand to include healthier, more active patients, more durable implants are necessary. Unlinked TEA has the theoretical advantage of increasing soft-tissue load bearing, which helps protect the implant-bone interface and may slow bearing wear and stem loosening.

The requirements for unlinked TEA include competency of both collateral ligaments and the dynamic stabilizers (elbow flexors and extensors) as well as preservation of the bony attachments of the ligaments. The radiocapitellar joint bears some of the load of the ulnohumeral joint, increases stability, and allows for balanced soft-tissue tension throughout the entire arc of elbow motion. Balanced loading of the ulnohumeral joint via adequate radiocapitellar alignment and intact muscle stabilizers may decrease stress on the ulnohumeral components, potentially reducing wear. Failure to restore radiocapitellar contact results in altered force vectors from the triceps and brachialis muscles and increases the risk of maltracking and instability.

A necessary prerequisite for unlinked TEA is the presence of intact brachialis and triceps muscle-tendon units. A preoperative assessment should focus on the clinical and radiologic evaluation of the disease, with particular attention given to articular alignment. If the native radial head cannot be retained and replacement is deemed impossible, the surgeon should be prepared to perform linked TEA. Severe bony deformity around the elbow may compromise inherent joint stability, thereby preventing the use of an unlinked TEA implant. Although TEA for the management of severe intra-articular distal humerus fractures has become common, the successful use of an unlinked implant may be difficult. Unlinked TEA is typically performed in younger patients with higher activity demands because of the relative success of linked TEA implants in older patients.

Many surgeons believe that unlinked TEA may be a better option for healthy, active patients because of the theoretical potential for longer implant survival. Currently, TEA with semiconstrained or older unconstrained implants in younger patients is associated with early aseptic loosening and accelerated wear. A recent review of the Norwegian

*Dr. King or an immediate family member has received royalties from and serves as a paid consultant to Wright Medical Technology and Tornier. Dr. O'Driscoll or an immediate family member has received royalties from Acumed, Tornier, and Aircast (DJO Global); is a member of a speakers' bureau or has made paid presentations on behalf of and serves as a paid consultant to Tornier; serves as an unpaid consultant to Acumed; and has received research or institutional support from Acumed and Tornier. Dr. Yamaguchi or an immediate family member has received royalties from Tornier and Zimmer Biomet. Neither Dr. Hebert-Davies nor any immediate family member has received anything of value from or has stock or stock options held in a commercial company or institution related directly or indirectly to the subject of this chapter.*

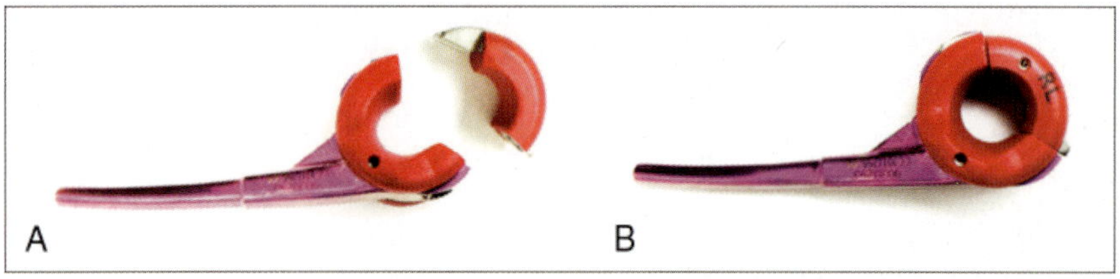


**Figure 1** Photographs of the Latitude EV Total Elbow Prosthesis (Tornier). The ulnar component is next to the linking cap, which is inserted and secured with a screw. Photographs show the ulnar component without the cap (unlinked; **A**) and the component "linked" around the humeral component (not shown; **B**).

Arthroplasty Register reported that patients who underwent TEA for the treatment of posttraumatic arthritis had a higher risk of early failure, regardless of TEA implant type.

Strict activity limitations are advised for all TEA implant designs. Conversely, most patients are unable or unwilling to fully comply with the recommended TEA postoperative limitations. The authors of this chapter advise patients to avoid stress on the elbow postoperatively, particularly varus stresses that are experienced during tasks such as lifting a container of milk out of the refrigerator.

Despite an adequate preoperative evaluation, insufficient intraoperative stability may be discovered in a patient who undergoes unlinked TEA. For this reason, the authors of this chapter recommend the use of a convertible TEA prosthesis (**Figure 1**). Alternatively, a surgeon can have two separate implant systems available during surgery.

## Contraindications

Absolute contraindications for unlinked TEA include ongoing local or systemic infection, insufficient soft-tissue coverage, gross instability, severely deficient bone stock, and deficient triceps or brachialis muscles. Relative contraindications for unlinked TEA include preoperative elbow instability, an inability to retain or restore the radiocapitellar joint, humeral epicondyle bone loss, and neuropathic destruction of the elbow. Previously infected elbows are evaluated preoperatively to rule out persistent infection. If any doubt remains, cultures are obtained intraoperatively and a one- or two-stage procedure is performed depending on the probability of persistent infection.

## Alternative Treatments

Alternative treatments for patients who have mild to moderate elbow arthritis include nonsurgical treatment, arthroscopic or open osteocapsular arthroplasty, and synovectomy. Interposition arthroplasty can be considered in younger patients; however, the results of interposition arthroplasty vary widely. Although elbow arthrodesis is an option, it is a disabling procedure and should be reserved only for patients in whom TEA is unacceptable but who require some form of treatment.

## Results

The complex anatomy and biomechanics of the elbow has led to challenges in the development of optimal TEA implant designs. As a result, many TEA implant designs have been developed, modified, and released in several iterations, making the comparison of outcomes extremely complicated. Furthermore, many TEA implants for which outcomes data have been published are no longer available for clinical use. The Capitellocondylar implant (Johnson & Johnson), the Souter-Strathclyde Elbow Replacement (Stryker), and the Kudo Elbow Replacement (Biomet; now the Instrumented Bone Preserving Elbow System [Biomet]) all had varying levels of success. Of these, only the Instrumented Bone Preserving Elbow System remains commercially available. The early Kudo Elbow Replacement implants were stemless and developed proximal subsidence in as many as 70% of patients, leading to early loosening and periprosthetic fractures. Improved results were reported with subsequent Kudo Elbow Replacement designs that incorporated stemmed components. Only two convertible linked/unlinked TEA implants have been developed: the Acclaim Total Elbow System (DePuy), which is no longer commercially available, and the Latitude EV Total Elbow Prosthesis (Tornier), which is discussed later (**Figure 2**).

The current literature on unlinked TEA consists of retrospective case series and joint registry results (**Table 1**). There are no current randomized trials comparing linked and unlinked TEA implants or unlinked devices with other unlinked devices. Overall outcomes of unlinked TEA are comparable with those of linked TEA. The revision surgery rate in some case series and joint registries is higher for some unlinked TEA implants, which may be caused by the higher demand younger patients place on these implants and the technical complexity of these implants compared with previous unlinked implants. In addition, patients who undergo TEA for the management of posttraumatic arthritis have inferior outcomes compared with patients with inflammatory arthritis who undergo TEA, even with linked implants (**Figure 3**). Furthermore, many revision surgeries for unlinked TEA are performed to manage postoperative instability, which, in the experience of the authors of this chapter, is uncommon

 

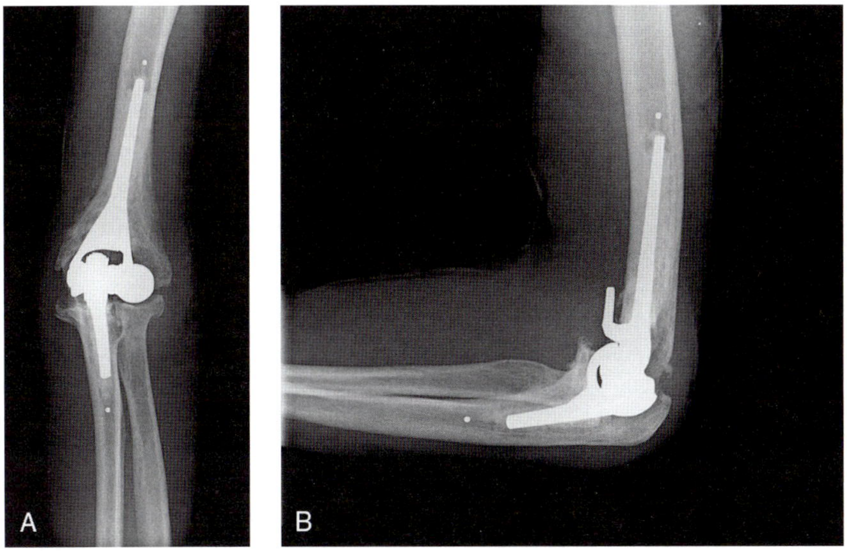


**Figure 2** AP (**A**) and lateral (**B**) radiographs of the elbow of a 60-year-old man who had primary osteoarthritis. The radiographs were obtained 18 months after unlinked total elbow arthroplasty with the Latitude EV Total Elbow Prosthesis (Tornier).

with current convertible unlinked TEA implants (**Figure 4**).

Although unlinked TEA has a theoretical biomechanical advantage of reducing implant-bone stress, studies have not yet demonstrated increased time to aseptic loosening. A retrospective cohort study compared linked TEAs and older-generation unlinked TEAs that were performed at a hospital over a 20-year period. At mean follow-up of 13 years, the researchers reported no significant differences with regard to loosening or functional outcomes. The overall revision surgery rate reported for unlinked implants was higher than that for linked implants (34% and 22%, respectively); however, the difference was not statistically significant. These results should be interpreted with caution because the revision surgery rates reported in the study were substantially higher than those reported in most studies.

Variability in the rate of aseptic loosening reported in the literature is believed to correspond with implant design. A study that compared linked and unlinked TEA implants reported no difference in aseptic loosening at 5-year follow-up. A systematic review reported varying rates of aseptic loosening in three different unlinked TEA implants, which were comparable with the rate of aseptic loosening of linked TEA implants. Although radiographic loosening is fairly common, there does not seem to be a direct correlation between radiographic loosening and short-term revision surgery. Revision surgery with the use of unlinked TEA implants can be difficult because of the bone loss and soft-tissue release that occurs during implant removal. A large retrospective study reported that patients who underwent revision TEA with unlinked implants had unacceptable survival rates compared with those who underwent TEA with linked implants (47% at 284 months and 84% at 271 months, respectively). The researchers concluded that unlinked TEA should be revised using linked TEA implants.

## Techniques

### Setup/Exposure

- The patient is placed under general anesthesia, and preoperative antibiotics are administered.
- The patient may be placed supine or in the lateral decubitus position, depending on the surgeon's preference. If the patient is positioned supine, the surgical arm is brought across the patient's chest with the use of an arm positioner or a sterile bolster. If the patient is placed in the lateral decubitus position, a padded support is placed under the patient's humerus just proximal to the elbow. It is important to ensure that patient positioning allows for full flexion of the elbow.
- The limb is exsanguinated, and a tourniquet is applied and inflated. Some surgeons prefer to use a sterile tourniquet.
- A posterior skin incision is made slightly medial to the olecranon. Minimal dissection is performed to the level of the triceps and forearm fascia.
- Medial dissection is performed to the level of the ulnar nerve. The ulnar nerve is isolated, carefully released through the entirety of the incision, and anteriorly transposed subcutaneously.
- Management of the triceps muscle is accomplished with either a preserving or a reflecting tongue approach. The authors of this chapter prefer to use either the recently described lateral paraolecranon approach (**Figure 5**) or the triceps tongue approach.
- The triceps insertion should be kept intact to improve triceps strength and accelerate rehabilitation. Although a complete triceps-on approach can be used, it makes preparation of the ulna slightly more difficult.
- An incision is made distally through the anconeus fascia, just lateral to the ulna, and is continued proximally through the triceps muscle just lateral to the olecranon (**Figure 5, A**).

**Table 1** Results of Unlinked Elbow Arthroplasty

| Authors (Year) | Number Treated | Procedure or Approach | Mean Patient Age in Years (Range) | Mean Follow-up in Months (Range) | Survival Rate (%) | Results | Level of Evidence |
|---|---|---|---|---|---|---|---|
| Little, Graham, Carr (2005) | 3,618 elbows | Capitellocondylar (Johnson & Johnson; 451), Kudo (Biomet; 258), Souter-Strathclyde (Stryker; 1,070), or Coonrad-Morrey (Zimmer; 302)[a] | 58 (NA) | Capitellocondylar: 61 (NA)<br>Kudo: 70 (NA)<br>Souter-Strathclyde: 60 (NA)<br>Coonrad-Morrey: 50 (NA) | Capitellocondylar: 95<br>Kudo: 89<br>Souter-Strathclyde: 85<br>Coonrad-Morrey: 90 | Good to excellent results in 85% (Capitellocondylar), 82% (Kudo), 85% (Souter-Strathclyde), and 88% (Coonrad-Morrey) | III |
| Little, Graham, Karatzas, et al (2005) | 92 patients | Triceps-off with Souter-Strathclyde (33), Kudo (29), or Coonrad-Morrey (30) | Souter-Strathclyde: 63 (NA)<br>Kudo: 60 (NA)<br>Coonrad-Morrey: 65 (NA) | Souter-Strathclyde: 61 (29-96)<br>Kudo: 67 (11-122)<br>Coonrad-Morrey: 68 (57-87) | Souter-Strathclyde: 85<br>Kudo: 93<br>Coonrad-Morrey: 90 | Mild to no pain in 95% (Souter-Strathclyde), 100% (Kudo), and 100% (Coonrad-Morrey) | III |
| Thillemann et al (2006) | 16 patients | Triceps split with Kudo type 3 (Biomet) | 60.3 (41-77) | 114 (NA) | 67.9 | MEPS: 7 excellent and 1 good | IV |
| Bassi et al (2007) | 36 patients | Triceps-off with Acclaim (DePuy) unlinked (34) or linked (2) | 64 (34-80) | 36 (24-49) | 94.5 | Mean MEPI score improved from 36 to 76<br>80.5% had no lucencies | IV |
| Fevang et al (2009) | 452 elbows | Norway (manufacturer unknown; 180), Kudo (161), IBP (Biomet; 111) | Norway: 60.8 (NA)<br>Kudo: 63.3 (NA)<br>IBP: 60.7 (NA) | 60 (NA) | Norway: 90<br>Kudo: 87.5<br>IBP: 90 | Not reported | II |
| Naqui et al (2010) | 11 patients | Triceps-off approach with Acclaim | 65.4 (51.1-80.9) | 57.6 (30-86.4) | 100 | MEPI score: 5 excellent, 4 good, and 2 fair<br>78% had no lucencies | IV |
| Park et al (2013) | 84 elbows | Triceps-off with unlinked (Pritchard ERS [DePuy; 18] or Kudo [17]) or linked (49) prostheses | 54.2 (34-74) | 156 (13-312) | Unlinked: 65.7<br>Linked: 77.6 | Mean 50-point increase in MEPS in linked and unlinked cohorts | III |
| Plaschke et al (2014) | 324 elbows | Unlinked with Souter-Strathclyde (90), Capitellocondylar (54), Pritchard ERS (23), or Kudo type 3 (5); or linked with Coonrad-Morrey (91), GSB III (Zimmer; 60) or Discovery (Biomet; 1) | 62 (25-91) | 105 (NA) | Unlinked: 90 at 5 yr, 77 at 10 yr<br>Linked: 90 at 5 yr, 88 at 10 yr | Not reported | III |

IBP = Instrumented Bone Preserving Elbow System, MEPI = Mayo Elbow Performance Index, MEPS = Mayo Elbow Performance Score, NA = not available.
[a] List of the more commonly used implants in the United Kingdom, not the totality of implants in the systematic review.

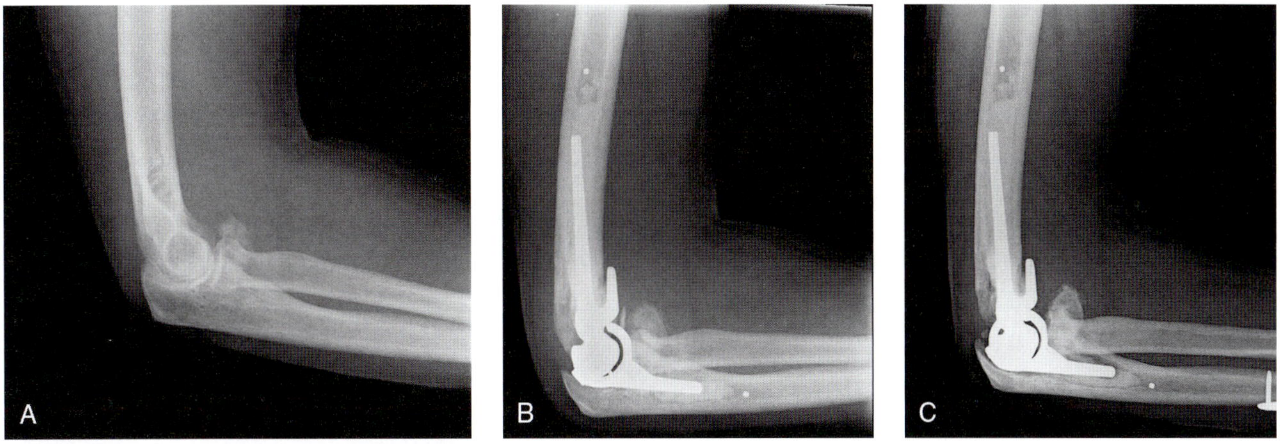

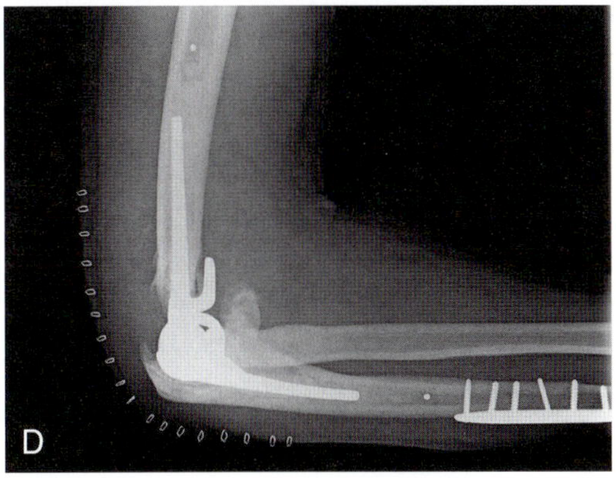

**Figure 3** Lateral radiographs of the elbow of a 57-year-old patient with posttraumatic arthritis who underwent unlinked total elbow arthroplasty (TEA). Radiographs obtained before (**A**) and 6 weeks after (**B**) unlinked TEA. **C,** Radiograph obtained 13 months after TEA demonstrates early loosening of the ulnar component. **D,** Radiograph obtained after revision to a linked ulnar component using a standard-length ulnar component rather than an extra-long stem.

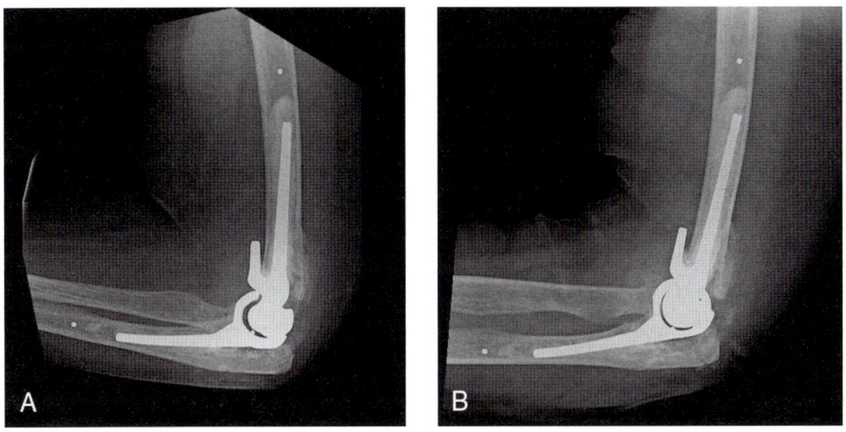

**Figure 4** Lateral radiographs of an elbow demonstrate residual instability after unlinked total elbow arthroplasty (**A**) and lack of residual instability after conversion to a linked implant (**B**).

- The triceps tendon is split centrally in a full-thickness fashion, leaving the entire olecranon insertion intact (**Figure 5**, **B** and **C**).
- There are two options for dislocating the joint. The first option includes radially elevating the extensor muscles and the lateral collateral ligament off the lateral condyle. The extensor muscles and lateral collateral ligament are tagged and retracted laterally. On the ulnar side, the medial collateral ligament and the flexor muscles are elevated directly off the medial epicondyle and tagged in a similar manner. The second option involves retaining the humeral muscle-tendon and ligament origins and releasing the ligament insertions from the ulna.
- The triceps origin is dissected off the distal humerus, revealing the joint capsule.
- The joint capsule is incised circumferentially around the humerus.
- The elbow is dislocated with the ulna retracted medially (**Figure 5, D**).

## Instruments/Equipment/ Implants Required

- Although many different unlinked TEA implants exist, this chapter specifically discusses a convertible TEA prosthesis (Latitude EV Total Elbow Prosthesis) that was designed by the three senior authors of this chapter (K.Y., S.W.O.,

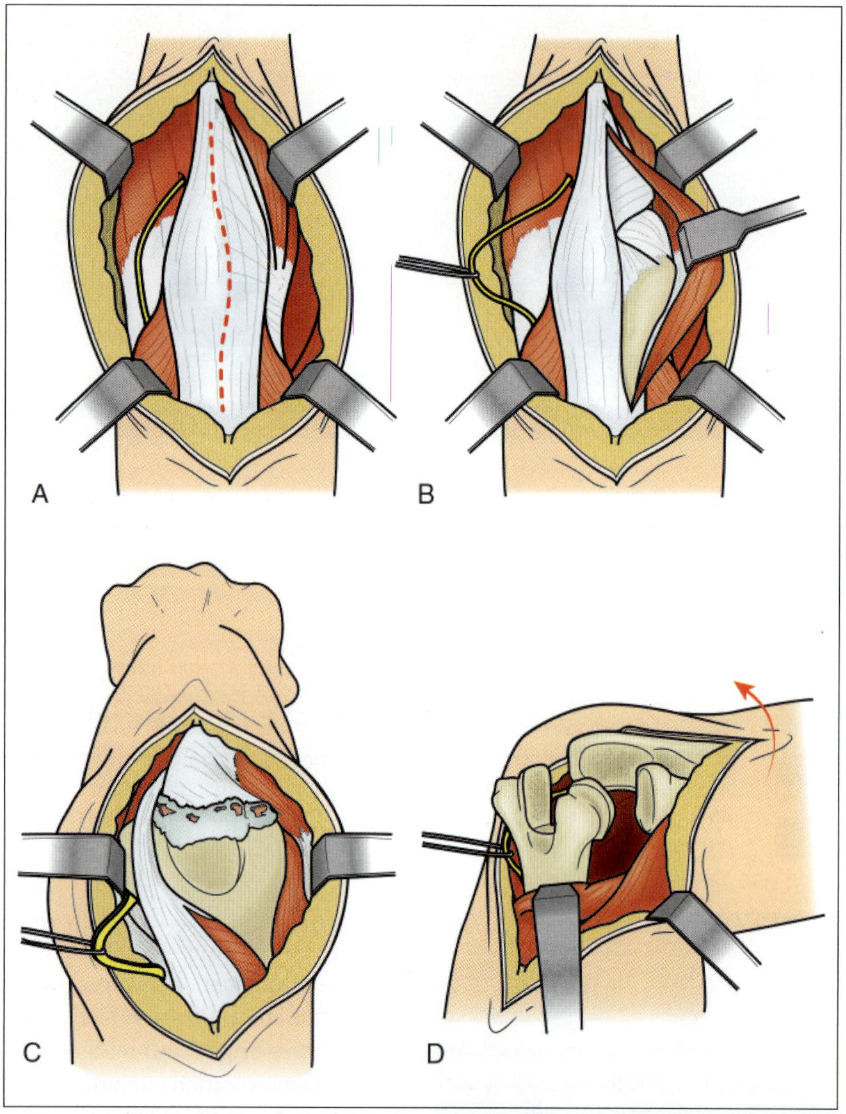


**Figure 5** Illustrations of the elbow show the paraolecranon approach for management of the triceps muscle-tendon unit in total elbow arthroplasty. An incision (dashed line) is made through the triceps immediately lateral to the olecranon (**A**), leaving the olecranon insertion intact (**B** and **C**). The ulnar nerve is identified and carefully retracted. **D,** The joint is dislocated, the humerus is delivered through the triceps, and the ulna is retracted medially. The direction of dislocation is indicated by the arrow. (Adapted with permission from Studer A, Athwal GS, MacDermid JC, Faber KJ, King GJ: The lateral para-olecranon approach for total elbow arthroplasty. *J Hand Surg Am* 2013;38[11]:2219-2226.e3.)

and G.J.W.K.). A convertible TEA implant differs from other TEA implant designs because it is anatomic and can re-create a balanced elbow via the retained or replaced radiocapitellar joint.

- A convertible TEA implant comes in four sizes (small, medium, large, and large-plus); the ulnar and humeral components must be size-matched.

## Procedure

- After full bony exposure, the component is sized using the appropriate trial spool (**Figure 6, A**). The trial spool should be superimposed on the trochlea and match the medial-lateral width of the distal humerus to allow radiocapitellar alignment.
- Sizing is confirmed by placing the trial spool into the trochlear notch and ensuring that the capitellar component is in line with the native radial head (**Figure 6, B** and **C**). If the native humerus size is between two trial spool sizes, the smaller spool size should be used.
- Preparation can begin on either the humeral or ulnar side; however, the humeral condyles may be susceptible to fracture after preparation. Therefore, beginning on the ulnar side can help reduce the risk of iatrogenic fracture.
- The trial spool is inserted in the trochlear notch, and a cutting jig is applied to the olecranon. If the radial head is deformed and cannot be retained, it is excised using a sagittal saw.
- The articular surface of the olecranon is resected using an appropriate bell saw. The ulnar nerve should be protected, and drilling should be accomplished from medial to lateral. In patients who have substantial bone loss, a barrel reamer can be used to prepare the ulna.
- A portion of the olecranon tip and the coronoid process are resected using a burr or rongeur to gain better access and avoid impingement in flexion and extension.
- A burr is used to open the medullary canal of the ulna.
- After correct rotational alignment is determined, broaching is performed. The dorsal aspect of the broach should be parallel with the dorsum of the ulna. The axis of rotation of the elbow, as it relates to the ulnar component, should intersect the radial head.
- Typically, a short-stemmed ulnar component is used if there is no

 

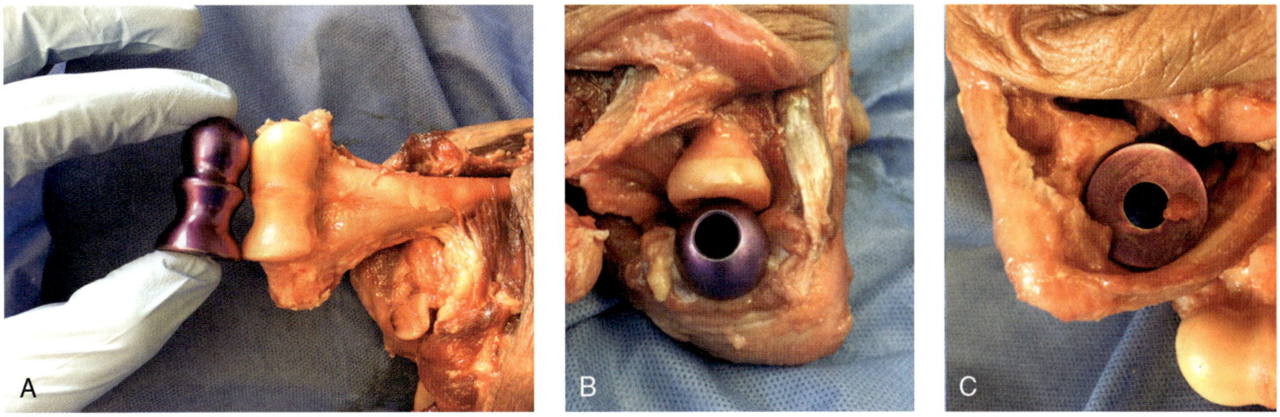


**Figure 6** Clinical photographs of a cadaver model show sizing of the humeral component in a convertible total elbow arthroplasty implant. **A,** The width of the distal humerus is matched to an appropriately sized trial spool. **B** and **C,** The trial spool is placed in the greater sigmoid notch to ensure alignment with the radial head. **B,** View from the lateral side shows correct sizing of the component compared with the native radial head. **C,** View of the medial elbow shows the correct fit of the spool within the olecranon.

plan to link the prosthesis. However, if a standard stem is used, the canal is prepared with flexible reamers over a guidewire.

- Holes are drilled on either side of the ulna at the insertions of the medial and lateral collateral ligaments. A transosseous No. 2 braided composite suture is placed through the ulna. If the ligaments were released from the ulna instead of the humerus, No. 1 synthetic absorbable sutures also are placed through the holes on either side.
- The radial canal is prepared using the provided rasps. The authors of this chapter do not recommend placement of a prosthetic radial head unless the surgeon is experienced with the procedure and understands the potential pitfalls of using a radial head component and how to prevent them.
- To prepare the humerus, an oscillating saw is used to remove the central portion of the trochlea; this is an initial cut that will be refined later with a cutting jig. The medullary canal is opened with a burr and broached. If the medullary canal is tight, it can be reamed sequentially over a guidewire.
- The humeral broaches are used sequentially, taking care to ensure the correct rotation and depth as determined by the axis indicator on the broach and the rotation pin. The patient's native flexion-extension axis, which is formed by a line running from the isometric point of the central capitellum to the anterodistal aspect of the medial epicondyle and is in approximately 15° of internal rotation compared with the dorsal aspect of the distal humerus, should be matched. A cutting guide is affixed to the final broach, and all definitive humeral cuts are completed.
- Final preparation of the canal with the gusset broach allows for placement of the antirotation fins of the implant.
- After the humeral trial is implanted, the elbow is reduced and evaluated for articular tracking and stability throughout motion. If substantial maltracking is present, either rotational positioning of the components must be verified and revised to correct the maltracking or the prosthesis should be converted to a linked prosthesis.
- All trial components are removed, and the medullary canals are occluded with cement restrictors or impacted bone, and then irrigated and dried. Definitive components are cemented in place with antibiotic-impregnated cement. Attention must be paid to ensure the correct position and rotation of the components.
- A cancellous bone fragment from the bone resected from the distal humerus is wedged between the humeral shaft and the anterior flange of the humeral component.
- After the cement has hardened, the elbow is reduced and moved through a range of motion to evaluate stability and tracking. If there are any concerns about stability, the ulnar cap may be inserted to link the joint.

## Wound Closure

- The tourniquet is released and careful hemostasis is obtained, after which the wound is copiously irrigated.
- Repair of the medial and lateral soft-tissue structures is achieved by placing a running No. 2 braided composite suture through the previously tagged medial and lateral ligaments. These sutures are then shuttled through the central

hole in the spool and tied to the contralateral soft tissues and on the medial or lateral side of the ulna.

- If the ligaments were released from the ulna instead of from the humerus, they are repaired with the sutures that were placed before implant insertion. The No. 2 braided composite suture that was placed through the ulna is then passed through the central hole in the spool of the prosthesis and tied as a temporary ligament to prevent joint subluxation.
- If the joint is unstable after soft-tissue repair, the TEA should be converted to a linked prosthesis.
- A drain is inserted, and the triceps and forearm fascia are closed with the use of inverted figure-of-8 No. 2 nonabsorbable braided sutures. If the triceps tongue was used, it is repaired with running No. 2 braided composite sutures.
- Subcutaneous closure is achieved with the use of 2-0 inverted sutures, and skin closure is achieved with the use of either 3-0 nylon sutures or staples.
- The elbow is splinted in the degree of extension obtained with the force of gravity, and an anterior slab is placed over a padded Robert-Jones bandage for 3 days postoperatively.

## Postoperative Regimen

Drains are removed on the first or second postoperative day, and elbow immobilization is maintained until adequate wound healing has been achieved. Elevation of the surgical arm in the early postoperative period is important to reduce swelling; however, the arm should be brought down from an elevated position for at least 5 minutes each hour to avoid problems with inadequate circulation, which could theoretically lead to compartment syndrome. Range of motion is begun with active flexion and progressive extension, depending on stability. If a triceps-off approach was used, active extension against resistance should be avoided and passive stretching in extension should be encouraged for the first 6 weeks postoperatively to protect the repair. Forearm pronation and supination is begun after range-of-motion exercises are commenced, with the elbow flexed to 90°. An extension splint may be used at night to minimize flexion contracture. Strengthening exercises are initiated at 8 weeks postoperatively.

## Limiting Adverse Events

Complications of TEA are substantial, approaching 20% after primary TEA. Complications are broadly categorized as intraoperative or postoperative. Intraoperative complications include neurovascular injury, periprosthetic fracture, and inadequate stability. Condyle fractures can be managed with plates or pins, and olecranon fractures can be managed with plates or tension-band wiring. Transient ulnar neuropathy is observed in as many as 25% of patients; however, it generally resolves within several weeks to months postoperatively.

Immediate and late postoperative complications include poor wound healing, hematoma, infection, triceps insufficiency, and complex regional pain syndrome. Hematoma, draining wounds, and skin breakdown should be managed aggressively with irrigation and débridement to avoid infection. The poor soft-tissue envelope around the elbow is unforgiving, and hardware can quickly become exposed with wound dehiscence. The deep infection rate after TEA is approximately 4% (range, 1% to 11%), which is considerably higher than the deep infection rates after other joint arthroplasties. Specific risk factors for infection include immunomodulation secondary to disease (such as diabetes) or medication (such as prednisone or methotrexate), smoking, wound drainage, hematoma, and revision elbow surgery. One of the senior authors of this chapter (S.W.O.) believes that the elevation of skin flaps is a major contributing factor to hematoma formation; therefore, he attempts to avoid skin flap elevation. Stiffness and heterotopic ossification are relatively common after TEA but rarely require surgical management. Extensor mechanism failure is associated with olecranon fracture and the triceps-off approach. To adequately recognize extensor mechanism failure, extension strength must be tested in extension rather than only in 90° of flexion.

Dislocation after unlinked TEA using the Latitude EV Total Elbow Prosthesis is rare. The sensation of instability or clicking without apparent instability may be more common; however, revision surgery for instability and conversion to linked TEA is rarely performed. In patients who have persistent instability, conversion to a linked TEA implant is indicated. If a convertible implant was used, conversion to a linked prosthesis can be achieved via a split through the triceps muscle.

 

## Bibliography

Alonso-Llames M: Bilaterotricipital approach to the elbow: Its application in the osteosynthesis of supracondylar fractures of the humerus in children. *Acta Orthop Scand* 1972;43(6):479-490.

An KN: Kinematics and constraint of total elbow arthroplasty. *J Shoulder Elbow Surg* 2005;14(1 suppl S):S168-S173.

Barlow JD, Morrey BF, O'Driscoll SW, Steinmann SP, Sanchez-Sotelo J: Activities after total elbow arthroplasty. *J Shoulder Elbow Surg* 2013;22(6):787-791.

Bassi RS, Simmons D, Ali F, et al: Early results of the Acclaim elbow replacement. *J Bone Joint Surg Br* 2007;89(4):486-489.

Bryan RS, Morrey BF: Extensive posterior exposure of the elbow: A triceps-sparing approach. *Clin Orthop Relat Res* 1982;(166):188-192.

Celli A, Arash A, Adams RA, Morrey BF: Triceps insufficiency following total elbow arthroplasty. *J Bone Joint Surg Am* 2005;87(9):1957-1964.

Choo A, Ramsey ML: Total elbow arthroplasty: Current options. *J Am Acad Orthop Surg* 2013;21(7):427-437.

De Vos MJ, Wagener ML, Hendriks JC, Eygendaal D, Verdonschot N: Linking of total elbow prosthesis during surgery: A biomechanical analysis. *J Shoulder Elbow Surg* 2013;22(9):1236-1241.

Fevang BT, Lie SA, Havelin LI, Skredderstuen A, Furnes O: Results after 562 total elbow replacements: A report from the Norwegian Arthroplasty Register. *J Shoulder Elbow Surg* 2009;18(3):449-456.

Gschwend N, Simmen BR, Matejovsky Z: Late complications in elbow arthroplasty. *J Shoulder Elbow Surg* 1996;5(2 pt 1):86-96.

Hildebrand KA, Patterson SD, Regan WD, MacDermid JC, King GJ: Functional outcome of semiconstrained total elbow arthroplasty. *J Bone Joint Surg Am* 2000;82(10):1379-1386.

Inagaki K, O'Driscoll SW, Neale PG, Uchiyama E, Morrey BF, An KN: Importance of a radial head component in Sorbie unlinked total elbow arthroplasty. *Clin Orthop Relat Res* 2002;(400):123-131.

Jenkins PJ, Watts AC, Norwood T, Duckworth AD, Rymaszewski LA, McEachan JE: Total elbow replacement: Outcome of 1,146 arthroplasties from the Scottish Arthroplasty Project. *Acta Orthop* 2013;84(2):119-123.

Kamineni S, O'Driscoll SW, Urban M, et al: Intrinsic constraint of unlinked total elbow replacements: The ulnotrochlear joint. *J Bone Joint Surg Am* 2005;87(9):2019-2027.

Kudo H, Iwano K: Total elbow arthroplasty with a non-constrained surface-replacement prosthesis in patients who have rheumatoid arthritis: A long-term follow-up study. *J Bone Joint Surg Am* 1990;72(3):355-362.

Labek G, Thaler M, Janda W, Agreiter M, Stöckl B: Revision rates after total joint replacement: Cumulative results from worldwide joint register datasets. *J Bone Joint Surg Br* 2011;93(3):293-297.

Leclerc A, King GJ: Unlinked and convertible total elbow arthroplasty. *Hand Clin* 2011;27(2):215-227, vi.

Levy JC, Loeb M, Chuinard C, Adams RA, Morrey BF: Effectiveness of revision following linked versus unlinked total elbow arthroplasty. *J Shoulder Elbow Surg* 2009;18(3):457-462.

Little CP, Graham AJ, Carr AJ: Total elbow arthroplasty: A systematic review of the literature in the English language until the end of 2003. *J Bone Joint Surg Br* 2005;87(4):437-444.

Little CP, Graham AJ, Karatzas G, Woods DA, Carr AJ: Outcomes of total elbow arthroplasty for rheumatoid arthritis: Comparative study of three implants. *J Bone Joint Surg Am* 2005;87(11):2439-2448.

Naqui SZ, Rajpura A, Nuttall D, Prasad P, Trail IA: Early results of the Acclaim total elbow replacement in patients with primary osteoarthritis. *J Bone Joint Surg Br* 2010;92(5):668-671.

O'Driscoll SW, An KN, Korinek S, Morrey BF: Kinematics of semi-constrained total elbow arthroplasty. *J Bone Joint Surg Br* 1992;74(2):297-299.

O'Driscoll SW, King GJ: Treatment of instability after total elbow arthroplasty. *Orthop Clin North Am* 2001;32(4):679-695, ix.

Park SE, Kim JY, Cho SW, Rhee SK, Kwon SY: Complications and revision rate compared by type of total elbow arthroplasty. *J Shoulder Elbow Surg* 2013;22(8):1121-1127.

Pierce TD, Herndon JH: The triceps preserving approach to total elbow arthroplasty. *Clin Orthop Relat Res* 1998;(354):144-152.

Plaschke HC, Thillemann TM, Brorson S, Olsen BS: Implant survival after total elbow arthroplasty: A retrospective study of 324 procedures performed from 1980 to 2008. *J Shoulder Elbow Surg* 2014;23(6):829-836.

Ramsey M, Neale PG, Morrey BF, O'Driscoll SW, An KN: Kinematics and functional characteristics of the Pritchard ERS unlinked total elbow arthroplasty. *J Shoulder Elbow Surg* 2003;12(4):385-390.

Sabo MT, Athwal GS, King GJ: Landmarks for rotational alignment of the humeral component during elbow arthroplasty. *J Bone Joint Surg Am* 2012;94(19):1794-1800.

Sanchez-Sotelo J: Total elbow arthroplasty. *Open Orthop J* 2011;5:115-123.

Spinner RJ, Morgenlander JC, Nunley JA: Ulnar nerve function following total elbow arthroplasty: A prospective study comparing preoperative and postoperative clinical and electrophysiologic evaluation in patients with rheumatoid arthritis. *J Hand Surg Am* 2000;25(2):360-364.

Studer A, Athwal GS, MacDermid JC, Faber KJ, King GJ: The lateral para-olecranon approach for total elbow arthroplasty. *J Hand Surg Am* 2013;38(11):2219-2226.e3.

Thillemann TM, Olsen BS, Johannsen HV, Søjbjerg JO: Long-term results with the Kudo type 3 total elbow arthroplasty. *J Shoulder Elbow Surg* 2006;15(4):495-499.

Venable CS: An elbow and an elbow prosthesis: Case of complete loss of the lower third of the humerus. *Am J Surg* 1952;83(3):271-275.

Wright TW, Wong AM, Jaffe R: Functional outcome comparison of semiconstrained and unconstrained total elbow arthroplasties. *J Shoulder Elbow Surg* 2000;9(6):524-531.

Yamaguchi K, Adams RA, Morrey BF: Infection after total elbow arthroplasty. *J Bone Joint Surg Am* 1998;80(4):481-491.

 

# Chapter 18
# Linked Total Elbow Arthroplasty

*Hill Hastings II, MD*

**Learning Objectives**

- Explain the indications and contraindications for linked total elbow arthroplasty (TEA).
- Describe the design principles of linked TEA implants.
- Describe the methods of surgical exposure for linked TEA.
- Explain the general expected outcomes and the short- and long-term complications of linked TEA.

## Indications

The design of total elbow implants has evolved over time, from the simple hinge total elbow implant of the early 1970s that resulted in high rates of early loosening to the resurfacing and linked total elbow (sloppy hinge) implants used today. Currently, total elbow implants are categorized as linked, unlinked, or convertible. The sloppy hinge total elbow implant allows for 8° of varus/valgus laxity. The potential advantage of unlinked total elbow implants is the reduction of forces at the bone-cement interface with diminished loosening; however, unlinked total elbow implants have experienced higher complication rates compared with linked designs and no advantage with respect to implant survivorship. Ulnohumeral instability is a particular risk of unlinked total elbow implants, particularly when the ligaments or the radial head are compromised. Convertible total elbow implants allow for conversion from an unlinked to a linked construct, which can be useful when an unlinked elbow is unstable. Currently, it is unclear whether the most recently designed convertible unlinked implants represent an advantage over current linked designs that warrants the increased risk of instability. Uncemented total elbow implants and hemiarthroplasty elbow implants currently are not cleared for use in the United States.

Historically, the most frequent and important indication for total elbow arthroplasty (TEA) was painful, limited motion secondary to inflammatory arthritis. Modern linked total elbow implant designs have expanded the indications for TEA to include fracture, nonunion, and instability. An emerging indication for TEA is a low, comminuted distal humerus fracture in older, low-demand patients. Compared with open reduction, TEA affords patients an expedient and initially more predictable method for treating distal humerus fractures. Linked TEA also is increasingly used to manage severe posttraumatic arthritis or end-stage primary osteoarthritis of the elbow in older, low-demand patients who are unsatisfied with the result of capsular release and débridement.

## Contraindications

As with any TEA, linked TEA is contraindicated in patients who have an acute infection or patients who have had an infection within the past 2 years. However, TEA may be considered in select patients after treatment of infection if multiple deep cultures and laboratory studies (white blood cell count, C-reactive protein level, and leukocyte esterase level) demonstrate negative results.

The most important relevant contraindications to linked TEA are good health (physiologically young age) and a high activity level as well as suspected patient noncompliance with regard to aftercare and implant-protective restrictions. Implant survivorship is better in low-demand patients in whom functional compromise from diffuse disease, such as rheumatoid arthritis, is present compared with patients with posttraumatic arthritis or osteoarthritis who have no considerable disabilities

*Dr. Hastings or an immediate family member has received royalties from, is a member of a speakers' bureau or has made paid presentations on behalf of, and serves as a paid consultant to Zimmer Biomet.*

**Table 1** Results of Linked Total Elbow Arthroplasty

| Authors (Year) | Number of Elbows | Implant | Mean Patient Age in Years (Range) | Mean Follow-up in Months (Range) | Results | Level of Evidence |
|---|---|---|---|---|---|---|
| Fevang et al (2009) | 562 | Norway (180)<br>Kudo (Biomet; 161)<br>iBP (Biomet; 111)<br>NES (implantcast; 45)<br>GSB III (Zimmer; 33)<br>Discovery (DJO Global; 24)<br>IBP Reconstruction (Biomet; 5)<br>Souter-Strathclyde (Stryker; 2)<br>Coonrad Morrey (Zimmer; 1) | 62 (NR) | 74.4 (34.8-106.8) | 92% survivorship at 5-yr follow-up (8% revision)<br>85% survivorship at 10-yr follow-up (15% revision)<br>3 patients underwent revision for deep infection<br>Noncemented ulnar components rendered inferior results<br>Higher risk of revision in patients with fractures | II |
| Giannicola et al (2014) | 24 | Discovery | 69 (45-89) | 41 (29-63) | Success rate, 83%<br>Mean flexion of 136°, mean extension of 17°, mean pronation of 80°, and mean supination of 83°<br>MEPI score: 20 excellent, 3 good, and 1 fair<br>No mechanical failures<br>2 patients with ulnar neuropathy<br>1 patient with wound infection<br>2 patients with epicondylar fracture<br>1 patient with progressive radiolucency | IV |
| Hastings et al (2014) | 99 | Discovery | 63.9 (33.4-88.7) | 49.2 (24-70.8) | Mean flexion-extension improved from 81° to 121°<br>Mean pronation-supination improved from 134° to 163°<br>Component survivorship: ulna and humerus, 100%; condyles, 97.8%; ulnar bearings, 95.7%; condylar locking screws, 95.7% | IV |

MEPI = Mayo Elbow Performance Index, NR = not reported.

that will limit force and repetitive use of the elbow. The author of this chapter prefers to defer TEA in patients who have posttraumatic arthritis or osteoarthritis until patients are at least age 60 years. Lower-demand patients in whom compromise from diffuse disease is present are considered candidates for TEA at a younger age if erosive bone loss precludes débridement or interposition arthroplasty. Patients should be advised that their elbow implant may not survive beyond 10 or 20 years and that revision surgery is less predictable and carries a higher risk for complications. Patients also should be advised that the risk for infection is higher for TEA compared with hip, knee, and shoulder arthroplasty, and that reimplantation after infection is problematic.

 

**Table 1** Results of Linked Total Elbow Arthroplasty *(continued)*

| Authors (Year) | Number of Elbows | Implant | Mean Patient Age in Years (Range) | Mean Follow-up in Months (Range) | Results | Level of Evidence |
|---|---|---|---|---|---|---|
| Alizadehkhaiyat et al (2015) | 100 | Discovery | 62 (22-86) | 48.5 (24-108) | Success rate, >90%<br>Mean flexion-extension improved from 72° to 93°<br>Mean pronation-supination improved from 86° to 111°<br>Percentage of pain-free patients increased from 7% preoperatively to 64% at final follow-up<br>Complications included deep infection (2%), osteolysis (4%), aseptic loosening requiring revision (primary, 5%; revision, 12%), ulnar neuropathy (3%), and prosthetic failure (1%) | IV |
| Wagener et al (2015) | 69 | Latitude convertible (Tornier) | 60 (23-87) | 43 (8-84) | 100% survivorship of humerus and ulna<br>31% of patients had disengagement of radial head component<br>Range of motion, pain, and function all improved<br>No loosening was reported | II |

MEPI = Mayo Elbow Performance Index, NR = not reported.

## Alternative Treatments

Advances in both surgical technique and implant design have improved the ability to achieve stable or rigid internal fixation of complex and comminuted distal humerus fractures that result from traumatic injury. In physically active patients and younger patients, all attempts at surgical repair should be pursued. A successfully united fracture that is complicated by stiffness may be salvaged via débridement and capsular release. Similarly, a clearer understanding of the primary and secondary contributors to elbow instability has improved the ability to manage complex, unstable elbow injuries. In patients who have fracture-dislocations of the elbow, TEA should be considered only if surgical attempts to restore stability have failed. In select patients, longstanding nonunion can be corrected via open reduction bone grafting and surgical repair.

If posttraumatic arthritis involves only a portion of the elbow articulation such as the radiocapitellar joint, correction may be achieved via radial head resection with or without radial head replacement. If stiffness and marginal osteophytes develop after trauma but the radiocapitellar and ulnohumeral joint surfaces remain intact, capsular release and excision of the marginal osteophytes often substantially improves comfort and motion. If trauma has led to considerable disruption of the articular surfaces, adequate subchondral bone often remains, which may allow for débridement and interposition arthroplasty. However, in patients who have single-column or major bone loss of the distal humerus or proximal ulna, allograft replacement and implant arthroplasty may be the only treatment options. Allograft hemiarthroplasty with TEA has not been a reliable treatment option because a Charcot joint and progressive deformity develop over time. Interposition arthroplasty should be considered in younger patients despite the higher complication rates and lower success rates compared with TEA. Interposition arthroplasty rarely results in satisfactory outcomes in patients with marked distal humerus bone loss.

## Results

The published results of linked TEA are summarized in **Table 1**. Most patients regain at least 100° of elbow flexion and extension after TEA and experience pain relief. Implant survivorship is better in low-demand patients with functional compromise from diffuse disease compared with patients with osteoarthritis

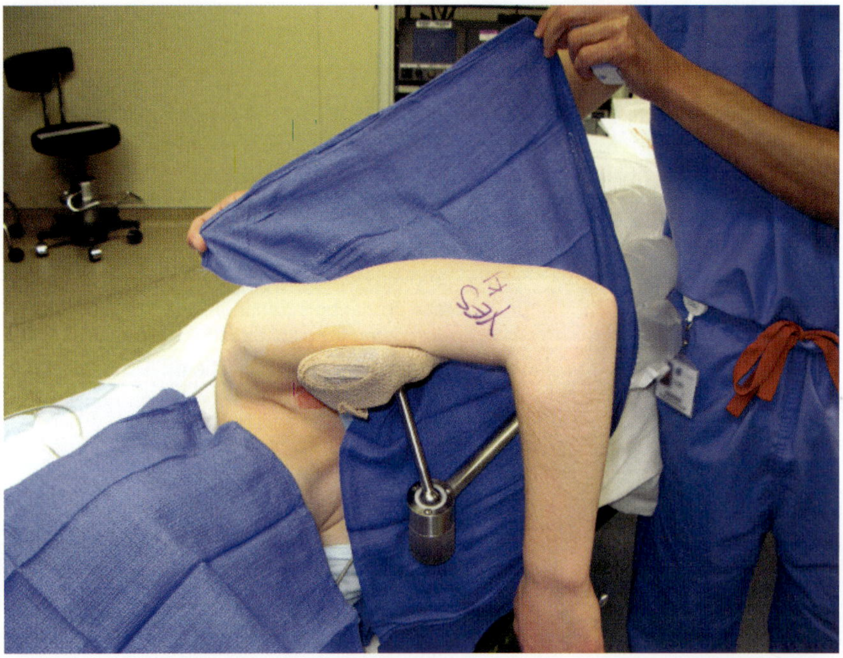

**Figure 1** Intraoperative photograph shows a patient placed in the lateral decubitus position with the affected arm in an arm holder for linked total elbow arthroplasty.

or posttraumatic arthritis. The results of TEA for the management of trauma have demonstrated better survivorship if at least one condyle or distal column of the humerus is preserved compared with if both columns are absent. Studies have not yet demonstrated an advantage to the use of unlinked total elbow implants compared with linked total elbow implants. The results of TEA for the management of a distal humerus fracture in older patients have shown more predictable early outcomes compared with open reduction and fixation, with little requirement for postoperative physical therapy. Late results—adverse events in particular—warrant an attempt at surgical fixation, if possible. TEA in younger, high-activity patients; patients with obesity; and patients with distal humerus nonunion has resulted in a higher incidence of complications and aseptic loosening that requires early revision. Similarly, TEA for the management of primary osteoarthritis is best reserved for older, low-demand patients.

**Video 18.1** Total Elbow Arthroplasty in a Rheumatoid Elbow. Hill Hastings II, MD (4 min)

## Techniques

### Setup/Exposure

- The author of this chapter prefers to use an ultrasonographic-guided infraclavicular block as well as general anesthesia.
- Intravenous antibiotics are administered at least 1 hour before skin incision.
- The patient is placed on a padded bean bag in the lateral decubitus position with an axillary roll.
- The lower extremities are carefully protected with pillows and foam padding.
- The affected elbow is positioned in an arm holder (**Figure 1**).
- The involved upper extremity is prepared and draped up to and including the shoulder.
- The patient's hand is covered with a sterile impervious stockinette, and a sterile tourniquet is applied to the upper brachium.
- Alternatively, the patient is rolled 30° toward the opposite side, and the prepared and draped arm is positioned over a bolster.
- A straight incision that passes just medial to the olecranon is marked on the posteromedial elbow.
- The exposed surgical area is covered with an antimicrobial adherent drape.
- Several surgical approaches to the elbow joint can be used to address the triceps muscle.
- Adequate exposure requires subluxation of the elbow as well as release of the anterior and posterior capsules and at least one collateral ligament.
- The most common surgical approaches include the paratricipital (triceps-on) approach for patients with a fracture and triceps-reflection (triceps-off) techniques for most all other patients. The best surgical approach for exposure is attained via a triceps-reflecting (triceps-off) technique, in which the triceps is detached and reflected from the ulna. Unless a surgeon is experienced in TEA, a triceps-off technique should be used to achieve easy access and optimal visualization of the ulna.
- Reflection of the triceps muscle is essential in all revision TEAs in which removal of the implant and cement demands perfect visualization of both the humerus and ulna.
- The ulnar nerve is decompressed from the midhumerus level proximally, through the cubital tunnel, and through the deep fascia of the flexor carpi ulnaris muscle and the origin of the flexor digitorum superficialis muscle.
- The intermuscular septum is excised, and the ulnar nerve is transposed anteriorly. Ulnar nerve

 

transposition protects the ulnar nerve from undue traction or torque during TEA.

- At the end of TEA, the ulnar nerve is assessed for stability and to ensure it remains in an anterior position through a full flexion-extension arc of elbow motion. The ulnar nerve often remains stable without the need for a formal sling. In the rare instance in which the ulnar nerve redisplaces posteriorly, it is stabilized with the use of a fascial sling that is elevated from the flexor-pronator fascia.

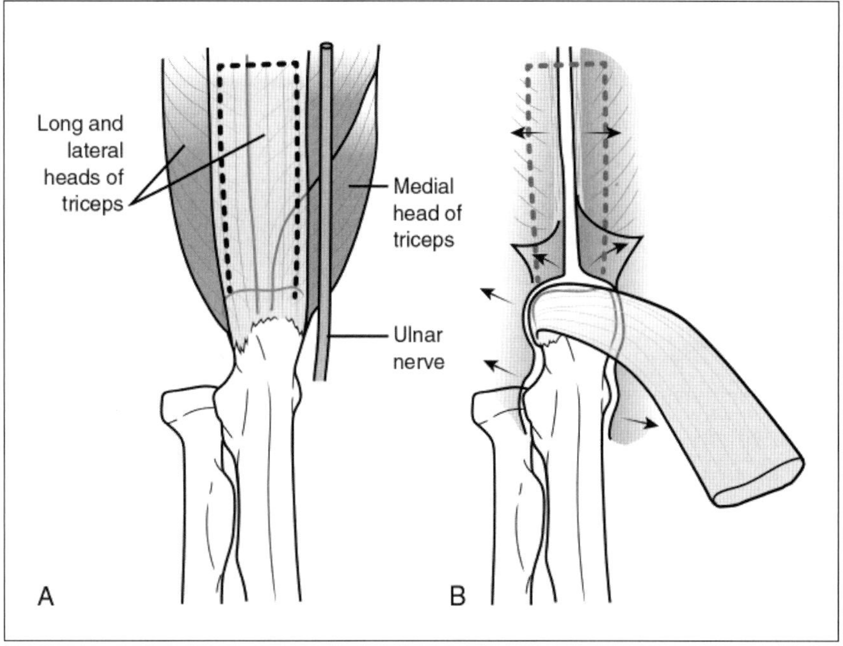


**Figure 2** Illustrations of an elbow show the steps used for the posterior triceps-off technique for linked total elbow arthroplasty. **A,** Exposure is attained via distal reflection of the triceps with preservation of the attachment to the ulna. The dotted lines indicate incision in the triceps fascia to create a distally based flap. **B,** The deep central triceps is incised longitudinally, with subperiosteal distal extension on the medial and lateral sides. The dotted lines indicate the area at which the distally based flap was raised. The arrows represent elevation and retraction of the deeper musculotendinous triceps mechanism along with subperiosteal release down the medial and lateral proximal ulna.

### POSTERIOR TRICEPS PROXIMAL REFLECTING TECHNIQUE (TRICEPS-OFF)

- The author of this chapter prefers to raise a 5- to 7-cm distal-based flap of triceps fascia with preservation of its Sharpey fibers of attachment to the ulna (**Figure 2, A**).
- The deep central triceps is split longitudinally from proximal to distal down through its tendinous long and lateral head to the olecranon (**Figure 2, B**).
- The medial portion of the long head of the triceps and the entire medial head of the triceps is subperiosteally dissected away from the medial olecranon and the proximal ulna distally to a point beyond the ulnar collateral ligament (UCL) attachment to the ulna.
- The medial subperiosteal dissection is continued up to the anteromedial coronoid.
- Similarly, the rest of the long and lateral heads of the triceps are sharply reflected in a subperiosteal manner from the lateral olecranon.
- Exposure is extended subperiosteally along the lateral proximal ulna to a point distal to the ulnar insertion of the lateral collateral ligament (LCL)/annular ligament complex.
- Healing of the collateral ligaments is more likely if they are released distally in this manner rather than released from their proximal origin. In this fashion, the flexor-pronator origin and collateral ligament attachment simply fall back into position at the end of TEA.

### TRICEPS-RETRACTING (TRICEPS-ON) AND UCL-SPARING TECHNIQUE

- If the surgeon has considerable experience performing TEA in thin, small patients, it is possible to gain adequate exposure without taking down the triceps or releasing the UCL (**Figure 3**).
- After the medial and lateral subcutaneous flaps have been reflected and the ulnar nerve has been transposed, an incision is made down the lateral triceps.
- The incision is extended distally in a subperiosteal fashion along the lateral ulna to a point distal to the LCL complex attachment on the ulna.
- The proximal-lateral collateral/extensor origin is released off the humerus, and the anterior and posterior capsules are completely excised.
- The elbow is dislocated via flexion and supination, hinged on the still-intact UCL and flexor-pronator origin. If subluxation of the elbow is insufficient, then subperiosteal release of the distal attachment of the UCL is performed.

### TRICEPS-ON TECHNIQUE FOR DISTAL HUMERUS FRACTURE OR NONUNION

- With a triceps-on approach, the triceps is left attached to the ulna. Preparation of the humerus with the triceps-on technique is easy;

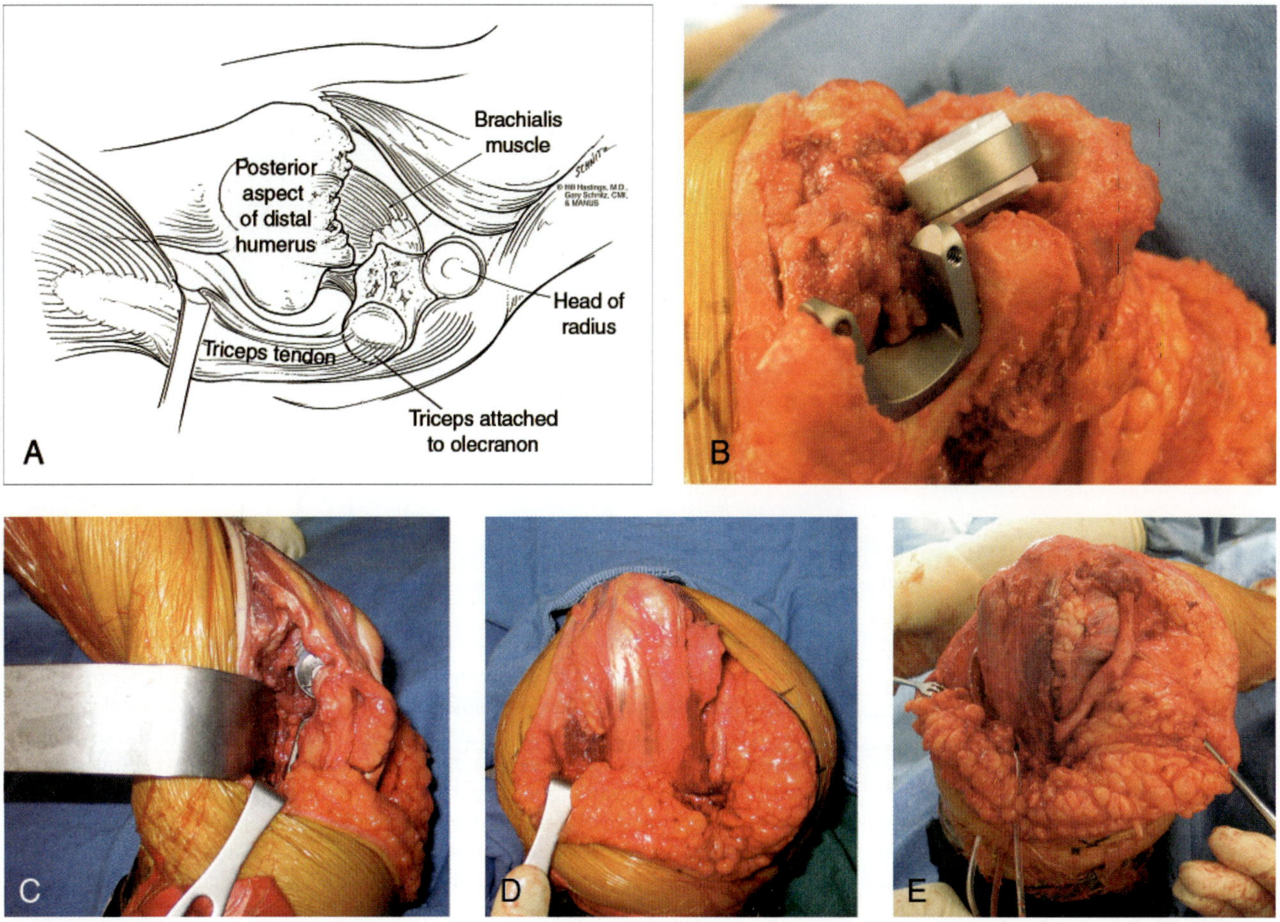


**Figure 3** Images of an elbow show the steps used for linked total elbow arthroplasty without takedown of the triceps or release of the ulnar collateral ligament (UCL). **A,** Illustration shows the surgical approach. **B,** Intraoperative photograph shows the position of the humeral and ulnar implants with the triceps and UCL still intact. **C,** Lateral-view intraoperative photograph shows the repositioned triceps mechanism after elbow reduction and before repair of the lateral collateral-extensor origin. Note that the anterior flange sits directly on the anterior cortex of the humerus. **D,** Posterior-view intraoperative photograph taken after elbow reduction. **E,** Posteromedial-view intraoperative photograph taken after elbow reduction shows the transposed ulnar nerve. (Panel A, copyright Hill Hastings, MD, and Gary Schnitz, Indiana Hand to Shoulder Center, Indianapolis, IN. Panels B through E, reproduced from Hastings H II: Linked total elbow arthroplasty: The Discovery Prosthesis, in Yamaguchi K, King GJW, McKee MD, O'Driscoll SWM, eds: *Advanced Reconstruction: Elbow.* Rosemont, IL, American Academy of Orthopaedic Surgeons, 2007, pp 229-239.)

however, visualization for preparation of the ulna is more difficult with the triceps attached.

- A posterior incision is made just medial to the olecranon.
- Thick medial and lateral subcutaneous flaps are elevated, with the plane of dissection immediately superficial to the fascial plane.
- The ulnar nerve is identified and transposed as previously described.
- An incision is made on the medial and lateral sides of the triceps and extended distally onto the ulna. In thin patients, the lateral incision extends from the humerus distally between the anconeus and extensor carpi ulnaris muscles.
- The anconeus muscle is elevated from the ulna to the subperiosteal border of the ulna. In most patients, it is easier to continue the triceps extension distally between the triceps fascia and the anconeus muscle; however, this can result in denervation of the anconeus muscle.
- On the lateral side, the extensor supinator and LCL origins are detached from the humeral condylar fracture fragments or nonunion.
- The UCL origin and flexor-pronator origin are detached medially, and the fractured distal humeral condyles are excised.
- The distal humerus is button-holed lateral to the triceps.
- The tip of the olecranon deep to the triceps attachment is exposed and excised.

 

- Preparation of the slot in the ulna is easier from the medial side, and reaming down the canal is easier and better aligned axially from the lateral side.

### TRICEPS-SPLITTING TECHNIQUE

- The author of this chapter no longer uses a triceps-splitting approach for primary surgery. However, the triceps-splitting approach is the preferred approach for revision surgery. It does not require exposure of a previously transposed ulnar nerve, and the surgical exposure can easily be extended proximally up to the radial nerve passage (**Figure 4**).
- The triceps mechanism is incised longitudinally from proximal to distal down to the center of the olecranon.
- To ensure anatomic reattachment of the triceps at the end of the TEA, a preplaced No. 2 braided Kevlar and polyester suture is passed through the lateral triceps attachment using an inside-out technique and advanced proximally using the Krackow technique.
- Similarly, a preplaced suture is passed through the medial portion of the triceps and advanced proximally using the Krackow technique.
- At the end of the procedure, each proximal suture will be brought back down distally, leap-frogging each of the preplaced suture locks and suturing together the split central triceps. The two medial and two lateral sutures will then be passed through drill holes through the olecranon and tied together along the medial or lateral side of the more distal ulna.
- The lateral portion of the triceps is released from the olecranon and the proximal ulna, and the dissection is extended subperiosteally along the lateral proximal ulna to a point distal to the ulnar insertion of the LCL ligament complex.
- Similarly, the medial portion of the triceps is subperiosteally released from the medial olecranon, and the subperiosteal dissection is extended distally to a point beyond the UCL attachment to the ulna.
- The medial subperiosteal dissection is continued up to the anteromedial coronoid.

### LATERAL REFLECTION TRICEPS-OFF TECHNIQUE (BRYAN-MORREY APPROACH)

- Historically, most surgeons were trained to use the lateral reflection triceps-off approach. The author of this chapter no longer uses this approach because it requires lateral retraction and torque on the triceps to maintain exposure and it cannot be easily extended proximally when needed. The author also believes that tendon healing back to the olecranon is less predictable than tendon-to-tendon healing as described previously in the section on posterior triceps proximal reflecting technique (**Figure 5**).
- The fascia is incised over the ulnar head of the flexor carpi ulnaris muscle from the cubital tunnel proximally to a point 7 to 10 cm distal to the olecranon.
- The fascia is elevated to expose the subcutaneous border of the ulna.
- The triceps is elevated from the humerus posteriorly to the medial intermuscular septum.
- From medial to lateral, the triceps fibers of insertion into the ulna are sharply detached from the ulna.
- To ensure accurate triceps tendon reattachment at the end of the procedure, a No. 2 braided Kevlar and polyester suture is placed using the Krackow technique.
- Reflection of the triceps and anconeus muscles is continued until the lateral condyle is reached.
- The proximal origin of the LCL is subperiosteally released from the humerus, and the anterior capsule is released and/or excised from lateral to medial. This step allows dislocation of the elbow via flexion and supination of the forearm with respect to the humerus.
- Typically, the UCL and the flexor-pronator origin are released from their proximal origins.

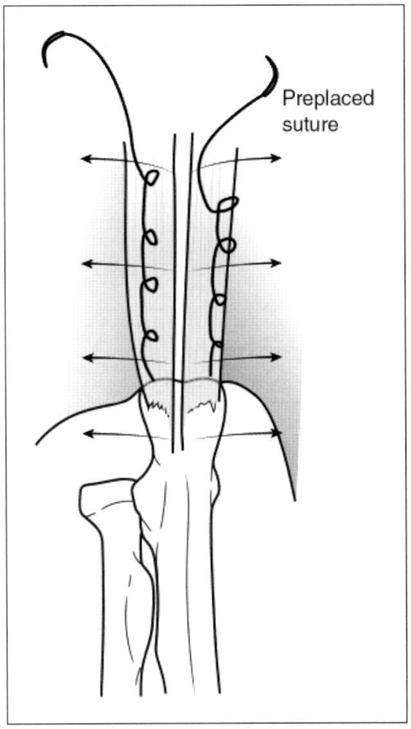


**Figure 4** Illustration of an elbow shows the triceps-splitting technique for linked total elbow arthroplasty, with braided suture passed through the lateral and medial triceps. The arrows indicate elevation and retraction of the split triceps mechanism.

### ANTERIOR CAPSULAR RELEASE/RESECTION

- The anterior capsule is released after subluxation of the elbow. Care is required to protect the radial nerve, which lies just anterior to the anterolateral capsule.
- A periosteal elevator is used to release the proximal capsule origin.
- A 1.5-inch malleable retractor is

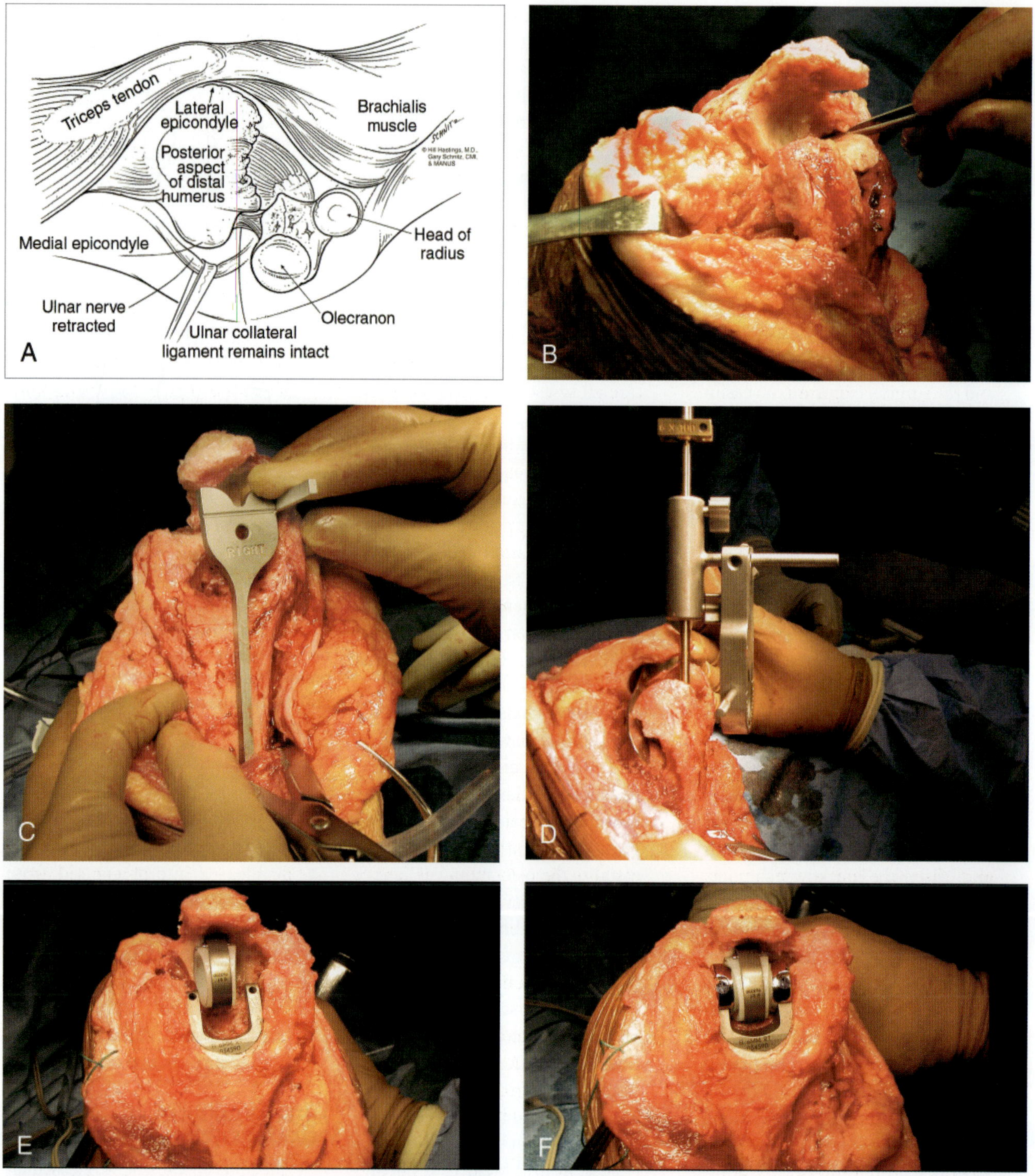


**Figure 5** Images of an elbow show steps in the lateral triceps-off technique for linked total elbow arthroplasty. **A,** Illustration shows the lateral triceps-off approach. **B,** Intraoperative photograph shows the exposed joint surfaces. **C,** Intraoperative photograph shows the application of the medial aspect of the exterior humeral cutting template to the medial aspect of the trochlea. **D,** Intraoperative photograph shows an alternative application of the external humeral cutting template to the humeral rasp. **E,** Intraoperative photograph shows the humeral and ulnar components after cement fixation and before implant coupling. **F,** Intraoperative photograph shows the coupling of the humeral and ulnar articular components with the use of cobalt-chromium condyles. (Reproduced from Hastings H II: Linked total elbow arthroplasty: The Discovery Prosthesis, in Yamaguchi K, King GJW, McKee MD, O'Driscoll SWM, eds: *Advanced Reconstruction: Elbow*. Rosemont, IL, American Academy of Orthopaedic Surgeons, 2007, pp 229-239.)

 

placed on the anterior humerus to protect the anterior soft tissues during preparation of the humerus.

## Instruments/Equipment/ Implants Required

- The Discovery Elbow System (DJO Global) is intended to limit bushing failures observed in other linked total elbow prosthesis designs, provide an accurate reproduction of the flexion-extension axis, and impart stability without the use of a true hinge (**Figure 6, A**). The humeral and ulnar stems closely match medullary morphology and, therefore, place the elbow joint in a correct anatomic location. The condylar projections of the humeral component allow for 5° of valgus laxity and 5° of internal rotation with respect to the humerus (**Figure 6, B**). The humeral stem is laterally offset to position the articulation in the center of the trochlea and allow for implantation with preservation of UCL mechanics (**Figure 6, C**). The humeral stem also incorporates an anatomic posterior bow (**Figure 6, D**). The juncture between the humeral stem and the condylar extensions is rounded and diminished in profile to preserve metaphyseal and condylar strength. The ulnar component uses a compression-molded, high-density polyethylene bearing that can be exchanged if wear occurs. The ulnar stem is laterally offset with respect to the bearing articulation, and incorporates a 23° anterior neck angle that allows for anatomic positioning of the joint axis (**Figure 6, E** and **F**). Complete modularity of size exists with respect to the humeral and ulnar implants. Extra-small implants are available for use in small-statured patients. The articulation includes two large cobalt-chromium hemispheric condylar surfaces that distribute contact forces and allow for 7° of varus-valgus laxity (**Figure 6, G** through **I**). The lateral condyle, which is the same size as the medial condylar surface, serves as a lateral buttress to valgus stress in the absence of a radial head. The humeral and ulnar components can be cemented without immediate coupling and without violation of the humeral condyles.
- A 1.5-inch malleable retractor is placed anterior to the humerus after exposure of the elbow is attained to protect the anterior soft tissues during preparation of the humerus.
- A large bone clamp is applied to the humeral distal diaphysis to help control rotation of the humerus during preparation.
- A power burr is used to enter and open the distal humeral and proximal ulnar canals, and to fine-tune the ultimate fit of the humeral and ulnar implants.
- Other tools used in humeral preparation include an oscillating saw and a barrel reamer.
- Appropriately sized cement restrictors should be available for use in the humeral and ulnar canals to contain the cement to the length of the implant stems and to facilitate better pressurization of the cement/implant interfaces. In the absence of smaller, appropriately sized restrictors for the ulnar canal, a plug of cancellous-only bone can be used. Alternatively, plugs can be made from a small amount of cement, which is injected separately.
- A cement gun with two injector nozzle sizes is used to fill the humeral and ulnar canals. The small size of the ulnar canal mandates the use of the smallest injector nozzle.
- Antibiotic powder, such as vancomycin, may be used just prior to wound closure.

## Procedure

### RESECTION OF THE RADIAL HEAD

- In the absence of arthrosis of the proximal radioulnar joint, resection of the radial head is not required.
- Correct anatomic medial placement of the ulnohumeral articulation as well as placement of an anterior flange directly on the anterior cortex prevents potential impingement of a retained radial head in flexion.
- The presence of arthrosis in the proximal radioulnar joint may limit forearm rotation and be a source of continued pain. In patients with arthrosis, the radial head should be excised.
- Retractors are placed around the junction of the radial head and neck, and the radial head is excised with the use of a 10- or 12-mm oscillating saw.
- The margins of resection should be checked to ensure that the level of resection is distal to the articular portion of the sigmoid notch and that the proximal radius does not contact the ulna.
- Patients with inflammatory disease may exhibit motion-limiting arthritis at the distal radioulnar joint, which may require that the distal radioulnar joint be addressed as well.

### PREPARATION OF THE HUMERUS

- To achieve resection of the intercondylar area of the distal humerus, the author of this chapter prefers to first remove a 1.5-cm section of the central trochlea with the use of an oscillating saw.
- A high-speed burr is used to gain entrance to the humeral canal, which is enlarged to 4 mm, at the proximal part of the olecranon fossa.
- The humerus is reamed with the use of a 3-mm starter rasp inserted with the posterior curve of the rasp matching the posterior bow of the humerus. Progressively larger rasps

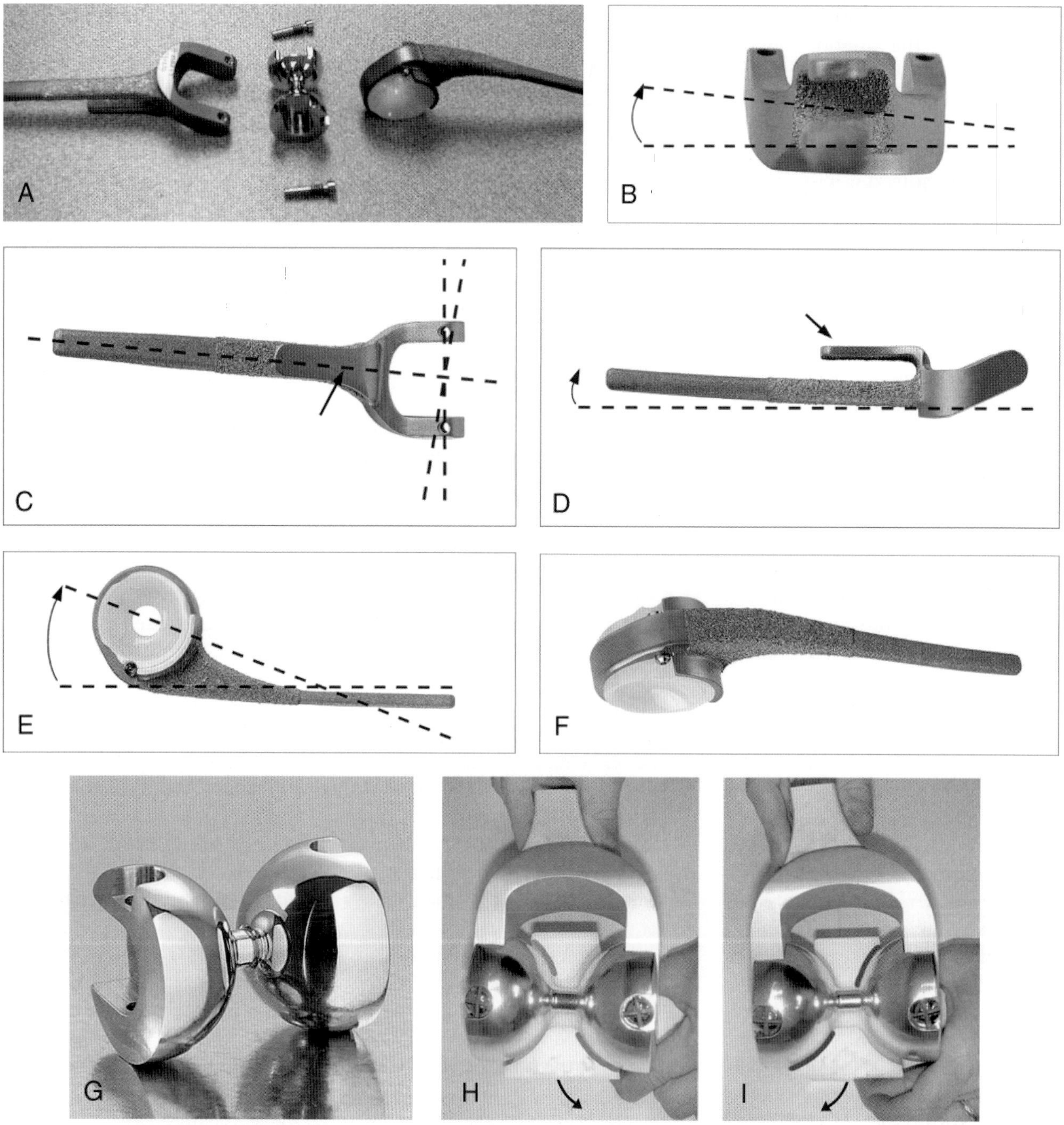


**Figure 6** Clinical photographs show the Discovery Elbow System (DJO Global). **A,** The components of the Discovery Elbow System. **B,** The humeral component incorporates 5° of internal rotation (arrow) with respect to the long axis of the stem. **C,** The humeral component incorporates 5° of varus alignment with respect to the long axis of the stem. Lateral offset of the humeral stem (arrow) places articulation in the center of the trochlea. **D,** The posterior anatomic bow of the humerus (horizontal dashed line shown for reference) matches the bow of the humerus in most patients. The anterior flange (arrow) is designed to sit directly on the anterior cortex of the humerus. **E** and **F,** The ulnar stem is laterally offset with respect to the articular component and incorporates a 23° anterior neck angle (arrow in panel E). **G,** Two cobalt-chromium hemispheric condyles simulate resurfacing/replacement of the trochlear surface. The size of the lateral condyle is equal to that of the medial condyle. Implant model depicts the large contact surfaces between the humeral and ulnar components, which distribute forces of varus (**H**) and valgus (**I**) motion. (Reproduced from Hastings H II: Linked total elbow arthroplasty: The Discovery Prosthesis, in Yamaguchi K, King GJW, McKee MD, O'Driscoll SWM, eds: *Advanced Reconstruction: Elbow.* Rosemont, IL, American Academy of Orthopaedic Surgeons, 2007, pp 229-239.)

 

are used until cortical resistance is attained.

- Because the humeral rasp has the same curvature and dimensions of the definitive implant, the application of a resection jig on the humeral rasp ensures that intercondylar resection coincides with that of the definitive implant.
- The resection guide is applied to the humeral rasp and adjusted so that the axis mark on the resection guide coincides with the flexion-extension axis of the elbow through the inferior-most portion of the medial epicondyle (**Figure 5, D**).
- After adjustment to the correct proximal-distal level is attained, the resection guide is locked in place.
- An oscillating saw is used to make four cuts through the resection jig.
- The humeral rasp and resection jig assembly are removed, the cuts are completed, and the intertrochlear area is removed.
- A barrel reamer (ulnar-based reamer) is used to round out the proximal part of the resection area.
- Alternatively, an external cutting template can be used in one of two ways to mark the area to be resected. For the first option, the humeral stem is aligned along the central exterior surface of the humeral shaft, with the medial-most portion of the distal cutting template aligned with the medial part of the trochlea (**Figure 5, C**). The medial and lateral margins of the cutting template are marked, and saw cuts are made to remove the trochlear portion of the joint. The second option uses a central hole in the exterior cutting template though which a drill can be passed, the template can be removed, and the centered tip of a step-cut reamer can be inserted. The step-cut reamer is advanced until it contacts the anterior cortex. An oscillating saw is used to complete the medial and lateral anterior margins of the resection. The humeral canal is then prepared as previously described.
- The supracondylar flare is rasped with the use of one of three rasps selected based on the size that corresponds with the last humeral shaft rasp used. The rasp is gently impacted until the axis mark on the rasp coincides with the level of the elbow axis that passes through the inferior-most aspect of the medial epicondyle. A burr may be used to fine-tune and finish the preparation of the metaphyseal flare.
- Any obstructions to complete insertion of the trial prosthesis are removed with the use of a small power burr.
- The holes on the condylar projections of the trial implant also identify the axis of flexion and extension. After complete insertion, these holes should coincide with the axis of flexion and extension through the inferior-most portion of the medial epicondyle (**Figure 5, E**).
- Complete seating of the prosthesis usually requires a small recession (notch) in the central anterior distal humeral cortex to accommodate the base of the anterior flange of the humeral component.

## PREPARATION OF THE ULNA

- Using a burr that is aimed 18° laterally and 55° posteriorly, a small window is made in the ulnar canal at the intersection of the olecranon and the coronoid.
- A starter awl is used to probe and identify the ulnar canal.
- Flexible ulnar reamers (either hand reamers or power reamers) are used to open the more distal ulnar canal to a depth of 75 or 100 mm, depending on the stem length of the ulnar implant.
- Reaming is continued until light cortical contact is attained. This step removes soft cancellous bone from inside the ulnar canal to enhance the strength of the subsequent cement mantle.
- A proper groove in the olecranon is essential to achieve proper axial reaming of the ulna. The end of a slot reamer is inserted in the ulnar canal and used as an anchor for drilling of a slot in the olecranon. The width of the slot is enlarged with the use of a burr.
- The ulna is serially reamed up to the chosen templated size of the implant, beginning with 3-, 4-, and/or 5-mm rasps. A barrel reamer can be used to round out the proximal ulna to ensure an appropriate fit with the curvature of the implant.
- The appropriately sized trial implant is tested. Fine-tuning with the use of a burr may be required.
- If the implant does not seat fully, then the surgeon should ensure the groove in the olecranon is deep enough before enlarging the anterior coronoid slot.

## TESTING THE TRIAL IMPLANT

- The provisional humeral and ulnar implants are inserted, and the elbow is taken through a full range of motion.
- If the motion is satisfactory, then the definitive implants are opened and tested to ensure that they also fully seat.

## CANAL PREPARATION, IMPLANT INSERTION, AND CEMENT FIXATION

- A cement restrictor is used in both the humeral and ulnar canals. Prefabricated cement restrictors are available with some total elbow implant systems. In the absence of appropriate cement restrictors, a small cancellous plug is used in the ulna, and a small amount of cement is injected at the appropriate depth in the humerus.
- The final components are cleaned and dried.

- The humeral canals are packed with thrombin-soaked surgical sponges.
- Low-viscosity cement that has been premixed with an antibiotic is delivered via an injection gun first into the humerus and then into the ulna. The cement should be freed of air bubbles with the use of either a prepackaged vacuum cement system or a centrifuge before delivery into the injection gun.
- One or two surgical sponges are packed around the distal humerus to absorb any cement spillage.
- The humeral component is inserted. The surgeon should ensure that on terminal insertion, the anterior flange sits flush with the anterior cortex of the humerus. A humeral impactor is used for complete seating.
- Cement is injected into the ulnar canal from distal to proximal, and the ulnar implant is seated. An ulnar impactor is used for complete seating.
- All extra cement is removed.

#### IMPLANT COUPLING

- After the cement has set, the tourniquet is deflated to ensure complete peri-implant hemostasis before articulation.
- After hemostasis is attained, the tourniquet is reinflated. The tourniquet is left deflated if minimal bleeding is present.
- Before articulation of the prosthesis, the wound is carefully irrigated and inspected to ensure that no fragments of cement or bone that may result in third-body wear of the high-density polyethylene interface are present.
- The definitive condylar bushings are applied to the ulna, and the articulation is distracted and rotated to fully seat both condyles on the humeral projections.
- Any screws necessary to lock the condyles in place are applied (**Figure 5, F**).

### Wound Closure

- The wound is irrigated and inspected both visually and on palpation to ensure that it is free of any debris that could result in wear of the polyethylene interface.
- The author of this chapter prefers to spread 2 g of an antibiotic powder, such as vancomycin, in the wound before closure, with one-half of the antibiotic powder applied to the deep wound and one-half of the antibiotic powder to the superficial wound.
- At the end of the posterior proximal-reflecting triceps-off technique, the longitudinal triceps split is repaired with the use of 2-0 resorbable monofilament suture. The distal extent of the tendon split on each side is sutured back to the base of the reflected triceps tendon flap. This flap is repositioned and sutured with the use of interrupted, running 2-0 resorbable monofilament suture. The stability of the transposed ulnar nerve is checked. In the unlikely instance that the ulnar nerve does not remain anterior during elbow flexion and extension, it is stabilized with the use of a fascial sling.
- At the end of the triceps-on and UCL-sparing technique, the extensor supinator origin is repaired back to the lateral triceps and the flexor-pronator is repaired back to the medial triceps with the use of 2-0 resorbable monofilament mattress sutures. The ulnar nerve almost always remains in a stable anterior position (**Figure 3, E**). One suction drain is placed in the deep wound, and one suction drain is placed in the subcutaneous space and brought out through the proximal skin. The subcuticular tissues are approximated with the use of 3-0 or 4-0 resorbable sutures, and the skin is closed with the use of staples or sutures. Meticulous suture closure is especially important at the level of the joint. Tissue glue is applied to seal the incision. A bulky dressing and splint are applied with the elbow positioned in 60° to 75° of flexion to minimize posterior wound tension.
- For the triceps-splitting technique, drill holes are placed in a crisscrossing fashion through the proximal olecranon at the side of the triceps insertion. The triceps split is repaired from proximal to distal with running suture, using the sutures that were placed early in the procedure. Large Keith needles are used to pass the two pairs of sutures through bone and tie the sutures distally on either the medial or lateral side of the ulna.
- At the end of the lateral triceps-off technique, the preplaced sutures are repaired back to the ulna in the same manner as that for the triceps-splitting technique.

## Postoperative Regimen

Antibiotics are continued for 24 hours postoperatively. The suction drains are removed 48 hours postoperatively or after they have stopped draining. Usually, the patient is discharged from the hospital on the second postoperative day. Between the third and fifth postoperative day, the dressing is removed and the wound is checked. If the wound is sealed and dry, active range of motion is initiated. Range-of-motion exercises should be deferred until the wound is dry and free of drainage. Regardless how the triceps was approached, the patient is instructed on active and passive flexion exercises. If the triceps was repaired, gravity-assisted active extension as well as passive extension are

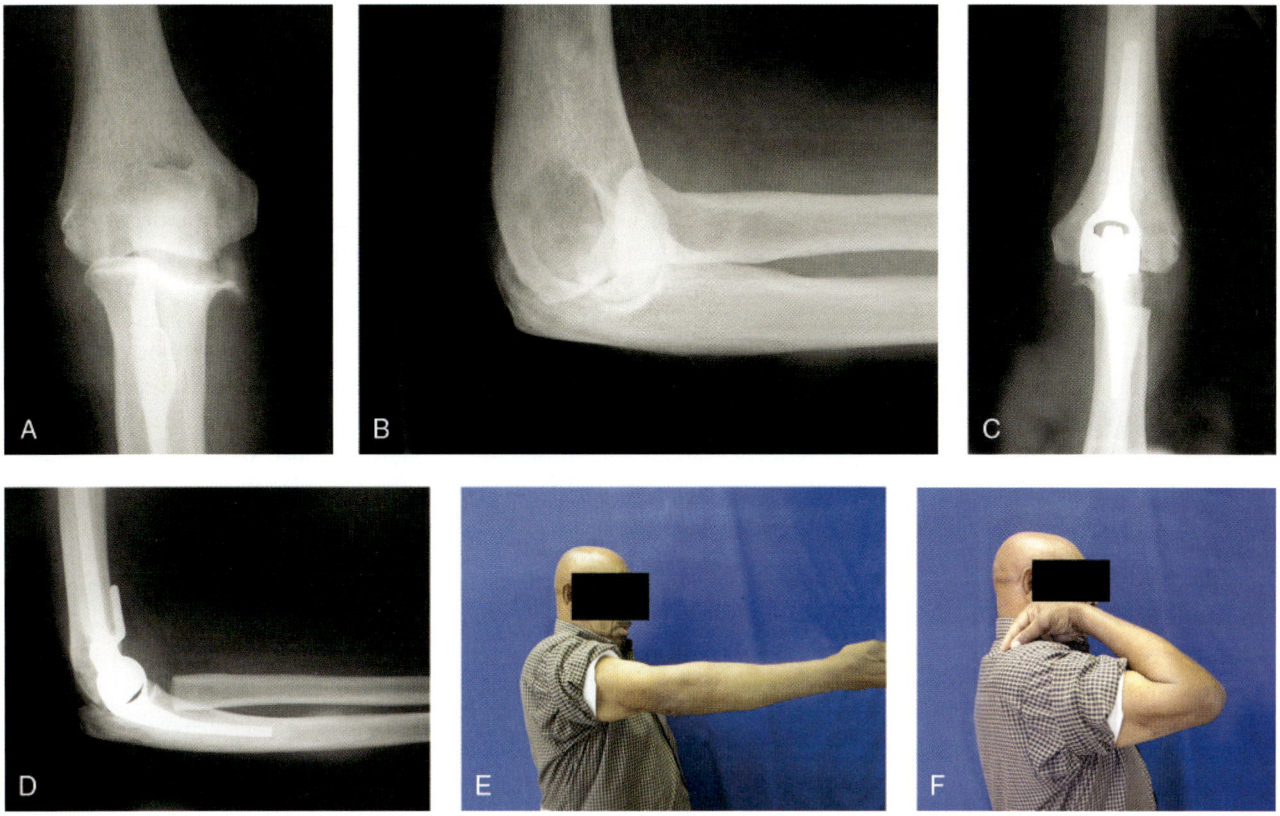


**Figure 7** Images of the right elbow of a 60-year-old man with destructive rheumatoid deformity of the elbow who underwent linked total elbow arthroplasty. Preoperative AP (**A**) and lateral (**B**) radiographs demonstrate diffuse severe, erosive elbow arthritis involving both the radiocapitellar and ulnotrochlear surfaces. AP (**C**) and lateral (**D**) radiographs obtained after total elbow arthroplasty. Clinical photographs of the patient show postoperative elbow extension (**E**) and flexion (**F**). (Reproduced from Hastings H II: Linked total elbow arthroplasty: The Discovery Prosthesis, in Yamaguchi K, King GJW, McKee MD, O'Driscoll SWM, eds: *Advanced Reconstruction: Elbow*. Rosemont, IL, American Academy of Orthopaedic Surgeons, 2007, pp 229-239.)

allowed. Extension against resistance, such as pushing up out of a chair, is deferred until 6 weeks postoperatively. If the triceps has not been detached, active and passive extension, even against resistance, is allowed. Any residual tightness in extension is corrected with the use of weighted extension exercises. A long-arm splint is used in full extension at night to maintain extension.

Sutures or staples are removed 10 to 14 days postoperatively, at which time routine radiographs are obtained (**Figure 7, A** through **D**). Normal light use and strengthening are initiated at 6 weeks postoperatively (**Figure 7, E** and **F**). Patients are advised to maintain a long-term weight restriction of 3 to 4 kg (6 to 9 lb); however, patients with restored function and reduced pain may not be willing or able to adhere to such weight restrictions. Participation in sports such as tennis and golf is not advised after TEA.

## Limiting Adverse Events

Most complications after TEA are related to either wound healing or neuritis of the ulnar nerve. Most wound complications result from poor skin quality, inadequate soft-tissue coverage, or hematoma.

Patients who have compromised immune function or who are being treated with immunosuppressive medications should discontinue the use of immune-compromising medications well before surgery, and a complete blood count should be obtained preoperatively. Cultures are obtained from the anterior nares of all patients preoperatively to rule out staphylococci. If cultures are positive, then the patient is treated with the use of an antistaphylococcal ointment preoperatively. Because of the superficial position of the elbow and its thin soft-tissue envelope, the author of this chapter prefers to premix antibiotics in the cement. Prophylactic antibiotics are used for 24 hours postoperatively. The wound should be carefully checked before range of motion is initiated. If any persistent drainage or erythema is present, then motion should be deferred until the wound is hemostatically sealed.

With the increasing age of the population, more patients are being treated with platelet-inhibiting and anticoagulant medications to manage cardiovascular disease. Platelet-inhibiting and anticoagulant medications should be carefully assessed preoperatively and discontinued at an appropriate point before surgery. The tourniquet should be deflated before wound closure (at least temporarily) to ensure a dry wound at closure. Suction drains are used for 24 to 48 hours postoperatively.

The preexisting incisions of patients with posttraumatic conditions should be carefully assessed and used if possible. If a decision is made to use a new incision, then an adequate skin bridge must be present between the new and preexisting incisions. Any new incision that has to cross a preexisting incision should cross at the largest angle possible. Older patients, particularly those who are being treated with steroids, have thin skin and subcutaneous tissue. Accurate closure of the skin edges is essential, particularly directly at the level of the elbow around the olecranon. Sutures rather than staples are preferred at this level to ensure perfect edge-to-edge closure. Splints, if used postoperatively, must have appropriate padding so they do not cause pressure necrosis.

Resection of the intercondylar area weakens the distal humerus to a certain extent; it may help to minimize the width of the condylar projection from the stem with maximal preservation of the supracondylar columns. Implant fixation does not depend on the presence, absence, or integrity of the medial and lateral condyles. Insertion and disimpaction of rasps with the use of a mallet should be done carefully without twisting or applying torque. Impediment to full insertion of the humeral component may require slight enlargement of the canal entrance with the use of a power burr. Fracture of the ulna can occur, particularly if the ulnar rasp is directed too posteriorly rather than axially down the canal. Correct axial reaming down the canal requires the creation of an adequate trough in the olecranon, which is easier to achieve with the use of the triceps-off technique.

In some semiconstrained total elbow implants, particulate-induced synovitis has been reported as early as 8 to 12 months postoperatively, particularly if the bushings are subject to a small-surface area and high-contact loading in combination with flexion and extension. Some studies suggest that particulate-induced synovitis is less common with newer total elbow implant designs. The surgeon should anticipate that the ulnar polyethylene component may experience wear with time. For some total elbow implant designs, new polyethylene components can be applied without revising the stem. Third-body wear can be prevented by carefully removing any particulate cement matter and bone fragments after implantation and copiously irrigating the wound before articulation and closure.

Prospective studies have not reported a significant difference in triceps strength between patients who undergo TEA with the triceps-off or triceps-on techniques. Triceps strength was manually tested but not measured by computerized instruments. The author of this chapter believes that there is always a consequence after triceps takedown. Most studies have noted occasional symptomatic triceps weakness or failure of the triceps repair after TEA with the triceps-off technique. Failure of triceps repair has not been observed in patients who undergo TEA with the posterior proximal reflecting triceps-off technique.

## Bibliography

Alizadehkhaiyat O, Al Mandhari A, Sinopidis C, Wood A, Frostick S: Total elbow arthroplasty: A prospective clinical outcome study of Discovery Elbow System with a 4-year mean follow-up. *J Shoulder Elbow Surg* 2015;24(1):52-59.

Baghdadi YM, Veillette CJ, Malone AA, Morrey BF, Sanchez-Sotelo J: Total elbow arthroplasty in obese patients. *J Bone Joint Surg Am* 2014;96(9):e70.

Dachs RP, Fleming MA, Chivers DA, et al: Total elbow arthroplasty: Outcomes after triceps-detaching and triceps-sparing approaches. *J Shoulder Elbow Surg* 2015;24(3):339-347.

Dalemans A, De Smet L, Degreef I: Long-term outcome of elbow resurfacing. *J Shoulder Elbow Surg* 2013;22(11):1455-1460.

Ducrot G, Ehlinger M, Adam P, Di Marco A, Clavert P, Bonnomet F: Complex fractures of the distal humerus in the elderly: Is primary total elbow arthroplasty a valid treatment alternative? A series of 20 cases. *Orthop Traumatol Surg Res* 2013;99(1):10-20.

 

Egol KA, Tsai P, Vazques O, Tejwani NC: Comparison of functional outcomes of total elbow arthroplasty vs plate fixation for distal humerus fractures in osteoporotic elbows. *Am J Orthop (Belle Mead NJ)* 2011;40(2):67-71.

Fevang BT, Lie SA, Havelin LI, Skredderstuen A, Furnes O: Results after 562 total elbow replacements: A report from the Norwegian Arthroplasty Register. *J Shoulder Elbow Surg* 2009;18(3):449-456.

Giannicola G, Scacchi M, Polimanti D, Cinotti G: Discovery elbow system: 2- to 5-year results in distal humerus fractures and posttraumatic conditions. A prospective study on 24 patients. *J Hand Surg Am* 2014;39(9):1746-1756.

Hastings H II, Lee DH, Pietrzak WS: A prospective multicenter clinical study of the Discovery elbow. *J Shoulder Elbow Surg* 2014;23(5):e95-e107.

Jeon IH, Morrey BF, Sanchez-Sotelo J: Ulnar component surface finish influenced the outcome of primary Coonrad-Morrey total elbow arthroplasty. *J Shoulder Elbow Surg* 2012;21(9):1229-1235.

Mansat P, Bonnevialle N, Rongières M, Mansat M, Bonnevialle P: Experience with the Coonrad-Morrey total elbow arthroplasty: 78 consecutive total elbow arthroplasties reviewed with an average 5 years of follow-up. *J Shoulder Elbow Surg* 2013;22(11):1461-1468.

Mansat P, Nouaille Degorce H, Bonnevialle N, Demezon H, Fabre T; SOFCOT: Total elbow arthroplasty for acute distal humeral fractures in patients over 65 years old: Results of a multicenter study in 87 patients. *Orthop Traumatol Surg Res* 2013;99(7):779-784.

Plaschke HC, Thillemann TM, Brorson S, Olsen BS: Implant survival after total elbow arthroplasty: A retrospective study of 324 procedures performed from 1980 to 2008. *J Shoulder Elbow Surg* 2014;23(6):829-836.

Pogliacomi F, Galavotti C, Cavaciocchi M, Corradi M, Rotini R, Ceccarelli F: Total elbow arthroplasty following traumas: Mid-term results. *Acta Biomed* 2013;84(3):212-218.

Schöni M, Drerup S, Angst F, Kyburz D, Simmen BR, Goldhahn J: Long-term survival of GSB III elbow prostheses and risk factors for revisions. *Arch Orthop Trauma Surg* 2013;133(10):1415-1424.

Smith GC, McCann PS, Simpson D, Blewitt N, Amirfeyz R: The effect of using a cement gun with a narrow nozzle on cement penetration for total elbow arthroplasty: A cadaveric study. *J Hand Surg Am* 2015;40(2):276-280.

Sørensen BW, Brorson S, Olsen BS: Primary total elbow arthroplasty in complex fractures of the distal humerus. *World J Orthop* 2014;5(3):368-372.

Toor AS, Jiang JJ, Shi LL, Koh JL: Comparison of perioperative complications after total elbow arthroplasty in patients with and without diabetes. *J Shoulder Elbow Surg* 2014;23(11):1599-1606.

Wagener ML, de Vos MJ, Hannink G, van der Pluijm M, Verdonschot N, Eygendaal D: Mid-term clinical results of a modern convertible total elbow arthroplasty. *Bone Joint J* 2015;97(5):681-688.

## Video Reference

Hastings H II: Video. *Total Elbow Arthroplasty in a Rheumatoid Elbow.* Telluride, CO, 2015.

 

# Chapter 19

# Revision Total Elbow Arthroplasty to Manage Aseptic Loosening

*David Stanley, MBBS, BSc, FRCS*

**Learning Objectives**

- Understand and avoid underestimating the difficulty that can be experienced in the removal of partially loose primary total elbow prostheses.
- Understand that appropriate revision total elbow arthroplasty instruments are essential to limit iatrogenic fractures.
- Be familiar with the creation of bone windows to facilitate the removal of a failed elbow arthroplasty prosthesis and cement mantle.
- Have the ability to decide if a direct-exchange arthroplasty can be undertaken (bone loss absent) or if bone reconstruction with or without a customized prosthesis will be necessary (bone loss present) based on preoperative radiographs and the intraoperative findings.

## Indications

The primary indication for revision total elbow arthroplasty (TEA) to manage aseptic loosening is the development of pain in a previously well-functioning elbow prosthesis. The pain is initially related to activity but progressively becomes constant. Pain results from movement of the prosthesis within the humeral (**Figure 1**) or ulnar (**Figure 2**) canal and is frequently associated with bone loss. If bone loss is substantial and likely to progress to a periprosthetic fracture, urgent revision TEA is indicated. Secondary indications for revision TEA include loss of elbow function, which is most frequently associated with elbow pain, and instability of the elbow as a result of gross component loosening.

## Contraindications

The only contraindications that preclude revision TEA are medical comorbidities that make the risks of surgery greater than the potential benefits. Because many patients with aseptic loosening have inflammatory arthritis, it is essential that patients are treated by a multidisciplinary team to mitigate any comorbidities.

## Alternative Treatments

Excision arthroplasty is an alternative treatment option; however, it rarely provides a functional outcome as good as that achieved with revision TEA. In particular, if either or both of the humeral columns are absent, the elbow is likely to be unstable. The author of this chapter has sometimes achieved reasonable function using cement ball spacers (the so-called "cue–ball" arthroplasty) to provide a fulcrum for elbow flexion, but has never found it to be as good as a successful revision TEA. Arthrodesis of the elbow is extremely difficult to perform after removal of a total elbow prosthesis and, even if successful, is poorly tolerated by most patients because of loss of function.

## Results

Although there are several published studies on the short-term to mid-term outcomes of revision TEA to manage aseptic loosening, the long-term outcomes of the technique are less clear (**Table 1**). The literature has demonstrated that revision TEA is a complex procedure and that surgeons must be familiar with a variety of surgical techniques including impaction grafting and the use of strut allografts, allograft-prosthetic composites, and customized implants to achieve a satisfactory elbow reconstruction. Surgeons must have the appropriate equipment available for all revision TEA procedures to facilitate the safe removal of a loose prosthesis as well as the cement mantle, and thereby reduce the risk for iatrogenic fractures and cortical bone perforations.

*Neither Dr. Stanley nor any immediate family member has received anything of value from or has stock or stock options held in a commercial company or institution related directly or indirectly to the subject of this chapter.*

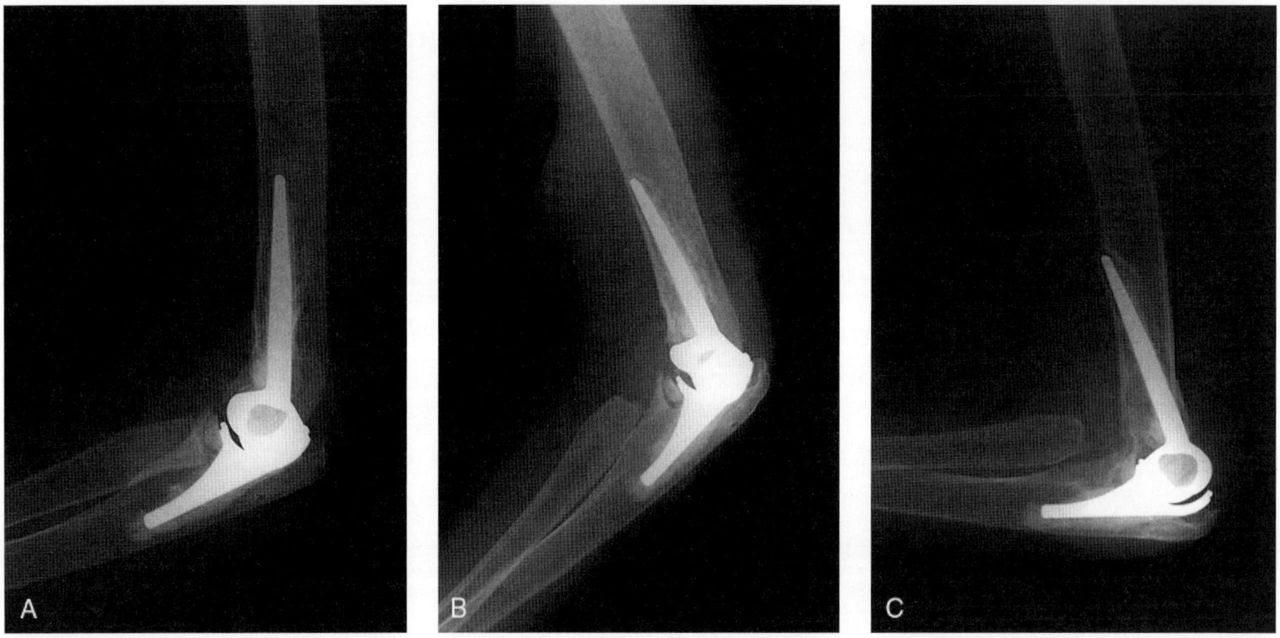


**Figure 1** **A-C,** Lateral radiographs of an elbow demonstrate progressive aseptic humeral component loosening of an unlinked prosthesis. Each sequential radiograph shows the tip of the humeral prosthesis migrating progressively more anteriorly and the axis displacing posteriorly. This is a result of the direction of resultant forces during elbow flexion and extension. The ulnar component remains well fixed in each image.

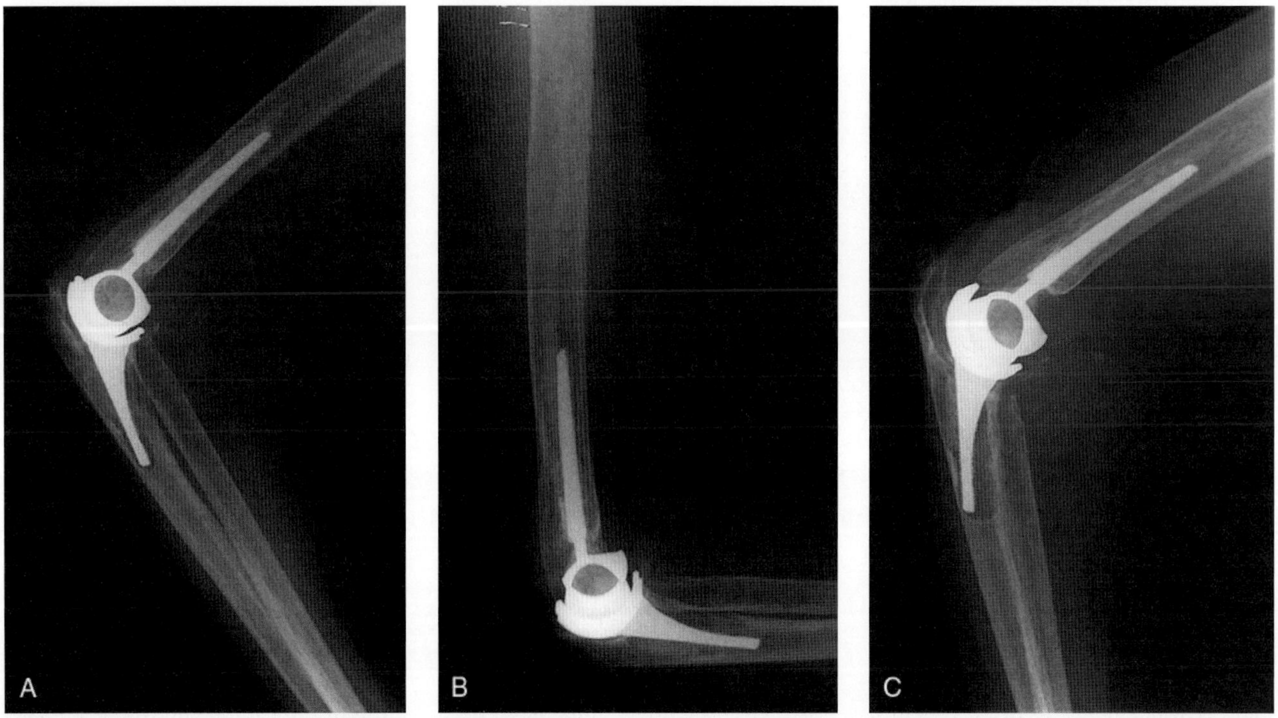


**Figure 2** **A-C,** Lateral radiographs of an elbow demonstrate progressive aseptic ulnar component loosening of an unlinked prosthesis. Each sequential radiograph shows increasing evidence of the ulnar component loosening. The humeral component remains well fixed in each image.

 

**Table 1** Results of Revision Total Elbow Arthroplasty to Manage Aseptic Loosening

| Authors (Year) | Number of Patients | Procedure or Approach | Mean Patient Age in Years (Range) | Mean Follow-up in Months (Range) | Results | Level of Evidence |
|---|---|---|---|---|---|---|
| Amirfeyz and Stanley (2011) | 10 | Allograft-prosthesis composite | 64 (40-84) | 75 (24-213) | Mean MEPI score improved from 9.5 to 74 | III |
| Malone et al (2012) | 52 | Exchange cementing | 59 (31-80) | 94.5 (26-266) | MEPS was good or excellent in 31 patients | III |
| Rhee et al (2013) | 16 | Impaction grafting | 58.4 (28-75) | 88.8 (49.2-134.4) | Mean MEPS improved from 41.0 to 82.8 | IV |
| Puskas et al (2014) | 711 | Revision with a 4- or 6-inch humeral stem | NA | 88 (0-260) | No significant difference in the revision rate between the two stem lengths | III |

MEPI = Mayo Elbow Performance Index, MEPS = Mayo Elbow Performance Score, NA = not available.

# Techniques

## Setup/Exposure

- The author of this chapter has found the lateral decubitus position, with the arm supported in a gutter and the forearm hanging vertically, to be the most useful patient position for revision TEA.
- Typically, a sterile high-arm tourniquet is applied. However, if a long-stem humeral component was used in primary TEA or there is a tail of cement that extends toward the shoulder, a tourniquet should not be used.
- Prophylactic antibiotics are administered in accordance with local protocols.
- Sterile preparation and draping are performed according to the surgeon's preference.

## Instruments/Equipment/Implants Required

- Revision TEA should be undertaken only by surgeons who have experience with primary TEA and have the appropriate equipment for revision TEA.
- Small-width fine osteotomes and cement splitters are essential for cement mantle removal.
- A range of curets for cement and membrane removal are necessary.
- Fine saw blades should be available.
- Power drills and a range of appropriately sized burrs should be available.
- If an implant extraction device is part of the arthroplasty tray for the implant that is being removed, it should be used; otherwise, a universal implant extraction device should be used (**Figures 3** and **4**).
- A membrane removal brush is useful.
- Revision total elbow implants are necessary. Depending on the implant that is being removed and the amount of bone loss present, a standard implant can possibly be used for revision TEA. If there is substantial bone loss and/or a periprosthetic fracture associated with aseptic loosening, a customized prosthesis may be required. The customized prosthesis should be obtained before the revision TEA is performed.
- If there is substantial medullary bone loss, impaction bone grafting may be indicated. Allograft bone should be obtained before revision TEA is performed.
- Allograft bone also may be necessary in patients in whom structural bone loss is present. Allograft bone should be obtained before revision TEA is performed.

## Procedure

- The skin incision usually involves the previous posterior incision; however, it often requires extension proximally and/or distally, depending on which component of the primary prosthesis is considered the more difficult to revise.
- If an incision other than a posterior incision was used for primary TEA, the surgeon should consider creating a new posterior incision that is centered at the level of the olecranon. A new incision should be undertaken only if it will not create a narrow skin flap that may subsequently undergo necrosis postoperatively.
- The ulnar nerve is identified and superficially decompressed. Whether the ulnar nerve is anteriorly transposed depends on the surgeon's preference. The author of this chapter does not routinely transpose the ulnar nerve; however, some surgeons transpose the ulnar nerve in every revision TEA without adverse effects. The author of this chapter

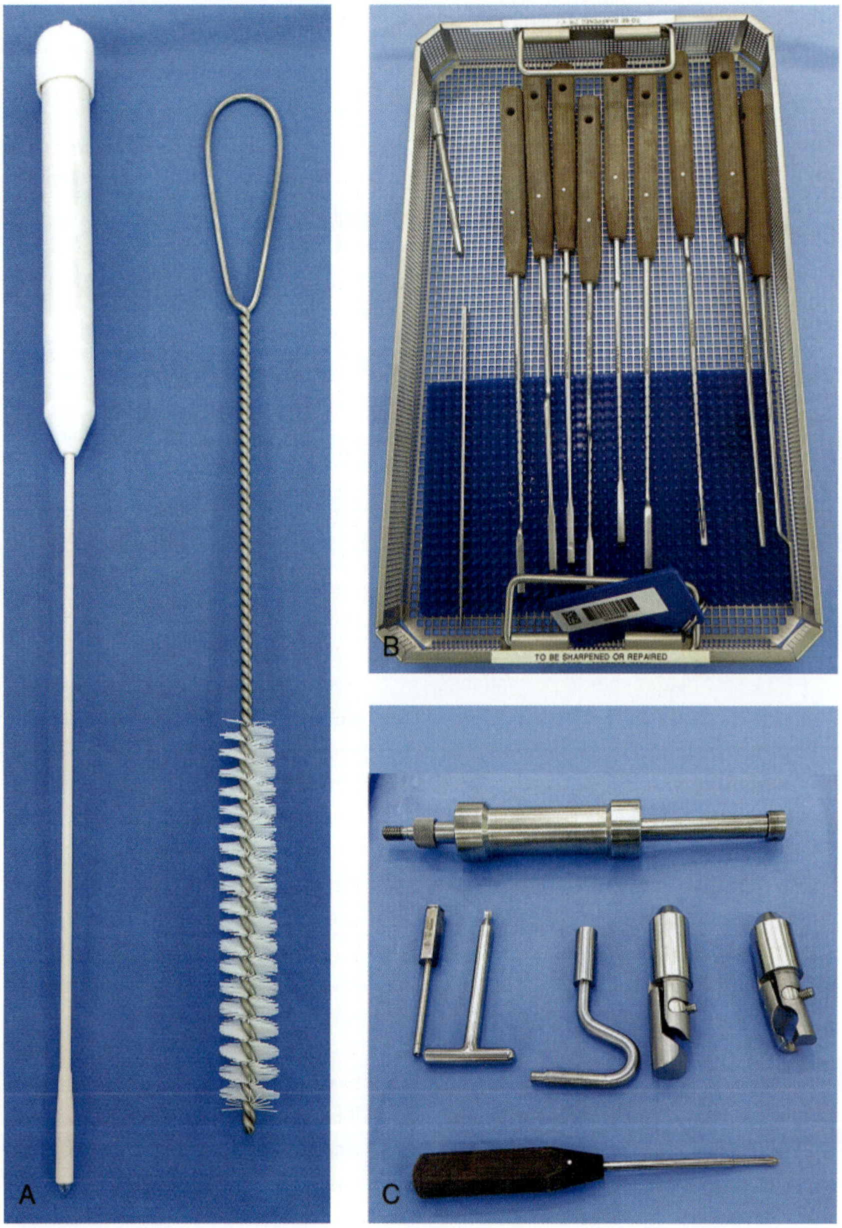


**Figure 3** Photographs show the specialized equipment necessary for revision total elbow arthroplasty (TEA). **A,** A brush (right) is useful for membrane removal and a flexible light (left) improves visualization in the humeral and ulnar canals. **B,** A range of small osteotomes and cement splitters is essential for cement mantle removal. **C,** An implant extraction device assists in the removal of primary TEA implants.

prefers to constantly check the position of the ulnar nerve throughout the surgical procedure by regularly visualizing the nerve at each stage of the procedure. Anything that may affect the vascularity of the ulnar nerve, such as excessive or prolonged retraction, is avoided. Slings are not placed around the ulnar nerve because of concerns for traction injury, particularly if clips are attached to the slings.

- The surgical approach to the elbow joint depends on the surgeon's experience and preference. The main options are triceps splitting, triceps reflecting, and triceps sparing. If it is clear from the surgical note what approach was originally used, the same approach should be used, if possible, to reduce the risk of additional triceps scarring, which in turn will decrease extension strength. The author of this chapter prefers to use the Shahane-Stanley approach, which allows for wide exposure of the elbow joint; mobilizes the ulnar nerve with its soft-tissue bed; facilitates soft-tissue tensioning after insertion of the revision total elbow prosthesis; and closes the soft tissues as a single envelope, thereby isolating the prosthesis from the superficial layers of the elbow.
- Fluid within the joint, if present, should always be sent for microscopy, culture, and sensitivity to confirm the absence of a low-grade infection, because infection may be the cause of loosening. In addition, and for the same reason, during exposure of the elbow joint and again after removal of the implant, multiple tissue samples—including membrane from the humeral and ulnar canals—should be sent for microscopy, culture, and sensitivity.
- Removal of the primary elbow prosthesis may be difficult unless both the humeral and ulnar components are loose. Unfortunately, this is rarely the case; more frequently, one component is loose and the other component either is well fixed or has partial radiolucent lines that are observed radiographically.
- The loose component is removed, after which attention is focused on the other component. It is reasonable to leave a truly well-fixed component in situ and simply revise the loose component. In this situation, however, a careful examination must be performed to identify and correct any impingement that may have contributed to the

 

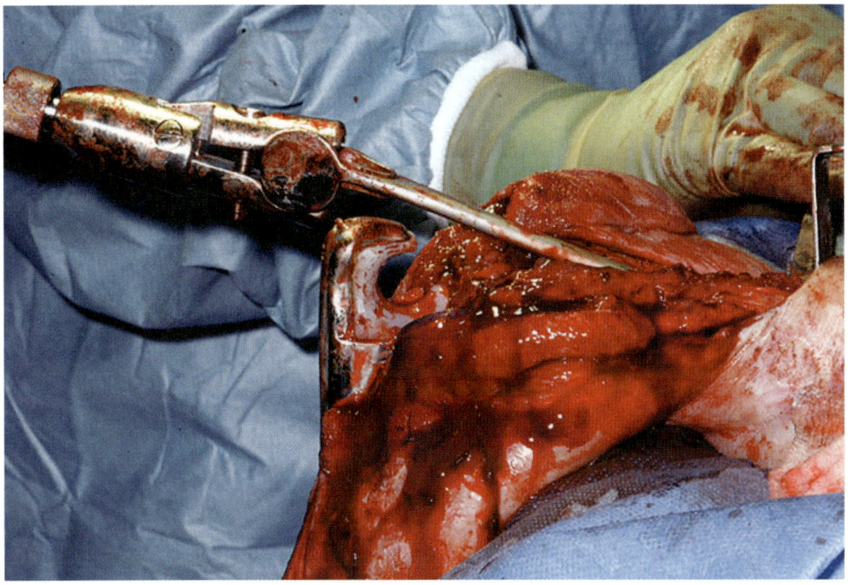

**Figure 4** Intraoperative photograph shows an implant extraction device attached to the humeral implant to assist in the removal of the humeral implant. The extraction device can only assist the removal. Typically, it is necessary to partially loosen the prosthesis with osteotomes before the extraction device can be successfully used.

loosening. The bushing mechanism of a linked prosthesis is changed to maximize the long-term survival of the prosthesis.

- In patients in whom either both components appear partially loose or one component is loose and the other component is partially loose, it is impossible to give a single technique description on how the implants should be removed. Rather, the steps in the procedure must be individualized to the patient. To assist in implant removal, the surgeon must have a full set of appropriate revision TEA instruments available to limit the potential for iatrogenic fracture.
- To reduce the risk for fractures, creation of a controlled window in the bony cortex should be considered. For the humerus, a rectangular window is made in the posterior lower one-third of the humeral shaft. The author of this chapter preserves the most distal posterior humeral cortex because this area of the humerus resists resultant forces during elbow movement (**Figure 5, A**). For the ulna, the author of this chapter usually makes a triangular window on the ulnar aspect of the proximal shaft. The use of bone windows facilitates safe implant removal and aids in cement mantle removal (**Figure 5, B** and **C**).
- After the implants have been removed, fine osteotomes, cement splitters, burrs, and curets are used to remove the cement mantle. In patients in whom the cement-bone interface is preserved and loosening has occurred at the implant-cement interface, it may be possible to leave the original cement in place and then cement the revision prosthesis into the existing cement mantle. In general, however, the author of this chapter prefers to remove all of the original cement before inserting the new prosthesis.
- After the cement has been removed, any soft-tissue membrane within the humeral and ulnar canals is excised. This can be achieved with the use of curets and a bone brush.
- After bone preparation is complete, any bone windows that were created are replaced (**Figure 6**), the trial implants are inserted, and impingement is corrected. A cement restrictor is then inserted in the humeral canal to prevent proximal migration of the cement.
- The definitive implants are inserted with cement pressurization.
- If possible, it is helpful to use a short-stemmed rather than long-stemmed revision total elbow prosthesis because short-stemmed prostheses preserve bone in the event that future revision TEA procedures are required. However, if bone windows were created or the humeral or ulnar shaft was perforated during the procedure, the implant stem should extend twice the medullary canal diameter beyond the bone window or perforation to reduce the risk of a postoperative periprosthetic fracture.
- If a triceps-reflecting surgical approach was used, the triceps should be securely reattached to the olecranon with the use of nonabsorbable sutures.
- For patients with loss of medullary bone as a result of movement of the implant within the canal, the surgeon should consider impaction grafting, which involves the use of morcellized allograft bone that is impacted into the bony canal before the prosthesis is inserted (**Figure 7**).
- Occasionally, a strut allograft may help reinforce and span a bone window or perforation in the humeral or ulnar shaft.
- If aseptic loosening is associated with substantial structural bone loss, an allograft-prosthetic composite reconstruction or a customized prosthesis should be considered (**Figures 8** and **9**).

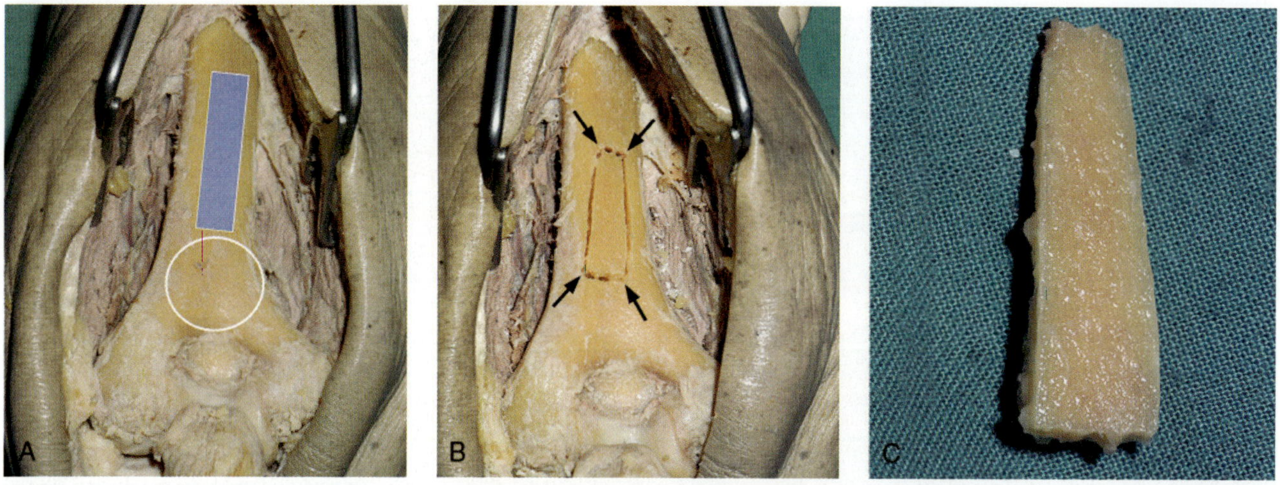


**Figure 5** **A,** Photograph of the humerus of a cadaver model shows planning of the position for a humeral window for removal of a well-fixed humeral implant. The blue rectangle indicates the planned site of the humeral window. The circle marked on the distal humerus indicates the posterior humeral bone that the surgeon will preserve because this section of the humerus resists resultant forces during elbow flexion and extension. **B,** Photograph shows the creation of a humeral window. Note the drill holes at the corners of the rectangle (arrows), which help reduce the risk for fractures that can result from the sharp corners of the bone window. **C,** Photograph shows the removed humeral window.

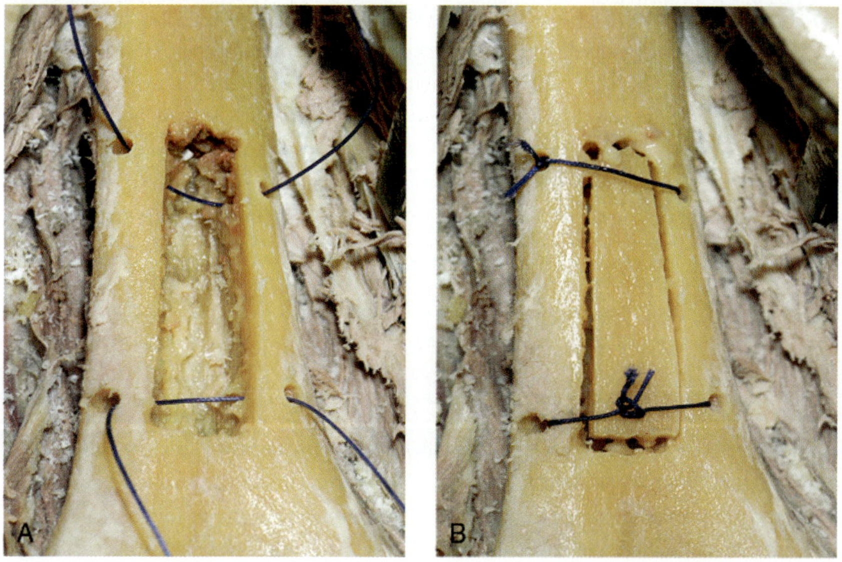


**Figure 6** Photographs of the humerus of a cadaver model show measures to prevent the humeral window from falling into the medullary space, which often occurs during humeral window replacement. Holes measuring 2 mm in diameter are drilled at the edges of the bone window, absorbable sutures are passed beneath the bone window (**A**), and the absorbable sutures are tied over the humeral window (**B**).

### Wound Closure

- A deep drain may be used if deemed appropriate by the surgeon.
- Wound closure depends to an extent on the previous surgical approach, but essentially, it is performed in layers with the use of absorbable sutures.
- The method of skin closure is based on the surgeon's preference. The author of this chapter uses an absorbable subcuticular suture for skin closure.
- A dressing of orthopaedic gauze and wool in combination with a plaster back slab is applied with the arm positioned as straight as possible.
- The arm is elevated on multiple pillows (at least 3) for 48 hours to allow soft-tissue swelling to reduce.

## Postoperative Regimen

In the experience of the author of this chapter, in the United Kingdom, adequate analgesic agents are administered postoperatively. In most patients, this is achieved via a preoperative nerve block. If a preoperative nerve block is not possible, a range of medications sufficient to control pain must be administered to the patient.

Adequate and safe pain relief are a priority. An opioid-centric model of pain control created an epidemic of diversion, misuse, and overdose death (as well as a resurgence of heroin use) in the United States and Canada of which every surgeon should be aware. Patients and surgeons living in countries not yet affected should be proactive and

 

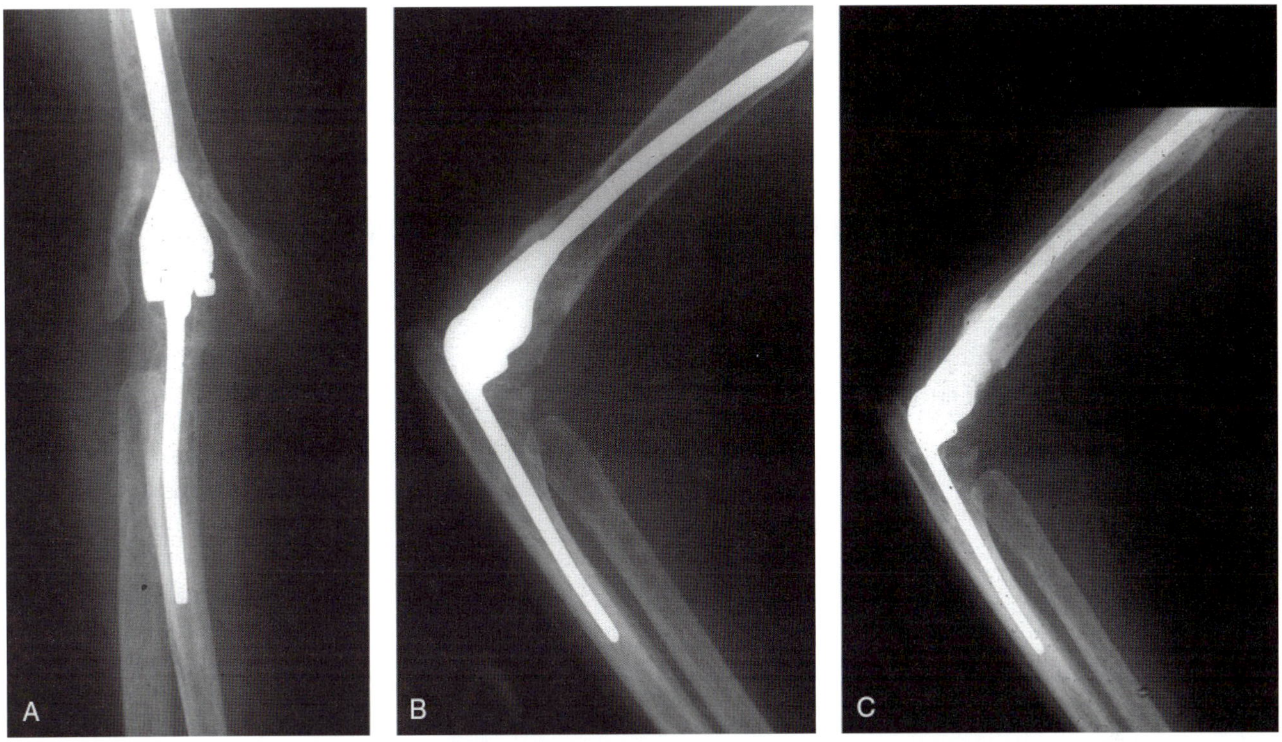


**Figure 7** AP (**A**) and lateral (**B**) radiographs of an elbow with a linked prosthesis demonstrate substantial intramedullary humeral bone loss as a result of aseptic loosening. **C,** Lateral radiograph of the same elbow shown in panels **A** and **B** obtained after revision total elbow arthroplasty with impaction bone grafting demonstrates restoration of intramedullary bone.

avoid the problems occurring in North America.

The surgeon should start with careful planning and preparation, and ask the patient what medications were taken after the previous injury or surgery. The message will be clear: surgery hurts; the surgeon cares; being pain free is not a reasonable goal; the surgeon should have a plan. Emphasize that the patient should be as comfortable and safe as possible. The surgeon should discuss the importance of understanding and preparing for the pain of surgery; the proper use of nonopioid pain relievers such as acetaminophen, NSAIDs, ice, heat, and elevation postoperatively; and the peace of mind that comes with pain relief. Nerve blocks can be helpful initially, but it can be unsettling when they wear off. The surgeon must ensure that every patient knows how to contact the team after surgery to make sure nothing is wrong and to avoid visits to urgent care. Practice or department limits on opioids should be determined to depersonalize difficult conversations and emphasize the risks of opioids. Patients must be instructed on and understand how to dispose of unused opioids in repositories (police station or pharmacy), flushed down the toilet, or mixed with something distasteful (for example, kitty litter) in the trash.

The wound is inspected 2 days postoperatively, and, if the swelling has subsided, a lighter dressing is applied and the patient is allowed to begin gentle flexion and extension exercises. If substantial swelling persists, a new dressing and plaster back slab are applied for an additional 7 days, after which a lighter dressing is applied and gentle flexion and extension exercises are begun. Progressive active elbow flexion and extension exercises are performed under the supervision of a physical therapist. Improvement in function is expected between 6 and 12 months postoperatively.

## Limiting Adverse Events

The worst pitfall of revision TEA is performing a single-stage revision for anticipated aseptic loosening if the cause of the loosening is a low-grade infection. Therefore, a surgeon must always consider the possibility of an infection if progressive radiolucency is observed on postoperative radiographs. To rule out infection, routine blood screenings should be performed, including hemoglobin level, complete blood count, erythrocyte sedimentation rate, and C-reactive protein level. In addition, the author of this chapter routinely performs elbow joint aspiration under radiographic visualization and sends the aspirate for microscopy, culture, and

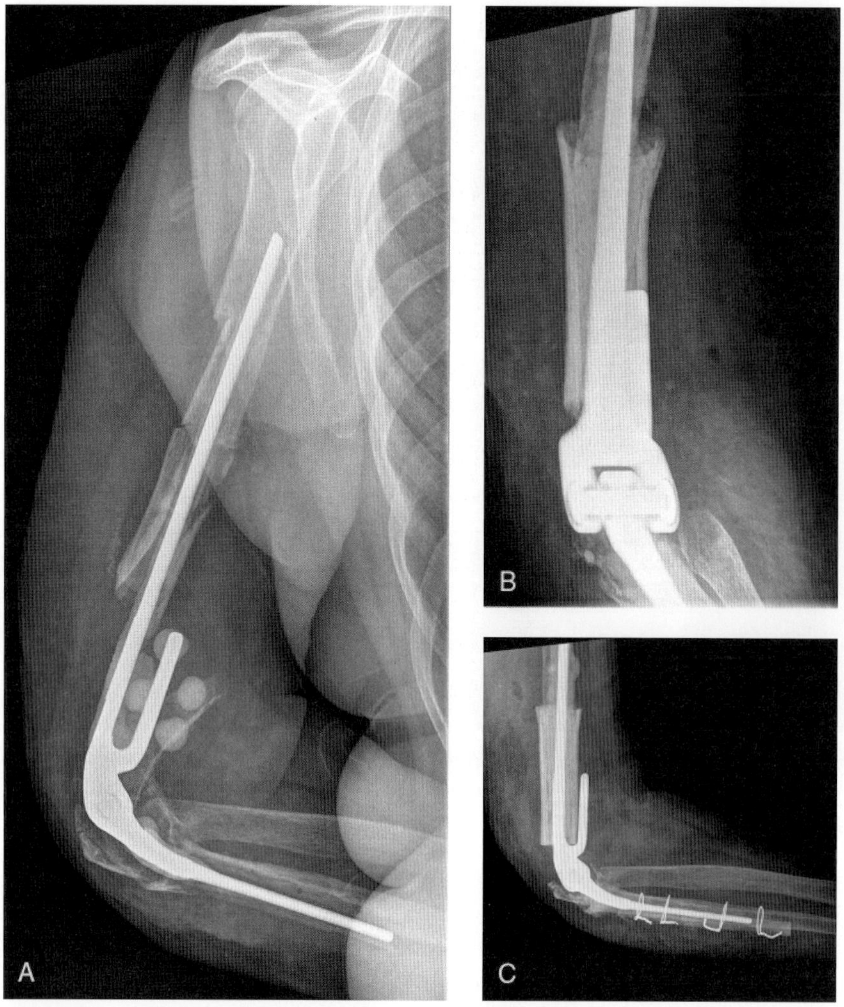


**Figure 8** Radiographs of the right elbow of a patient who underwent four previous total elbow arthroplasties (TEAs) to manage aseptic loosening. **A,** Lateral view demonstrates loss of distal humeral bone, antibiotic beads, and an ulnar fracture. AP (**B**) and lateral (**C**) views obtained immediately after revision TEA. The absent distal humerus was reconstructed with the use of a proximal humeral allograft. The surgeon identified the appropriate length of proximal humeral allograft necessary for distal humerus reconstruction, and the proximal humeral allograft was inverted, which allowed the bone to be inserted such that it overlapped the patient's humeral shaft, providing rigid fixation between host and allograft bone. A strut graft was used to reinforce the ulnar reconstruction.

sensitivity. Only if the findings of all of these tests are normal or, in the case of patients with inflammatory arthritis, consistent with a patient's baseline results, does the author of this chapter confirm that a patient has aseptic loosening. Performing a single-stage revision TEA in patients with a low-grade infection is associated with a high risk for recurrent loosening caused by infection.

Both the ulnar and radial nerves are at risk during revision TEA. The ulnar nerve must always be identified, superficially decompressed, and protected throughout revision TEA. Whether the ulnar nerve is routinely anteriorly transposed at the end of the procedure usually depends on the surgeon's preference; however, there is one situation in which transposition of the ulnar nerve is essential. The ulnar nerve must be transposed if it appears to be stretched during passive flexion of the elbow after insertion of the revision prosthesis. The radial nerve is at risk if a long-stemmed humeral component is being revised or if a long tail of cement has to be removed before insertion of the revision prosthesis. In these patients, the radial nerve should be exposed and protected throughout the revision TEA.

The removal of partially loose total elbow implants can be surprisingly difficult and may be associated with iatrogenic fractures and bone perforations. To minimize the risk for iatrogenic fractures and bone perforations, a wide range of appropriately sized revision instruments must be available. The risk of iatrogenic fracture also can be reduced by creating a bone window to facilitate implant removal. Replacing and maintaining the bone window in a satisfactory position before insertion of the revision prosthesis may be difficult but can be aided with the use of absorbable sutures (**Figure 6**).

Postoperative periprosthetic fractures are more likely to occur if the tip of either the humeral or the ulnar implant ends at the level of a bone window or perforation. To reduce the risk for postoperative periprosthetic fractures, the tip of the prosthesis should extend twice the medullary canal diameter beyond any bone window or perforation.

The anatomic axis of flexion and extension of the elbow should be determined as accurately as possible during revision TEA. If the anatomic axis of flexion and extension of the elbow is not achieved, the forces across the elbow during functional movement will result in early loosening of the prosthesis. Identification of the anatomic axis is often difficult, however, particularly in patients who have structural bone loss. The technique the author of this chapter uses involves passive flexion and extension of the elbow with the trial implants in place. If either the humeral or ulnar

 

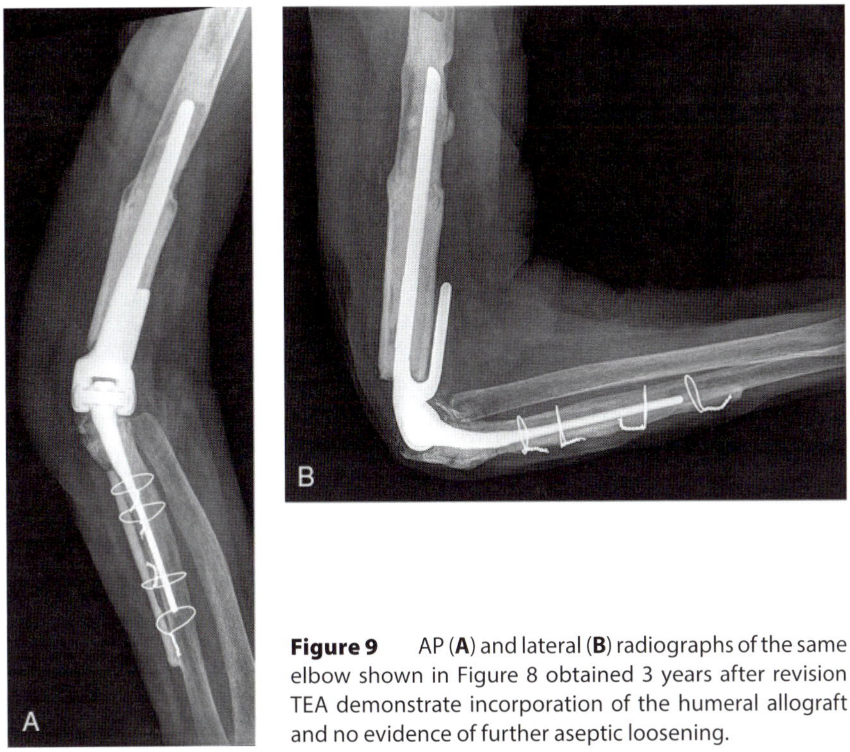

**Figure 9** AP (**A**) and lateral (**B**) radiographs of the same elbow shown in Figure 8 obtained 3 years after revision TEA demonstrate incorporation of the humeral allograft and no evidence of further aseptic loosening.

implant pistons within the bony canal of the humerus or ulna, the author of this chapter attempts to reposition the prosthesis to minimize or avoid pistoning of the humeral or ulnar implants within the bony canal of the humerus or ulna.

Impingement during elbow flexion and extension must be avoided because it will cause premature loosening of the prosthesis. A careful examination for impingement should be made at the time of the trial reduction and again after insertion of the definitive prosthesis. Impingement during elbow flexion is most frequently caused by either a prominent coronoid process or a prominent radial head. Impingement during elbow extension usually is caused by prominence of the tip of the olecranon. Prominent bone that results in impingement should be resected before surgical closure.

## Bibliography


Amirfeyz R, Stanley D: Allograft-prosthesis composite reconstruction for the management of failed elbow replacement with massive structural bone loss: A medium-term follow-up. *J Bone Joint Surg Br* 2011;93(10):1382-1388.

Loebenberg MI, Adams R, O'Driscoll SW, Morrey BF: Impaction grafting in revision total elbow arthroplasty. *J Bone Joint Surg Am* 2005;87(1):99-106.

Malone AA, Sanchez JS, Adams R, Morrey B: Revision of total elbow replacement by exchange cementing. *J Bone Joint Surg Br* 2012;94(1):80-85.

Mansat P, Adams RA, Morrey BF: Allograft-prosthesis composite for revision of catastrophic failure of total elbow arthroplasty. *J Bone Joint Surg Am* 2004;86(4):724-735.

Morrey BF, Bryan RS: Revision total elbow arthroplasty. *J Bone Joint Surg Am* 1987;69(4):523-532.

Presnal BP, Chillag KJ: Radiohumeral arthrodesis for salvage of failed total elbow arthroplasty. *J Arthroplasty* 1995;10(5):699-701.

Puskas GJ, Morrey BF, Sanchez-Sotelo J: Aseptic loosening rate of the humeral stem in the Coonrad-Morrey total elbow arthroplasty: Does size matter? *J Shoulder Elbow Surg* 2014;23(1):76-81.

Rhee YG, Cho NS, Parke CS: Impaction grafting in revision total elbow arthroplasty due to aseptic loosening and bone loss. *J Bone Joint Surg Am* 2013;95(11):e741-e747.

Shahane SA, Stanley D: A posterior approach to the elbow joint. *J Bone Joint Surg Br* 1999;81(6):1020-1022.

Sneftrup SB, Jensen SL, Johannsen HV, Søjbjerg JO: Revision of failed total elbow arthroplasty with use of a linked implant. *J Bone Joint Surg Br* 2006;88(1):78-83.

Throckmorton TW, Zarkadas PC, Sanchez-Sotelo J, Morrey BF: Radial nerve palsy after humeral revision in total elbow arthroplasty. *J Shoulder Elbow Surg* 2011;20(2):199-205.

 

# Chapter 20

# Management of the Infected Total Elbow Arthroplasty

*Varun Kashyap Gajendran, MD*
*Xavier C. Simcock, MD*
*William H. Seitz, Jr, MD*

**Learning Objectives**

- Recognize the presentation of and major risk factors for periprosthetic infection after total elbow arthroplasty.
- Integrate data from the history, physical examination, and laboratory studies to identify patients with a high probability of infection who may benefit from surgical treatment.
- Evaluate the various treatment options for total elbow arthroplasty periprosthetic infection, including long-term antibiotic suppressive therapy, resection arthroplasty, one-stage exchange, and two-stage exchange; include the advantages and drawbacks of each treatment.
- Explain the techniques used in the surgical treatment of total elbow arthroplasty periprosthetic infection, including resection arthroplasty, one-stage exchange, and two-stage exchange, including how to recognize and manage wound complications.
- Explain the important elements of postoperative care, including working with interdisciplinary teams and planning for future reconstructions when appropriate.

## Indications

Infection after total elbow arthroplasty (TEA) is more common than infection after total hip and total knee arthroplasty (3% to 11% compared with 1% to 2%, respectively). Several risk factors are associated with higher rates of infection. TEA is often performed on older patients with multiple medical comorbidities, including severe rheumatoid arthritis, posttraumatic arthritis, and, more recently, comminuted intra-articular distal humerus fractures. Rates of wound complications are higher for patients undergoing immunosuppressive therapy for rheumatoid arthritis or who have undergone multiple previous surgeries, resulting in a compromised soft-tissue envelope around the elbow. Many patients also have diabetes, which is an independent risk factor for wound complications and infections of other organ systems.

It can be challenging to diagnose periprosthetic joint infection after TEA. Recent studies have attempted to validate the algorithms used for hip and knee prosthetic joint infection, with limited success. The clinical findings of wound dehiscence and drainage, sinus tracts communicating with the joint, and visible purulence on aspiration are clearly indicative of infection. However, the clinical presentation is not generally obvious. Therefore, the history, examination, and laboratory results (including inflammatory markers, preoperative and intraoperative cultures, and histology) should be considered together to arrive at a probability of periprosthetic elbow infection.

Unlike total hip and total knee arthroplasty, in which diagnostic test results indicate sensitivities and specificities exceeding 90%, these same tests are not as accurate for the elbow. To date, no definitive diagnostic test exists for periprosthetic elbow infection. The most reliable diagnostic data come from the intraoperative histology and cultures. However, because of the indolent

*Dr. Seitz or an immediate family member serves as a paid consultant to or is an employee of Kapp Surgical Instruments, Materialise, and Stryker; and serves as a board member, owner, officer, or committee member of the American Academy of Orthopaedic Surgeons, the Academy of Medicine Education Foundation, the Academy of Medicine of Cleveland & Northern Ohio, the American Orthopaedic Association, and the American Society for Surgery of the Hand. Neither of the following authors nor any immediate family member has received anything of value from or has stock or stock options held in a commercial company or institution related directly or indirectly to the subject of this chapter: Dr. Gajendran and Dr. Simcock.*

growth of coagulase-negative staphylococcus and *Propionibacterium acnes*, two of the most common organisms causing periprosthetic elbow infections, results of cultures often are unreliable for the first 14 days of incubation. Sonication of explanted prostheses has been shown to be more sensitive than cultures for detecting biofilm-producing bacteria. However, use of sonication requires that the surgeon be committed to removing the prosthesis. Intraoperative histology has been shown to provide more reliable real-time results compared with sonication during revision surgery, which can influence surgical decision making. However, the sensitivity of histology remains low (approximately 50%). Furthermore, the absence of acute inflammation on histology does not definitively rule out infection, particularly in patients with low-virulence organisms or immunosuppressed patients.

A 2008 study comprehensively detailed the organisms detected during resection arthroplasty and reimplantation. The most common infecting organism was *Staphylococcus epidermidis* in 45% of elbows, followed by methicillin-sensitive *Staphylococcus aureus* in 24% and *Klebsiella pneumoniae* in 7%. Negative cultures were encountered in 10% of elbows. The incidence of *P acnes* infections also has increased with improved diagnostic techniques and awareness for detection of organisms.

Because of the difficulty of eradicating periprosthetic elbow infections, the authors of this chapter think that surgical treatment is indicated for any patient with a suspected TEA infection. The presence of any of the following primary criteria warrants consideration for surgical intervention: wound breakdown, active drainage, or deep sinus tract formation on physical examination; elevated C-reactive protein level later than the acute inflammatory postoperative period of 3 weeks without any other obvious cause; or joint aspirate showing a cell count greater than 25,000/mm$^3$, a differential greater than 75% neutrophils, or positive intraoperative cultures after incubation for at least 3 weeks. To diagnose an infection, the authors of this chapter also use intraoperative histology demonstrating greater than five neutrophils per high-powered field and positive intraoperative cultures in any of the samples. Although a single positive intraoperative culture can be a result of contaminant from skin flora, these same organisms commonly cause indolent infections in the elbow. Therefore, the authors of this chapter treat any patient with suspected periprosthetic elbow infection aggressively with formal irrigation and débridement at minimum. The exact procedure indicated in each situation is outlined later in this chapter.

## Contraindications

Before discussing the surgical treatment of periprosthetic infection with the patient, the surgeon must take into consideration the patient's functional capacity, overall health, and general expectations for postoperative function. Contraindications to a two-stage exchange of a TEA can be divided by stage.

The first-stage exchange consists of irrigation and débridement with or without explantation and placement of an antibiotic cement spacer. Any and all operations may be contraindicated if the patient has severe medical comorbidities that place him or her at high risk for perioperative complications, particularly for a patient with low physical demands preoperatively without any physiologic compromise resulting from the infection. In these patients, even a single-stage irrigation and débridement with resection arthroplasty may be contraindicated, and long-term antibiotic suppression may be the best and safest treatment option.

The second-stage exchange consists of a revision TEA. This procedure is contraindicated if there is evidence that the infection has not been completely eradicated, which places the patient at high risk for reinfection. Repeated irrigation and débridement with antibiotic cement spacer replacement may be the best treatment option until all objective evidence indicates that the infection has been eradicated and all devitalized or foreign tissue has been removed. Other contraindications include lack of adequate bone stock to support a prosthesis and a poor or inadequate soft-tissue envelope that is unlikely to withstand another operation; these factors also place a patient at risk for wound complications and reinfection.

## Alternative Treatments

Depending on the goals of the patient, a variety of treatments may be appropriate to suppress or eliminate periprosthetic joint infections in the elbow. These treatments include serial débridement, resection arthroplasty, arthrodesis, and implant removal followed by staged reimplantation. Treatment varies depending on the chronicity of the infection, the suspected organism, and the patient's overall status.

Some surgeons prefer to perform débridement and retain the implant. If an infection occurs within 3 weeks of the index procedure or an event occurred that caused hematogenous seeding and ultimately periprosthetic joint infection, then it may be reasonable to retain the implants. Although implant retention produces good outcomes after total hip and total knee arthroplasty, the outcomes of this strategy are not as good following TEA. A study published in 1998 observed high rates of reinfection with *S epidermidis* when infected TEA was managed with irrigation and débridement alone.

Resection arthroplasty is a good option for older patients with low physical demands or severe medical comorbidities. Resection arthroplasty also may be a good option for patients with extremely poor bone stock or an inadequate soft-tissue envelope and for patients with a high risk of reinfection. For patients with poor bone stock, arthrodesis may be an option after the infection has been eradicated. For patients who cannot tolerate any surgical procedure, lifelong antibiotic suppression of the infection or simply letting the sinus drain without antibiotic suppression may be the safest option.

## Results

Published results from current and/or significant studies on management of infection after TEA are summarized in **Table 1**. The decision to proceed with a particular surgical treatment is based on several factors, including patient history, physical examination findings, serum inflammatory markers, joint aspiration results, and intraoperative findings. A dilemma arises when a patient demonstrates clinical evidence of infection without positive culture data. Overall, the diagnostic tests do not have enough specificity to reliably rule out infection when adequate clinical suspicion exists. In these situations, the literature supports proceeding with a two-stage revision to optimize the odds of eradicating the infection.

## Techniques

### Setup/Exposure

- Information about the implanted prosthesis should be obtained before the procedure to ensure that the necessary extraction tools are readily available. The surgical report from the patient's previous operation should be studied to determine the condition of the ulnar nerve and whether it has been transposed.
- If any concern exists that the skin may not close easily after the débridement, then a preoperative plastic surgery consultation is advised. Plans should be made for the use of local, regional, or distant flaps with the help of the plastic surgeon, as needed, to achieve robust wound coverage.
- The patient may be placed in the supine position with the arm across the chest, the lateral decubitus position on a beanbag, or the prone position, depending on surgeon preference. The authors of this chapter prefer to place the patient in the lateral decubitus position to facilitate the procedure and intraoperative imaging, and to allow the anesthesiologist unencumbered access to the patient's airway.
- A sterile tourniquet is generally preferred to allow proximal extension of the incision, if necessary.
- Antibiotics are withheld until the intraoperative aspiration is performed and tissue cultures are obtained, and then the appropriate antibiotics are administered and re-dosed as necessary.
- Gravity exsanguination by elevation is performed, and the tourniquet is inflated.
- Whenever possible, existing incisions are used to preserve the vascularity of the flaps, and any necrotic skin is sharply excised.
- Full-thickness flaps should be elevated down to the fascial level, and the integrity of the triceps mechanism should be carefully examined.
- The elbow joint can be aspirated at this time and the aspirate sent for a cell count with differential, as well as aerobic, anaerobic, fungal, and acid-fast bacillus cultures.
- The ulnar nerve is identified and carefully dissected out from the arcade of Struthers proximally to the first anterior motor branch to the flexor carpi ulnaris muscle distally, tagged with a vessel loop passed around the nerve, and tied to itself.

### Instruments/Equipment/Implants Required

- Small and large curettes, both straight and curved, are used.
- Rongeurs, including pituitary rongeurs, are used for cement removal.
- A Cobb elevator is used during anterior release.
- Straight and curved osteotomes are used.
- A microsagittal saw and high-speed burrs are used in implant removal.
- Flexible cannulated reamers are used.
- Pulse lavage irrigation equipment with a long, narrow tip is used.
- A canal brush is used in irrigation and débridement.
- Cement restrictors are used.
- Cerclage wires and cables are used for stabilization.
- TEA instruments specific to removal of the implanted prosthesis are used.
- Fragment plates and distal humerus periarticular plates (small and large) are used.
- Long, smooth Steinmann pins are used.
- Antibiotic-impregnated cement with 4 g of vancomycin and 3.6 g of tobramycin is used.
- The total elbow implant of choice is used.

### Procedure

- After exposure of the triceps muscle and tendon, the authors of this chapter prefer a tongue approach in which a distally based, inverted V–shaped incision in the triceps aponeurosis is made with the apex located proximally and the triceps tendon left attached to the olecranon tip distally. The muscle fibers of the underlying deep head of the triceps are divided longitudinally at

**Table 1** Results of Management of Infected Total Elbow Arthroplasty

| Authors (Year) | No. of Patients | Procedure or Approach | Mean Patient Age in Years (range) | Mean Follow-up in Months (range) | Success Rate | Results | Level of Evidence |
|---|---|---|---|---|---|---|---|
| Yamaguchi et al (1998) | 25 | Group 1: irrigation and débridement with implant retention (14)<br>Group 2: two-stage revision (6)<br>Group 3: resection alone (5) | 57.5 (42-89) | 71 (24-189) | Group 1: 50%<br>Group 2: 67%<br>Group 3: 100% | Irrigation and débridement was unsuccessful in the 4 patients infected with *Staphylococcus epidermidis*<br>Reimplantation as part of two-stage exchange was unsuccessful in the 2 patients with infected *S epidermidis* | IV |
| Cheung et al (2008) | 29 | Reimplantation after resection arthroplasty | 61.6 (28-78) | 89 (26-103) | 3-yr survival: 77%<br>8-yr survival: 48% | 28% reinfection rate<br>Mean MEPS improved from 35.5 to 66.3 ($P < 0.001$)[a] | IV |
| Spormann et al (2012) | 19 (20 elbows) | Irrigation and débridement versus two-stage revision | 61.2 (41-82) | 60.2 (25-136) | 89% | Success rate based on eradication of infection with irrigation and débridement in 8 of 9 elbows with early infection (<3 mo)<br>Mean MEPS improved from 48.3 to 91.7[a] | IV |
| Ahmadi et al (2013) | 139 | Intraoperative histology to predict infection | 62.1 (31-95) | 4.4 (0-10.4) | Success rate not reported<br>Sensitivity, 51.3% (20/39)<br>Specificity, 93.1% (175/188)[b] | Sensitivity for *S epidermidis*, 36.4%; 14 false negatives and 8 true positives | I |

MEPS = Mayo Elbow Performance Score.

[a] Excellent, ≥90 points; good, 75-89 points; fair, 60-74 points; poor, <60 points.

[b] Sensitivity and specificity reported based on number of arthroplasties, not number of patients; 139 patients underwent 227 procedures.

the midline and elevated to either side to completely expose the posterior aspect of the distal humerus (**Figure 1**).

- The triceps is assessed to determine whether it appears compromised. If either a triceps split or a Bryan-Morrey approach, in which the triceps is sharply detached from the bone, was used during the previous operation, then the same approach should be considered during the revision surgery to avoid imparting trauma to the triceps in a different location.
- A complete and thorough synovectomy is then performed and the synovium sent for cultures.

 

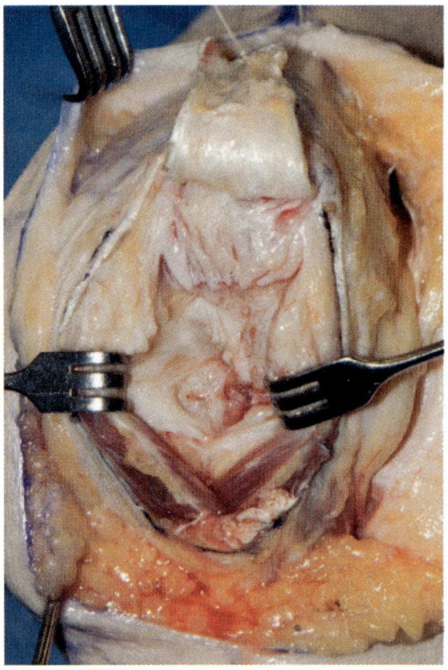

**Figure 1** Intraoperative photograph shows complete exposure of the posterior elbow after the triceps has been taken down during the tongue approach.

- The collateral ligaments, if present, are taken down completely.
- The locking mechanism of the humeral and ulnar components is disengaged and the bushing removed to uncouple the components.
- An anterior release is performed by sliding up the anterior humeral shaft using a Cobb elevator and sharply releasing the capsular attachments to the anterior humerus.
- A complete débridement of the olecranon and coronoid fossae is performed. Osteophytes from the coronoid or olecranon tip may be removed if they are causing limitations to flexion or extension, respectively.
- In patients with acute infections (<3 weeks after the previous procedure or after a hematogenous seeding event) in whom the components are well fixed and the causative organism is not *S epidermidis*, it may be sufficient to replace the bushing, retain the humeral and ulnar components, and perform thorough irrigation and débridement. However, failure rates as high as 50% to 90% have been described after irrigation and débridement alone.
- In patients with acute infections (<3 weeks) caused by *S epidermidis* or subacute or chronic infections (>3 weeks) caused by any other organism, a two-stage exchange yields the highest probability of eradicating the infection, although even then there is no guarantee of clearing the infection because of the biofilm-forming capacity of *S epidermidis*. (Although one-stage exchange has been reported in the literature, the authors of this chapter do not recommend it.) Stage one consists of cement and implant removal, thorough irrigation and débridement of the surgical site and removal of any infected or necrotic bone, and insertion of an antibiotic-impregnated cement spacer. Intravenous antibiotics are also administered. After the erythrocyte sedimentation rate and C-reactive protein level have normalized (6 weeks postoperatively), the intravenous antibiotics are discontinued. Oral antibiotics are administered for an additional 2 weeks, then discontinued for a 6-week interval, after which the elbow joint is aspirated. Provided the infection has been cleared, second-stage surgery is performed, in which new implants are inserted, if the patient is an appropriate candidate for reimplantation. A 3-month infection-free interval before reimplantation has been recommended, and the authors of this chapter agree with this conservative approach. If there is any concern for persistent infection, the patient should be returned to the operating room for another formal irrigation and débridement, and the process of antibiotic administration should be repeated until the infection is cleared. In patients with high risk of reinfection, older patients with low physical demands, or patients with severe medical comorbidities, resection arthroplasty may be the best treatment option. In resection arthroplasty, the antibiotic cement spacer is left in place permanently and is supported externally by a hinged elbow brace.

**IMPLANT REMOVAL**

- In many patients, the periprosthetic infection causes gross loosening of the implants, and the implants may simply be removed using the available extractor tools.
- In a less common scenario, the implants are well fixed. In these patients, an attempt can be made to break up and undermine the cement mantle around the visible end of the implants using high-speed burrs and osteotomes, and then the extractors can be used to remove the implants if they are sufficiently loose (**Figure 2**). If this method is unsuccessful, then limited longitudinal periprosthetic osteotomies may be performed.
- A microsagittal saw can be used to create a cortical window along the entire length of the cement mantle and involving one-third to one-half of the circumference of the bone (**Figure 3, A** through **C**).
- The cortical window is opened, allowing direct access to the cement all around the stem of the prosthesis, which can then be removed with high-speed burrs and osteotomes.
- After sufficient cement has been removed along the entire length of the prosthetic stem, the prosthesis is extracted. All the cement can be removed through the cortical window as well.
- The cortical window is replaced and fixed with multiple cerclage wires; a

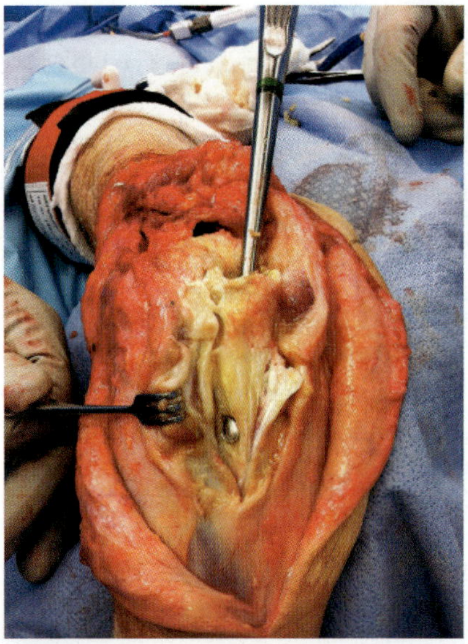

**Figure 2** Intraoperative photograph shows an elbow after removal of an infected ulnar implant. High-speed burrs and osteotomes were used to undermine the cement mantle proximally. The ulnar component was then extracted without requiring an osteotomy; however, the ulnar diaphyseal cortex was perforated during cement extraction from the canal.

strut allograft may be used for augmentation if the surgeon is confident that the wound is completely clean and free of infection. However, the authors of this chapter generally do not recommend using allograft in the setting of infection (**Figure 3**, **D** and **E**).

#### CEMENT REMOVAL

- When the implants are removed, much of the cement may come out with them.
- All remaining traces of cement should be removed in an attempt to eliminate the infection. This step is most safely accomplished by inserting guidewires for the cannulated flexible reamers, confirming the position of the guidewires under fluoroscopic visualization, and then inserting the reamers, starting with the smallest and advancing in size incrementally until chatter from cortical contact is heard.
- Curettes, flexible osteotomes, and a high-speed burr may also be used for cement removal; however, with all of these methods, great care must be taken to avoid cortical perforation.
- The authors of this chapter do not perform ultrasonic cement fragmentation because it can generate high heat levels, which in turn can injure adjacent nerves.
- After the cement mantle has been broken up, it can be irrigated and suctioned out. Pituitary rongeurs are also useful for removing the pieces of the cement mantle.

#### IRRIGATION AND DÉBRIDEMENT

- Thorough débridement may be the most critical part of the procedure.
- After all the hardware and cement have been evacuated, all devitalized or infected tissue including bone is removed sharply with a knife or rongeur until only healthy tissue remains. Osteomyelitic bone that does not bleed should be removed down to a healthy, bleeding bed with a rongeur, saw, and/or burr. For the most severe infections, it may be necessary to remove the periarticular bone, including the humeral condyles and the proximal ulna at the triceps insertion, to eradicate the infection, resulting in a flail elbow (**Figure 4**).
- The canals are then irrigated with at least 6 L of sterile normal saline using a pulsatile lavage irrigator and cleaned with a bristled brush or cannulated flexible reamers. Care must be taken to avoid cortical fracture or cortical perforation. After irrigation and débridement, new drapes are placed over the old drapes and all surgeons' gloves are changed.

#### CREATION AND PLACEMENT OF THE ANTIBIOTIC-IMPREGNATED CEMENT SPACER

- After irrigation and débridement in the first stage of a two-stage exchange, an antibiotic-impregnated cement spacer is inserted. The advantage of creating a cement spacer is that it allows some motion at the elbow joint and may serve as the final construct in a patient who is infirm or at high risk for recurrence of infection after reimplantation. The authors of this chapter recognize that the cement spacer may need to be left in place indefinitely in some patients.
- One packet of cement, 4 g of vancomycin, and 3.6 g of tobramycin are mixed together in a bowl.
- The cement is first applied in the distal humerus so that some cement is packed into the canal. In a patient in whom the condyles have been resected, the remaining cement outside the canal is molded to form two condyles with a gap in the middle to allow the ulna to articulate with this gap.
- The cement is then applied to the proximal ulna so that some cement is inserted into the canal. The remaining cement is molded to fit into the gap created between the two condyles of the distal humerus.
- Alternatively, a static spacer can be created by bending a smooth Steinmann pin approximately 90° and inserting it into the humeral and ulnar canals, applying cement around the pin in the space between the two bones, and packing cement into the canals as well (**Figure 3**, **C**; **Figure 4**, **C** and **D**).

#### TRICEPS REPAIR AND IMPLANT INSERTION

- In a single-stage exchange, the infected implants and cement are removed, and new implants are

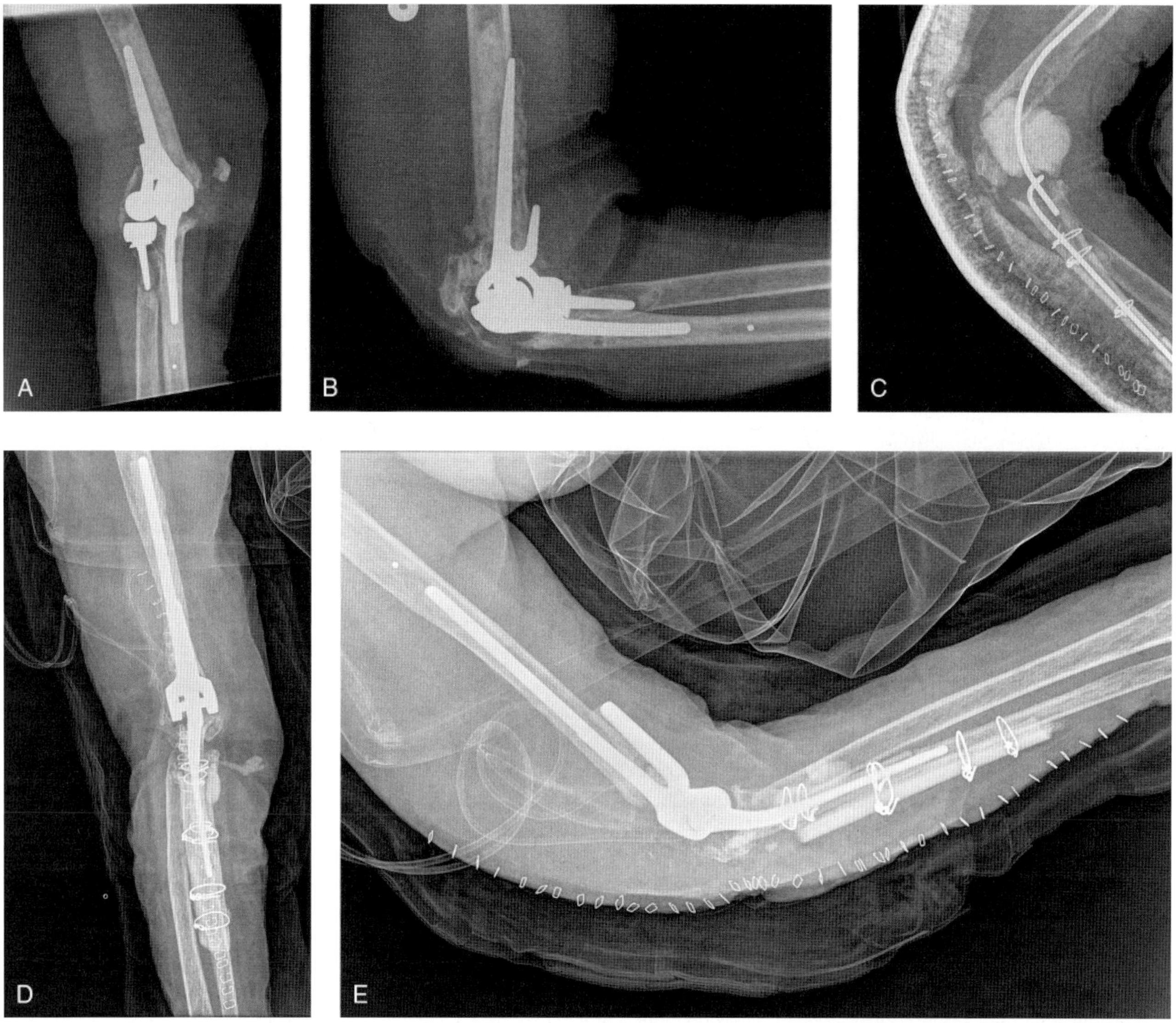


**Figure 3** Postoperative AP (**A**) and lateral (**B**) radiographs from a 68-year-old woman with advanced rheumatoid arthritis in whom a chronic periprosthetic infection and proximal ulna nonunion developed after primary total elbow arthroplasty. During revision surgery to manage the infection and proximal ulna nonunion, the loose humeral implant was easily removed. However, the ulnar implant was well fixed, which required cutting the ulna along its medial and lateral borders as well as anteriorly at the level of the distal stem tip to create a cortical window to extract the implant and cement. This step resulted in iatrogenic completion of the fracture at the distal end of the cortical window. **C,** Intraoperative lateral radiograph demonstrates the ulnar corticotomy stabilized with cerclage wires and a long Steinmann pin incorporated into the antibiotic-impregnated cement spacer. AP (**D**) and lateral (**E**) immediate postoperative radiographs obtained after second-stage revision arthroplasty demonstrate implant position and fixation as well as strut allograft augmentation of the proximal ulna. The patient was pleased with her elbow function despite a fibrous union of the proximal ulna.

inserted immediately after irrigation and débridement.

- In the second stage of a two-stage exchange, the antibiotic cement spacer is removed and the new implants are inserted after intramedullary reaming.
- Insertion of new implants is performed using the principles of revision TEA, a description of which is beyond the scope of this chapter.
- The authors of this chapter prefer a tongue approach to take down and repair the extensor mechanism. The tendon is repaired first at the apex with a figure-of-8 No. 2 braided nonabsorbable composite stitch, which also allows the length of the triceps tendon to be adjusted and set. To complete the repair, the suture is run from proximal to distal and then from distal to proximal to create a double, baseball-style stitch

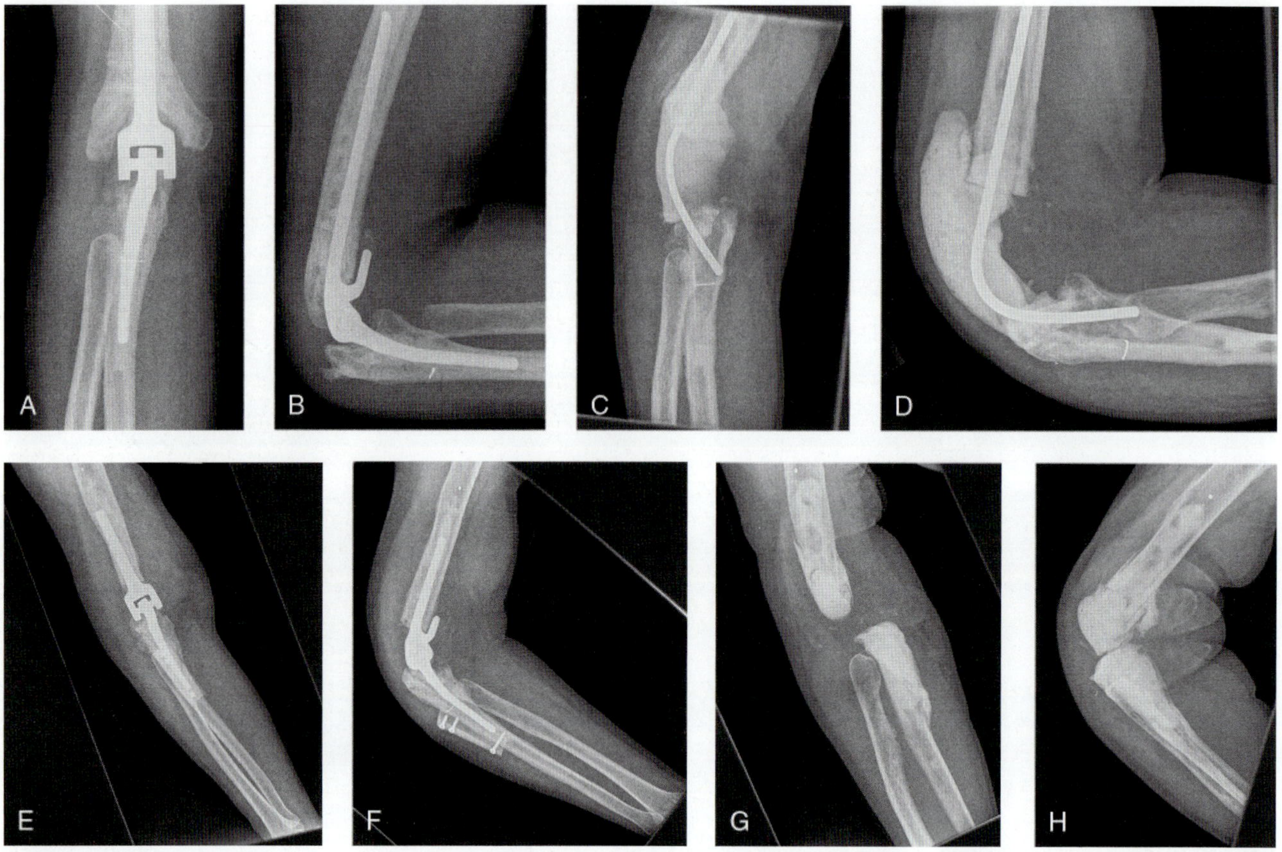

**Figure 4** Postoperative AP (**A**) and lateral (**B**) radiographs from a 55-year-old man with diabetes who underwent total elbow arthroplasty (TEA). The deep infection with distal humerus osteomyelitis that subsequently developed were initially treated with irrigation and débridement, resection of the osteomyelitic distal humerus, and placement of the antibiotic-impregnated cement spacer. AP (**C**) and lateral (**D**) radiographs demonstrate placement of the spacer. AP (**E**) and lateral (**F**) radiographs obtained after revision TEA with allograft augmentation of a proximal ulna defect. The infection was eradicated before the revision surgery. However, another deep infection, this time with osteomyelitis of the proximal ulna, subsequently developed, requiring treatment with resection arthroplasty. Postoperative AP (**G**) and lateral (**H**) radiographs demonstrate the elbow after resection of the proximal ulna osteomyelitis and placement of an antibiotic-impregnated cement spacer. This procedure ultimately resulted in a flail elbow with good hand function and a reasonable amount of elbow control aided by a locking hinged brace.

on both the radial and ulnar sides of the apex.

- When a different approach is used as dictated by the previous procedure, the appropriate repair is performed. Most commonly, the triceps is taken directly off its insertion on the olecranon at the Sharpey fibers.

## Wound Closure

- An intracapsular drain is routinely used to prevent infection. The drain may be removed 24 to 48 hours postoperatively.
- The wound is meticulously closed in a layered fashion. The use of nonbraided, monofilament sutures is preferred in patients with previous infection.
- The skin is loosely approximated with interrupted, nonabsorbable, monofilament sutures or staples.
- Incisional negative-pressure wound therapy can be used to keep the wound sterile and decrease postoperative swelling and drainage. The vacuum pump can be set to deliver low-pressure, continuous suction at 75 mm Hg and removed 5 to 7 days postoperatively.
- Negative-pressure wound therapy also can be used to manage an acutely or chronically infected wound that has been débrided but cannot be closed primarily. Early coverage with a flap is recommended in these patients.
- A bulky, supportive soft dressing is placed, and the tourniquet is deflated at the conclusion of the procedure.
- After a reimplantation procedure, a long arm splint with medial and lateral slabs is fashioned with the elbow in 30° to 45° of flexion to rest the wound and allow early healing before beginning motion.

 

## Postoperative Regimen

The patient is evaluated clinically 2 weeks postoperatively. If sufficient healing has occurred, the sutures or staples are removed and the splint is discontinued. Gentle active and passive flexion as well as passive extension exercises are begun with the elbow in a hinged brace that is unlocked under the supervision of a physical therapist. Active extension is begun 6 weeks postoperatively, when the triceps has sufficiently healed. Gentle strengthening is begun 3 months postoperatively. The patient has a lifetime weight-bearing restriction of 10 lb (4.5 kg); however, often patients are unable or unwilling to comply with this restriction.

If the patient has undergone a resection arthroplasty, then follow-up is coordinated with the infectious diseases team to manage long-term antibiotic treatment and determine when the patient is ready for the second-stage exchange. Patients who have successfully cleared the infection and are candidates for reimplantation are offered surgery and are counseled extensively. If the patient has undergone a definitive resection arthroplasty or the second-stage exchange, then clinical and radiographic follow-up is subsequently performed at 2 weeks, 6 weeks, 3 months, 6 months, 1 year, and annually thereafter. The authors of this chapter recommend that patients indefinitely receive antibiotic prophylaxis for dental and other minor medical procedures as prescribed by the most recent clinical practice guideline from the American Academy of Orthopaedic Surgeons.

## Limiting Adverse Events

The surgeon should become familiar with the implant that needs to be removed as well as the available extraction tools. A preoperative consultation with the plastic surgeon should be considered if there is any concern about soft-tissue quality or wound closure. The soft-tissue envelope around the elbow can be compromised by repeated surgical procedures, so it is imperative to develop full-thickness flaps and use existing scars when possible to avoid wound complications. Local advancement flaps can be easily created by undermining the full-thickness skin flaps so that the wound is not under any undue tension after closure. In addition, the position of the ulnar nerve can be unpredictable. A meticulous dissection should be performed, and as many of the feeding vessels as possible should be preserved. Antibiotics should be withheld until the synovial fluid has been aspirated and the cultures have been sent for analysis. The triceps should be managed in the same manner as in the previous operation if possible, so it is important to be familiar with multiple methods of managing the triceps.

All hardware, cement, and infected bone and soft tissues must be completely removed to increase the chance of successfully eliminating the infection. During the process of implant removal, the surgeon should plan for the possibility of extended osteotomies or fixation of iatrogenic fractures. Although unstable iatrogenic fractures require fixation, the use of hardware should be limited given the previous infection.

When shaping the antibiotic-impregnated cement spacers, a space should be left between the condyles in the humeral spacer to articulate with the ulnar spacer. Should it be necessary to leave the spacer in situ indefinitely, this step ensures that some motion can be obtained through the articulation. During reimplantation, linked semiconstrained implants should be used. The use of unlinked implants should be avoided.

To complete the procedure, a meticulous, layered wound closure is performed and a deep drain is placed in the wound. The use of incisional negative-pressure wound therapy and/or prolonged immobilization is acceptable to avoid soft-tissue and healing complications. Elbow stiffness can be managed with physical therapy or surgical releases. Typically, stiffness is easier to address than another deep infection with soft-tissue breakdown.

*S epidermidis* infections can be difficult to eradicate with retained implants even in the acute setting; thus, a two-stage exchange or a resection arthroplasty may be the most effective treatment option. High rates of failure are associated with two-stage exchanges, however. Resection arthroplasty should be considered in older patients, medically frail patients, and patients with low physical demands.

## Bibliography


Achermann Y, Vogt M, Spormann C, et al: Characteristics and outcome of 27 elbow periprosthetic joint infections: Results from a 14-year cohort study of 358 elbow prostheses. *Clin Microbiol Infect* 2011;17(3):432-438.

Ahmadi S, Lawrence TM, Morrey BF, Sanchez-Sotelo J: The value of intraoperative histology in predicting infection in patients undergoing revision elbow arthroplasty. *J Bone Joint Surg Am* 2013;95(21):1976-1979.

Aldridge JM III, Lightdale NR, Mallon WJ, Coonrad RW: Total elbow arthroplasty with the Coonrad/Coonrad-Morrey prosthesis: A 10- to 31-year survival analysis. *J Bone Joint Surg Br* 2006;88(4):509-514.

American Academy of Orthopaedic Surgeons: *Clinical Practice Guideline on Prevention of Orthopaedic Implant Infection in Patients Undergoing Dental Procedures.* Rosemont, IL, American Academy of Orthopaedic Surgeons, December 2012. http://www.aaos.org/uploadedFiles/PreProduction/Quality/Guidelines_and_Reviews/PUDP_guideline.pdf.

Bauer TW, Parvizi J, Kobayashi N, Krebs V: Diagnosis of periprosthetic infection. *J Bone Joint Surg Am* 2006;88(4):869-882.

Cheung EV, Adams RA, Morrey BF: Reimplantation of a total elbow prosthesis following resection arthroplasty for infection. *J Bone Joint Surg Am* 2008;90(3):589-594.

Gill DR, Morrey BF: The Coonrad-Morrey total elbow arthroplasty in patients who have rheumatoid arthritis: A ten to fifteen-year follow-up study. *J Bone Joint Surg Am* 1998;80(9):1327-1335.

Gille J, Ince A, González O, Katzer A, Loehr JF: Single-stage revision of peri-prosthetic infection following total elbow replacement. *J Bone Joint Surg Br* 2006;88(10):1341-1346.

Howe CR, Gardner GC, Kadel NJ: Perioperative medication management for the patient with rheumatoid arthritis. *J Am Acad Orthop Surg* 2006;14(9):544-551.

Jeon IH, Morrey BF, Anakwenze OA, Tran NV: Incidence and implications of early postoperative wound complications after total elbow arthroplasty. *J Shoulder Elbow Surg* 2011;20(6):857-865.

Kim JM, Mudgal CS, Konopka JF, Jupiter JB: Complications of total elbow arthroplasty. *J Am Acad Orthop Surg* 2011;19(6):328-339.

Lawrence TM, Ahmadi S, Morrey BF, Sánchez-Sotelo J: Wound complications after distal humerus fracture fixation: Incidence, risk factors, and outcome. *J Shoulder Elbow Surg* 2014;23(2):258-264.

Morrey BF, An K-N: Functional evaluation of the elbow, in Morrey BF, ed: *The Elbow and its Disorders, ed 3.* Philadelphia, PA, WB Saunders, 2000, pp 74-83.

Morrey BF, Bryan RS: Infection after total elbow arthroplasty. *J Bone Joint Surg Am* 1983;65(3):330-338.

Parvizi J, Ghanem E, Menashe S, Barrack RL, Bauer TW: Periprosthetic infection: What are the diagnostic challenges? *J Bone Joint Surg Am* 2006;88(suppl 4):138-147.

Sanchez-Sotelo J, Morrey BF: Total elbow arthroplasty. *J Am Acad Orthop Surg* 2011;19(2):121-125.

Spormann C, Achermann Y, Simmen BR, et al: Treatment strategies for periprosthetic infections after primary elbow arthroplasty. *J Shoulder Elbow Surg* 2012;21(8):992-1000.


 

Toor AS, Jiang JJ, Shi LL, Koh JL: Comparison of perioperative complications after total elbow arthroplasty in patients with and without diabetes. *J Shoulder Elbow Surg* 2014;23(11):1599-1606.

Vergidis P, Greenwood-Quaintance KE, Sanchez-Sotelo J, et al: Implant sonication for the diagnosis of prosthetic elbow infection. *J Shoulder Elbow Surg* 2011;20(8):1275-1281.

Wolfe SW, Figgie MP, Inglis AE, Bohn WW, Ranawat CS: Management of infection about total elbow prostheses. *J Bone Joint Surg Am* 1990;72(2):198-212.

Yamaguchi K, Adams RA, Morrey BF: Infection after total elbow arthroplasty. *J Bone Joint Surg Am* 1998;80(4):481-491.

Yamaguchi K, Adams RA, Morrey BF: Semiconstrained total elbow arthroplasty in the context of treated previous infection. *J Shoulder Elbow Surg* 1999;8(5):461-465.

Zimmerli W, Trampuz A, Ochsner PE: Prosthetic-joint infections. *N Engl J Med* 2004;351(16):1645-1654.

# Chapter 21

# Management of Periprosthetic Fractures

Emilie V. Cheung, MD

**Learning Objectives**

- Classify periprosthetic fractures about the elbow and decide which fracture types need to be treated surgically.
- Learn about the technical aspects of fracture fixation, implant revision, and preserving periprosthetic bone stock.
- Learn how to avoid pitfalls and complications, such as nerve injury and infection.

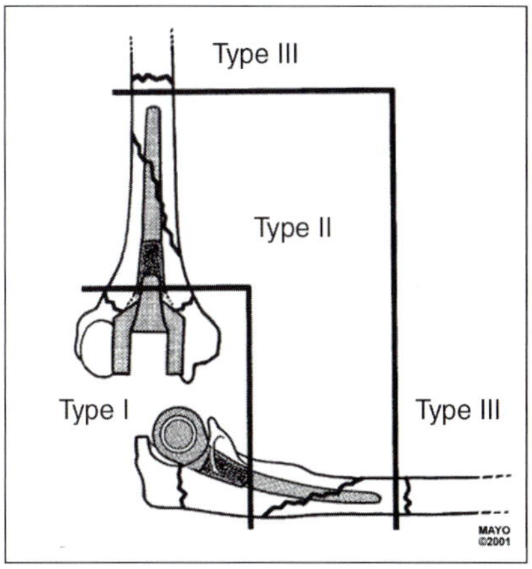


**Figure 1** Illustration depicts the Mayo classification of periprosthetic fractures of the humerus and the ulna. Fractures are classified according to the region of bone involved relative to the implant. Type I, periarticular fracture. Type II, shaft fracture around the stem. Type III, shaft fracture beyond the tip of the stem. (Reproduced with permission from the Mayo Foundation for Medical Education and Research, Rochester, MN.)

## Indications

Historically, total elbow arthroplasty (TEA) was performed in patients with rheumatoid arthritis and in low-demand patients with posttraumatic conditions of the elbow. Multiple studies have shown that 5% to 36% of primary TEAs are complicated by periprosthetic fractures intraoperatively or postoperatively. In a recent prospective study, the use of a total elbow prosthesis that mimics the anatomic characteristics and kinematics of the elbow joint resulted in periprosthetic fracture in 7% of primary surgeries and 8% of revisions.

Intraoperative fractures occur during bone preparation (such as a cortical breach during reaming), during implantation, or as the result of torsional forces on the bone during limb positioning. Displaced humeral condyle fractures can be excised and the soft-tissue envelope repaired to the triceps fascia. Intraoperative fractures of the olecranon should be fixed to secure the integrity of the extensor mechanism.

The Mayo classification of periprosthetic fractures about the elbow categorizes fractures into one of three types based on fracture location, implant fixation, and associated bone loss (**Figure 1**; **Table 1**). Type I fractures are most common and involve the humeral condyle or the olecranon. In the patient with a functional elbow and a stable implant, a type I fracture may be managed nonsurgically with immobilization. However, type I fractures associated with a loose-fitting stem may benefit from fixation or implant revision.

Type II fractures are shaft fractures that occur around the stem of the prosthesis. Type II fractures are subclassified into types 1, 2, and 3, depending on the fixation of the stem and the quality of the bone about the implant. If the fracture is associated with a loose stem, then revision arthroplasty may be necessary. The quality of bone stock available also dictates the treatment of type II fractures. Treatment options include a long-stem prosthesis, strut allograft, and impaction bone grafting or locked compression plating with cerclage wires or screws.

Type III fractures are located outside the margin of the stem and usually occur in the postoperative period.

Meticulous preoperative planning is imperative for the management of periprosthetic elbow fractures. The prostheses, equipment, and bone graft

*Dr. Cheung or an immediate family member serves as a paid consultant to Exactech and serves as a board member, owner, officer, or committee member of the American Academy of Orthopaedic Surgeons.*

**Table 1** Mayo Clinic Classification of Periprosthetic Fractures of the Elbow

| Fracture Type | Description |
|---|---|
| Humeral fractures | |
| H-I | Fracture of the columns or condyles |
| H-II | Fracture around the stem |
| H-II1 | Implant well fixed |
| H-II2 | Implant loose with acceptable bone stock |
| H-II3 | Fracture proximal to the stem |
| Ulnar fractures | |
| U-I | Fracture of the olecranon |
| U-II | Fracture around the stem |
| U-II1 | Implant well fixed |
| U-II2 | Implant loose with acceptable bone stock |
| U-II3 | Implant loose with severe bone loss |
| U-III | Fracture proximal to the stem |

Reproduced with permission from Sanchez-Sotelo J, O'Driscoll S, Morrey BF: Periprosthetic humeral fractures after total elbow arthroplasty: Treatment with implant revision and strut allograft augmentation. *J Bone Joint Surg Am* 2002;84(9):1642-1650.

materials used are not readily available in most hospitals and must be ordered in advance. For example, if cement extraction is required, then instruments such as disposable long, flexible osteotomes that are commercially available for the humerus must be ordered. The surgeon should identify the type of prosthesis implanted during previous surgery and the exact year in which it was implanted. Implant designs have changed, and different generations of specific linkage mechanisms exist. Each implant system has unique nuances and limitations, such as the coupling mechanisms, and these must be understood before surgery. If an unlinked prosthesis was implanted originally, then the anatomic requirements for stability must be well understood. Bone loss may preclude the use of an unlinked implant in the revision setting, and the surgeon must be prepared to revise the implant completely to a linked design. If this is the case, then the surgeon should be experienced in implant extraction with bone preservation techniques, such as the use of osteotomies.

## Contraindications

Contraindications for surgical treatment include infection, infirmity, and patient noncompliance. Patients who fall frequently may not be good candidates for surgery. Intraoperative humeral shaft fractures result from torsional forces applied to the arm during positioning and intramedullary broaching and reaming. These fractures compromise implant stability and should be managed by using a longer stem that spans the defect to bypass the cortical breach. Supplemental strut allograft augmentation with cerclage wires is used if bone quality is weak.

## Alternative Treatments

The application of a fracture brace is usually sufficient to manage periprosthetic fractures that do not affect implant stability, such as minimally displaced type III fractures located distant to the stem of the prosthesis. Patients with a type III fracture typically have osteopenia, and bone stimulators may be used to augment healing and optimize the time to fracture union.

## Results

Published results of the surgical management of periprosthetic fractures are summarized in **Table 2**. In a small study on implant revision and strut allograft augmentation to manage humeral periprosthetic fractures about loose humeral components, almost 30% of the patients treated experienced major complications, consisting of triceps insufficiency, permanent ulnar nerve injury, olecranon fracture, humeral fracture, and nondisplaced humeral periprosthetic fracture. However, all but one patient achieved clinical and radiographic fracture union.

In a 2004 study on strut allograft reconstruction of the proximal ulna as an adjunct to revision TEA in patients with aseptic failure, including periprosthetic fracture, the mean Mayo Elbow Performance Score improved markedly, and greater than 50% incorporation of the strut allograft was achieved. In approximately one-third of the patients, soft-tissue and bony complications developed that required additional surgery.

More recently, satisfactory outcomes were seen in a 2011 study after revision of the ulnar component for ulnar periprosthetic fractures in semiconstrained elbow arthroplasties. Fracture healing occurred in all patients, and most patients had no or minimal pain. However, three deep infections and one implant loosening occurred, which highlights the concern for serious complications during ulnar component revision.

A two-stage reconstruction for type II fractures was described in a 2006 case report. In the initial stage, iliac crest bone graft with compression plating is performed to achieve fracture union. After radiographic evidence of bony union,

 

**Table 2** Results of the Management of Periprosthetic Fractures[a]

| Authors (Year) | No. of Patients | Procedure or Approach | Mean Patient Age in Years (Range) | Mean Follow-up in Years (Range) | Success Rate (%) | Results |
|---|---|---|---|---|---|---|
| Sanchez-Sotelo et al (2002) | 11 | Implant revision and strut allograft augmentation | 66 (42-85) | 3 (0.75-7.8) | 90.9 (fracture union) | 4 patients had one major complication, and 2 patients had two major complications |
| Kamineni and Morrey (2004) | 21 | Proximal ulnar reconstruction with strut allograft in revision TEA | 57 (37-79) | 4 (2-11) | 86 (>50% incorporation of the strut graft) | MEPS improved from 34 to 79 points |
| Foruria et al (2011) | 21 | Ulnar component revision | 64 (24-84) | 5 | 100 (fracture healing) | Complications included 3 deep infections and 1 implant loosening |

MEPS = Mayo Elbow Performance Score, TEA = total elbow arthroplasty.

[a] All studies are level IV evidence.

the second stage commences, consisting of revision to a longer stem and impaction bone grafting to achieve pain relief and improved range of motion (ROM).

Bone loss may develop after multiple failed revisions and periprosthetic fractures, resulting in technical problems with prosthesis fixation during reconstruction. The amount of viable bone is graded based on humeral bone stock. Up to 8 cm of segmental bone loss may be accommodated when using a noncustom, longer component with an extended anterior flange. Treatment options for excessive bone loss include flail elbow, amputation, arthrodesis, and endoprosthetic arthroplasty. However, endoprosthetic arthroplasty has been associated with poor outcomes and high complication rates.

# Techniques

## Setup/Exposure

- The patient is positioned supine with a bump placed under the scapula.
- The arm is prepped and draped, and a sterile tourniquet is applied.
- The locations of scars are noted and used, especially if they are near the midline.
- Full-thickness skin flaps are developed medially and laterally.
- The triceps-sparing approach is preferred at the level of the elbow joint.
- Medially, the ulnar nerve is identified and protected during bone preparation.
- Laterally, the interval between the extensor carpi ulnaris and the anconeus muscle is developed along the subcutaneous border of the ulna and continued proximally to enable exposure of the linkage mechanism.
- If component revision is required, the prosthesis is disarticulated.
- For humeral shaft fractures that require strut allograft augmentation or plating, a modified posterior approach is preferred. This approach involves elevating the entire triceps off the lateral intramuscular septum. This approach is muscle sparing, and less bleeding occurs than with a triceps muscle-splitting approach. The modified approach also allows for proximal extensile exposure. The radial nerve is identified as it crosses the lateral intermuscular septum approximately 14 cm proximal to the lateral epicondyle. The triceps muscle is retracted medially, and the humeral shaft is exposed.
- For ulnar shaft fractures, the author of this chapter prefers to use a posterior approach, with extension along the subcutaneous border of the ulna.

## Procedures

### TYPE I FRACTURES

- Symptomatic condylar fractures occurring around a linked implant can be excised by releasing the flexor-pronator or common extensor muscles by using subperiosteal dissection and then repairing the soft tissue to the adjacent triceps fascia.
- If fixation is tenuous, the author of this chapter prefers to excise the fragments, which results in little functional consequence. Fragment excision is preferable to painful nonunion.

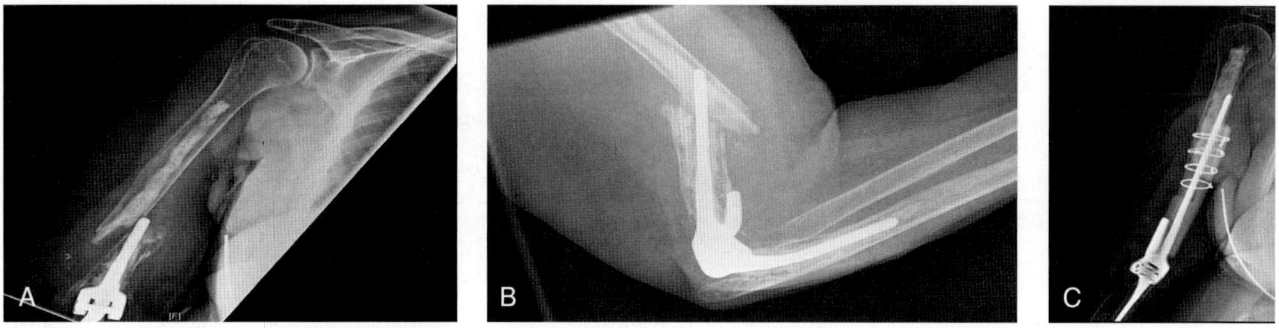


**Figure 2** Radiographs from a 64-year-old woman who had undergone total elbow arthroplasty 9 years previously. **A,** AP view demonstrates a periprosthetic humerus fracture resulting from a mechanical fall. **B,** Lateral view demonstrates insufficient humeral bone stock. **C,** AP view after placement of an allograft-prosthetic composite with bulk femoral allograft and revision to a long-stemmed humeral component. The patient experienced healing and achieved a satisfactory result.

- Periarticular fractures of the olecranon are repaired to maintain the integrity of the extensor mechanism. The author of this chapter prefers to manage displaced fractures of the olecranon with tension-band wiring. The presence of the ulnar component precludes the use of standard tension-band techniques.
- Smooth Kirschner wires are placed along the dorsal aspect of the ulna, engaging the cement mantle adjacent to the prosthesis.
- The figure-of-8 tension band is placed in standard AO fashion over the dorsum of the olecranon.

#### TYPE II2 FRACTURES

- Type II2 fractures of the humerus or ulna that occur in the presence of a loose prosthesis without associated bone loss are managed with implant revision and strut graft augmentation.
- The fracture is circumferentially exposed to allow complete visualization of the proximal and distal fragments.
- The loose implant is removed carefully to avoid further damage to the bone. Loose cement and the relative membrane are removed.
- The canal is prepared to receive an implant with a longer stem that will extend beyond the fracture site.
- Trial reduction is performed to approximate the allograft length and ensure adequate elbow flexion and extension. For humeral fractures, shorter anterior and longer posterior struts are preferred. For ulnar fractures, a dorsal strut is placed laterally under the anconeus muscle or medially under the flexor carpi ulnaris muscle to prevent subcutaneous prominence.
- It is preferable to cement the revision stem before the struts are placed to monitor for cement extravasation. Cement extrusion underneath the allograft may limit allograft incorporation, cause nerve damage, or impinge on ROM.
- The cerclage wires are secured.
- Intraoperative fluoroscopy is used to visualize hardware placement, any cement penetration, and the construct itself.

#### TYPE II3 FRACTURES

- Fractures around the stem of a loose prosthesis with associated bone loss (type II3 fractures) are the most technically challenging. Periprosthetic fractures can occur after progressive osteolysis around the stem.
- The loose prosthesis is revised, the fracture is reduced, and the bone is reconstructed.
- Ultrasonic cement removal tools can aid in removing cement within the canal; however, these tools are known to cause thermal injury to nerves. Care should be taken to identify the radial nerve and protect it during placement of an ultrasonic device within the humeral canal. The ulnar nerve should be identified and protected if an ultrasonic device is placed in the proximal ulna. Manual cement removal with ultrasonic devices, reamers, curets, or osteotomes is associated with cortical perforation and possible cement extravasation at the time of final cementing.
- Bone grafting may be done using bulk allograft or strut allograft. Bulk allograft is used in patients in whom intramedullary bone loss from a loose prosthesis results in insufficient bone for the placement of a new prosthesis. The allograft is fashioned with a long structural step cut that is intended to mate with the remaining bone. The allograft is fixed to the native host bone with cerclage wires or a plate, and the new implant is implanted into the allograft-native bone construct. Allograft struts stabilize the fracture and provide biologic reconstitution of cortical bone (**Figure 2**).

#### TYPE III FRACTURES

- In the patient with a well-fixed humeral stem and good native bone

 

stock, strut allograft with cerclage wires and a plate-and-screw construct are used to achieve fracture fixation.
- The radial nerve is mobilized and protected.
- Typically, the plate and screws are placed along the posterior surface of the humerus. Bicortical fixation is achieved above the prosthesis.
- Fixation along the humeral implant is achieved with unicortical screws supplemented with cerclage wires or cables.
- Posterior and anterior strut allograft may be needed to align and stabilize the fracture (**Figure 3**).
- Shaft fractures beyond the tip of the stem can be managed in the same way as shaft fractures without TEA. Immobilization and early conversion to a functional brace is the recommended treatment.
- Open reduction and internal fixation is recommended if satisfactory alignment cannot be maintained with closed techniques.

### Wound Closure

- If a triceps-reflecting exposure was used, then the triceps is repaired back to the olecranon through cruciate drill holes and a supplemental drill hole.
- The wound is closed in layers over a drain.
- To optimize healing, the author of this chapter often uses a vacuum-assisted wound closure device to keep the wound dry, minimize drainage, and encourage early epithelialization (**Figure 4**).

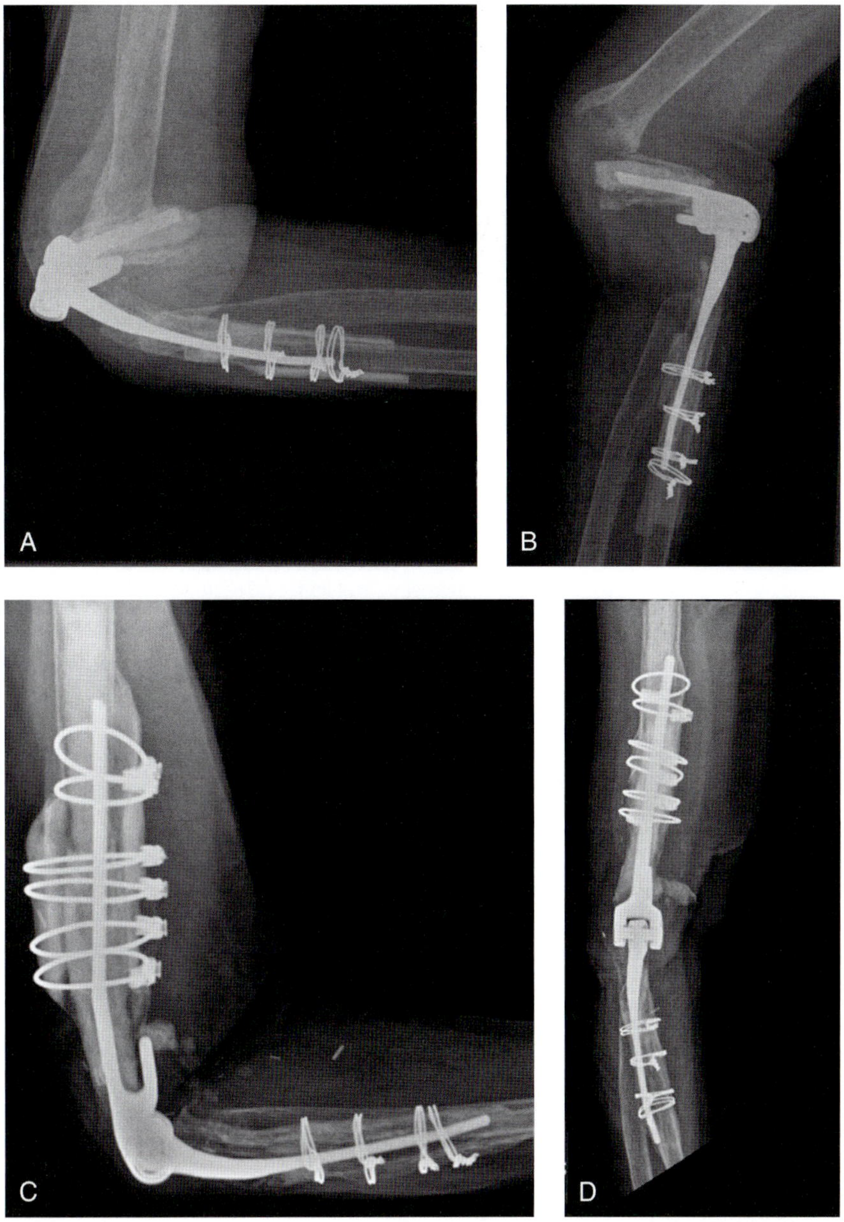


**Figure 3** Radiographs from a 60-year-old woman who sustained a periprosthetic fracture of the ulna. Lateral (**A**) and AP (**B**) views demonstrate the appearance of a periprosthetic humeral fracture resulting from a mechanical fall. Lateral (**C**) and AP views (**D**) obtained after strut allograft fixation and revision of the humeral component. The patient experienced healing and achieved a satisfactory result.

## Postoperative Regimen

The arm is immobilized in extension with an anterior splint to remove tension on the posterior skin incision. The arm is kept elevated to minimize postoperative edema. The author of this chapter recommends leaving the dressings in place for 1 week. At 1 week postoperatively, active ROM is initiated. Sutures are removed after the second postoperative week.

## Limiting Adverse Events

Adverse events associated with the management of periprosthetic fractures include transient and permanent nerve injury, infection, and wound

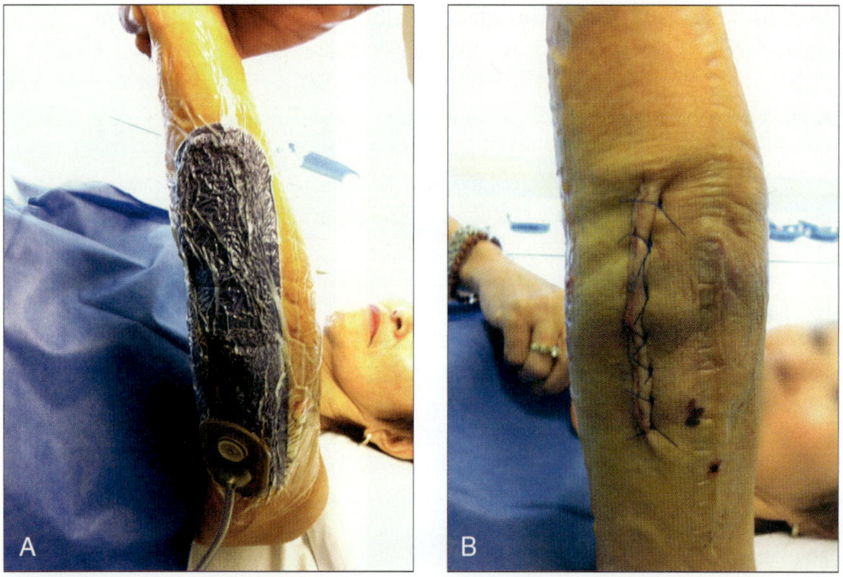


**Figure 4** **A,** Intraoperative photograph shows the placement of a vacuum-assisted wound closure device along the posterior incision to facilitate wound closure. **B,** Clinical photograph shows the wound 2 weeks postoperatively. The wound is epithelialized and dry and exhibits minimal edema.

complications. These adverse events can be limited by achieving adequate exposure. The ulnar and radial nerves, respectively, must be identified when performing open reduction and internal fixation of ulnar and humeral fractures. The judicious use of a drain and a wound vacuum device in addition to immobilization of the elbow in extension may be warranted to reduce the risk of wound complications and infection. Stabilization of the arm with strut allograft or allograft-prosthetic composites may allow restoration of a functional limb.

## Bibliography

Alizadehkhaiyat O, Al Mandhari A, Sinopidis C, Wood A, Frostick S: Total elbow arthroplasty: A prospective clinical outcome study of Discovery Elbow System with a 4-year mean follow-up. *J Shoulder Elbow Surg* 2015;24(1):52-59.

Bassi RS, Simmons D, Ali F, et al: Early results of the Acclaim elbow replacement. *J Bone Joint Surg Br* 2007;89(4):486-489.

Choo A, Ramsey ML: Total elbow arthroplasty: Current options. *J Am Acad Orthop Surg* 2013;21(7):427-437.

Foruria AM, Sanchez-Sotelo J, Oh LS, Adams RA, Morrey BF: The surgical treatment of periprosthetic elbow fractures around the ulnar stem following semiconstrained total elbow arthroplasty. *J Bone Joint Surg Am* 2011;93(15):1399-1407.

Hildebrand KA, Patterson SD, Regan WD, MacDermid JC, King GJ: Functional outcome of semiconstrained total elbow arthroplasty. *J Bone Joint Surg Am* 2000;82(10):1379-1386.

Jensen CH, Jacobsen S, Ratchke M, Sonne-Holm S: The GSB III elbow prosthesis in rheumatoid arthritis: A 2- to 9-year follow-up. *Acta Orthop* 2006;77(1):143-148.

Kamineni S, Morrey BF: Proximal ulnar reconstruction with strut allograft in revision total elbow arthroplasty. *J Bone Joint Surg Am* 2004;86(6):1223-1229.

Kim JM, Mudgal CS, Konopka JF, Jupiter JB: Complications of total elbow arthroplasty. *J Am Acad Orthop Surg* 2011;19(6):328-339.

O'Driscoll SW, Morrey BF: Periprosthetic fractures about the elbow. *Orthop Clin North Am* 1999;30(2):319-325.

Ross AC, Sneath RS, Scales JT: Endoprosthetic replacement of the humerus and elbow joint. *J Bone Joint Surg Br* 1987;69(4):652-655.

 

Sanchez-Sotelo J, O'Driscoll S, Morrey BF: Periprosthetic humeral fractures after total elbow arthroplasty: Treatment with implant revision and strut allograft augmentation. *J Bone Joint Surg Am* 2002;84(9):1642-1650.

Schneeberger AG, Hertel R, Gerber C: Total elbow replacement with the GSB III prosthesis. *J Shoulder Elbow Surg* 2000;9(2):135-139.

Tokunaga D, Hojo T, Ohashi S, et al: Periprosthetic ulnar fracture after loosening of total elbow arthroplasty treated by two-stage implant revision: A case report. *J Shoulder Elbow Surg* 2006;15(6):e23-e26.

Torbert JT, Fox EJ, Hosalkar HS, Ogilvie CM, Lackman RD: Endoprosthetic reconstructions: Results of long-term followup of 139 patients. *Clin Orthop Relat Res* 2005;438:51-59.

# SECTION 4
## *Posttraumatic Reconstruction*

# Chapter 22

# Ulnar Neuropathy

*Ryan P. Calfee, MD, MSc*

**Learning Objectives**

- Understand the management of posttraumatic ulnar neuropathy.
- Understand the expected outcome of posttraumatic ulnar neuropathy.

## Indications

The ulnar nerve is vulnerable during the surgical management of elbow trauma, in particular for fractures of the distal humerus. The ulnar nerve is identified and protected during the fixation of distal humerus fractures, the fixation of coronoid fractures, and medial-sided soft-tissue procedures for elbow instability. The techniques used to protect the ulnar nerve during surgical management of a traumatized elbow vary by surgeon. Many surgeons unroof the ulnar nerve so that it can be visualized and, essentially, decompressed in situ. Alternatively, the ulnar nerve may be elevated with the surrounding soft tissues during subperiosteal dissection under the medial elbow capsule, allowing for retraction during fracture fixation. Other surgeons unroof and circumferentially dissect around the ulnar nerve during exposure to allow for transposition into the subcutaneous tissues for the remainder of the procedure. Regardless of the initial management of the ulnar nerve, there is no consensus as to whether the ulnar nerve should be transposed anteriorly or left in its native position at the conclusion of the procedure.

Although preoperative ulnar nerve dysfunction, which is uncommon, warrants transposition, routine transposition of an asymptomatic ulnar nerve during acute distal humerus fracture fixation is controversial. The author of this chapter universally decompresses and usually transposes the ulnar nerve except in patients in whom the ulnar nerve does not come in contact with the internal fixation and does not appear to be under tension. During revision fracture surgery about the elbow, such as that performed for the management of distal humerus nonunion, transposition of the ulnar nerve is routinely performed.

Symptoms of ulnar neuropathy include paresthesia in the little finger, ulnar half of the ring finger, and ulnar half of the dorsal hand. Results of the two-point discrimination test and the Semmes-Weinstein monofilament test are used to quantify sensory function. Provocative physical examination maneuvers include the Tinel test to detect an irritable ulnar nerve and the elbow flexion test (with or without external nerve compression) to detect compression or tension on the ulnar nerve with flexion. Weakness attributable to the ulnar nerve typically affects the intrinsic musculature of the hand, including the interossei (finger abduction and adduction), the lumbricals (interphalangeal extension), and the adductor pollicis. Visible atrophy is most readily appreciated because the dorsal bulk of the first web space is lost secondary to atrophy of the first dorsal interossei. Weakness of the flexor digitorum profundus to the little and ring fingers also occurs. Although several grading systems exist, the hallmark of advanced neuropathy is muscle atrophy and weakness that typically is present in combination with substantial loss of two-point sensibility.

Surgical intervention for posttraumatic ulnar neuropathy may be indicated in patients with ulnar nerve dysfunction that is recalcitrant to nonsurgical treatment. Before ulnar nerve surgery is recommended, consideration should be given to the pathologic lesion and whether ulnar nerve function will be improved by surgical dissection and changed positioning of the nerve.

Immediate surgical exploration should be strongly considered in patients who have marked ulnar nerve dysfunction after any elbow surgery during which the ulnar nerve was not

*Dr. Calfee or an immediate family member serves as a paid consultant to DePuy Synthes, has received research or institutional support from Medartis, and serves as a board member, owner, officer, or committee member of the American Society for Surgery of the Hand.*

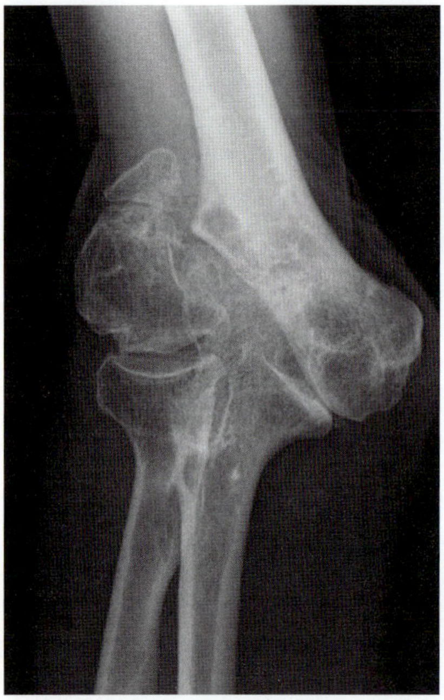

**Figure 1** AP radiograph of an elbow demonstrates a chronic lateral condyle nonunion complicated by tardy ulnar neuropathy.

completely visualized. Surgery also is considered in patients in whom dense or worsening ulnar nerve function developed subacutely or chronically after trauma or elbow surgery without prior ulnar nerve transposition (**Figure 1**). In these patients, electrodiagnostic testing may be considered to attempt to locate areas of compression. Although scarring is often considered the cause of evolving ulnar nerve dysfunction, imperfect documentation or early postoperative examinations limited by pain contribute to the difficulty in distinguishing persistent ulnar nerve dysfunction from worsening nerve function.

Patients who experience pain over the course of the ulnar nerve and paresthesias in the little and ring fingers during elbow flexion may have difficulty flexing the elbow to more than 90° and may have a compressive ulnar neuropathy, which may occur in the absence of distal neurologic symptoms in the hand. In these patients, if the irritable section of the ulnar nerve is clearly localized on physical examination, electrodiagnostic testing may be used to provide confirmatory data; however, nerve irritability must be carefully distinguished from more generalized pain in patients attempting to regain motion after elbow trauma.

## Contraindications

Relative contraindications to the surgical management of posttraumatic ulnar neuropathy include ulnar nerve dysfunction after elbow surgery in which the ulnar nerve was visually confirmed as intact and transposed. In these patients, re-exploration offers limited benefit because ulnar nerve dysfunction is likely secondary to blunt injury (that is, stretch or compression) or temporary vascular compromise that will not benefit from revision surgery. Alternatively, patients with long-standing advanced ulnar neuropathy with chronic muscular denervation and complete loss of two-point discrimination are unlikely to substantially improve after surgical management at the cubital tunnel; however, some ulnar nerve recovery is possible. In one study, improved nerve function was reported in 10 patients with advanced ulnar nerve dysfunction after neurolysis and transposition during posttraumatic reconstructive surgery; however, whether ulnar nerve dysfunction was improving or worsening before reconstructive surgery was unclear.

Before considering ulnar nerve surgery during posttraumatic reconstructive surgery, the surgeon must discuss with the patient the expected recovery potential of the ulnar nerve. Notably, the surgical management of advanced neurologic dysfunction is more likely to provide benefit if neuropathic changes are of recent onset or occur in a younger patient. If mild neuropathic changes persist after submuscular transposition, reliable improvement of ulnar nerve function may not be attainable during subsequent revision surgery. If an ulnar nerve dysfunction about the elbow is not amenable to direct surgical management, some surgeons may consider distal transfer of the anterior interosseous nerve to the motor branch of the ulnar nerve in an attempt to restore intrinsic muscle function, or offer tendon transfers to reduce clawing or improve pinch.

## Alternative Treatments

Nonsurgical management options for posttraumatic ulnar neuropathy are similar to those for idiopathic cubital tunnel syndrome. These options include cessation of triceps strengthening exercises, avoidance of direct external pressure on the ulnar nerve, avoidance of prolonged daytime elbow flexion, and use of a nighttime splint to maintain the elbow in a semi-extended position. Although the author of this chapter has found that these nonsurgical interventions may calm the ulnar nerve, no evidence exists to show that these nonsurgical management options are disease modifying. Nerve gliding exercises are hypothesized to improve ulnar nerve excursion; however, their effectiveness has not been substantiated in clinical series. Low-dose gabapentin administered in the evening is sometimes used for patients who have painful ulnar dysfunction, despite no evidence that it is effective. The dose can be increased based on symptom relief and patient tolerance of the medication. Such use of gabapentin is an off-label application, however.

## Results

Although the surgical management of posttraumatic ulnar nerve dysfunction may improve ulnar nerve function, the subjective gains may exceed the

**Table 1** Results of Surgical Management of Posttraumatic Ulnar Nerve Dysfunction

| Authors (Year) | No. of Patients | Procedure or Approach | Mean Patient Age in Years (Range) | Mean Follow-up in Months (Range) | Success Rate (%) | Results | Level of Evidence |
|---|---|---|---|---|---|---|---|
| Barrios et al (1991) | 53 | Decompression and anterior transposition | NA | ≥36 | 73 | Patients who had posttraumatic ulnar neuropathy were less likely to completely recover<br>Success was defined by an excellent result | III |
| McKee et al (1994) | 13 | Subcutaneous transposition | 39.7 (17-62) | 25 (12-60) | 100 | Improved monofilament sensibility and intrinsic muscle strength<br>All patients experienced decreased symptoms | IV |
| McKee et al (1998) | 20 | Decompression | 48.3 (23-75) | 32.1 (24-67) | 85 | 16 of 17 patients recovered intrinsic strength<br>Success rate was based on 21 elbows | IV |
| Kang et al (2013) | 13 | Subcutaneous transposition | 41 (22-56) | 33 (24-52) | 92 | 12 patients with subjectively improved ulnar nerve function | IV |

NA = not available.

objective findings (**Table 1**). Similar to idiopathic cubital tunnel syndrome, the surgical management of chronic advanced neuropathy is expected to yield limited improvement. Painful neuropathy reliably improves, whereas the loss of intrinsic hand musculature and sensibility may persist in patients with chronic advanced neuropathy. Although no consensus exists on an optimal surgical management option for posttraumatic ulnar neuropathy, a case-control study reported that previous elbow trauma increased the risk of patient dissatisfaction (defined as the need for revision surgery) after ulnar nerve decompression. Currently, the author of this chapter prefers to transpose the ulnar nerve in patients who have posttraumatic ulnar neuropathy and to perform submuscular transposition in patients who have advanced neuropathy.

# Techniques

## Ulnar Nerve Transposition

### SETUP/EXPOSURE

- The patient is placed in the supine position on a surgical stretcher or table with the affected arm abducted on an arm table.
- A tourniquet is placed on the patient's upper arm. Some surgeons prefer to use a sterile tourniquet.
- The skin is incised directly over the course of the ulnar nerve centered posteroinferior to the medial epicondyle. After trauma, the original posterior incision is used.
- The superficial subcutaneous tissues are sharply dissected as the cross veins are cauterized.
- The superficial fascia is defined at the distal and proximal extents of the incision, the location at which the ulnar nerve is always deep to the fascia and the subcutaneous fibrotic bands are minimal compared with those overlying the Osborne fascia.
- As dissection approaches the fascial level, blunt dissection is used to identify and protect the branches of the medial antebrachial cutaneous nerve that course the fascial surface distal to the medial epicondyle.
- The subcutaneous fat is elevated off the medial flexor-pronator mass and the medial epicondyle in preparation for transposition.

- Multiple perforating vessels near the medial epicondyle are cauterized.

### INSTRUMENTS/EQUIPMENT/IMPLANTS REQUIRED

- Soft-tissue instrumentation is sufficient for the management of ulnar neuropathy.
- Access to an electrocautery device and a bipolar electrocautery device is beneficial.
- Many surgeons use a Penrose drain to help retract the ulnar nerve.
- To limit the risk of traction neurapraxia, the author of this chapter does not use a loop for ulnar nerve retraction.

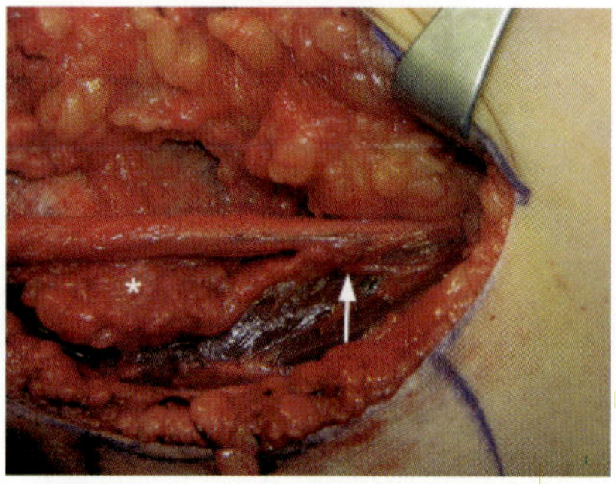

**Figure 2** Intraoperative photograph of an elbow shows the inferior ulnar collateral artery (arrow), which has been protected with the ulnar nerve during circumferential dissection, providing longitudinal vasculature. The asterisk indicates the medial epicondyle.

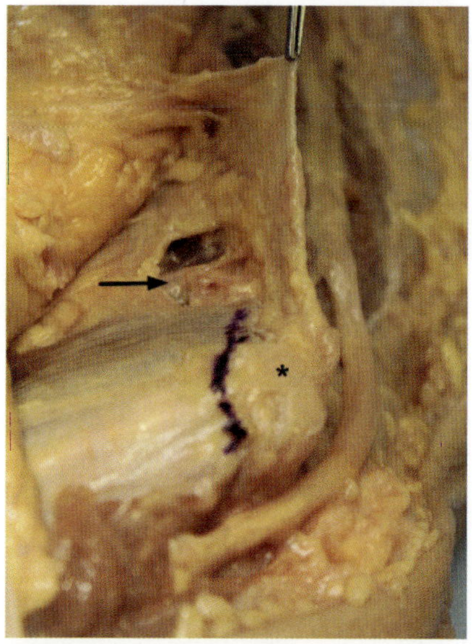

**Figure 3** Photograph of the elbow of a cadaver model shows the medial intermuscular septum held with forceps before excision. The asterisk indicates the medial epicondyle. The arrow indicates the inferior ulnar collateral artery traversing the medial intermuscular septum.

### PROCEDURE

- The fascia is incised just posterior to the medial intermuscular fascia to directly visualize the ulnar nerve. The ulnar nerve may be surrounded by fat or obscured by triceps muscle.
- The overlying fascia directly over the ulnar nerve is divided as it courses posterior to the medial epicondyle and into the forearm between the humeral and ulnar heads of the flexor carpi ulnaris (FCU) muscle.
- The Osborne ligament is divided, and the superficial fascia over the FCU is divided approximately 8 cm distal to the medial epicondyle. Blunt retraction in line with the fascial incision can help split the FCU muscle fibers to expose the deep fascia overlying the ulnar nerve.
- The deep fascia over the ulnar nerve is carefully and sharply divided to avoid the longitudinal nerve branches that variably exit the proper ulnar nerve and pass obliquely under this translucent fascia.
- If the ulnar nerve subluxates over the medial epicondyle with elbow flexion preoperatively, elevation of the subcutaneous fat off the flexor-pronator fascia and the medial epicondyle is performed only after complete visualization of the ulnar nerve is attained to minimize the risk for iatrogenic nerve injury.
- The first motor branch is protected. If the surgeon believes that one of the early posterior branches is a motor branch, it can be mobilized either by dissecting it out of the proper ulnar nerve, incising the FCU fascia overlying the motor branch, or mobilizing the origin of the ulnar head of the FCU. Articular nerve branches are divided in preparation for transposition.
- In the arm, the inferior ulnar collateral artery is identified as it traverses the medial intermuscular septum 25 mm proximal to the medial epicondyle. The inferior ulnar collateral artery and its longitudinal vessels are protected and dissected to remain with the ulnar nerve during circumferential dissection (**Figure 2**). The longitudinal vessels are cauterized distally at the location at which they routinely diverge posteriorly from the ulnar nerve as it curves around the medial epicondyle.
- The medial intermuscular septum is completely excised down to the medial humerus and the inferior ulnar collateral artery so that the ulnar nerve is not kinked after transposition (**Figure 3**).
- The author of this chapter prefers subcutaneous transposition in patients with greater amounts of subcutaneous fat and mild to moderate ulnar neuropathy.
- After confirming that the ulnar nerve is resting tension-free without any abrupt turns proximally or distally, a sling of superficial fascia measuring approximately 3 cm long and 2 cm wide is raised off the flexor-pronator fascia. The base of the fascial sling should be 1 to 3 cm anterior to the medial epicondyle to ensure that the ulnar nerve will not rest directly over the medial epicondyle and parallel to the anticipated course of the ulnar nerve to prevent ulnar nerve compression at the edge of the sling (**Figure 4**).

 

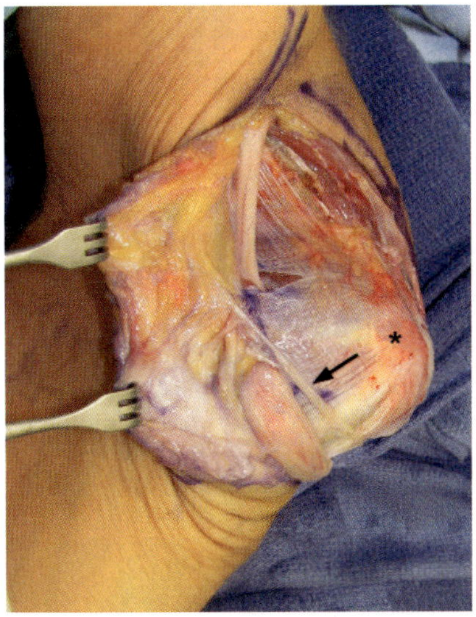

**Figure 4** Intraoperative photograph of an elbow shows subcutaneous ulnar nerve transposition. A fascial sling is used to keep the overlying medial antebrachial cutaneous nerve (arrow) and the ulnar nerve well anterior to the medial epicondyle (asterisk).

- The wound is irrigated, and the fascial sling is sutured to the subcutaneous fat posterior to the ulnar nerve with the use of three simple 3-0 braided nonabsorbable sutures (one in each corner and one in the center).
- The author of this chapter prefers submuscular transposition in patients who have advanced neuropathy such as muscular atrophy, weakness, or two-point discrimination greater than 15 mm, as well as in very thin patients.
- After preparing the ulnar nerve for transposition, the bicipital aponeurosis is incised along the superior border of the pronator teres. The median nerve is identified via longitudinal spreading with tenotomy scissors (**Figure 5, A** and **B**).
- A large, blunt curved clamp is passed deep to the flexor-pronator mass to isolate it medial to the median nerve and anterior to the ulnar nerve (**Figure 5, C**).
- The flexor-pronator mass is completely released from the medial epicondyle, leaving a 0.5- to 1.0-cm rim of tissue for subsequent repair. The flexor-pronator mass is peeled off the ulnar collateral ligament and down to the brachialis fascia, which is visualized running longitudinally with a distinct white tendinous surface (**Figure 5, D**).
- The longitudinal fascia bands between the ulna and humeral head of the FCU are released to allow the ulnar nerve to transpose deeply without an abrupt turn distally (**Figure 5, E**).
- The ulnar nerve is transposed onto the brachialis fascia, medial to the median nerve (**Figure 5, F**).
- The flexor-pronator mass is repaired back to the fibrous tissue on the medial epicondyle with the use of multiple No. 1 or No. 2 braided nonabsorbable sutures that are inverted to ensure the knots are not palpable.
- The longitudinal split between the heads of the FCU is closed with the use of a running No. 0 or No. 2 braided nonabsorbable sutures starting distally and proceeding proximally until approximation is not possible with the elbow in flexion greater than 90°.
- The repaired muscle should not gap or separate with full elbow extension or wrist motion.
- Direct repair of the flexor-pronator mass does not create undue tension or compression on the transposed ulnar nerve; therefore, no step-cut or Z-lengthening is required (**Figure 5, G**).

## In Situ Decompression

- If in situ decompression of the ulnar nerve is selected, then the entire procedure is performed via a smaller incision made directly over the ulnar nerve centered just distal to the medial epicondyle.
- The author of this chapter only considers in situ decompression in patients with idiopathic ulnar neuropathy.
- Superficial dissection is unchanged, and the fascia is identified at the location at which the muscle fibers of the humeral and ulnar heads of the FCU diverge; the ulnar nerve courses just deep to this location.
- The fascial layers are incised as previously described, starting in the forearm, and the ulnar nerve is decompressed.
- Circumferential dissection is avoided to minimize the likelihood of creating ulnar nerve hypermobility.
- The adherence of the skin and the subcutaneous tissue to the medial epicondyle is not disturbed.
- After ulnar nerve decompression, the elbow is moved through a range of motion from extension to full flexion with visualization of the ulnar nerve to determine if the ulnar nerve is snapping over the medial epicondyle during flexion. If the ulnar nerve subluxates, the author of this chapter transposes the ulnar nerve as previously described.

## Second Ulnar Nerve Surgery

- If surgery is performed in a patient in whom the ulnar nerve was transposed subcutaneously, the surgeon should anticipate difficulty identifying the ulnar nerve within the scarred subcutaneous bed.
- The author of this chapter prefers submuscular transposition if a patient requests a second ulnar nerve surgery after subcutaneous transposition or in situ decompression.
- The ulnar nerve is dissected proximal to the prior surgical field before it is removed from the scar across the elbow.
- To most safely dissect the ulnar nerve, the author of this chapter recommends working from proximal to distal first and using additional

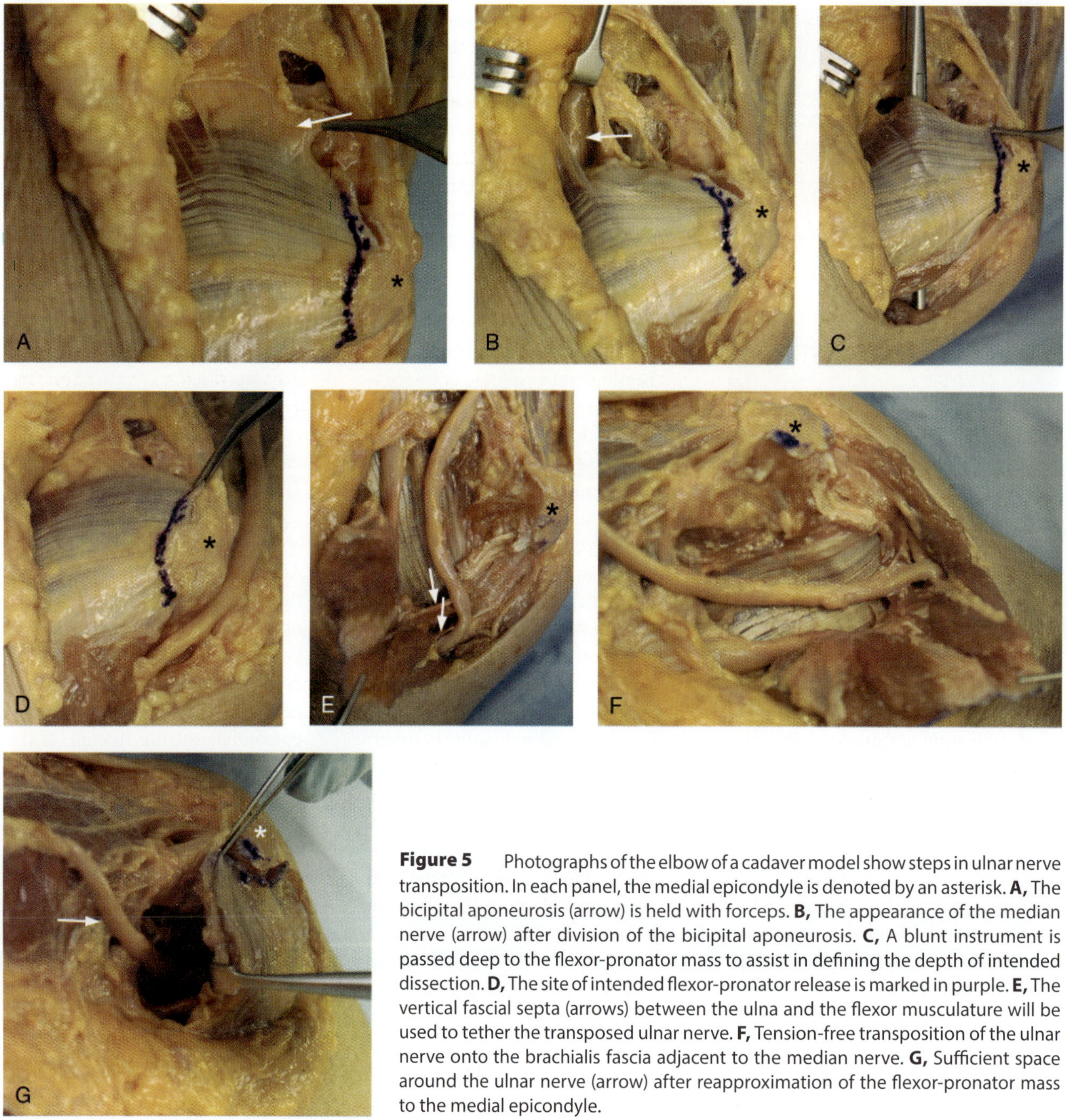


**Figure 5** Photographs of the elbow of a cadaver model show steps in ulnar nerve transposition. In each panel, the medial epicondyle is denoted by an asterisk. **A,** The bicipital aponeurosis (arrow) is held with forceps. **B,** The appearance of the median nerve (arrow) after division of the bicipital aponeurosis. **C,** A blunt instrument is passed deep to the flexor-pronator mass to assist in defining the depth of intended dissection. **D,** The site of intended flexor-pronator release is marked in purple. **E,** The vertical fascial septa (arrows) between the ulna and the flexor musculature will be used to tether the transposed ulnar nerve. **F,** Tension-free transposition of the ulnar nerve onto the brachialis fascia adjacent to the median nerve. **G,** Sufficient space around the ulnar nerve (arrow) after reapproximation of the flexor-pronator mass to the medial epicondyle.

dissection from distal to proximal only if a severe scar is encountered.

### Wound Closure

- Before wound closure, the tourniquet is deflated and hemostasis is confirmed.
- The subcutaneous tissues are closed with 3-0 absorbable sutures, and the skin is closed with 4-0 nylon sutures in an interrupted horizontal mattress pattern.
- After submuscular transposition, the arm is placed in a long-arm plaster splint with the elbow positioned in 90° of flexion.

## Postoperative Regimen

Patients are clinically evaluated approximately 10 days postoperatively. If an elbow splint was used, it is removed at that time. Sutures also are removed, and thin adhesive strips are placed. Full active elbow range-of-motion exercises are begun at that clinical visit. Patients who undergo submuscular transposition are instructed to avoid heavy lifting and forceful gripping until 6 weeks after surgery, during which time a removable wrist brace is worn to serve as a reminder to protect the surgical arm. A formal physical therapy regimen is rarely required.

## Limiting Adverse Events

Multiple branches of the medial antebrachial cutaneous nerve may cross the surgical field, and laceration should be avoided to prevent painful neuroma formation. The branches of the medial antebrachial cutaneous nerve course directly superficial to the fascial layer. A careful preoperative assessment of ulnar nerve stability minimizes the risk for iatrogenic ulnar nerve injury at the level of the medial epicondyle. If the ulnar nerve subluxates over the medial epicondyle with elbow flexion, the ulnar nerve is substantially more superficial during exposure; the safest dissection identifies the ulnar nerve proximally in the arm before following it distally. Elevation of the subcutaneous fat off the flexor-pronator fascia is delayed until the ulnar nerve is visualized. Alternatively, the hypermobile ulnar nerve is approached at the level of the epicondyle with the elbow in relative extension to ensure that the ulnar nerve is posterior to the epicondyle. During transposition, the surgeon must ensure that the ulnar nerve is no longer compressed and that no new sites of compression have been created. During subcutaneous transposition, the base of any fascial sling should be kept 1 to 3 cm anterior to the medial epicondyle so the ulnar nerve does not rest directly over the bony medial epicondyle.

## Bibliography

Aleem AW, Krogue JD, Calfee RP: Outcomes of revision surgery for cubital tunnel syndrome. *J Hand Surg Am* 2014;39(11):2141-2149.

Antuña SA, Morrey BF, Adams RA, O'Driscoll SW: Ulnohumeral arthroplasty for primary degenerative arthritis of the elbow: Long-term outcome and complications. *J Bone Joint Surg Am* 2002;84(12):2168-2173.

Barrios C, Ganoza C, de Pablos J, Cañadell J: Posttraumatic ulnar neuropathy versus non-traumatic cubital tunnel syndrome: Clinical features and response to surgery. *Acta Neurochir (Wien)* 1991;110(1-2):44-48.

Ehsan A, Hanel DP: Recurrent or persistent cubital tunnel syndrome. *J Hand Surg Am* 2012;37(9):1910-1912.

Kang HJ, Koh IH, Jeong YC, Yoon TH, Choi YR: Efficacy of combined osteotomy and ulnar nerve transposition for cubitus valgus with ulnar nerve palsy in adults. *Clin Orthop Relat Res* 2013;471(10):3244-3250.

Krogue JD, Aleem AW, Osei DA, Goldfarb CA, Calfee RP: Predictors of surgical revision after in situ decompression of the ulnar nerve. *J Shoulder Elbow Surg* 2015;24(4):634-639.

McGowan AJ: The results of transposition of the ulnar nerve for traumatic ulnar neuritis. *J Bone Joint Surg Br* 1950;32(3):293-301.

McKee MD, Jupiter JB, Bosse G, Goodman L: Outcome of ulnar neurolysis during post-traumatic reconstruction of the elbow. *J Bone Joint Surg Br* 1998;80(1):100-105.

McKee M, Jupiter J, Toh CL, Wilson L, Colton C, Karras KK: Reconstruction after malunion and nonunion of intra-articular fractures of the distal humerus: Methods and results in 13 adults. *J Bone Joint Surg Br* 1994;76(4):614-621.

Robinson CM, Hill RM, Jacobs N, Dall G, Court-Brown CM: Adult distal humeral metaphyseal fractures: Epidemiology and results of treatment. *J Orthop Trauma* 2003;17(1):38-47.

Shin R, Ring D: The ulnar nerve in elbow trauma. *J Bone Joint Surg Am* 2007;89(5):1108-1116.

Vazquez O, Rutgers M, Ring DC, Walsh M, Egol KA: Fate of the ulnar nerve after operative fixation of distal humerus fractures. *J Orthop Trauma* 2010;24(7):395-399.

Yamaguchi K, Sweet FA, Bindra R, Gelberman RH: The extraneural and intraneural arterial anatomy of the ulnar nerve at the elbow. *J Shoulder Elbow Surg* 1999;8(1):17-21.

 

# Chapter 23

# Soft-Tissue Coverage Options for the Elbow

*L. Scott Levin, MD, FACS*
*Milan Stevanovic, MD*

**Learning Objectives**

- Understand the treatment algorithm for reconstruction of soft-tissue defects about the elbow.
- Understand the concepts of pedicle flap versus microvascular composite tissue transplant for soft-tissue and bone defects of the elbow.

## Introduction

The elbow has an anatomically unique soft-tissue envelope that includes substantial anterior skin, muscle, and fascia, all of which protect the median and radial nerves as well as the brachial vessels. The ulnar nerve is immediately subcutaneous and vulnerable at the medial epicondyle. The lateral and medial epicondyles and the olecranon are covered only by skin. The posterior skin of the elbow is particularly prone to soft-tissue breakdown after fracture treatment or olecranon bursitis. Timely intervention to address soft-tissue defects can help restore function and limit adverse events.

In general, the simplest wound closure method should be considered first. For example, a burn eschar can often be treated with débridement and a split-thickness skin graft (STSG). In contrast, an exposed olecranon without periosteum may be better addressed with a muscle pedicle flap or a microvascular tissue transfer, such as an anterolateral thigh flap. Some techniques, such as a muscle flap and a skin graft, can be used together. Soft-tissue reconstruction of the elbow increases in complexity as follows: primary closure, healing by secondary intention, skin grafts, dermal substitutes, tissue expansion, local flaps (skin or muscle, such as fascial subcutaneous, anconeus, brachioradialis, flexor carpi ulnaris [FCU], and distally based lateral arm flaps), regional flaps (latissimus dorsi flaps and variations, including abdominal-based flaps), soft-tissue free flaps (perforator flaps), and microvascular free flaps with bone (such as fibula or medial geniculate artery). If less toxic methods for allograft immune tolerance are developed, vascularized composite allotransplantation may be a useful alternative in patients who have bone and soft-tissue elbow defects.

Skin that is scarred and adherent to bone, skin and muscle that are tight and noncompliant, and any areas prone to abrasion or breakdown merit special attention. Treatment should include prophylactic augmentation of the soft-tissue envelope, often with full-thickness flaps. The goals of soft-tissue coverage for the elbow are wound closure, limited risk of infection, and mobilization of the elbow. The soft-tissue coverage option selected should be based on the size and etiology of a defect as well as a patient's general health and functional demands. The authors of this chapter favor soft-tissue coverage within 5 days of elbow injury, if possible.

## Types of Soft-Tissue Coverage

### Primary Closure

Primary closure or delayed primary closure is often used for patients who have defects with no underlying bone, joint, dead space, or implant. Whether primary closure can be performed is dictated by the size of the defect as

*Dr. Levin or an immediate family member has received royalties from Mavrek Medical; has received research or institutional support from AxoGen; and serves as a board member, owner, officer, or committee member of the American College of Surgeons, the American Society for Reconstructive Microsurgery, the American Society for Surgery of the Hand, the International Hand and Composite Tissue Allotransplantation Society, the United Network for Organ Sharing, the Vascularized Composite Allograft Transplantation Committee, and the World Society for Reconstructive Microsurgery. Neither Dr. Stevanovic nor any immediate family member has received anything of value from or has stock or stock options held in a commercial company or institution related directly or indirectly to the subject of this chapter.*

well as the mobility, compliance, and vascularity of the surrounding skin. Excessive tension must be avoided because of the risk for skin-edge necrosis, wound breakdown, and a defect larger than the original defect.

## Healing via Secondary Intention

Wound healing via secondary intention may be considered if structural integrity is preserved and there is no exposed bone, joint, neurovascular structure, or tendon without paratenon. Wound healing via secondary intention can be achieved with the use of serial wet-to-moist dressing changes or a wound closure system, such as a negative-pressure dressing system.

## Skin Grafts and Dermal Substitutes

STSGs or full-thickness skin grafts are appropriate for any size defect with a tissue bed that will accept a graft. Skin grafts provide reliable coverage for exposed subcutaneous tissue, muscle, tendon with paratenon, and bone with periosteum. Although skin grafts will heal to paratenon or periosteum, this usually results in an unstable scar that is susceptible to breakdown. Skin grafts will not provide durable coverage sufficient to withstand repeated flexion and extension at the dorsal surface of the elbow. With the advent of skin substitutes, such as bilaminar dressings, wounds that are not immediately amenable to skin grafting can be treated with an artificial skin substitute, which generates a dermal surface that can provide a vascularized tissue bed capable of accepting a skin graft. After débridement, a skin substitute is applied and secured with staples or sutures. The skin substitute is left in place for 2 to 3 weeks to allow for vascular ingrowth of the collagen matrix. The patient's elbow must be immobilized during this 2- to 3-week period in which the collagen substrate of the dermal substitute inoculates. In the second stage, the outer plastic membrane is removed and an STSG is applied. The elbow is then immobilized for approximately 5 days to allow the STSG to take. The results of this two-stage procedure are favorable for improved wound healing compared with primary skin grafting on a less-than-optimal wound bed.

## Tissue Expansion

Tissue expansion is another option for soft-tissue restoration about the elbow. The advantages of tissue expansion are that distal donor sites are not required and local tissue is modified to provide additional surface area for reconstruction. The disadvantages of tissue expansion are the need for a two-stage procedure (expander insertion and subsequent removal) and the risk for extrusion or infection of an implant. Because of the risk for infection, tissue expanders, which are most often used to replace unstable areas of scar tissue with pliable, normal skin before reconstructive surgery, cannot be used to resurface traumatic wounds. Recent techniques that use balloon dissectors to create pockets for tissue expansion have minimized the risk for expander extrusion through the incisions used to place the expander and have facilitated more rapid tissue expansion. Expanders are designed with either remote ports for filling or ports within the expander itself. Selection of a tissue expander is based on its width, length, shape, and total fill volume.

After an expander is placed, sterile saline is used to inflate the expander. The rate of expansion depends on the give of the skin over the expander, the comfort of the patient with regard to skin stretch, and, most importantly, maintenance of skin perfusion after a particular volume of saline is added. It may take several weeks to achieve fill of an expander. After the maximal volume of the expander is attained, the expander is removed during a second procedure. The resultant redundant skin can then be advanced or transposed over abnormal areas in preparation for reconstructive surgery or to improve the cosmetic appearance of a scarred area. During the process of expansion, a capsule may form around the expander, which can limit excursion of expanded tissue. A capsulotomy may help increase excursion; however, if performed too aggressively, it may compromise vascular supply to the overlying skin. Tissue expansion has been used in patients who have burn scar contractures about the elbow, which obviates the need for distant donor tissue and skin grafts.

## Local Random Flaps

Local random flaps are perfused through the dermal plexus and subdermal plexus. They are not based on any particular vascular pattern or pedicle. Small defects can be closed with local skin flaps, such as transposition flaps, if the primary closure creates excessive tension on the tissue margins or if skin grafting is not a suitable option. Local random flaps are advantageous because they allow for wound closure with similarly textured skin. The use of local random flaps in the upper extremity is limited because of relatively poor vascularity and limited tissue mobility.

## Axial Fasciocutaneous Flaps

Axial fasciocutaneous flaps are based on anatomically named arteriovenous systems, which provide vascular supply to a defined area of skin and subcutaneous tissue. Axial fasciocutaneous flaps can be harvested as island flaps or as wide-based peninsular flaps, in which the vascular pedicle is fully mobilized. Island flaps provide greater versatility in coverage because of the increased arc of rotation. Most axial fasciocutaneous flaps can be harvested as free flaps. Among the axial fasciocutaneous flaps found in the arm and forearm are the lateral arm flap, posterior interosseous flap, ulnar artery flap, and the radial forearm flap.

### Distant Pedicle Flaps: Two-Stage Flaps

Distant pedicle flaps provide reliable coverage for large soft-tissue defects if recipient vessels are not available or if a patient is a poor candidate for other types of soft-tissue reconstruction. Although distant pedicle flaps can cover defects as large as 22 cm in length, they do not convey a permanent independent blood supply to the defect. Distant pedicle flaps are seldom used, but they are an important reconstructive option in select patients. The main limitations of distant pedicle flaps relate to the prolonged immobilization required for the two-stage procedure, which may affect final elbow motion. Problems of stiffness and contracture at the shoulder and fingers can be minimized if patients maintain mobility of the unaffected joints. Another potential source of morbidity is secondary surgery for flap division and subsequent flap contouring. Distant pedicle flaps also are criticized for donor site cosmesis, bulk, and need for secondary surgery. Examples of distant pedicle flaps include the use of abdominal-based flaps on either the inferior or superior epigastric systems. In the experience of the authors of this chapter, the arm must remain attached to the chest or abdomen for at least 3 weeks to ensure ingrowth of vessels from the periphery of the wound bed. This process of inosculation depends on host characteristics and local wound conditions.

### Local Muscle Pedicle Flaps

Local muscle rotational flaps can be used to cover small defects around the elbow. In general, the arc of rotation of local muscle rotational flaps allows for anterior and posterior wound coverage. The use of several local muscle rotational flaps, including the brachioradialis, the extensor carpi radialis longus, the anconeus, and the FCU, have been described in small series but often only as case reports. The brachioradialis, extensor carpi radialis longus, anconeus, and FCU muscles often lie within the zone of injury, which limits their use. Local muscle rotational flaps may be useful for steroid-induced fat atrophy that results in thin skin and chronic pain. The anconeus and brachioradialis are effective for steroid-induced fat atrophy that results in thin skin and chronic pain because the volume of muscle is small but will provide improved vascularity and bulk to compromised areas.

### Distant Muscle Pedicle Flaps

For patients with moderate to large soft-tissue defects about the elbow, the latissimus dorsi rotational flap is the only distant pedicle muscle rotational flap that can provide adequate coverage. The latissimus dorsi and its neurovascular pedicle lie well away from the elbow and are generally outside the zone of injury. The latissimus dorsi rotational flap is a one-stage procedure, and motion and stretching exercises can begin within 7 to 10 days after surgery.

### Free-Tissue Transfer

In patients in whom local muscle rotational flaps or distant one-stage pedicle muscle rotational flaps are not suitable for soft-tissue reconstruction, excellent functional outcomes and cosmesis can be achieved with free-tissue transfer. Free-tissue transfer as a single-stage reconstruction allows for elbow exercises within a few days after the risk for vascular compromise is decreased. The donor site is selected based on a variety of factors, including defect size and location, underlying structural or functional deficits, the presence of exposed or prominent implants, and a patient's overall health status. Fascial, fasciocutaneous, muscle, musculocutaneous, and osteocutaneous flaps are options for free-tissue transfer. In general, the authors of this chapter prefer free muscle flap with a skin graft over musculocutaneous flap. However, the defect size dictates the preferred flap. The authors of this chapter prefer to use the gracilis muscle for defects of moderate size and the latissimus for larger defects. Free fascial flaps can be used to manage defects for which filling of a dead space is not required. Commonly used fascial flaps include radial forearm, parascapular, and temporoparietal fascial flaps; all of these flaps provide thin, pliable coverage and allow tendon gliding. Free lateral arm, and radial and ulnar forearm flaps can be harvested from the contralateral limb as sensory flaps. These sensory flaps provide protective sensation over areas that are subject to pressure breakdown; however, there is some donor site morbidity, with reports of deformity and dysesthesia.

### Perforator Flaps

Perforator flaps are defined as tissue territories based on a single perforator vessel that originates from a source artery. The anterolateral thigh flap is a perforator flap. Almost all of the skin of the thigh can be harvested on one or two perforators that originate from the descending branch of the lateral femoral circumflex artery and vein. Currently, perforator flaps are in vogue and provide excellent coverage. An advantage of perforator flaps is the ability to lift the flap for secondary reconstruction (**Figures 1** and **2**).

## Results

Results of rotational flaps for soft-tissue coverage are reported in **Table 1**. Data on soft-tissue coverage procedures are difficult to find. Most techniques are reported in small series or case reports. In many patients, the underlying pathology has a greater impact on functional outcomes than any particular soft-tissue coverage technique. In larger series, soft-tissue coverage procedures are often performed for a variety of underlying pathologies. A 2011 study reported that anconeus rotational flaps provided reliable coverage of soft-tissue defects,

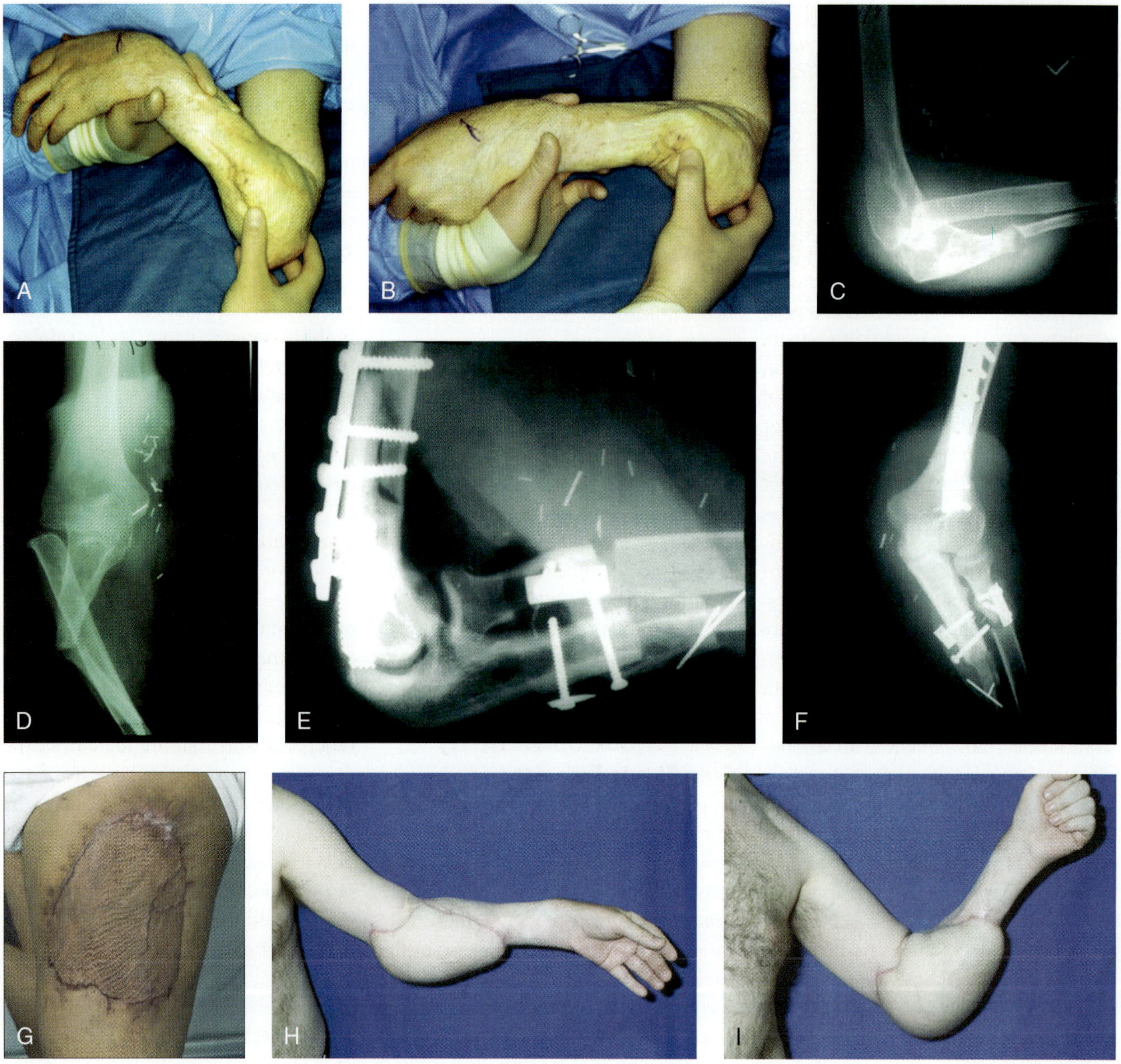


**Figure 1** Images from a man who underwent an anterolateral thigh flap procedure. Preoperative clinical photographs show a painful, unstable elbow in flexion (**A**) and extension (**B**). **C,** Preoperative lateral radiograph of the elbow in flexion. **D,** Preoperative AP radiograph of the elbow in extension. Lateral radiograph of the elbow in flexion (**E**) and AP radiograph of the elbow in extension (**F**) demonstrate two-stage reconstruction with the use of an anterolateral thigh flap, which was followed by elbow allograft. **G,** Clinical photograph of the thigh shows the donor site. Clinical photographs show the elbow in extension (**H**) and flexion (**I**) 1 year postoperatively.

most of which were the result of chronic draining olecranon bursitis, with a mean size of 4 × 3 cm.

The outcomes of using FCU rotational flaps have been reported in a few small series. A 2008 cadaver model study reported that the FCU provided reliable coverage of soft-tissue defects with a width of 2 to 4 cm at the olecranon. In both clinical and cadaver model dissections, the authors of this chapter have been able to use the FCU to cover soft-tissue defects with a width of 2 to 5 cm. Fan-folding of the FCU offers a greater width for soft-tissue coverage. Without fan-folding, the FCU can reach 8 to 9 cm proximal to the olecranon tip with the elbow in 90° of flexion.

Although a high rate of antegrade radial forearm flap survival and healing has been reported, rates of donor site

 

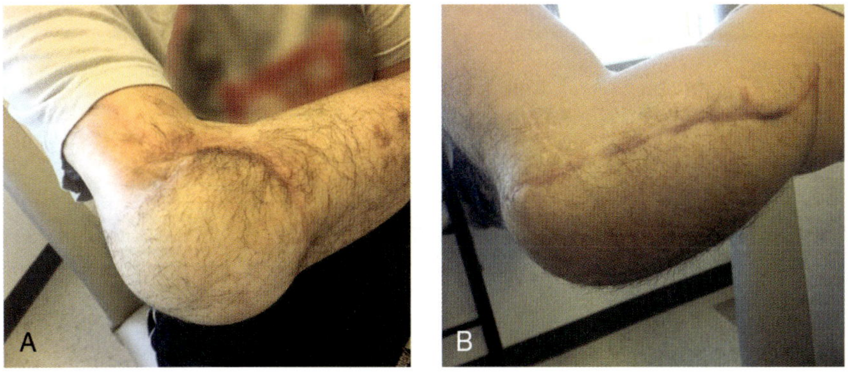


**Figure 2** Clinical photographs of the elbow from a man who sustained a traumatic injury at age 14 years. The patient underwent radial head replacement as an adult, which resulted in ankylosis of the elbow (**A**). The soft-tissue envelope was deficient, which precluded elbow contracture release. A free anterolateral thigh flap was used to provide adequate soft tissue for contracture release. **B,** Appearance of the elbow after placement of the thigh flap but before contracture release.

morbidity are mixed. Concerns at the donor site are related to cosmesis, dysesthesia, wrist flexion contracture, pinch and grip strength, and radial fractures if it is taken as an osteocutaneous flap. The most common donor site complications are cosmesis and dysesthesia, with reported rates between zero and 25%. Prophylactic plating of the radius can be performed to reduce the risk for radial fracture in a patient in whom an osteocutaneous flap is harvested.

A 1987 cadaver model study reported that the latissimus dorsi rotational flap consistently reached the olecranon and often was able to provide soft-tissue coverage to the proximal forearm. Similar results were reported in a 1999 clinical study on the use of a latissimus dorsi pedicle rotational flap for complex soft-tissue defects about the elbow. Complications included hematoma from loss of a ligating clip on a branch to the serratus and partial flap necrosis at the distal flap if soft-tissue coverage farther than 8 cm distal to the olecranon tip was attempted.

In a comprehensive study on soft-tissue coverage options for the elbow published in 2007, pedicle flaps accounted for 65% of the soft-tissue coverage procedures. Of these procedures, the radial forearm flap was the most common, followed by the latissimus dorsi flap. The highest complication rate was reported with the use of latissimus dorsi rotational flaps to cover defects distal to the olecranon tip.

## Most Commonly Used Rotational Flaps

The procedures used most frequently by the authors of this chapter are described below, and the authors believe these procedures are reliable and durable in patients who have consistent anatomy. No microsurgical techniques are required in performing these procedures, and they are relatively quick to perform.

### Local Muscle Rotational Flaps

#### ANCONEUS

The anconeus is a small, triangular muscle that crosses the lateral elbow. The anconeus originates on the posterior surface of the lateral humeral epicondyle and inserts on the lateral proximal olecranon. Blood supply is through two constant arterial pedicles—the medial collateral artery and the recurrent posterior interosseous artery—both of which anastomose within the muscle belly of the anconeus. The medial collateral artery is a terminal branch of the profunda brachii artery, which always travels with the radial nerve branch to the anconeus and enters the anconeus on its proximal deep surface. Although the anconeus can be mobilized on either its proximal or distal pedicle, mobilization on the distal pedicle requires sacrifice of the nerve, which leads to atrophy and flap scarring. The anconeus is approximately 2.5 cm wide and 7 cm long. The anconeus functions as a minor elbow extensor and may augment lateral elbow stability.

The anconeus is useful for soft-tissue coverage of small defects on the posterior and lateral elbow, including the lateral radiocapitellar joint, the distal triceps tendon at its insertion, and the olecranon. The anconeus can reliably cover a soft-tissue defect measuring 5 to 7 cm$^2$. The anconeus can be harvested without measurable functional deficit. There are no specific contraindications for use of the anconeus other than the size of the soft-tissue defect and involvement of the muscle in the area of injury. Instability of the lateral elbow is a relative contraindication to the use of the anconeus, although concomitant collateral ligament reconstruction can aid in preventing such instability.

Particular attention should be paid to certain steps in the surgical technique. Dissection should be carried to the distal-most insertion of the anconeus, approximately 10 cm from the lateral epicondyle. The interval between the anconeus and the extensor carpi ulnaris is best identified distally. The anconeus should be elevated from distal to proximal. The lateral ulnar collateral ligament complex and radiocapitellar joint capsule should be protected. The anconeus origin can be released to increase the arc of rotation of the flap. Rotation on the proximal pedicle preserves the radial nerve innervation to the anconeus, which improves flap suppleness.

**Table 1** Results of Rotational Flaps for Soft-Tissue Coverage Procedures

| Authors (Year) | Number of Patients | Flap Type | Mean Patient Age in Years (Range) | Mean Follow-up in Months (Range) | Results |
|---|---|---|---|---|---|
| Jutte et al (1987) | 4 | Latissimus dorsi | 64 (55-76) | 6 (1-12) | Coverage >6 cm from tip of olecranon on posterior elbow not recommended |
| Stevanovic et al (1999) | 9 | Latissimus dorsi pedicle | 34 (17-75) | 28 (18-51) | Complications in 2 patients (1 hematoma and 1 partial flap necrosis) |
| Choudry et al (2007) | 96 (99 flaps) | Latissimus dorsi (21), radial forearm (24), random fasciocutaneous (15), other pedicled (20)[a] | 45 (5-90) | 32 (4-150) | 31% overall complication rate (30 minor complications that did not require additional reconstruction and 12 major complications that required additional reconstruction)<br>55% complication rate for latissimus dorsi flap used to cover the olecranon tip; mean defect size, 147 cm$^2$<br>20% complication rate for radial forearm rotational flap; mean defect size[2], 66 cm$^2$<br>25% complication rate for random fasciocutaneous flap; mean defect size, 46 cm$^2$ |
| Wysocki et al (2008) | 17 | Flexor carpi ulnaris pedicle | N/A | N/A | Cadaver model study<br>Reliable coverage of defects with a width of 2 to 4 cm at the olecranon<br>Width of coverage correlated with forearm circumference |
| Elhassan et al (2011) | 20 | Anconeus | 57 (36-88) | 17 (15-20) | Reliable coverage of defects with a mean size of 4 × 3 cm<br>Mean time to wound healing was 3 wk<br>Wound dehiscence developed in 2 patients; healing was achieved with local wound care |
| Sharpe et al (2014) | 7 | Flexor carpi ulnaris pedicle | 42 (20-76) | ≥24 | Cadaver (25 specimens) and clinical (7 patients) study<br>5.7 cm mean distance from proximal pedicle to medial epicondyle (range, 3-10 cm)<br>All flaps healed by 3 wk postoperatively<br>No additional procedures were required for soft-tissue coverage |

N/A = not applicable, NR = not reported.

[a] 19 free tissue transfers.

**BRACHIORADIALIS**

The brachioradialis is the most superficial muscle on the lateral forearm. The origin of the brachioradialis lies between the brachialis and triceps muscles. The brachioradialis arises from the upper two-thirds of the lateral supracondylar ridge of the humerus and from the anterior aspect of the lateral intermuscular septum. The brachioradialis tendon inserts on the radial styloid. The muscle belly of the brachioradialis extends to the mid-forearm, at which point it becomes a thin flat tendon. The brachioradialis acts as a weak elbow flexor that is strongest with the forearm in mid-pronation. The brachioradialis can initiate both pronation and supination. The brachioradialis is innervated above the elbow joint by a branch of the radial nerve. The dominant pedicle of the brachioradialis is a branch of the radial recurrent artery that is close to its origin from the radial artery. The pedicle of the brachioradialis measures approximately 3 cm in length and 1 mm in diameter. Minor pedicles arise as branches more distal from the radial recurrent artery, but they are smaller and less consistent.

The brachioradialis rotational flap is best suited for small soft-tissue defects along the anterolateral or posterolateral border of the distal arm and proximal forearm. The brachioradialis can be sacrificed with minimal donor site morbidity and functional loss. The brachioradialis can be used as a muscle flap and a musculocutaneous flap. The authors of this chapter prefer not to use the brachioradialis as a musculocutaneous flap because it commonly results in a bulky, disfigured appearance of the forearm. The brachioradialis should not be sacrificed in the absence of the dominant elbow flexors.

Particular attention should be paid to certain steps in the surgical technique. The superficial radial nerve and the radial artery are located volar and deep to the brachioradialis and should be protected. The brachioradialis should be released distally near the musculotendinous junction to leave a cuff of tendon for insetting. The entire brachioradialis should be harvested, if necessary, for triceps tendon or ligament reconstruction. Several perforating branches from the radial artery enter the brachioradialis. Ligation of these branches improves the arc of rotation of the muscle. The radial recurrent artery branches off of the radial artery near the bicipital tuberosity of the radius. The origin of the brachioradialis may be released to increase the range of soft-tissue coverage. Subcutaneous tunnels can be used to reach the area of soft-tissue defect; however, this may compress and compromise the brachioradialis flap. The authors of this chapter prefer to place a skin graft over the exposed muscle belly.

#### FLEXOR CARPI ULNARIS

The FCU is the most ulnar superficial flexor of the forearm. One head of the FCU originates at the medial epicondyle of the distal humerus, and the other head originates from the proximal ulna. The dominant pedicle of the FCU comes from the ulnar artery or the ulnar recurrent artery, which is a branch of the ulnar artery. Typically, the FCU is supplied by several pedicles along the length of the muscle; however, it is well perfused by the most proximal one to two pedicles, which are small, 1- to 2-mm vessels. A branch of the ulnar nerve innervates the FCU. This branch enters the proximal FCU immediately distal to the medial epicondyle. The muscle belly of the FCU has a mean width of 5 cm and a mean length of 20 cm. In most patients, the muscle belly of the FCU extends to the wrist flexion crease.

FCU flaps are local muscle rotational flaps, and as with most such flaps for the elbow, the size and arc of rotation limits their use to small- to medium-size defects on the anterior, posterior, or medial elbow. A 6- × 8-cm soft-tissue defect is the largest soft-tissue defect the authors of this chapter have covered on the posterior elbow with an FCU flap. The FCU also can be used to cover neurovascular structures, arteriovenous shunts, and vascular prosthetic grafts. The FCU is the preferred rotational flap of the authors of this chapter for prophylactic coverage in an elbow that has undergone multiple surgeries and has a poor soft-tissue envelope. The tendinous FCU can be used for reconstruction of the triceps or collateral ligament. The FCU should not be sacrificed if soft-tissue coverage options with a lower morbidity are available. For patients who expect to return to their preoperative level of function and require a strong wrist flexor, the FCU may not be the best option. Specific contraindications for use of the FCU flap for soft-tissue coverage are an absent ulnar artery, absent innervation to the FCU, and involvement of the FCU in the zone of injury. The use of the FCU flap for soft-tissue coverage is controversial because donor site morbidity is potentially associated with use of the dominant wrist flexor and ulnar deviator.

Particular attention should be paid to certain steps in the surgical technique. A preoperative Allen test and/or Doppler or color Doppler ultrasonography is used to assess the radial and ulnar arteries before dissection of the FCU. In general, there are five to seven pedicles to the FCU from the ulnar artery. A relatively distal proximal pedicle can limit the arc of rotation of the FCU flap. The proximal pedicles should be evaluated before ligation of the distal pedicles. The FCU is usually well perfused by the proximal two perforators and, often, only the most proximal perforator. The area of soft-tissue coverage by the FCU is maximized by transecting the FCU at the level of the wrist flexion crease, using longitudinal and transverse fascial incisions to spread the FCU to cover the soft-tissue defect or fan-folding the FCU to cover a wider soft-tissue defect. FCU flap durability is optimized by maintaining innervation to the flap. Harvesting the FCU with an overlying skin paddle can result in poor donor site cosmesis.

### Radial Forearm Flap

The radial forearm flap is perhaps the most versatile and reliable rotational flap for soft-tissue reconstruction of the hand and elbow. As mentioned previously, the radial forearm flap provides thin, durable soft-tissue coverage. The incorporation of the medial or lateral antebrachial cutaneous nerve can make this a sensate flap that provides sensory protection to large areas of reconstructed soft tissue about the elbow. If a large skin flap is required, it can be harvested alone or with vascularized tendon and/or bone graft. Alternately, vascularized fascia alone can be taken as free-flap or rotational soft tissue. The wide arc of rotation afforded by the long pedicle of the radial forearm flap allows easy circumferential soft-tissue coverage. Depending on the distance to the soft-tissue defect, it is possible to trace the radial artery and its venae comitantes proximally as far as the bifurcation of the brachial artery to maximize the arc of rotation. Thus, the radial forearm flap is indicated for any size soft-tissue defect about the elbow. Because it is possible to harvest vascularized bone and tendon with the radial forearm flap, this flap is uniquely suited for small bone defect and/or collateral ligament reconstruction in conjunction with soft-tissue coverage. Portions of the flexor carpi radialis, brachioradialis, and/or palmaris longus tendons may be included in the radial forearm flap and used for triceps tendon reconstruction or augmentation, or for vascularized medial or lateral ligament reconstruction. For bone reconstruction of the distal humerus or proximal forearm, bone may be harvested from the radial aspect of the radial metaphysis.

The flap is harvested from the volar surface of the forearm. The donor site location is determined by the size of the soft-tissue defect and the length of the pedicle required to rotate the radial forearm flap to the defect site. The radial artery and its fascial perforators supply the radial forearm flap, and use of this flap sacrifices the radial artery supply to the hand. In the proximal forearm, the radial artery lies proximally between the brachioradialis muscle and the pronator teres. Distally, the radial artery lies between the tendons of the brachioradialis and the flexor carpi radialis. The radial muscles of the forearm are supplied by numerous branches along the course of the radial artery. In addition, there are branches that perforate the fascia, which supply the antebrachial fascia and its overlying subcutaneous tissue and skin. The radial forearm flap is based on these perforating branches, which must be protected throughout the dissection. There are numerous perforating branches in the distal forearm; however, there are fewer perforating branches in the proximal forearm. Inadvertent injury to the perforators in the proximal forearm can result in loss of the proximal portion of the distal forearm flap. The venae comitantes of the radial artery provide venous outflow for the distal forearm flap. The cephalic vein may be included in the distal forearm flap; however, neither its course nor quality is predictable, and it is not critical for flap outflow. Donor site cosmesis is the main concern with the radial forearm flap; it is reported to be a substantial source of patient dissatisfaction, particularly in women. Functional outcomes data are mixed with respect to grip and pinch strength as well as loss of dorsiflexion at the wrist.

Suprafascial dissection of the radial forearm flap may decrease donor site morbidity. Injection studies have reported that the dominant subcutaneous vessels and their anastomosing vessels lie superficial to the fascia. Nevertheless, dissection in the subfascial plane is preferred because it may provide protection to the longitudinal vessels and protect the radial forearm flap from shear stresses.

Absolute contraindications for a radial forearm flap are incomplete or inadequate perfusion of the hand through the ulnar artery or previous injury to the radial artery. Hand circulation must be carefully evaluated preoperatively. An Allen test and/or Doppler ultrasonography should be performed. Radial forearm flaps are contraindicated in patients with an incomplete superficial arch or an absent ulnar artery. Relative contraindications include previous volar forearm surgery, history of peripheral vascular disease or other vascular disorders, and donor site cosmesis that would negatively affect a patient's self-image or profession. Patients should be counseled on the cosmetic appearance of the donor site, the potential for cold intolerance, and the low risk for vascular compromise of the hand. Patients also should be aware of the sensory deficits associated with harvesting a sensate flap.

Particular attention should be paid to certain steps in the surgical technique. Dissection is most commonly performed in the subfascial plane, staying superficial to the paratenon. Suprafascial harvest, which may minimize donor site morbidity, also can be performed. Dissection should begin on the ulnar side, continuing toward the radial artery. After encountering the radial artery, the intermuscular septum between the brachioradialis and flexor carpi radialis should be preserved. Next, dissection is performed toward the radial artery from radial to ulnar. Eversion of the medial edge of the brachioradialis allows for better visualization of the radial artery and its pedicles. The pedicle should not be kinked when rotating the radial forearm flap to cover the soft-tissue defect. Donor site cosmesis is better with a non-meshed STSG. If paratenon has been harvested with the flap, the surgeon should attempt to cover the tendon with adjacent muscle. If this is not possible, resection of noncritical portions of tendon should be considered.

## Distant Muscle Rotational Flap

### LATISSIMUS DORSI MUSCLE FLAP

The latissimus dorsi is a strong pennate muscle. It originates from the thoracodorsal fascia and inserts on the proximal medial humerus between the insertions of the pectoralis major and teres major. The muscle is innervated by the thoracodorsal nerve and is supplied by the thoracodorsal artery. The latissimus dorsi can be harvested as a muscle or musculocutaneous flap. The proximal location of the neurovascular pedicle allows for a wide arc of rotation for soft-tissue coverage of the head, neck, shoulder, arm, and elbow. For coverage about the elbow, anatomic and clinical studies have reported that the latissimus dorsi rotational flap can reach 6 to 8 cm distal to the olecranon. The latissimus dorsi rotational flap is particularly useful if a patient's zone of injury prevents the use of local tissue for soft-tissue coverage and for large soft-tissue defects. Because of its neurovascular supply, the

 

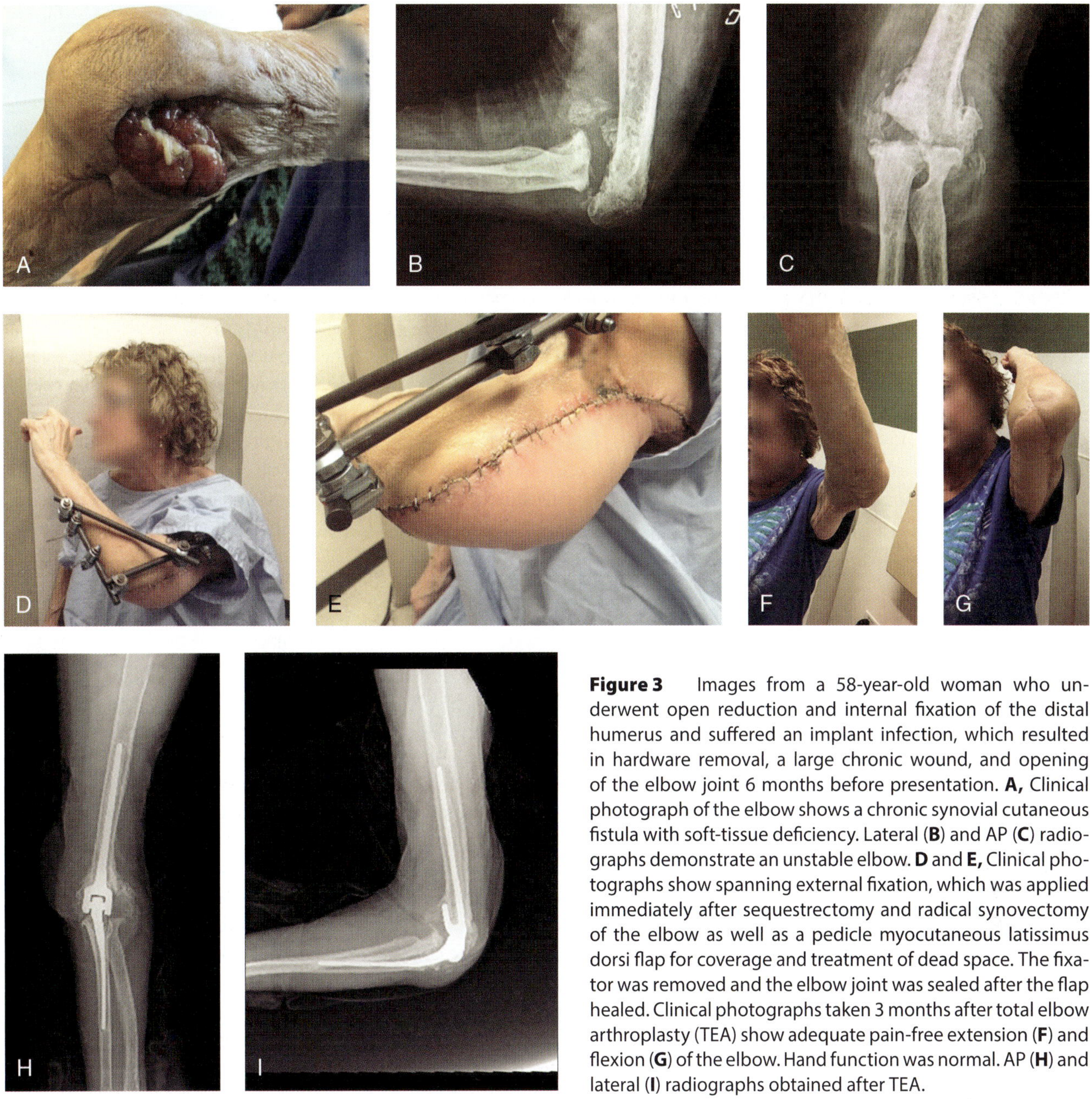


**Figure 3** Images from a 58-year-old woman who underwent open reduction and internal fixation of the distal humerus and suffered an implant infection, which resulted in hardware removal, a large chronic wound, and opening of the elbow joint 6 months before presentation. **A,** Clinical photograph of the elbow shows a chronic synovial cutaneous fistula with soft-tissue deficiency. Lateral (**B**) and AP (**C**) radiographs demonstrate an unstable elbow. **D** and **E,** Clinical photographs show spanning external fixation, which was applied immediately after sequestrectomy and radical synovectomy of the elbow as well as a pedicle myocutaneous latissimus dorsi flap for coverage and treatment of dead space. The fixator was removed and the elbow joint was sealed after the flap healed. Clinical photographs taken 3 months after total elbow arthroplasty (TEA) show adequate pain-free extension (**F**) and flexion (**G**) of the elbow. Hand function was normal. AP (**H**) and lateral (**I**) radiographs obtained after TEA.

latissimus dorsi can be rotated as a functional muscle transfer to restore biceps or triceps function independently or in combination with soft-tissue coverage. A latissimus dorsi rotational flap cannot be performed in patients who use crutches or a wheelchair. Paraplegia, severe lower extremity injuries, ipsilateral shoulder girdle weakness, previous surgery about the shoulder girdle, previous trauma to the subclavian or axillary artery, and tumor resection or lymph node dissection in the area of the thoracodorsal artery and nerve are contraindications to latissimus dorsi rotational flap. Relative contraindications include patients with a family history of breast cancer who may require future reconstruction (**Figure 3**).

Particular attention should be paid to certain steps in the surgical technique. The latissimus dorsi may be tightly adhered to the chest wall origin of the serratus anterior and/or to the scapular origin of the teres major. Electrical stimulation of the muscle fibers can help distinguish the latissimus dorsi from adjacent muscles. The humeral insertion of the latissimus dorsi is often conjoined with the teres major. Only the humeral insertion of the latissimus dorsi should be released and not the teres major. A portion (approximately 20%) of the latissimus dorsi insertion should be maintained on the humerus to prevent traction injury to the pedicle. Complete release of the humeral insertion of the latissimus dorsi allows for greater mobilization of the muscle. The fascia around the neurovascular pedicle should be released and the branches to the serratus as well as the more proximal perforators should be ligated to increase length and mobility of the pedicle. There should be no kinking of or tension on the pedicle at the time of insetting. The color of the vena comitantes is monitored during insetting. Darkening of the venous return suggests possible venous obstruction. The surgeon should check for kinking of the pedicle, which most commonly occurs at the axilla. The innervation to the latissimus dorsi should be preserved to limit some of the fibrotic changes that are seen in completely denervated flaps.

#### LATISSIMUS DORSI MUSCULOCUTANEOUS FLAP

In general, the authors of this chapter prefer to transfer the latissimus dorsi as a muscle flap rather than a musculocutaneous flap. A skin paddle for soft-tissue coverage of the elbow should be included in patients with a massive soft-tissue defect that requires more distal coverage or with a muscle that is to be used as a functional transfer. Muscle and tendon gliding is improved and muscle adhesion may be prevented with inclusion of a skin paddle in functional transfers.

During transposition, the authors of this chapter recommend not tunneling the latissimus dorsi below a subcutaneous bridge to prevent compression of the muscle and/or pedicle, which can result in myonecrosis. After the latissimus dorsi is completely inset, a Doppler ultrasonography probe is used to check the patency of the vessel with the elbow in full extension and 90° of flexion. Obliteration of a patient's pulse with the elbow in 90° of flexion indicates that the latissimus dorsi is stretched too far distally and should be re-inset. If these potential areas of vascular compromise are not recognized, partial or complete flap necrosis can occur. If the entire latissimus dorsi is used, the portion of the latissimus dorsi flap that closes to the origin may not be adequately perfused on the proximal pedicle. The portion of the latissimus dorsi flap that closes to the origin should be assessed after the latissimus dorsi is rotated; if perfusion is questionable, the portion of the latissimus dorsi flap that closes to the origin should be resected. A dressing is applied, and the arm is placed in 30° to 40° of shoulder abduction and 40° to 60° of elbow flexion. Such positioning reduces the likelihood that swelling about the axilla will cause compression of the vascular pedicle. Gentle passive range of motion may be initiated 1 week postoperatively. In patients in whom the latissimus dorsi is used for simultaneous soft-tissue coverage and functional reconstruction, the elbow should be immobilized for a minimum of 8 weeks postoperatively, after which a gentle remobilization program may begin.

Particular attention should be paid to certain steps in the surgical technique. A musculocutaneous latissimus dorsi flap can improve muscle tendon gliding in a functional transfer. The arm should be placed in full forward flexion and abduction when marking the resting length of the latissimus dorsi. Marking sutures are placed in the muscle belly of the latissimus dorsi at 5-cm intervals, beginning at the musculotendinous junction and working caudad (toward the origin). The humeral insertion should be released as close to bone as possible. Reconstruction of elbow flexion includes transfer of the latissimus dorsi insertion to the coracoid below the pectoralis major tendon, insertion of the latissimus dorsi origin into the residual stump of the biceps tendon, restoration of resting length with the elbow in full extension, and immobilization of the elbow in 90° of flexion. Reconstruction of elbow extension includes transfer of the latissimus dorsi insertion to the scapular spine, anchoring of the latissimus dorsi origin to the olecranon, restoration of resting length with the elbow in maximum flexion, and immobilization of the elbow in full extension.

## Bone Defects

There are unique patients who have both bone and soft-tissue deficiencies about the elbow. Vascularized bone flaps, such as the osteocutaneous fibular flap or the medial femoral condyle (MFC) flap, can be used to simultaneously reconstruct skeletal defects and provide coverage for deficient soft-tissue. The osteoseptocutaneous fibular flap has been a mainstay of treatment for patients who have multiple long bone defects. Use of the osteoseptocutaneous fibular flap in the humerus has been well described. The skin island can be large (up to 10 × 20 cm) based on perforating vessels from the peroneal artery to the overlying skin of the lateral compartment of the leg. The donor site usually requires closure with an STSG. Donor site morbidity includes scarring from the skin graft and occasional contracture of the flexor hallucis longus muscle. In patients who have suspected peripheral vascular disease, preoperative vascular studies can help ensure patency of the peroneal artery. Nonunion of the distal humerus, which often occurs as a result of hardware failure or infection, has been effectively managed with the osteoseptocutaneous fibular flap.

The MFC and overlying skin based on perforating vessels of the descending branch of the medial geniculate artery have been shown to augment bone healing in patients who have smaller bone defects or refractory supracondylar humeral nonunion (**Figure 4**). The MFC is a rich source of vascularized periosteum, cortical bone, and cancellous bone. The periosteum can be taken by itself and wrapped around areas of

 

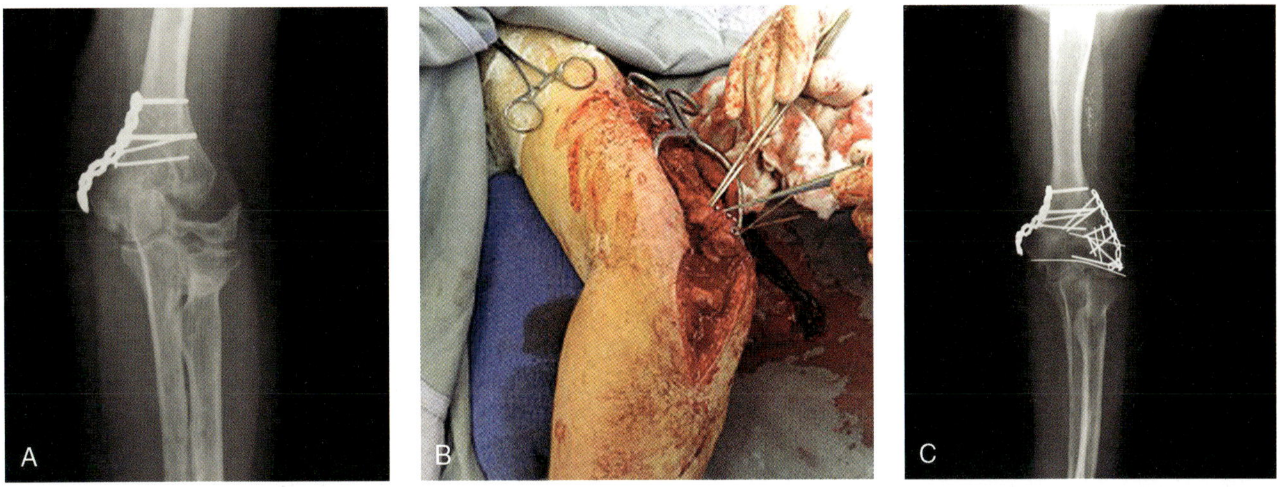


**Figure 4** Images of the elbow of a 47-year-old woman who underwent open reduction and internal fixation of the distal humerus. **A,** Preoperative AP radiograph demonstrates resorption of bone in the medial column with preservation of a small articular fragment. **B,** Intraoperative photograph shows anastomosis of the posterior radial collateral artery to the pedicle of the medial geniculate artery. The elbow was salvaged with a medial femoral condyle vascularized bone flap. The inflow vessel was the posterior radial collateral artery and vena comitantes. **C,** Postoperative AP radiograph obtained 6 months postoperatively demonstrates healing of the humerus.

nonunion to promote healing. The MFC flap is advantageous because it allows for customization of the soft-tissue and bone components, and donor site morbidity is minimal.

## Vascularized Composite Allotransplantation

The future of soft-tissue reconstruction about the elbow may include vascularized composite allotransplantation. Arm transplants, including elbow transplants, from deceased donors have been performed at several surgical centers around the world. Compared with prosthetic use, transfer of the elbow joint and the surrounding muscle and skin results in improved upper extremity function. Patients who undergo vascularized composite allotransplantation require lifelong immunosuppression, which is a complex risk/reward decision that patients and surgeons must make. In the future, it may be possible to procure elbow replacement parts, including bone, joint, and soft tissue, that are designed for a given need.

## Limiting Adverse Events

Hand ischemia is the most serious complication that may occur after soft-tissue coverage procedures for the elbow. Acute hand ischemia, although extremely rare, can occur with the use of the radial forearm flap; affected patients must undergo emergent arterial reconstruction. The next most serious complication of soft-tissue coverage procedures is loss of the flap, whether partial or complete. In the early recovery period, partial or complete loss of the flap results from arterial inflow or venous outflow problems. Later, partial or complete loss of the flap may result from infection. To reduce the risk for infection, necrotic and poorly vascularized tissue must be aggressively débrided, infected or contaminated wounds must be treated appropriately before soft-tissue coverage, and adequate antibiotic therapy must be administered. Seroma formation is not uncommon at large donor sites. The surgeon must select the procedure that offers optimal soft-tissue coverage, taking into account the cosmetic and functional losses related to the specific donor tissue.

Limitations of vascularized allotransplantation include the need to provide the patient with immunosuppression, which can increase the risk of infection and, in the long term, lead to compromised kidney function. Appropriate flap selection, careful attention to pedicle positioning, and close postoperative monitoring help reduce the risk for complications after any carefully performed soft-tissue coverage procedure that is appropriately sized to a particular defect.

## Bibliography

Choudry UH, Moran SL, Li S, Khan S: Soft-tissue coverage of the elbow: An outcome analysis and reconstructive algorithm. *Plast Reconstr Surg* 2007;119(6):1852-1857.

Coessens B, Vico P, De Mey A: Clinical experience with the reverse lateral arm flap in soft-tissue coverage of the elbow. *Plast Reconstr Surg* 1993;92(6):1133-1136.

Elhassan B, Karabekmez F, Hsu CC, Steinmann S, Moran S: Outcome of local anconeus flap transfer to cover soft tissue defects over the posterior aspect of the elbow. *J Shoulder Elbow Surg* 2011;20(5):807-812.

Fleager KE, Cheung EV: The "anconeus slide": Rotation flap for management of posterior wound complications about the elbow. *J Shoulder Elbow Surg* 2011;20(8):1310-1316.

Govila A, Sharma D: The radial forearm flap for reconstruction of the upper extremity. *Plast Reconstr Surg* 1990;86(5):920-927.

Harvey E, Aponte R, Levin L: Application of the island pedicle latissimus dorsi flap for soft tissue coverage of the elbow. *Can J Plast Surg* 1999;7:23-26.

Jones NF, Jarrahy R, Kaufman MR: Pedicled and free radial forearm flaps for reconstruction of the elbow, wrist, and hand. *Plast Reconstr Surg* 2008;121(3):887-898.

Jutte DL, Rees R, Nanney L, Bueno R, Lynch JB: Latissimus dorsi flap: A valuable resource in lower arm reconstruction. *South Med J* 1987;80(1):37-40.

Lalikos JF, Fudem GM: Brachioradialis musculocutaneous flap closure of the elbow utilizing a distal skin island: A case report. *Ann Plast Surg* 1997;39(2):201-204.

Mordick TG II, Britton EN, Brantigan C: Pedicled latissimus dorsi transfer for immediate soft-tissue coverage and elbow flexion. *Plast Reconstr Surg* 1997;99(6):1742-1744.

Orgill DP, Pribaz JJ, Morris DJ: Local fasciocutaneous flaps for olecranon coverage. *Ann Plast Surg* 1994;32(1):27-31.

Rohrich RJ, Ingram AE Jr: Brachioradialis muscle flap: Clinical anatomy and use in soft-tissue reconstruction of the elbow. *Ann Plast Surg* 1995;35(1):70-76.

Schmidt CC, Kohut GN, Greenberg JA, Kann SE, Idler RS, Kiefhaber TR: The anconeus muscle flap: Its anatomy and clinical application. *J Hand Surg Am* 1999;24(2):359-369.

Sharpe F, Barry P, Lin SD, Stevanovic M: Anatomic study of the flexor carpi ulnaris muscle and its application to soft tissue coverage of the elbow with clinical correlation. *J Shoulder Elbow Surg* 2014;23(1):82-90.

Stevanovic M, Sharpe F: Soft-tissue coverage of the elbow. *Plast Reconstr Surg* 2013;132(3):387e-402e.

Stevanovic M, Sharpe F, Thommen VD, Itamura JM, Schnall SB: Latissimus dorsi pedicle flap for coverage of soft tissue defects about the elbow. *J Shoulder Elbow Surg* 1999;8(6):634-643.

 

Tizian C, Sanner F, Berger A: The proximally pedicled arteria radialis forearm flap in the treatment of soft tissue defects of the dorsal elbow. *Ann Plast Surg* 1991;26(1):40-44.

Wysocki RW, Gray RL, Fernandez JJ, Cohen MS: Posterior elbow coverage using whole and split flexor carpi ulnaris flaps: A cadaveric study. *J Hand Surg Am* 2008;33(10):1807-1812.

# Chapter 24

# Open Capsular Release to Manage Elbow Contracture

*Mark S. Cohen, MD*

**Learning Objectives**

- Understand the etiology of elbow stiffness.
- Appreciate the nonsurgical measures that can be used to successfully manage posttraumatic stiffness of the elbow.
- Understand the anatomy and surgical principles and techniques used to manage the stiff elbow.

## Indications

Several anatomic factors make the elbow prone to stiffness after traumatic injury, including the congruity of the joint, the presence of three articulations in a synovium-lined cavity, and the close relationship of the joint capsule and intracapsular ligaments to the surrounding muscles. After even relatively minor trauma, the joint capsule can thicken and become noncompliant. Prolonged immobilization after trauma is a risk factor for stiffness.

Patients are candidates for contracture release if they have a flexion contracture of at least 25° to 30°, flexion of less than 110° to 115°, or a combination of the two findings. It is helpful for patients to continue with a course of stretching exercises (with or without supervision by a therapist and with or without static progressive splinting) until they can perform the exercises confidently and effectively and have done so for many months. Additional requirements for a simple release of the stiff elbow include adequate soft tissue to ensure good coverage of the surgical site and a congruous elbow with an adequate ulnohumeral joint space, at least centrally. Joint congruency usually can be determined radiographically. However, CT may be helpful, especially in the posttraumatic setting. Imaging (including three-dimensional CT) can facilitate preoperative planning. To allow for resolution of posttraumatic inflammation, surgery should be delayed until at least 3 to 4 months after the injury. Patients can continue to improve for many months after trauma, and it is best to delay surgery until recovery of motion plateaus.

## Contraindications

Surgery for elbow stiffness is contraindicated in a patient who is deemed unable or unwilling to stretch the elbow after surgery. This is especially true in adolescents, who may not be dedicated to improving their elbow motion. An incongruous ulnohumeral joint is a contraindication because a simple release of the joint may not improve motion and might worsen pain. In fact, although pain at the extremes of motion is common in patients who are candidates for simple surgical release, the elbow typically is not very painful within the allowable arc of motion. In this setting, the surgeon should evaluate for other causes of pain, such as ulnar nerve dysfunction, more advanced arthritis within the joint, or stress or ineffective coping strategies (such as catastrophic thinking or reactive depression). Patient selection for this procedure is not influenced by the severity of the contracture, the number of previous surgical procedures, or the presence of minor heterotopic ossification.

## Alternative Treatments

Alternative measures to improve elbow stiffness include nonsurgical modalities to decrease joint swelling and inflammation and to relax or stretch contracted soft tissues. To manage protracted swelling, compression sleeves, ice, elevation, active motion (including the forearm, wrist, and hand), and oral agents such as NSAIDs may be useful. A short-term tapered course of oral prednisone can be effective in difficult cases. In addition,

*Dr. Cohen or an immediate family member has received royalties from Integra LifeSciences and serves as a paid consultant to Acumed and Integra LifeSciences.*

an intra-articular cortisone injection to decrease inflammation and joint synovitis may be useful.

Historically, dynamic splints were used that applied constant tension to the soft tissues over long periods (for example, 23 hours per day). In the management of elbow contracture, however, patient-adjusted static braces may be more effective (**Figure 1**). The use of a static progressive elbow brace enables passive progressive stretching of the contracted elbow capsule and muscles. The static braces are applied for much shorter periods and are preferred by many patients.

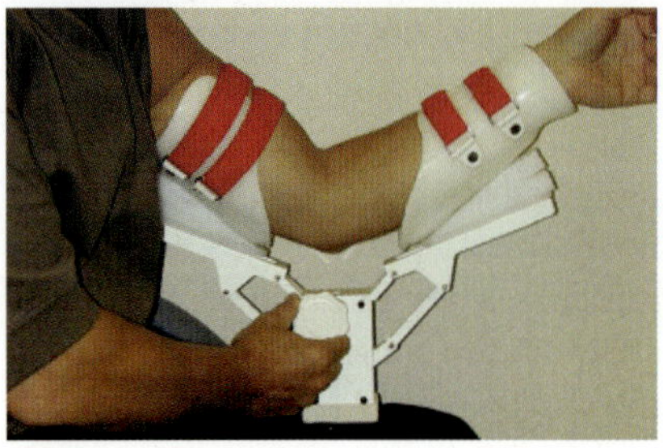

**Figure 1** Clinical photograph shows a patient-adjusted static elbow brace used in the nonsurgical management of soft-tissue contracture of the elbow. (Copyright Mark S. Cohen, MD, Chicago, IL.)

## Results

In carefully selected patients, release of the contracted elbow leads to reliable and satisfactory outcomes (**Table 1**). In one study, motion and pain improved in all 22 patients treated for posttraumatic elbow stiffness by means of a soft-tissue release of the elbow through a lateral approach. The three instances of transient ulnar sensory neuropathy and one instance of median sensory neuropathy resolved over several months. In a study in which 38 elbows in 37 patients were managed surgically for joint stiffness using a similar lateral approach, 33 patients had substantial improvement in motion and pain. Two patients had hematomas, and two had transient ulnar paresthesia that resolved spontaneously.

## Techniques

To improve elbow flexion, posterior soft-tissue tethers are released. The posterior joint capsule is divided or resected, and adhesions of the triceps muscle and tendon are released from the humerus. In addition, anterior bony or soft-tissue impingement is removed, including osteophytes off the coronoid process and any bony or soft-tissue overgrowth in the coronoid and radial fossae (**Figure 2, A**). For full flexion to occur, there must be a concavity above the humeral trochlea and capitellum to accept the coronoid centrally and the radial head laterally. To improve elbow extension, posterior impingement between osteophytes off the olecranon tip and bone overgrowth in the olecranon fossa are removed. Anteriorly, the anterior joint capsule is excised, and any adhesions between the brachialis and the humerus are released (**Figure 2, B**).

### Setup/Exposure

- The author of this chapter prefers to use regional anesthesia with a long-acting brachial plexus block, in part because it allows for postoperative muscular relaxation and pain control. An indwelling catheter is favored by some surgeons.

### Procedure

- The stiff elbow can be released by using a medial or lateral approach. Advantages of the lateral exposure

**Table 1** Results of Open Capsular Release for Soft-Tissue Contracture of the Elbow

| Authors (Year) | No. of Patients (Elbows) | Procedure or Approach | Mean Patient Age in Years (Range) | Mean Follow-up in Months (Range) | Results |
|---|---|---|---|---|---|
| Cohen and Hastings (1998) | 22 (22) | Lateral collateral ligament sparing | 35 (15-72) | 29 (15-73) | Mean ulnohumeral joint motion improved from 74° to 129°<br>Mean forearm rotation improved from 135° to 159°<br>Pain and function improved significantly ($P < 0.001$)<br>Transient ulnar sensory neuropathy in 3 patients<br>Median sensory neuropathy in 1 patient |
| Mansat and Morrey (1998) | 37 (38) | Column procedure | 41 (5-68) | 43 (24-74) | Mean ulnohumeral joint motion improved from 49° to 94°<br>82% satisfactory<br>89% improved at latest follow-up<br>11% had 24° loss of motion compared with preoperative measurement<br>Hematoma in 2 patients<br>Transient ulnar paresthesia in 2 patients |

 

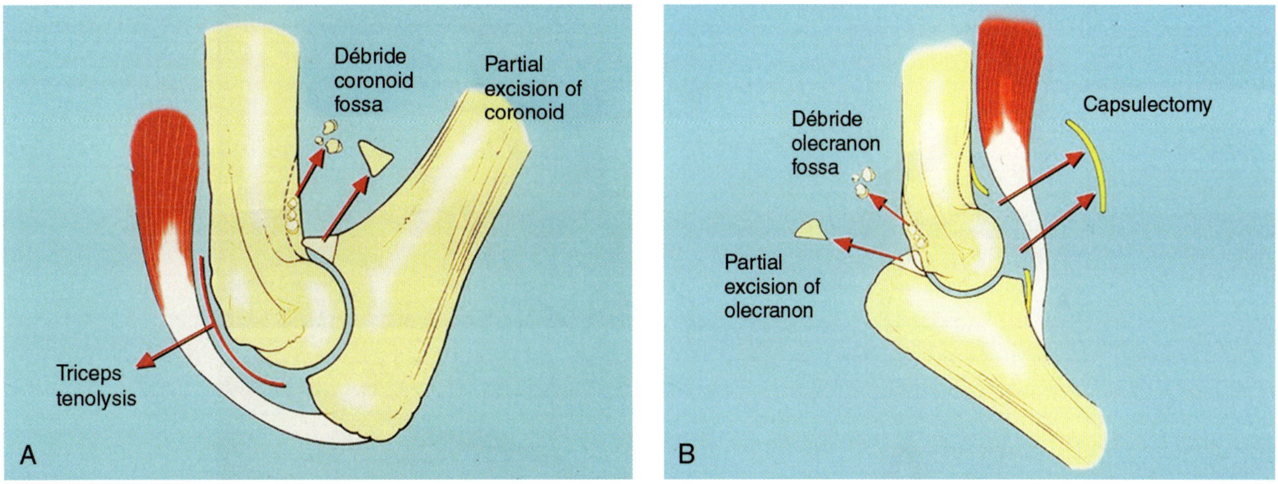


**Figure 2** Illustrations depict the surgical principles involved in improving flexion and extension in the stiff elbow. **A,** To improve elbow flexion, posterior soft-tissue tethers, including the joint capsule and triceps, are released, and anterior impingement is removed between the coronoid and coronoid fossa of the humerus. As shown here, there must also be a concavity above the capitellum laterally to accept the radial head (radial fossa). **B,** To improve elbow extension, posterior impingement is removed at the olecranon tip, and the anterior capsule and brachialis are released. (Courtesy of Hill Hastings II, MD, Telluride, CO.)

include its simplicity, use of an internervous subcutaneous plane, the potential for reduced muscle damage, and access to all three elbow articulations (ulnohumeral, radiocapitellar, and proximal radioulnar). The main disadvantage of the lateral exposure is that it does not allow access to the ulnar nerve.

- A medial approach can be used instead of or in addition to the lateral approach. Advantages of the medial approach include the ability to decompress the ulnar nerve, esthetics (a medial scar is less conspicuous than a lateral scar), and the ability to release the posteromedial ulnohumeral joint capsule, which some surgeons think might assist regaining flexion in the setting of severe stiffness. The main disadvantage of the medial approach is that it does not allow the surgeon to address lateral joint pathology, namely, the radiocapitellar joint.
- Patients with ulnar neuropathy and lateral intra-articular pathology (or other similar combinations) might benefit from a combined medial and lateral release.

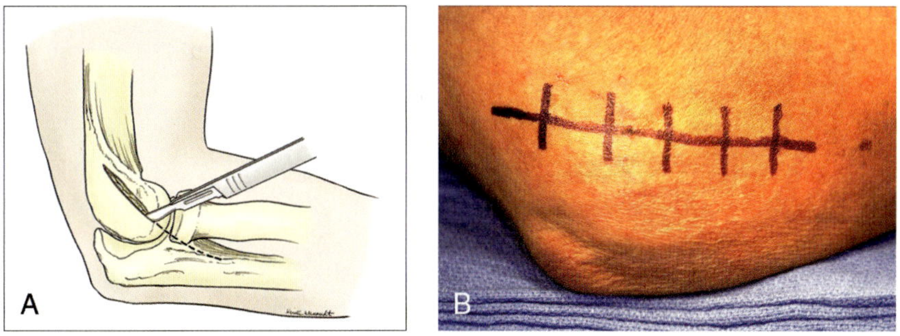


**Figure 3** Illustration (**A**) and intraoperative photograph (**B**) show the skin incision typically used for the lateral deep approach. The incision begins along the supracondylar ridge of the humerus, courses approximately over the epicondyle, and continues down toward the ulna. (Copyright Mark S. Cohen, MD, Chicago, IL.)

- A long posterior skin incision that allows access both medially and laterally is favored by some surgeons; however, this does increase the risk of postoperative seroma formation.
- Scars from previous skin incisions must be considered in preoperative planning.
- The type of skin incision used is less important than is the deep approach chosen for joint release.

**LATERAL APPROACH**

- After a sterile tourniquet is applied to the upper arm and inflated, the skin incision is begun along the supracondylar ridge of the humerus, passing at or just anterior to the epicondyle and down toward the ulna (**Figure 3**).
- For the posterior exposure, the proximal anconeus is reflected posteriorly and dissection is carried proximally beneath the humeral epicondyle and along the supracondylar ridge of the humerus, reflecting the anconeus and the triceps posteriorly.
- A triceps tenolysis is performed with an elevator to release adhesions

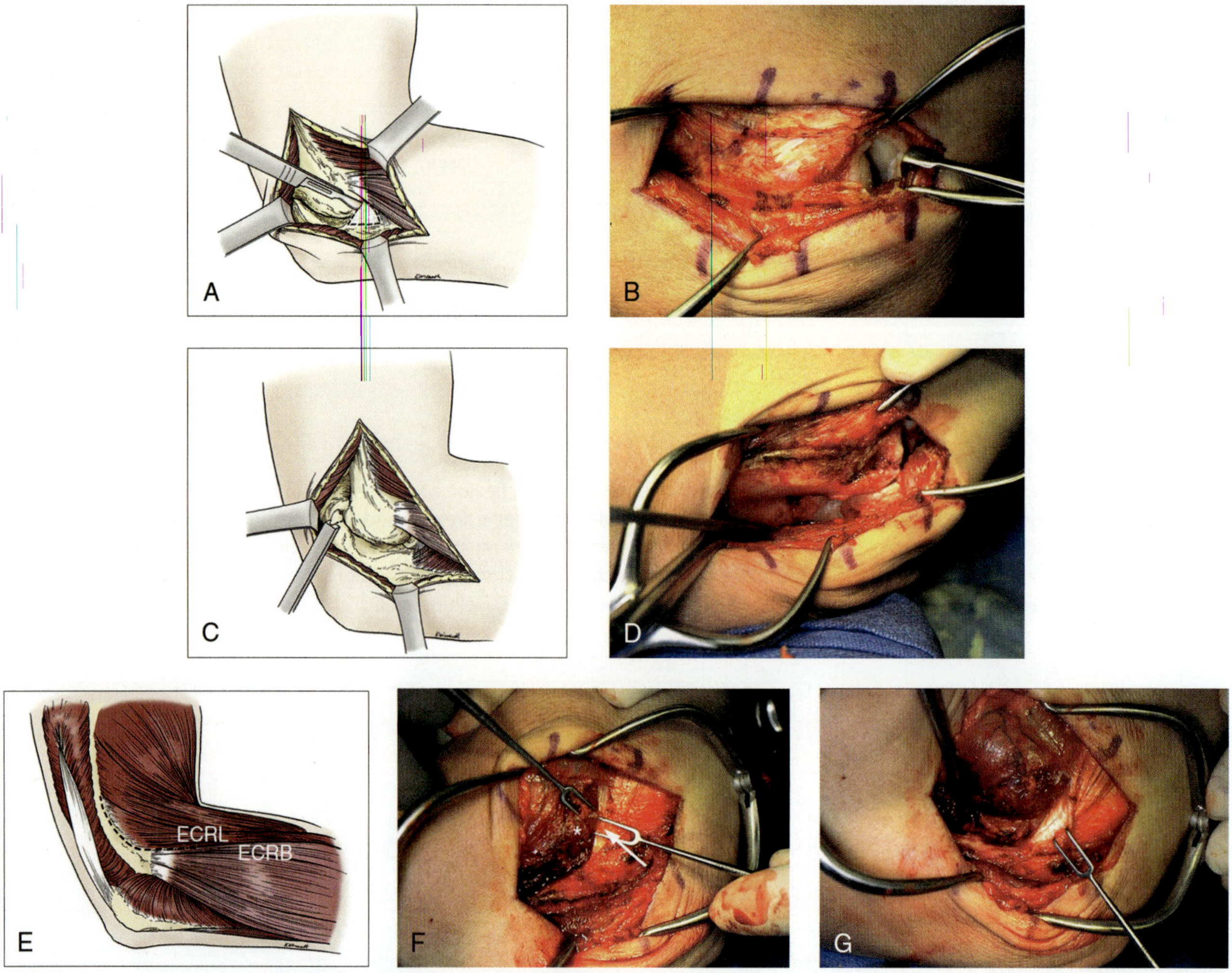


**Figure 4** Images depict steps in the deep lateral approach to release of elbow contracture, from initial exposure through the point of reaching the level of the anterior joint through the muscular extensor carpi radialis longus (ECRL) anteriorly and the fascia-covered extensor carpi radialis brevis (ECRB) posteriorly. Illustration (**A**) and intraoperative photograph (**B**) show the exposure of the lateral gutter and the posterior radiocapitellar joint. Deep to the anconeus/extensor carpi ulnaris interval, the posterolateral soft-spot capsule can be excised up to the proximal margin of the radial head without violating the lateral collateral ligament complex. The posterior capitellum and the radial head are exposed. Illustration (**C**) and intraoperative photograph (**D**) depict the exposure of the lateral and posterior ulnohumeral joint. The anconeus and triceps are reflected posteriorly, exposing the posterior capsule, olecranon tip, and olecranon fossa, to allow visualization and débridement of the posterior joint to remove any bony impingement. Illustration (**E**) and intraoperative photograph (**F**) depicting the lateral collateral ligament–sparing approach to the anterior joint through the muscular ECRL anteriorly (asterisk) and the fascia-covered ECRB posteriorly (arrow). **G,** Intraoperative photograph shows how the deep approach through this interval courses from anterolateral to posteromedial as the ECRL is swept off the undersurface of the ECRB tendon.

between the muscle and the posterior humerus.

- The posterior aspect of the radiocapitellar joint (including the lateral gutter) can be inspected by excising the elbow capsule just proximal to the conjoined lateral collateral and annular ligament complex through the so-called soft spot of the lateral elbow (**Figure 4, A** and **B**). The proximal edge of this complex lies along the proximal border of the radial head; thus, the capsule can be safely excised proximal to the radial head without compromising lateral elbow stability. Loose bodies and proliferative synovitis are often found in this sulcus.
- The anconeus is reflected posteriorly until the ulnohumeral joint is identified (**Figure 4, C** and **D**). Any lateral osteophytes are resected.
- Posteriorly, the olecranon fossa is cleared of its fat pad and any fibrous tissue or scarring that might inhibit terminal extension. A burr can be helpful for débridement of the olecranon fossa.
- If there is evidence of overgrowth or impingement of the tip of the

 

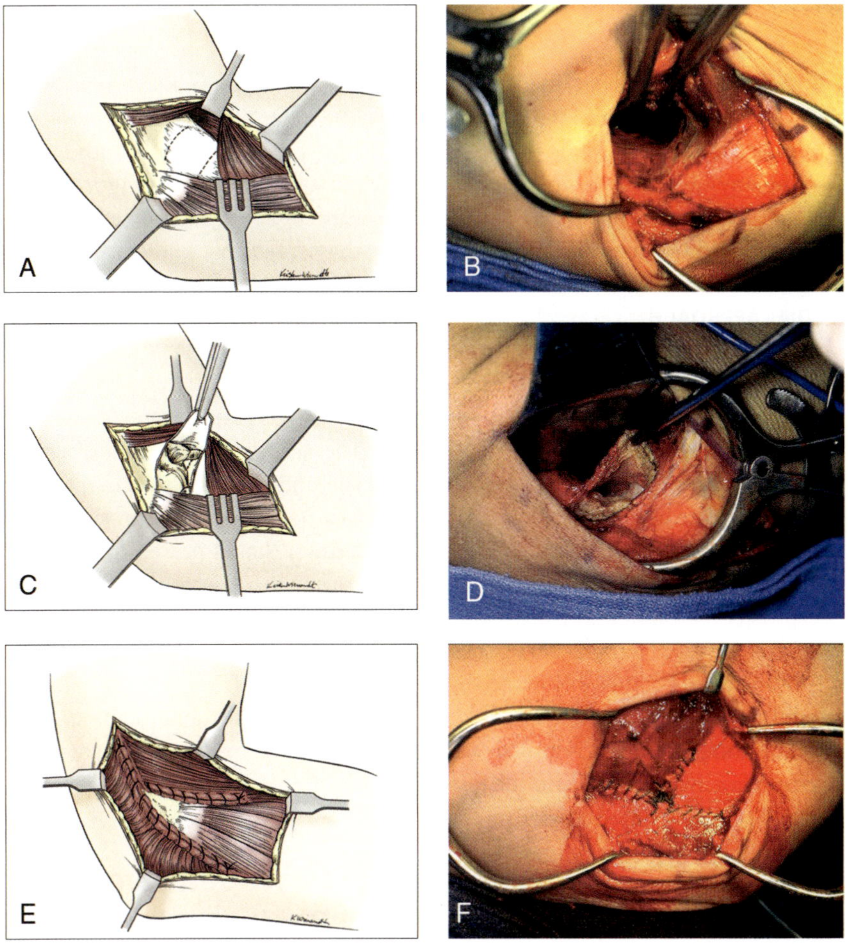


**Figure 5** Images depict steps in the deep lateral approach to release of elbow contracture, beginning with exposure of the anterior elbow capsule by elevation and retraction of the extensor carpi radialis longus and brachialis (**A** and **B**) to achieve visualization of the capsule extending to the medial joint with all muscle reflected anteriorly. Illustration (**C**) and intraoperative photograph (**D**) show the isolation of the anterior joint capsule, which is thickened and adherent to the anterior humerus and the joint. The capsule was excised by removing a thick strip from lateral to medial to expose the joint proper. Débridement was then performed. Illustration (**E**) and intraoperative photograph (**F**) depict the closure of the lateral deep approach. The Y-shaped split in the lateral fascia is closed over a drain. (Copyright Mark S. Cohen, MD, Chicago, IL.)

olecranon, a large retractor is used to reflect the triceps, and the tip of the olecranon proximal to the triceps insertion is removed with an osteotome. Care is taken not to plunge medially because the ulnar nerve lies adjacent to the medial border of the olecranon. A burr can be used as well to sculpt the olecranon tip.

- Any osteophytes or bony overgrowth behind the capitellum that might limit recovery of elbow extension are removed. This completes the posterior débridement and release.
- Dissection is carried anteriorly along the anterior supracondylar ridge of the humerus. Proximally, the brachialis is reflected anteriorly, exposing the anterior humerus.
- As was done posteriorly, tenolysis is performed anteriorly, using an elevator to release any adhesions between the brachialis muscle and the bone.
- Distally, dissection is continued in a muscle-splitting fashion between the extensor carpi radialis longus (ECRL) and the extensor carpi radialis brevis (ECRB) (**Figure 4, E** through **G**). This interval can be identified by noting that a thin white fascia covers the ECRB, whereas the ECRL lies more anteriorly and is predominantly muscular at this level. Sliding from proximal to distal along the anterior slope of the lateral humeral column helps define the distal plane for the extensor tendon split. The plane between the ECRL and the ECRB is not perpendicular to the wound but courses from the anterolateral to the posteromedial aspect down to the joint capsule. In this way, the ECRL is reflected off the undersurface of the ECRB tendon.
- It is often easiest to elevate the brachialis and ECRL off the humeral ridge and anterior joint capsule with a blunt scissors. This ensures an extracapsular reflection of the muscles anteriorly.
- Dissection is continued to expose the entire anterior joint capsule (**Figure 5, A** and **B**). This allows for a collateral ligament–preserving approach that avoids disturbing the more posterior extensor tendon origins (ECRB, extensor digitorum communis, and extensor carpi ulnaris) and the underlying lateral collateral ligament complex at the humeral epicondyle.
- After the capsule is exposed, dissection is performed sharply along the anterolateral humerus, releasing its lateral origin.
- The capsule is elevated and defined between the joint and the brachialis. The capsule is typically thickened and often adherent to the underlying humerus, especially in posttraumatic cases.

- A capsulectomy is performed, excising a thick strip of capsule to the medial joint to expose the radiocapitellar and ulnohumeral joints anteriorly (**Figure 5, C** and **D**).
- The radial and coronoid fossae are cleared of any fibrous tissue, the tip of the coronoid is removed if impingement exists in flexion, and any loose bodies are removed. A burr can be used to remove bony overgrowth within the coronoid and radial fossae that would limit terminal flexion of the elbow.
- If forearm rotation is limited, the radiocapitellar and proximal radioulnar joints are inspected. Occasionally, spurs can be resected at the radioulnar articulation. Adhesions between the radial head and the overlying annular ligament anteriorly can be released as well.
- After complete anterior and posterior capsular release and débridement, the elbow is extended by applying firm pressure to the forearm under direct visualization. This normally brings the joint out to almost full extension. Flexion is obtained by careful manipulation as well. In patients with long-standing contracture, the brachialis and/or triceps muscles may be tight, inhibiting full terminal elbow extension or flexion. This myostatic contracture can be stretched for several minutes during the procedure and must be overcome with stretching after surgery.
- Tendon lengthening is not required or helpful.
- Optimally, motion is limited only by muscular contracture with soft end points. In severe cases, contracture of the posteromedial joint capsule (that is, the posterior bundle of the medial collateral ligament) may limit recovery of elbow flexion. A separate medial approach, described later, may be necessary to transpose the ulnar nerve and release this joint capsule.
- Typically, the tourniquet is deflated and hemostasis is obtained.
- The lateral Y-shaped fascial split is closed over a drain without imparting any instability to the joint because the lateral ligament has been preserved (**Figure 5, E** and **F**).

#### MEDIAL APPROACH

- A deep medial approach that is analogous to the ligament-sparing lateral approach is typically performed through a medial or posterior incision along with exposure of the entire flexor-pronator muscle origins (**Figure 6, A** and **B**).
- Care must be taken to identify and protect the branches of the medial antebrachial cutaneous nerve; these branches are commonly found distal to the epicondyle.
- The ulnar nerve is released well proximally and distally to the joint and retracted anteriorly for protection (**Figure 6, C**).
- The triceps is elevated posteriorly off the intermuscular septum and the humerus, exposing the medial and posterior ulnohumeral joint.
- The posterior joint is released and débrided as described previously for the lateral approach.
- The posteromedial joint capsule can be sharply incised as well.
- Dissection continues along the supracondylar ridge of the humerus and distally through approximately the posterior one-third of the flexor-pronator muscle origin (**Figure 6, D**). This approach protects the anterior band of the medial collateral ligament, which lies beneath the flexor carpi ulnaris humeral head (analogous to the lateral ligament–sparing approach).
- The flexor-pronator and brachialis muscles are reflected anteriorly, exposing the anterior joint capsule.
- The capsule is released and excised, allowing visualization and débridement of the anterior joint, including the coronoid and radial fossae (**Figure 6, E**).
- The ulnar nerve is most commonly transposed anteriorly into a subcutaneous position (**Figure 6, F**). Care must be taken to ensure that the nerve is not kinked proximally or distally.
- The intermuscular septum is typically resected.

### Wound Closure

- The deep fascia, subcutaneous tissue, and skin are closed in the usual manner. The author prefers to use a drain that is passed through the triceps posteriorly.
- A soft-tissue compressive dressing is applied to the upper extremity.
- The anterior dressing and padding over the antecubital fossa may be removed to permit adequate elbow flexion postoperatively.

## Postoperative Regimen

Although several rehabilitation programs may be effective, the author of this chapter thinks continuous passive motion that is begun immediately in the recovery room and used until the following morning helps maintain the motion gained at surgery. The day after surgery, the dressing and drain are removed; a physical or occupational therapist teaches and provides coaching for the patient in active, self-assisted stretching exercises; and the arm is fitted with a compression sleeve or elastic bandage in an attempt to limit swelling. Active and gentle passive elbow motion is combined with intermittent continuous passive motion. Many protocols exist, but the author typically prescribes continuous passive motion twice per day for approximately 30 minutes each time. To help maintain extension, weighted passive stretches using a 2-lb wrist weight

 

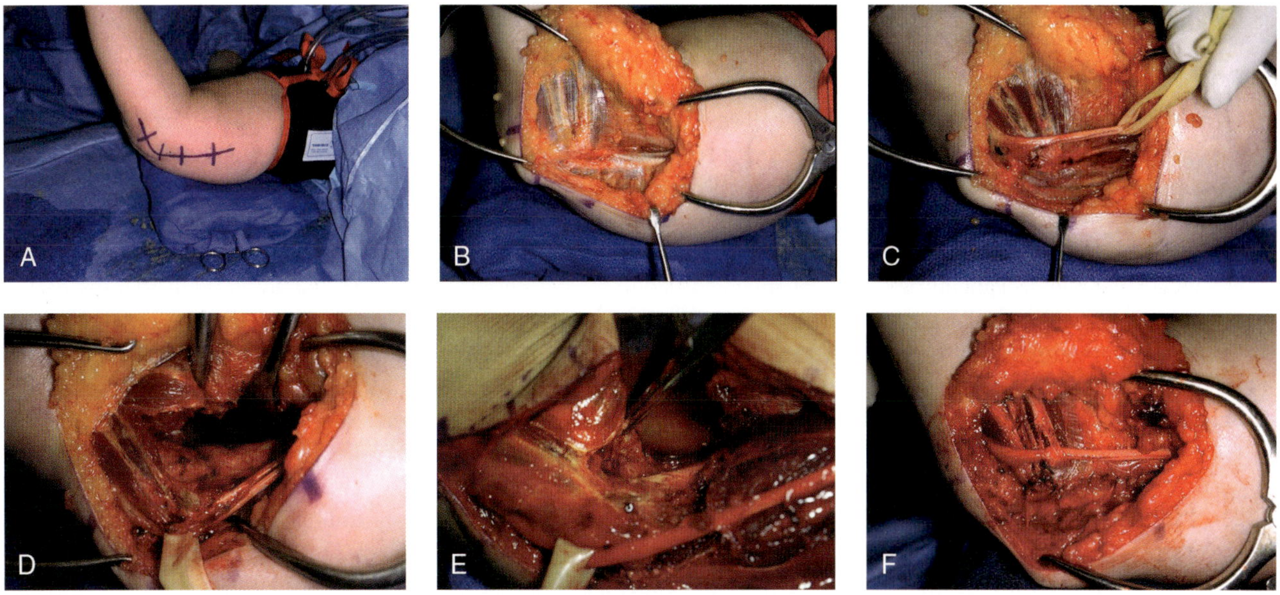


**Figure 6** Intraoperative photographs show the deep medial approach to the elbow. **A,** The medial incision typically used for the deep medial approach for release of the stiff elbow is marked. **B,** The skin and subcutaneous tissue are reflected, revealing the view of the entire flexor-pronator origin, medial triceps, and brachialis fascia. **C,** The ulnar nerve is decompressed and retracted anteriorly to allow for posterior joint exposure. The triceps is easily elevated off of the intermuscular septum and reflected posteriorly to reveal the posterior ulnohumeral joint. The posteromedial joint capsule is released under direct visualization. **D,** The entire anterior joint capsule is exposed by elevation of the brachialis and the anterior flexor-pronator muscular origins from the humeral epicondyle. **E,** The anterior capsule is dissected from medial to lateral off the humerus. The capsule is excised, allowing visualization and débridement of the anterior joint. **F,** Closure of the medial soft tissues is shown. The flexor-pronator release is repaired, as is the triceps to the brachialis fascia. Note the anterior transposition of the ulnar nerve, held here by a strip of fascia. (Copyright Mark S. Cohen, MD, Chicago, IL.)

with the arm extended over a bolster are performed for 10 to 15 minutes several times per day.

Static progressive elbow bracing is also begun immediately after surgery. The brace is worn for approximately 30 minutes, two or three times per day. Flexion and extension are alternated, based on the preoperative deficit and progress. An NSAID is commonly prescribed as prophylaxis against heterotopic ossification for several weeks postoperatively. In the opinion of the author of this chapter, NSAID prophylaxis can also help limit inflammation of the joint and soft tissues during rehabilitation.

Patients are typically discharged home on postoperative day 1 with instructions to perform exercises several times per day thereafter, including active, self-assisted stretches; continuous passive motion; weighted stretches; and patient-adjusted bracing. Formal outpatient therapy is helpful to provide patients with guidance and monitor their progress. Continuous passive motion is typically discontinued 3 to 4 weeks after surgery, but bracing is continued for several months according to the patient's preferences.

## Limiting Adverse Events

Ulnar neuropathy is the most common complication after surgical release of elbow contracture. Occasionally, ulnar neuropathy caused by compression contributes to posttraumatic limitation of elbow flexion, which places the nerve under tension and compression. Symptoms of ulnar neuropathy may include tingling and numbness in the ulnar digits, intrinsic muscle weakness, and medial joint pain in flexion. The author of this chapter recommends that the ulnar nerve be released in patients who present with signs of neuropathy preoperatively or with signs of nerve irritability such as a positive Tinel sign or a positive result of an elbow flexion test. Ulnar nerve decompression is also considered when release is performed for a substantial elbow extension contracture because the marked increase in flexion may reveal or precipitate nerve compression. Although a precise criterion has yet to be determined, it is often recommended that ulnar nerve release be considered in patients with preoperative elbow flexion of less than approximately 90° to 105°. Over time, the threshold of the author of this chapter to decompress the ulnar nerve during surgery to manage elbow stiffness has lowered. In patients in whom a lateral approach is chosen, the author of this chapter might add a limited medial exposure and in situ ulnar nerve decompression in most cases.

Careful patient selection and education is essential because gains made in surgery may be lost if the patient does not adhere to the extensive postoperative rehabilitation program required after elbow capsular release. Patients must therefore be motivated and understand the commitment required after surgery. It can take 1 year or longer for patients to stretch their elbows as well as possible.

## Heterotopic Ossification

The elbow is uniquely predisposed to heterotopic ossification, and heterotopic bone can be an independent factor leading to joint stiffness. Heterotopic ossification should not be confused with periarticular calcification, in which amorphous calcium deposits form most often in the capsule or collateral ligaments after injury. Periarticular calcification is common and of minimal clinical significance.

Heterotopic ossification of the elbow occurs most commonly after direct joint trauma and seems, in part, to be related to the severity of the injury. It is reported in approximately 3% of simple elbow dislocations and in up to 20% of fracture-dislocations. Heterotopic ossification is next most often seen in neural axis trauma, occurring below the level of spinal cord injuries. It also forms in 5% to 10% of patients with isolated closed head trauma, most commonly on the side of involvement in patients with hemiplegia. The individuals at greatest risk are those with combined head injury and elbow trauma, in whom heterotopic ossification develops at a rate of 75% to 90%. In addition, heterotopic bone occurs in the elbow in 1% to 3% of burn patients; it is related to the degree and severity of the burn, not to the location in the upper extremity.

Historically, heterotopic ossification was attributed to vigorous passive motion of the elbow performed in therapy. Although this relationship is not scientifically proved and is no longer believed to be clinically relevant, forceful and repeated manipulation of the stiff elbow should probably be avoided because this mechanism has led to the development of heterotopic bone in experimental models. In addition, a 2- to 3-day delay in surgical intervention after elbow trauma was traditionally thought to be an independent risk factor for heterotopic ossification. This association with surgical delay is not scientifically supported. However, multiple surgical insults in the first 7 to 14 days after trauma seems to be associated with a higher risk of the development of ectopic bone.

After the process of heterotopic ossification begins, there is no effective medical management. Thus, prophylaxis is essential in high-risk patients. Whereas diphosphonates only delay bone mineralization, NSAIDs are effective if administration begins within approximately 3 to 5 days of the inciting event. Indomethacin, ibuprofen, naproxen, and plain aspirin have all been shown to be beneficial for this purpose in patients who have undergone hip surgery. These agents disrupt the prostaglandin pathway and experimentally inhibit the migration and differentiation of stem cells that are required for ectopic bone formation. The optimal duration of treatment is unknown; the courses reported to be effective range from 5 days to 6 weeks.

The standard management for heterotopic bone prophylaxis is low-dose external beam radiation, which is thought to be effective because it inhibits the differentiation of stem cells, which are particularly radiosensitive. This radiation can be given as a single dose of 600 to 700 cGy with limited field technique decreasing soft-tissue exposure. As with oral medication, radiation should be administered within 2 to 4 days of injury to be effective. Radiation-induced sarcoma has not been reported with doses lower than 3,000 cGy.

An additional prophylactic modality is early active mobilization of the elbow after an inciting event. Clinical experience supports this benefit, although the mechanism is not entirely clear. Instituting active joint therapy earlier seems to lessen the likelihood of ectopic ossification and allows for a more rapid functional recovery after trauma. It is uncertain whether the same benefit is provided by passive joint mobilization.

Clinically, heterotopic ossification presents as local soft-tissue swelling, tenderness, warmth, and progressive loss of elbow motion. This is an inflammatory-mediated condition not uncommonly mistaken for infection, especially in the perioperative period. Pain is not usually the predominant symptom but is observed at the extremes of motion. Although the actual process begins at the time of the initial insult, it can manifest at any time between 2 and 12 weeks thereafter. Although laboratory studies and technetium Tc-99m bone scanning were historically used in the evaluation and treatment of heterotopic ossification about the elbow, use of both methods has been discontinued because neither has been shown to provide prognostic information.

Radiography is the most effective method for evaluating heterotopic ossification and monitoring its progression. Within several weeks of the initial trauma, a fluffy, ill-defined periarticular density can be identified radiographically (**Figure 7**). In time, the margins become more distinct with trabeculation. Radiographic maturity, defined as the ability to identify sharp cortical margins, commonly takes 3 to 5 months, at which point surgical intervention can safely proceed. In children, it may be prudent to wait longer because nonbridging heterotopic bone may resorb over time in skeletally immature individuals.

 

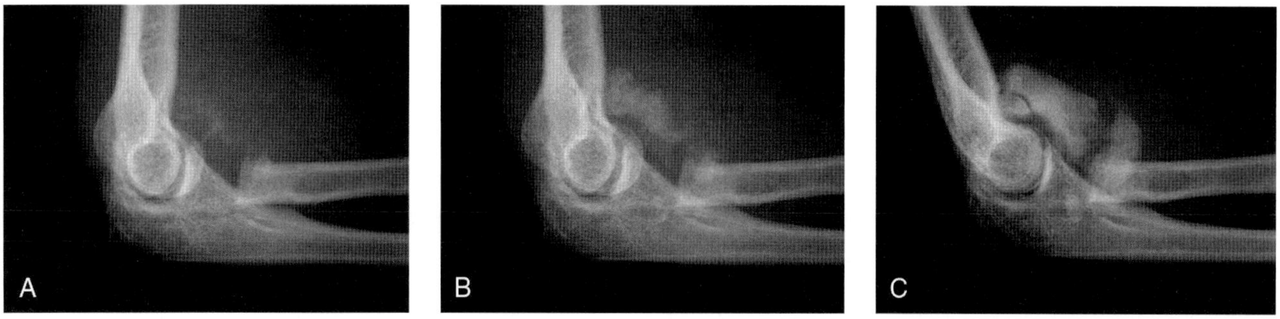


**Figure 7** Radiographs of a right elbow. **A,** Lateral view obtained 4 weeks after trauma demonstrates the typical appearance of heterotopic ossification as a fluffy, ill-defined density. **B,** Lateral view obtained 8 weeks after trauma demonstrates consolidation of the ectopic bone with poorly defined borders. **C,** Lateral view obtained 16 weeks after trauma demonstrates a mature ossification with sharp cortical margins. (Copyright Mark S. Cohen, MD, Chicago, IL.)

Heterotopic bone formation can develop in a localized or a more diffuse pattern and does not necessarily follow anatomic tissue planes. Furthermore, its development does not necessarily imply a loss of motion or function. Surgical resection is indicated only for functional impairment. When heterotopic ossification develops anteriorly, the process most commonly forms beneath the brachialis muscle and is separated from the anterior articular surface by an area of radiolucency. Posterior heterotopic bone, which often forms in continuity with the joint beneath the triceps, is the most common pattern leading to complete ankylosis.

In most cases, radiographs are adequate for following the development of heterotopic bone and preoperatively planning surgical resection. However, CT (particularly three-dimensional reconstruction) may be helpful to define the status of the ulnohumeral joint and the geometry of the ectopic bone. Advantages of early resection after radiographic maturity include limiting capsular and ligamentous contracture, muscle atrophy, and cartilage degeneration, as well as allowing a more rapid return of function. Early surgical intervention may also be technically easier than late intervention.

The appropriate surgical approach for resection depends, in part, on the location and extent of the ectopic bone. Surgical technique includes bony resection with burrs, curets, osteotomes, and rongeurs, with identification and protection of the radial, median, and ulnar nerves when indicated. Posterior heterotopic ossification requires elevation of the triceps from the olecranon, either in part or completely. With posteromedial involvement (typical in patients with severe burns), the ulnar nerve can be totally encased in a shell of bone without preoperative neurologic symptoms. There is often no demonstrable difference in the quality and appearance of the heterotopic bone and the host cortex; thus, resection is facilitated by the use of intraoperative fluoroscopy.

Anterior heterotopic ossification is most commonly approached from the medial or lateral side, or from both in more extensive cases. Ectopic bone location dictates the approach. The lateral approach described previously allows access to the radiocapitellar and proximal radioulnar joints, whereas the medial approach allows decompression of the ulnar nerve and ulnohumeral exposure. Postoperatively, patients with heterotopic ossification are typically treated with the exercise program outlined previously. Although there is some evidence to suggest that it may not be necessary in all cases, it is common to use some form of prophylaxis (an NSAID or low-dose radiation) in most patients to decrease the potential for recurrence.

Resection of heterotopic bone about the elbow can be gratifying. Results are, in part, related to the initial severity of the heterotopic bone development and the preoperative functional limitations. However, a functional arc of joint motion can be obtained even in elbows with long-standing ulnohumeral joint ankylosis. Negative predictive factors after resection include residual spasticity and incomplete neurologic recovery of the upper extremity, both of which correlate with a higher recurrence rate. Although limited partial regrowth of heterotopic bone can occur, this is clinically significant only if it limits elbow motion, and functionally limiting recurrence is rare.

## Bibliography

Cohen MS: Heterotopic ossification of the elbow, in Jupiter JB, ed: *The Stiff Elbow.* Rosemont, IL, American Academy of Orthopaedic Surgeons, 2006, pp 31-40.

Cohen MS, Hastings H II: Operative release for elbow contracture: The lateral collateral ligament sparing technique. *Orthop Clin North Am* 1999;30(1):133-139.

Cohen MS, Hastings H II: Post-traumatic contracture of the elbow: Operative release using a lateral collateral ligament sparing approach. *J Bone Joint Surg Br* 1998;80(5):805-812.

Cohen MS, Hastings H II: Rotatory instability of the elbow: The anatomy and role of the lateral stabilizers. *J Bone Joint Surg Am* 1997;79(2):225-233.

Gates HS III, Sullivan FL, Urbaniak JR: Anterior capsulotomy and continuous passive motion in the treatment of post-traumatic flexion contracture of the elbow: A prospective study. *J Bone Joint Surg Am* 1992;74(8):1229-1234.

Jupiter JB, O'Driscoll SW, Cohen MS: The assessment and management of the stiff elbow. *Instr Course Lect* 2003;52:93-111.

Kasparyan NG, Hotchkiss RN: Dynamic skeletal fixation in the upper extremity. *Hand Clin* 1997;13(4):643-663.

Mansat P, Morrey BF: The column procedure: A limited lateral approach for extrinsic contracture of the elbow. *J Bone Joint Surg Am* 1998;80(11):1603-1615.

Modabber MR, Jupiter JB: Reconstruction for post-traumatic conditions of the elbow joint. *J Bone Joint Surg Am* 1995;77(9):1431-1446.

Ring D, Adey L, Zurakowski D, Jupiter JB: Elbow capsulectomy for posttraumatic elbow stiffness. *J Hand Surg Am* 2006;31(8):1264-1271.

Ring D, Jupiter JB: Operative release of complete ankylosis of the elbow due to heterotopic bone in patients without severe injury of the central nervous system. *J Bone Joint Surg Am* 2003;85(5):849-857.

Summerfield SL, DiGiovanni C, Weiss A-PC: Heterotopic ossification of the elbow. *J Shoulder Elbow Surg* 1997;6(3):321-332.

 

# Chapter 25

# Radial Head Excision and Prosthetic Replacement

*David Ring, MD, PhD*
*Neal C. Chen, MD*

**Learning Objectives**

- Identify the indications for radial head arthroplasty.
- Identify the advantages and disadvantages of different types of prostheses.
- Describe the surgical exposures that can be used for radial head arthroplasty.

## Indications

The goal of radial head arthroplasty is to restore the radiocapitellar relationship and enhance ulnohumeral and forearm stability. Radial head arthroplasty is indicated for patients in whom a radial head fracture is reparable but has tenuous fixation in the setting of acute ulnohumeral joint instability or longitudinal forearm instability (Essex-Lopresti injury) and for patients with radial head insufficiency, nonunion, or malunion in the setting of ulnohumeral joint subluxation or dislocation or longitudinal forearm instability.

Radial head arthroplasty is usually performed in patients with traumatic elbow instability. Restoration of the radiocapitellar relationship helps prevent subluxation or repeated dislocation of the elbow. Radial head repair (open reduction and internal fixation) is preferred if it provides adequate stability and a high likelihood of union and if implant prominence is manageable. Radial head arthroplasty is a useful option if fixation is tenuous, there are missing fragments or metaphyseal comminution, and substantial internal fixation that may restrict motion is necessary. These decisions are based on a patient's preferences as well as the surgeon's judgment and preferences during surgery. If the elbow or forearm is unstable, the authors of this chapter recommend erring on the side of prosthetic radial head replacement.

Radiography and CT are performed to aid in preoperative planning. If tenderness at the wrist and forearm is present—after the forearm has been stabilized during the examination so that pain from the radial head fracture does not confuse the examination—a radiograph of the wrist is obtained. Proximal subsidence of the radius (positive ulnar variance at the wrist) suggests a longitudinal forearm dissociation (injury to the interosseous ligament) and may alter management. The radial head fracture may have multiple fragments that can be identified on radiographs. Occasionally, radial head fragments may be entrapped in the lateral soft tissues posterior to the ulnohumeral joint or within the joint itself. Radial head fractures may occur in the setting of proximal ulnar fractures. If possible, radiographs should be obtained to determine other associated fractures. Small bony fragments that are present anteriorly and do not appear to be part of the radial head may be part of the coronoid, which indicates a more unstable injury pattern. A CT scan can be obtained to demonstrate the number, size, and shape of the fracture fragments; any impaction (fractured but stable segments that are misaligned); and the amount of radial head involvement. CT also can help identify and characterize associated fractures. Radiographs of the contralateral elbow may be obtained for templating purposes. For example, they may indicate the size of a patient's uninjured lateral ulnotrochlear articulation to allow assessment for overstuffing. However, radiographic evaluation of the unaffected elbow is not routine.

*Dr. Ring or an immediate family member has received royalties from Zimmer Biomet, Medartis, Skeletal Dynamics, and Wright Medical Technology; serves as a paid consultant to or is an employee of Acumed and Zimmer Biomet; has stock or stock options held in IlluminOss; and serves as a board member, owner, officer, or committee member of the American Shoulder and Elbow Surgeons and the American Society for Surgery of the Hand. Dr. Chen or an immediate family member serves as a board member, owner, officer, or committee member of the American Association for Hand Surgery.*

There are three general designs for radial head arthroplasty components: fixed monopolar, fixed bipolar, and loose monopolar. If the fracture extends distal to the radial neck, a longer stem or partial fracture fixation of the radial neck may be necessary. If concern exists regarding later revision surgery that involves prosthesis removal, a loose monopolar prosthesis may be preferable. Removal of an ingrown or a cemented stem can be difficult in patients who undergo revision surgery for infection. In some patients, osteotomy of the proximal radius may be the only option for removal of a well-fixed stem.

Preoperative imaging, even with CT, may not accurately identify the number, size, and shape of fracture fragments; therefore, preoperative plans may change as a result of intraoperative findings. Fractures with more than three parts—defined as two articular segments and a shaft fragment—have an increased likelihood of early fixation failure, nonunion, and limited range of motion (ROM). Unstable partial articular fractures of the radial head that are associated with ulnohumeral instability often have multiple small fragments that are accompanied by metaphyseal impaction or comminution and are difficult to repair. Even if there are more than three fragments, a solidly repaired radial head fracture can help stabilize the ulnohumeral joint until the ligaments heal (approximately 4 weeks postoperatively) and can be removed later if there are complications, such as nonunion or restricted motion. A repaired radial head can serve as a biologic spacer, even if it will ultimately be removed. In a setting in which radial head arthroplasties are not routinely available, a prosthesis can be made from methyl methacrylate cement (occasionally using a small screw to help form the neck of the prosthesis). Cement spacers are an inexpensive, readily available option for a loose, smooth spacer prosthesis.

## Contraindications

Radial head arthroplasty is contraindicated in patients who have an acutely or chronically colonized or infected elbow and in patients who have an elbow with a poor soft-tissue envelope that is at risk for colonization and infection.

## Alternative Treatments

Patients with a radial head malunion or nonunion in the setting of a stable elbow and forearm may undergo radial head excision without prosthetic replacement. Before small screws for internal fixation were developed, a fractured radial head was often excised without prosthetic replacement. Excision without radial head replacement is an option; however, it is best limited to patients who have multifragmented displaced fractures and elbow or forearm instability (an uncommon occurrence that typically is seen in older patients). Excision without radial head replacement also is a reasonable option for patients who have an elbow dislocation and a radial head fracture, provided no coronoid fracture exists.

There is a long-standing debate regarding the effect of excision without radial head replacement. Concerns that have been raised include proximal migration of the radius (usually just a few millimeters), valgus alignment of the elbow (uncommon), and more rapid arthrosis of the ulnohumeral joint (some arthrosis is inevitable, particularly if the elbow is dislocated). Several studies have reported remarkably good results in patients who underwent radial head excision decades earlier. Therefore, it is unclear whether the presence of a metal articulation with the capitellum leads to better long-term results compared with no radiocapitellar articulation. The excision of a malunited or ununited radial head fracture and the removal of a problematic prosthesis without radial head replacement are effective treatments, and radial head replacement in the absence of clear elbow and forearm instability may not prove better than radial head excision alone. Radial head excision predictably restores excellent forearm rotation provided no pathology of the forearm (such as heterotopic bone or distal radioulnar joint malalignment) exists and is an excellent salvage procedure. Given the excellent long-term outcomes reported in patients who undergo radial head resection alone, the role of radial head replacement as a way to protect the ulnohumeral joint or allow for a higher level of function is debatable.

If radial head fixation is tenuous but radial head healing is desired, a rationale exists for protecting the radial head fixation with the use of temporary static or hinged external fixation of the elbow. There are no data on the effectiveness of this approach, and the morbidity and cumbersome nature of external fixation make this approach less appealing.

## Results

Several notable trends have been observed at midterm follow-up after radial head arthroplasty (**Table 1**). Risk factors for revision surgery include the use of Silastic implants and younger patient age. (Approximate patient age cannot be estimated because of the uncertainty of the longevity of the arthroplasty.) Capitellar wear is common to all implant designs and is associated with a prosthesis that is too long, too wide, or both. Stress shielding of the proximal radius, which is common in cemented or press-fit prostheses, usually is radiographically evident approximately 1 year postoperatively. Whether stress shielding has any consequences for patients is unknown.

Prostheses that are intended to have a tight fit with bone ingrowth into the prosthesis often are unsuccessful. Loose

 

**Table 1** Results of Radial Head Excision and Prosthetic Replacement[a]

| Authors (Year) | No. of Patients | Procedure or Approach | Mean Patient Age in Years (Range) | Mean Follow-up in Years (Range) | Results |
|---|---|---|---|---|---|
| Harrington and Tountas (1981) | 17 | Monopolar, loose fit | 52 (20-77) | 6.9 (NA) | 8 excellent, 6 good, 2 fair, and 1 poor |
| Harrington et al (2001) | 20 | Monopolar, loose fit | 46 (21-75) | 12.1 (6-29) | 9 patients with radiographically detectable arthrosis |
| Doornberg et al (2007) | 27 | Monopolar | 52 (22-71) | 3.3 (2-4.6) | 17 patients with radiolucencies about the prosthetic stem |
| Popovic et al (2007) | 51 | Bipolar | 51 (21-69) | 8.4 (4-13) | Mean MEPI score, 83<br>Progressive osteolysis in 37 patients |
| Shore et al (2008) | 32 | Monopolar, loose fit | 54 (32-93) | 8 (2-14) | Mean MEPS, 83<br>14 patients demonstrated capitellar osteopenia |
| Burkhart et al (2010) | 17 | Bipolar | 44.1 (25-60) | 8.8 (6.5-11.6) | Mean MEPS, 90.8<br>Mean DASH score, 9.8<br>2 dislocations |
| Flinkkilä et al (2012) | 37 | Monopolar, press fit | 56 (23-85) | 4.2 (1-8.9) | Mean MEPS, 86<br>Mean DASH score, 23<br>9 prostheses removed for loosening |
| Chanlalit et al (2012) | 26 | Cemented/press fit | NA | 2.8 (1.1-5.8) | 17 patients with stress shielding |
| Duckworth et al (2014) | 105 | Various | 50 (16-93) | 6.7 (1.8-18) | Mean Broberg and Morrey score, 80<br>29 revisions<br>Risk factors for revision: younger patient age, Silastic implants |

DASH = Disabilities of the Arm, Shoulder and Hand; MEPI = Mayo Elbow Performance Index; MEPS = Mayo Elbow Performance Score; NA = not available.

[a] All studies are level IV evidence.

prostheses that have a rough finish, grooves, fins, or a curve can lead to substantial loss of bone in the neck of the radius. In a study of 37 patients who had acute unstable elbow injuries, nine press-fit modular radial head prostheses were removed as a result of symptomatic prosthetic loosening, which occurred at a mean of 11 months after implantation. Of the 25 well-fixed prostheses, 12 demonstrated radiolucencies.

Lucency around the proximal radius and stem are common in loose, smooth monopolar prostheses. One study noted radiolucencies around the prosthetic stem in 17 of 27 patients who underwent radial head arthroplasty with a smooth monopolar prosthesis; however, these changes were not associated with increased pain. Radiolucencies were observed in 16 of 31 elbows that underwent radial head arthroplasty with a smooth monopolar prosthesis in another study; however, no change in lucent areas was noted radiographically on comparison of 2-year and 8-year follow-up images, and the areas did not seem to be symptomatic. Bipolar prostheses are subject to wear debris and osteolysis caused by an inflammatory response similar to that which occurs in other prostheses. The initial short-term follow-up of patients who undergo bipolar radial head arthroplasty has been clinically encouraging, with few radiolucencies reported; however, midterm results warrant careful study. In a study of 51 patients who underwent radial head arthroplasty with a biopolar prosthesis, osteolysis was reported in 37 patients and progressive radiographic lucency was reported in 16 patients during the 8-year follow-up period. Although the observed clinical results were similar to those of short-term reports, the authors of the study expressed concern regarding further bony loss and eventual clinical deterioration.

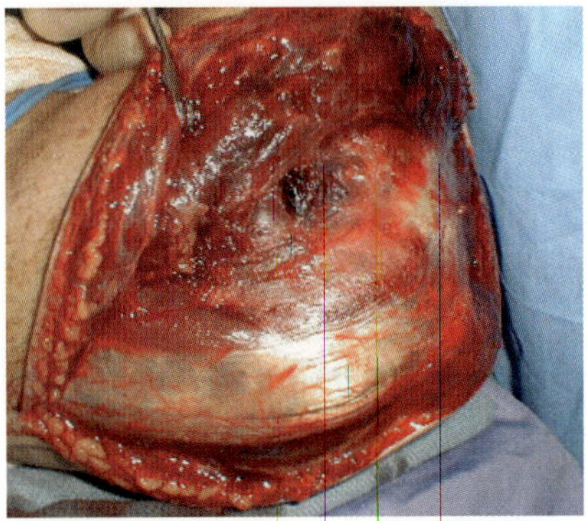

**Figure 1** Intraoperative photograph shows the lateral approach to the elbow. In radial head fractures that are associated with an ulnohumeral dislocation, as seen in this photograph, the common extensor mass is often avulsed from the epicondyle, and the damaged muscle provides an interval to access the radial head. (Copyright David Ring, MD, PhD, Austin, TX.)

**Video 25.1** Radial Head Arthroplasty. Graham J.W. King, MD (17 min)

# Techniques

## Setup/Exposure

- The setup for radial head replacement is often dictated by associated injuries.
- Associated injuries include radial head fracture with elbow dislocation, Essex-Lopresti injury and radial head fracture with medial collateral ligament (MCL) rupture, and posterior olecranon fracture-dislocation.

### RADIAL HEAD FRACTURE WITH ELBOW DISLOCATION

- The patient is placed in the supine position, and a hand table is used.
- A sterile tourniquet is used.
- Either a posterior skin incision with elevation of a skin flap or a direct lateral skin incision can be used. For a lateral skin incision, the lateral epicondyle is identified, and an incision approximately 10 cm long is centered over the lateral epicondyle.
- Full-thickness flaps are raised anteriorly and posteriorly, and the fascia over the extensor mass and anconeus muscle are identified.
- If the elbow has dislocated, the origins of the medial and collateral ligaments are usually avulsed from the epicondyles, as are the origins of some or all of the common flexor and extensor muscles. On the lateral side, there is usually a rent in the fascia near the lateral epicondyle (**Figure 1**). This rent usually provides an interval at or near the division between the extensor carpi radialis brevis and the extensor digitorum muscle tendons. This interval can be extended distally and proximally.
- The avulsion of the lateral collateral ligament (LCL) and the common extensors from the lateral epicondyle provides good access to the radial head.
- The elbow can be subluxated or dislocated to improve access to the radial neck for preparation of prosthesis insertion.
- The supinator can be partially divided and the extensor carpi radialis longus origin can be elevated off the supracondylar ridge for additional exposure, if necessary.
- As the split in the supinator extends distally, the radial nerve lies in close proximity to the dissection and, in general, approximately 4 cm distal to the native radiocapitellar joint.
- Displaced, fragmented radial head fractures may not have an associated LCL/common extensor avulsion in patients who have a forearm fracture-dislocation with an interosseous ligament injury, a fracture-subluxation with MCL rupture but no dislocation, or a posterior olecranon fracture-dislocation.

### ESSEX-LOPRESTI INJURY AND RADIAL HEAD FRACTURE WITH MCL RUPTURE

- If the ulnohumeral joint has not dislocated, the LCL origin often remains intact, which makes exposure more challenging. The authors of this chapter usually use the interval between the extensor carpi radialis brevis muscle and the extensor digitorum muscle for exposure. The key is to split the common extensor musculature so that the posterior one-half of the lateral epicondyle and the LCL origin are not disrupted.
- Access to the radial head can be improved by placing a small, stout osteotome inferiorly between the radius and ulna and then using the osteotome to lever the radius anteriorly and laterally away from the ulna.
- In addition, to make insertion easier the radial head prosthesis can be downsized (in particular, the diameter of the neck of a loose, smooth monopolar prosthesis).
- If necessary, the origin of the LCL may be reflected off the lateral epicondyle or removed with a piece of bone and reattached later.

### POSTERIOR OLECRANON FRACTURE-DISLOCATION

- In patients who have a posterior olecranon fracture-dislocation or a posterior Monteggia injury, the radial head may be approached via the damage created by the injury.
- The patient is often placed in the lateral decubitus position.
- A posterior incision is made over the olecranon and the ulna, and skin flaps are raised medially and laterally.
- Typically, rents in the muscles on either side of the olecranon fracture can be extended slightly; however, some surgeons believe that the extent of dissection between the proximal radius and the ulna

 

correlates with the risk of radioulnar synostosis.

- Release and/or transposition of the ulnar nerve may be performed if desired, although this is not usually necessary, and the proximal olecranon fragment is elevated proximally.
- Re-creating and exaggerating the apex posterior deformity of the ulnar fracture delivers the proximal radius through the traumatic defect in the muscle, and the joint is exposed by mobilizing the proximal olecranon fragment and removing the blood clot.
- Occasionally, a displaced fragment of the ulna that contains the distal supinator crest or the sublime tubercle may be mobilized to improve visualization of the ulnohumeral joint and the radial head. Such mobilization should be done selectively and only for displaced, unstable fractures because it risks devitalization of important fracture fragments.
- If the ulnar fracture is too distal to safely mobilize the olecranon fragment proximally for visualization of the joint, the radial head may be best approached via a separate lateral muscle interval as previously described. Other surgeons favor an exposure between the radius and the ulna that is similar to the Speed and Boyd approach; however, this approach risks detaching the distal insertion of the LCL at the supinator crest and may increase the risk of proximal radioulnar synostosis.

## Instruments/Equipment/ Implants Required

- A hand table should be used if the patient is positioned supine.
- A bean bag or kidney rests should be used if the patient is positioned laterally.
- An elbow positioner or a bump is necessary if the patient is positioned laterally or prone and management of proximal ulnar fracture is planned.
- A sagittal saw is necessary to remove radial head fragments at the neck of the radius.
- An image intensifier should be available.
- Suture anchors or, alternatively, sutures that can be placed through drill holes are necessary.
- A drill is required.
- A plate and screws should be available for radial head repair.
- A radial head arthroplasty set is necessary.

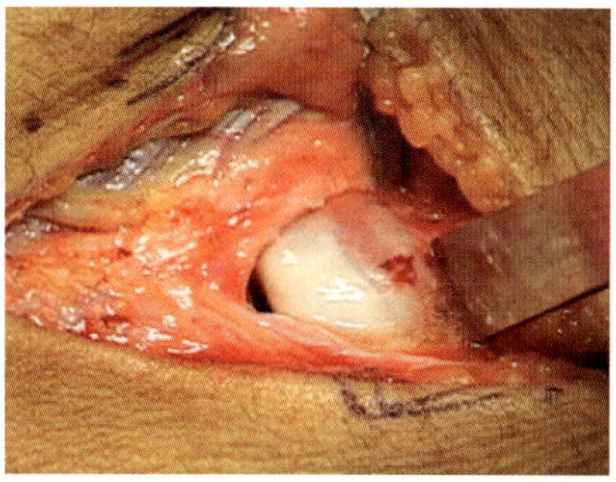

**Figure 2** Intraoperative photograph of an elbow shows an osteotomy at the radial head-neck junction, which is performed if necessary during radial head excision and replacement. (Copyright David Ring, MD, PhD, Austin, TX.)

## Procedure

- The fracture is examined, and a decision on whether to repair the radial head is made.
- Fracture fragments with little or no soft-tissue attachments can be reassembled on the back table and then brought back to the elbow and reattached to the intact radius with a plate and screws. If a part of the radial head is either lost or too small or fragmented to repair, the authors of this chapter prefer to perform radial head arthroplasty because even small anterolateral fragments have important contributions to elbow stability.
- If the radial head will be replaced with a prosthesis, the fracture fragments are excised.
- A retractor can be placed over the anterior surface of the distal humerus to improve exposure.
- Care should be taken not to place excessive force on the anterior retractor to prevent injury to the posterior interosseous nerve.
- A sagittal saw and/or an osteotome is used to cut the radial neck at the junction of the radial head to the shaft (**Figure 2**).
- The radial head fragments are reassembled to ensure that no fragments are left in the elbow. Occasionally, a small fragment may be missing, and the surgeon must ensure that it is not in the ulnohumeral joint.
- The largest fragments are used to template the radial head prosthesis. Sizing of the prosthesis varies by manufacturer. In general, a smaller diameter prosthesis is selected if the radial head diameter is between available sizes.
- In some patients, the fracture may extend distal to the radial neck. One notable pattern is a head-neck fracture that results in a triangular wedge of bone that is missing from the radial shaft. This problem can be conceptualized as missing a percentage of the 360° arc of the radial shaft (**Figure 3**). Additional radial neck resection decreases the percentage of the arc of the radial shaft that is missing and theoretically improves stability. A longer prosthetic stem also can provide additional stability.
- Finally, the location of the arc of the radial shaft is important. If the missing wedge of bone is associated with a radial head fragment that articulates with the proximal radioulnar joint, the prosthetic articulation with the proximal ulna will also help provide stability.

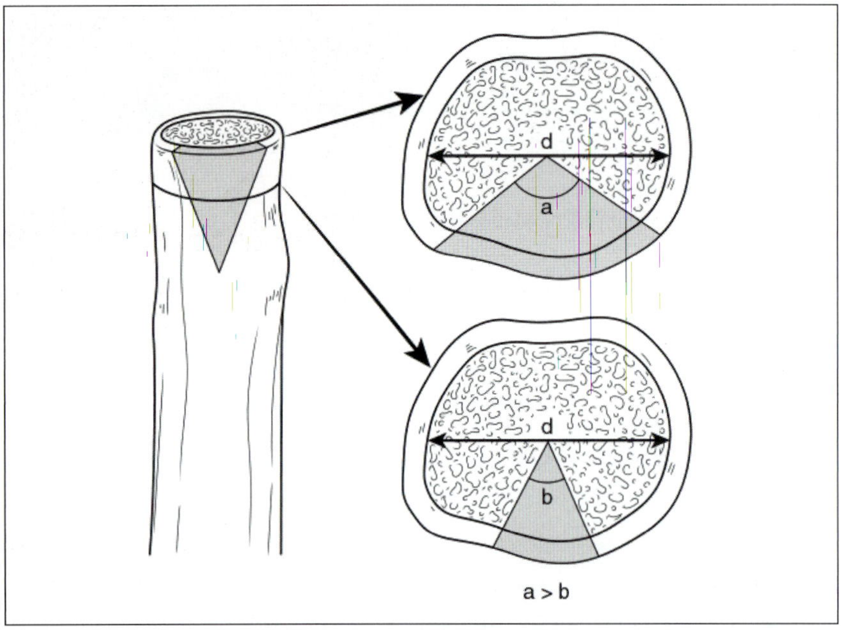


**Figure 3** Illustration shows a triangular wedge of bone missing from the radial neck. Shortening of the radial neck can decrease the amount of missing bone relative to the radial neck diameter (*d*). The arc of bone loss is represented by angle *a*. If the radial neck is shortened, the radial neck diameter remains relatively constant, but the arc of bone loss (angle *b*) is decreased.

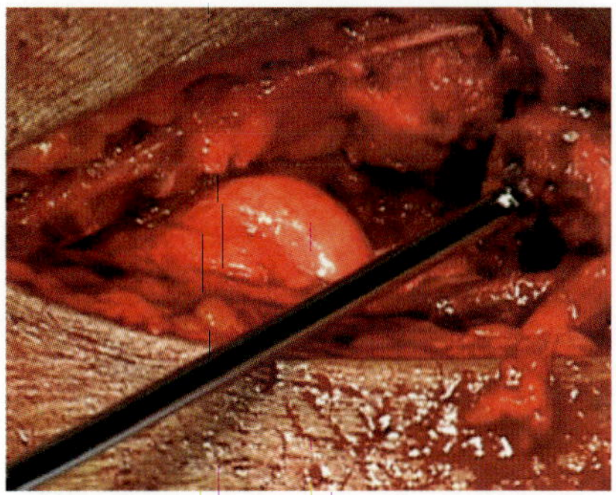

**Figure 4** Intraoperative photograph of an elbow shows broaching of the radial stem. (Copyright David Ring, MD, PhD, Austin, TX.)

- If the radial head fragment is large, the fragment can be plated and then the stem can be downsized.
- The radial neck is serially reamed (**Figure 4**). The broaching instrument varies by implant system.
- After the starting reamer is placed down the radial shaft, marrow elements should extrude from the neck. If the reamer does not feel right and visualization is poor, either radiographs should be obtained or visualization should be improved before further reaming is performed.
- The shaft is progressively reamed until gentle resistance and chatter are evident.
- The neck cut can be planned to match the shaft based on the final reamer that is used.
- A trial head is selected and inserted. If the trial head is difficult to insert, the prosthesis can be downsized or the anterior capsule can be freed off its lateral edge of the distal humerus. Alternatively, as a last resort, the LCL can be released off the lateral epicondyle or an osteotomy of the lateral epicondyle can be performed and repaired later if necessary.
- The elbow is flexed, extended, supinated, and pronated to ensure that there are no hard blocks to motion.
- If the trial head is acceptable, it is removed, and the actual prosthesis is brought into the surgical field (**Figure 5**).
- Some prosthetic designs require assembly before implantation, whereas other prosthetic designs allow for in situ assembly.
- After the final implant is in place, the examination is repeated as previously described.
- If the LCL has been injured or released, it is repaired. One method of repair involves placing suture anchors into the lateral epicondyle and passing sutures through the soft tissues at two levels. The sutures are tied down without cutting the needles. The remaining suture tails from the inferior anchor are used to close the extensor split or the extensor digitorum muscle/anconeus split and are tied distally. The remaining suture tails from the superior anchor are used to close the proximal soft-tissue split.
- The arm is examined for stability with the use of a gravity stress test. The humerus is placed over a bump with the forearm in supination, and a lateral fluoroscopic image is obtained. If the ulnohumeral joint remains concentric, then the elbow is considered stable (**Figure 6**).

### Wound Closure

- The subcutaneous tissues are closed with resorbable sutures.
- The skin is closed with staples, nylon sutures, or buried resorbable sutures.

## Postoperative Regimen

The postoperative regimen after isolated radial head arthroplasty without ligament reconstruction involves early active motion on postoperative day 1, if possible. If the LCL has been repaired, either for injury or for takedown to allow access, varus loads (that is, shoulder

 

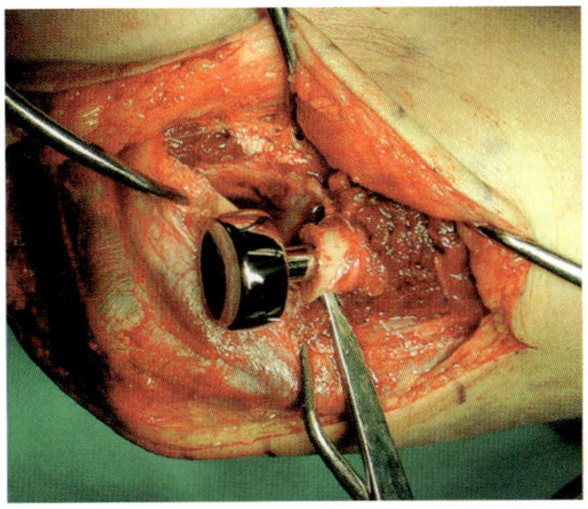

**Figure 5** Intraoperative photograph of an elbow shows implantation of the final radial head replacement prosthesis. (Copyright David Ring, MD, PhD, Austin, TX.)

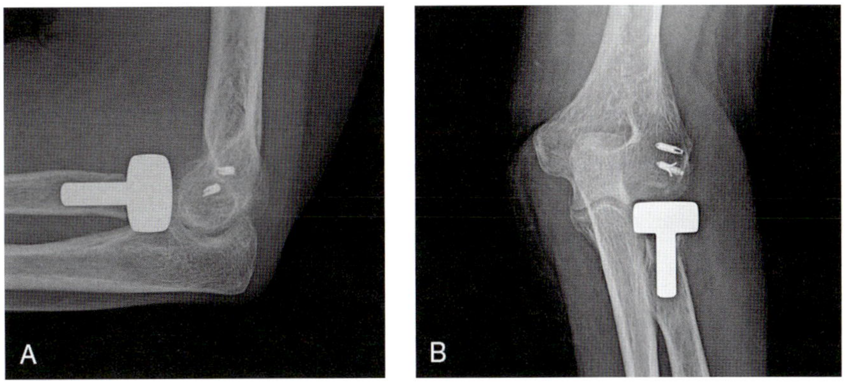


**Figure 6** Lateral (**A**) and AP (**B**) radiographs of an elbow demonstrate a stable radial head prosthesis. The lateral extensor mass was repaired with the use of suture anchors.

abduction) are avoided for 4 weeks postoperatively. In addition, performing ROM exercises in a supine position with the arm overhead (gravity-assisted exercises) can help protect the reconstruction/repair because gravity tends to locate the elbow. The authors of this chapter progress their patients from protected supine ROM to upright motion at 4 weeks postoperatively. Force is allowed beginning 6 weeks postoperatively.

If the elbow is stiff, dynamic splinting or static progressive splinting may be initiated after any associated bony injuries demonstrate radiographic healing, and splinting may be continued for up to 1 year postoperatively to improve ROM. If the patient demonstrates signs of ulnar neuropathy or heterotopic bone formation that limits ROM, the nerve or ectopic bone is surgically removed.

## Limiting Adverse Events

Radial head arthroplasty with a prosthesis that is too long may result in an overstuffed joint, which can lead to pain and limited ROM. To avoid overstuffing, the surgeon can template the prosthesis to the native radial head fragments. Most surgeons prefer to insert an undersized prosthesis in an effort to avoid this problem. The following guidelines can help prevent overstuffing. If the elbow cannot be fully extend intraoperatively, the joint may be overstuffed. The proximal edge of the prosthesis should not lie more than 1 mm proximal to the lateral edge of the coronoid as observed on an AP radiograph. The relationship between the coronoid and the trochlea should be congruent and the joint space should be relatively even as observed on an AP radiograph. In vitro studies suggest that overstuffing may not be detected radiographically until the radial head is overlengthened by 6 mm or more.

In patients with a radial head fracture who undergo radial head excision, a radius pull test should be performed. If the interosseous ligament is divided in vitro, the radius can be pulled 3 mm proximally; if there is a complete dissociation of the radius and the ulna, the radius can be pulled 6 mm proximally. If the radius migrates proximally during a radius pull test, longitudinal forearm instability may be present, and radial head arthroplasty should be considered.

## Bibliography

Alolabi B, Studer A, Gray A, et al: Selecting the diameter of a radial head implant: An assessment of local landmarks. *J Shoulder Elbow Surg* 2013;22(10):1395-1399.

Burkhart KJ, Mattyasovszky SG, Runkel M, et al: Mid- to long-term results after bipolar radial head arthroplasty. *J Shoulder Elbow Surg* 2010;19(7):965-972.

Chanlalit C, Shukla DR, Fitzsimmons JS, An KN, O'Driscoll SW: Stress shielding around radial head prostheses. *J Hand Surg Am* 2012;37(10):2118-2125.

Charalambous CP, Stanley JK, Siddique I, Powell E, Alvi F, Gagey O: The Wrightington approach to the radial head: Biomechanical comparison with the posterolateral approach. *J Hand Surg Am* 2007;32(10):1576-1582.

Doornberg JN, Linzel DS, Zurakowski D, Ring D: Reference points for radial head prosthesis size. *J Hand Surg Am* 2006;31(1):53-57.

Doornberg JN, Parisien R, van Duijn PJ, Ring D: Radial head arthroplasty with a modular metal spacer to treat acute traumatic elbow instability. *J Bone Joint Surg Am* 2007;89(5):1075-1080.

Duckworth AD, Wickramasinghe NR, Clement ND, Court-Brown CM, McQueen MM: Radial head replacement for acute complex fractures: What are the rate and risks factors for revision or removal? *Clin Orthop Relat Res* 2014;472(7):2136-2143.

Flinkkilä T, Kaisto T, Sirniö K, Hyvönen P, Leppilahti J: Short- to mid-term results of metallic press-fit radial head arthroplasty in unstable injuries of the elbow. *J Bone Joint Surg Br* 2012;94(6):805-810.

Frank SG, Grewal R, Johnson J, Faber KJ, King GJ, Athwal GS: Determination of correct implant size in radial head arthroplasty to avoid overlengthening. *J Bone Joint Surg Am* 2009;91(7):1738-1746.

Guitton TG, van der Werf HJ, Ring D: Quantitative three-dimensional computed tomography measurement of radial head fractures. *J Shoulder Elbow Surg* 2010;19(7):973-977.

Harrington IJ, Sekyi-Otu A, Barrington TW, Evans DC, Tuli V: The functional outcome with metallic radial head implants in the treatment of unstable elbow fractures: A long-term review. *J Trauma* 2001;50(1):46-52.

Harrington IJ, Tountas AA: Replacement of the radial head in the treatment of unstable elbow fractures. *Injury* 1981;12(5):405-412.

Popovic N, Lemaire R, Georis P, Gillet P: Midterm results with a bipolar radial head prosthesis: Radiographic evidence of loosening at the bone-cement interface. *J Bone Joint Surg Am* 2007;89(11):2469-2476.

Ring D, Quintero J, Jupiter JB: Open reduction and internal fixation of fractures of the radial head. *J Bone Joint Surg Am* 2002;84(10):1811-1815.

Shore BJ, Mozzon JB, MacDermid JC, Faber KJ, King GJ: Chronic posttraumatic elbow disorders treated with metallic radial head arthroplasty. *J Bone Joint Surg Am* 2008;90(2):271-280.

Smets S, Govaers K, Jansen N, Van Riet R, Schaap M, Van Glabbeek F: The floating radial head prosthesis for comminuted radial head fractures: A multicentric study. *Acta Orthop Belg* 2000;66(4):353-358.

Smith AM, Urbanosky LR, Castle JA, Rushing JT, Ruch DS: Radius pull test: Predictor of longitudinal forearm instability. *J Bone Joint Surg Am* 2002;84(11):1970-1976.

## Video Reference

King GJ: Video. *Radial Head Arthroplasty.* London, ON, Canada, 2013.

 

# Chapter 26

# Treatment of Refractory Elbow Dislocation and Detection of the Elbow at Risk

*Aaron Daluiski, MD*

*Robert N. Hotchkiss, MD*

**Learning Objectives**

- Identify the features of an elbow at risk for redislocation.
- Understand the detection, preemption, and management of elbow redislocation.

## Indications

Most elbow dislocations, even those with associated fractures, can be effectively managed by following a treatment algorithm that includes reduction of the elbow joint, fracture alignment and stabilization, and protection of the ligaments during motion throughout the healing phase. However, in some patients with elbow dislocation, redislocation may occur. If the redislocation is undetected and left untreated, the elbow quickly becomes stiff, and the cartilage of the elbow joint rapidly deteriorates and is permanently lost. Identification of the individual anatomic features of an elbow at risk for redislocation and recognition of other factors that cause a failure of detection and lack of recognition may help prevent or minimize permanent consequences.

Optimal surgical care depends on recognition of the anatomy of the injury, specifically which crucial bony and ligamentous structures are injured and require repair or reconstruction, and a treatment strategy that takes into account how much time has passed since the initial injury occurred. Patient age and body habitus are other factors that directly influence management choices and outcome. Even with the best efforts and early recognition, some elbow redislocations will result in unsatisfying outcomes for both the patient and the orthopaedic surgeon. The treatment goal of the authors of this chapter is to minimize the incidence of refractory elbow dislocation and offer treatment guidance for patients in whom it occurs.

For the purposes of this chapter, the elbow at risk for redislocation is a traumatically dislocated elbow (with or without fracture) that either cannot be easily reduced or, after relocation, cannot be maintained in a reduced position with the use of a splint or sling. If elbow dislocation goes unrecognized or is treated with an insufficient repair or protection strategy, the elbow can slip back into a dislocated or subluxated position. A refractory dislocation usually occurs more than 2 to 3 weeks after the initial injury and cannot be reduced nonsurgically. The elbow can redislocate in a splint, brace, or cast, and the patient may not be able to sense the redislocation. There are patients in whom a dislocation is not appreciated for months. Associated fractures of the olecranon/proximal ulna, coronoid process, and radial head are common and often disguise ulnohumeral dislocations (**Figure 1**). Subluxation or dislocation that continues for many months causes damage to the articular cartilage, presumably because of a lack of boundary lubrication and a lack of nutrition to the chondrocytes. With complete dislocation, the cartilage is usually adequate; however, with subluxation, damage may be sufficient for consideration of interposition arthroplasty or total elbow arthroplasty (TEA).

Refractory dislocation is not posterolateral rotatory instability (PLRI) or recurrent instability. A patient with PLRI that develops weeks or months after a dislocation or near-dislocation experiences intermittent and infrequent episodes of subluxation as a result of isolated insufficiency of the posterolateral ligamentous complex. In patients with PLRI, the elbow is fully reduced after injury and easily moves through

*Dr. Daluiski or an immediate family member serves as a board member, owner, officer, or committee member of the American Board of Orthopaedic Surgery and the American Society for Surgery of the Hand. Dr. Hotchkiss or an immediate family member has received research or institutional support from Auxilium Pharmaceuticals.*

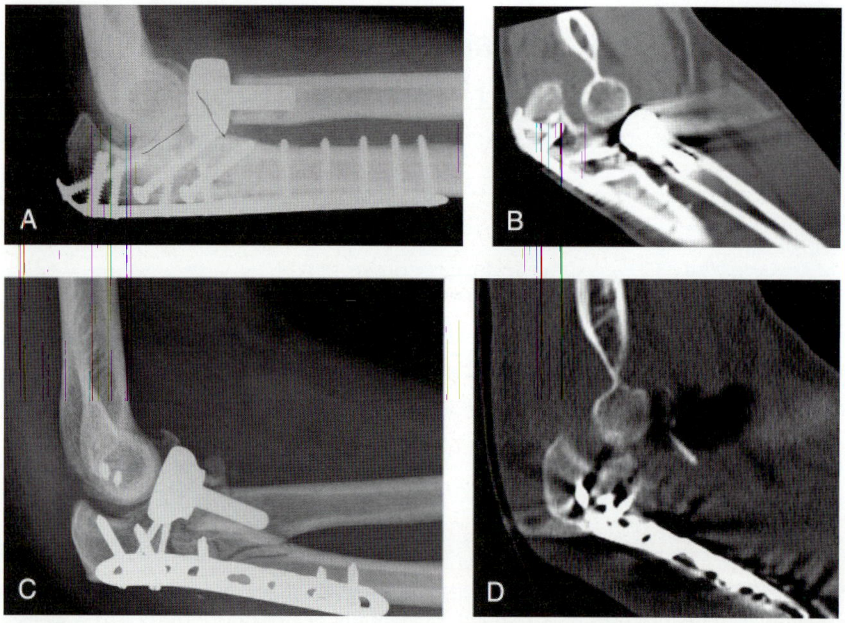


**Figure 1** Lateral radiograph (**A**) and sagittal CT scan (**B**) of the elbow from one patient and lateral radiograph (**C**) and sagittal CT scan (**D**) of the elbow from a different patient demonstrate complex fractures with dislocation that were initially reduced but had subluxation/dislocation confirmed on CT. Both patients underwent open reduction and internal fixation for an ulnar fracture (Monteggia fracture) and replacement of the prosthetic radial head, and had subtle residual subluxation postoperatively. (Copyright Robert Hotchkiss, MD, New York, NY.)

flexion and extension in most circumstances. However, if the elbow joint is moved into a position of vulnerability (often with extension of the elbow and supination of the forearm), it begins to subluxate and the patient experiences momentary pain and varying degrees of dysfunction until he or she can restore alignment by repositioning the elbow joint. In effect, an elbow with PLRI occasionally and momentarily slips into a subluxated position. In contrast, in a refractory dislocation the elbow resides in a subluxated position and appears to be reduced only occasionally and in certain positions.

## Factors That Can Lead to Dislocation

Anatomic factors that place a patient at risk of dislocation are high-energy injuries with wide displacement of dislocation, medial facet fractures of the coronoid, terrible triad injury, and Monteggia variant injuries with radial head fracture. In a high-energy injury with wide displacement of dislocation observed on prereduction radiographs, the wide separation and displacement indicates that the entire distal humerus has been stripped of soft tissue. In a medial facet fracture of the coronoid, if the medial facet alone is displaced, the elbow joint will tend to dislocate with shoulder abduction and the resultant varus load. This same defect often is evident in comminuted fracture of the proximal ulna; however, the dorsal surface of the fractured ulna, olecranon, and shaft are more readily observed. Without recognition and stabilization of a medial facet fracture of the coronoid, the elbow is at risk for refractory dislocation (**Figure 2**).

An elbow dislocation accompanied by fractures of the coronoid and radial head (terrible triad injury) is very unstable. The soft tissues are detached, and the constraint normally provided by the radial head and coronoid is lost. The coronoid fracture in patients with a terrible triad injury usually involves the tip or the lateral aspect, which is an important finding because repair of the coronoid fragment may not be as important as repair of a medial facet fragment; small coronoid fragments do not require repair. The presence of a large coronoid fragment, however, should prompt an effort for repair. Repair or replacement of the radial head and repair of the lateral collateral ligament (LCL) should be strongly considered.

A fracture of the ulnar shaft (Monteggia fracture) in combination with a radial head fracture can result in subtle refractory dislocation (**Figure 1**). Often, dislocation of the ulnohumeral joint is not readily apparent. The treatment strategy for Monteggia fractures usually involves reduction of the ulnar shaft, alignment of the radial head with repair or replacement, and repair of the ligament.

Obesity and polytrauma are patient factors that can lead to refractory dislocation. Elbow dislocations in patients with obesity are difficult to manage for many reasons. The distance from the skin to the bone and the thickness of the soft tissue in patients with obesity decreases the mechanical effectiveness of splints. The panniculus and the lower trunk pushes the shoulder into abduction in patients with obesity, which places a varus load on an already unstable elbow. Imaging after reduction also is a challenge in patients with obesity. Radiographs are difficult to interpret with the elbow in a splint or brace, and some CT scanners cannot accommodate very large patients. If the alignment of the ulnohumeral joint is uncertain, fluoroscopic imaging with the patient placed in the supine position may be required. An examination under anesthesia also may be useful.

In the presence of thoracic, abdominal, or multilimb injuries, elbow

 

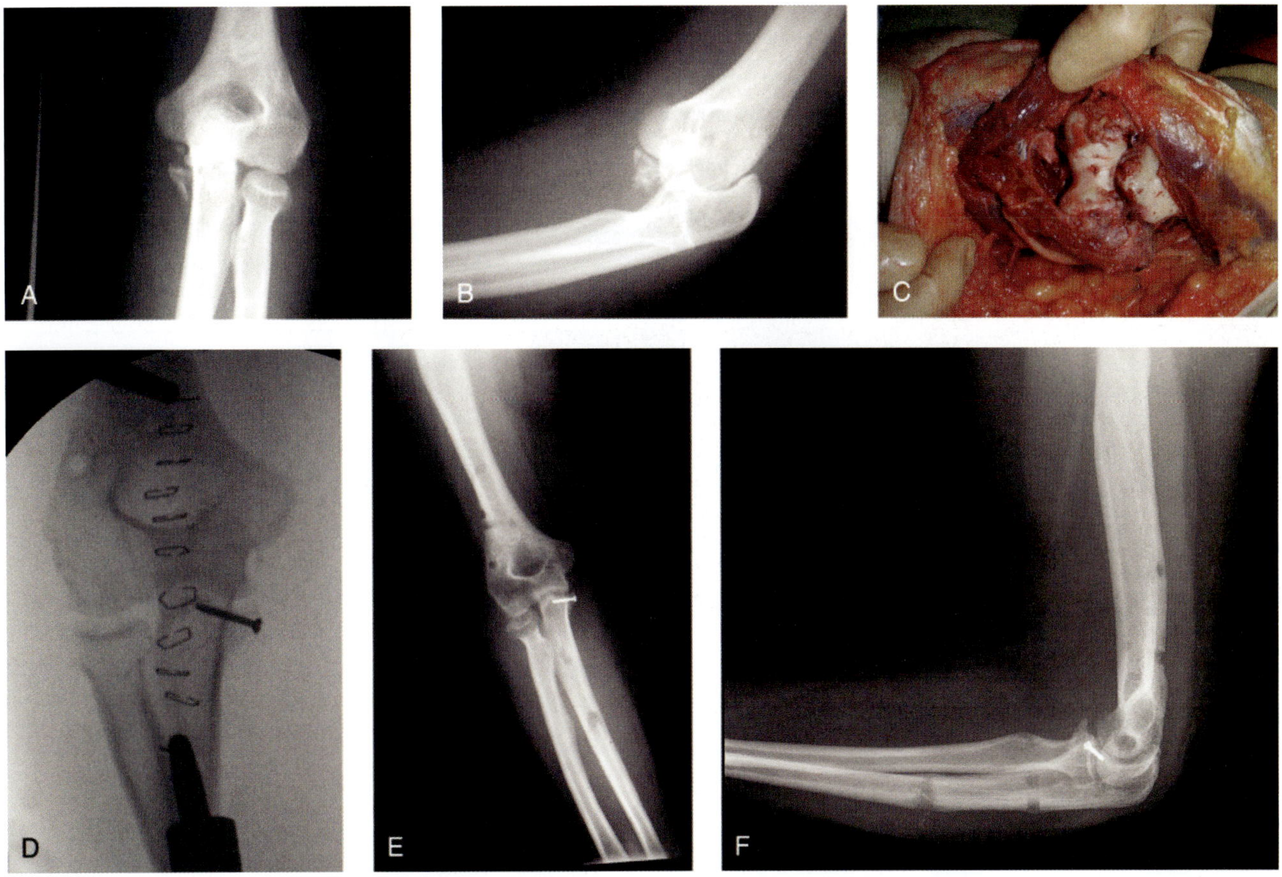


**Figure 2** Images of the elbow of a 41-year-old woman who sustained an elbow dislocation after a fall on ice 8 weeks prior. The elbow was reduced and placed in a splint in the emergency department, and radiographs confirmed reduction. The patient was seen 10 days after injury and 5 weeks after injury, and no signs of subluxation or dislocation were noted on physical examination or radiographs. Seven weeks after injury, numbness and pain suddenly developed in the ulnar nerve distribution, and elbow dislocation was observed on AP (**A**) and lateral (**B**) radiographs. The medial facet fracture of the coronoid demonstrated in panel A rendered the elbow at risk for refractory dislocation. **C,** Intraoperative photograph shows the status of the articular cartilage of the elbow at the time of open reduction and coronoid fixation. **D,** AP intraoperative fluoroscopic image demonstrates concentric reduction, hinged external fixation, and screw fixation of the medial facet of the coronoid. AP (**E**) and lateral (**F**) radiographs obtained 6 months after injury demonstrate good alignment of the elbow joint. The patient reported no additional instability and the coronoid fragment healed. (Copyright Robert Hotchkiss, MD, New York, NY.)

injuries—including dislocations—initially can be missed. Treatment of life-threatening injuries is paramount, and discovery and definitive treatment of elbow injury may be delayed. A dislocation can be temporized with the use of a static external fixation frame, which is applied to hold the joint in a reduced position and protect the articular cartilage. After a patient's condition stabilizes, repair of fractures and soft tissue can be undertaken.

## Patient Monitoring After Initial Treatment

The first 3 weeks after initial treatment require vigilance. Even if surgery was performed to repair the ligaments and internally stabilize the fractures, a substantial risk for redislocation exists. In most patients, the elbow has been placed in a position of flexion, usually greater than 90° as tolerated and as much as the swollen limb permits. The position of the forearm is dictated by the position of vulnerability. Usually, protection of the lateral ligaments is the priority and pronation is the position of choice. If the medial side is equally disrupted, which usually is the case, the forearm is placed in a neutral position. If supervised rehabilitation is begun, the overhead protocol may decrease the likelihood of subluxation. Commercially fabricated hinged braces with mechanical blocks to extension do not guarantee maintenance of reduction. The extent to

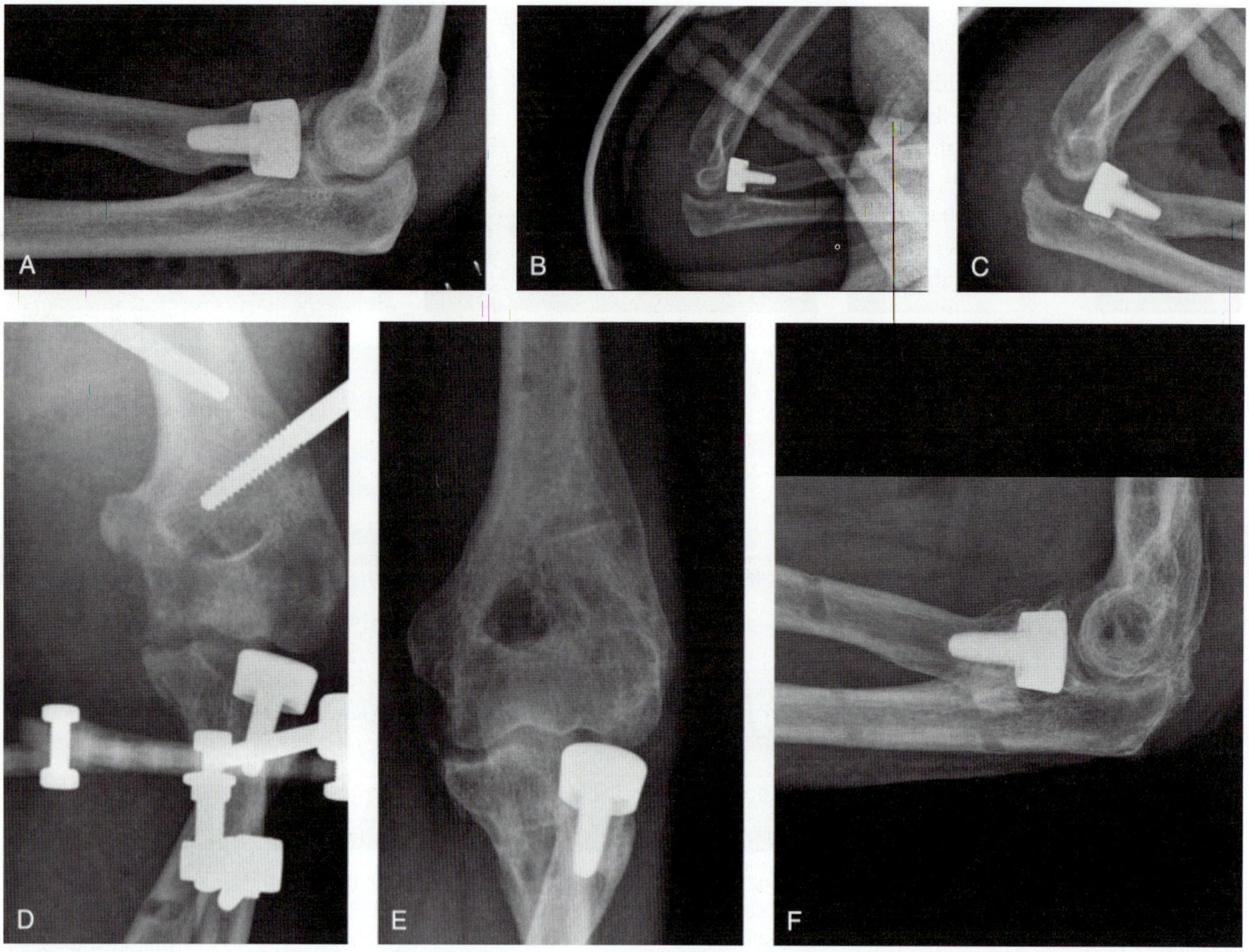


**Figure 3** Images of the elbow from a 40-year-old man who fell and sustained an elbow dislocation, a radial head fracture, and a coronoid fracture. **A,** Lateral radiograph obtained immediately after radial head replacement, with both medial and lateral ligament repair; the coronoid was not repaired. **B,** Lateral radiograph obtained 3 weeks postoperatively demonstrates subluxation; based on this finding, the elbow was splinted in approximately 110° of flexion. **C,** Lateral radiograph obtained 7 weeks postoperatively demonstrates persistent subluxation into the coronoid defect. The patient underwent a second surgery, in which the elbow was located, the collateral ligaments were reattached, and hinged external fixation was applied. **D,** AP radiograph obtained 12 weeks after initial injury demonstrates an external fixation frame, which was used to maintain reduction. AP (**E**) and lateral (**F**) radiographs obtained 4 years postoperatively demonstrate a stable elbow and minimal arthrosis. The patient experienced painless motion from 30° to 125° of flexion. (Copyright Robert Hotchkiss, MD, New York, NY.)

which maximal flexion limits redislocation is unclear. The first few weeks of the rehabilitation program are intended to restore coaptive muscle tension and improve proprioception. It may be useful to observe the patient during a portion of a rehabilitation session to assess progress and examine joint tracking.

Imaging, especially a well-positioned lateral view, is crucial. A cross-table lateral view obtained with the patient in a standing position helps avoid the varus-loaded position. If the patient has difficulty positioning the joint, supporting the limb for a spot fluoroscopic image may be more productive.

## Signs of Impending Dislocation or Loss of Reduction

There are three key signs of impending dislocation or loss of reduction: the patient reports a shift of position and/or new mechanical pain with attempted motion (dislocations can occur in a splint or brace); radiographic evidence of loss of alignment (**Figure 3**); and lack of smooth elbow joint tracking. Nonsurgical management may occasionally be used to treat patients with minimal bony involvement if the elbow can be reduced in a closed manner a second time. In these patients, especially those who have small coronoid tip fractures and no other evidence of bony instability, the simple application of greater flexion of the elbow to a degree that is comfortable—typically 115° of flexion—can restore congruence (**Figure 4**). These patients are treated with the use of a thermoplastic posterior elbow shell positioned in 115° of flexion, after which congruence is verified radiographically. If complete congruity can be achieved with this method, which is often the case, overhead motion rehabilitation protocol consisting of gravity-assisted reduction of the elbow joint can begin, continuing for 2 to 3 weeks, after which the patient can be graduated to a seated position for range-of-motion (ROM) exercises (**Figure 5**). If this method is unsuccessful based on follow-up and imaging, the patient may require revision surgery. Delaying revision surgery, especially if the fracture fragments are losing their reduction or the elbow joint is drifting to redislocation, only increases the stiffness of the tissue and the extent of exposure necessary for revision surgery.

Before revision surgery is planned, the surgeon should consider several factors, including whether any of the repairs require graft augmentation for additional immediate and long-term strength, whether the fractures require re-exploration and bone grafting with added fixation, whether external fixation needs to be added to neutralize the deforming forces, whether external fixation should be accomplished with the use of an axis-based hinged fixator or a simple static fixator, and whether the external fixation frame or device should support the medial and lateral sides. The surgeon also should consider whether there is a role for transarticular pinning and whether the necessary team and equipment are available. Revision surgery in these patients can be daunting, even if performed only days after the initial procedure. Finding, mobilizing, and protecting the neurovascular elements, especially the ulnar nerve, can be time-consuming; however, revision surgery is best performed with deliberate speed.

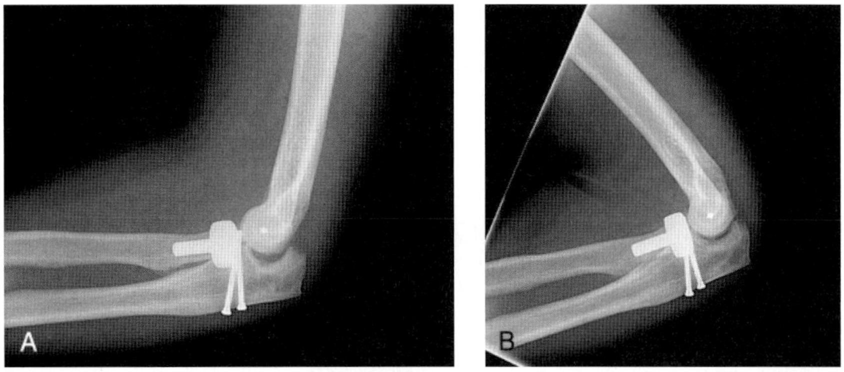


**Figure 4** Lateral radiographs of the elbow from a patient who underwent radial head replacement and coronoid fracture fixation. **A,** The elbow is positioned in approximately 80° of flexion. **B,** Note the subtle increase in ulnohumeral distraction and incongruity (the so-called drop sign) that is restored on elbow flexion to 100°. (Copyright Aaron Daluiski, MD, New York, NY.)

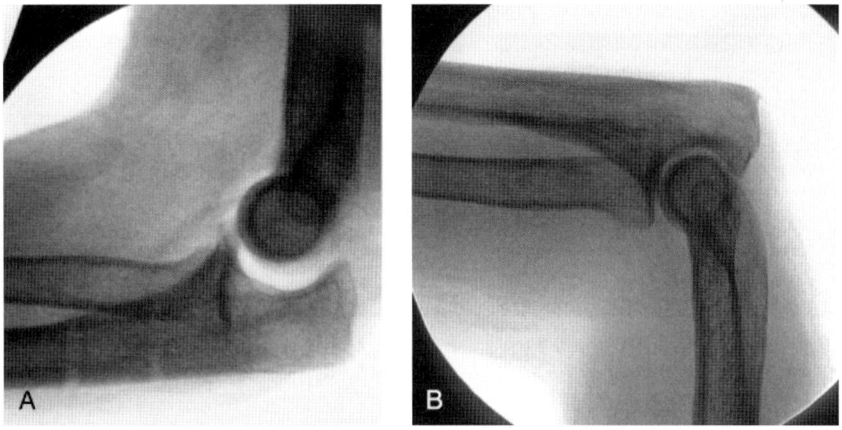


**Figure 5** **A,** Lateral fluoroscopic image of a cadaver elbow demonstrates ulnohumeral incongruity induced with the weight of the forearm, resulting in distraction of the elbow joint. This occurs during seated, upright range of motion (ROM). **B,** Lateral intraoperative fluoroscopic image of a cadaver elbow demonstrates elbow joint reduction when it is placed in the so-called overhead position (supine); this motion converts the distraction force to a compression force. (Copyright Aaron Daluiski, MD, New York, NY.)

In hindsight, revision surgery can be regarded as preventable; however, most of these patients can be and are managed successfully without the use of external fixation on initial discovery. Thus, the automatic use of external fixation is not indicated. Usually, patients who understand the reason for vigilance and recognize impending instability or frank redislocation understand that additional surgery is required to protect the irreplaceable cartilage and joint surfaces. Most patients will have a better understanding of the decision not to use an external fixation device after it is in place and they witness the complexity and inconvenience associated with its use.

For infirm and less active patients, TEA with a constrained implant may be the best solution (**Figure 6**). The recovery after TEA is rapid, and there is no concern for half-pin infections or further instability. The decision to perform TEA with a constrained implant should be made before external fixation is used

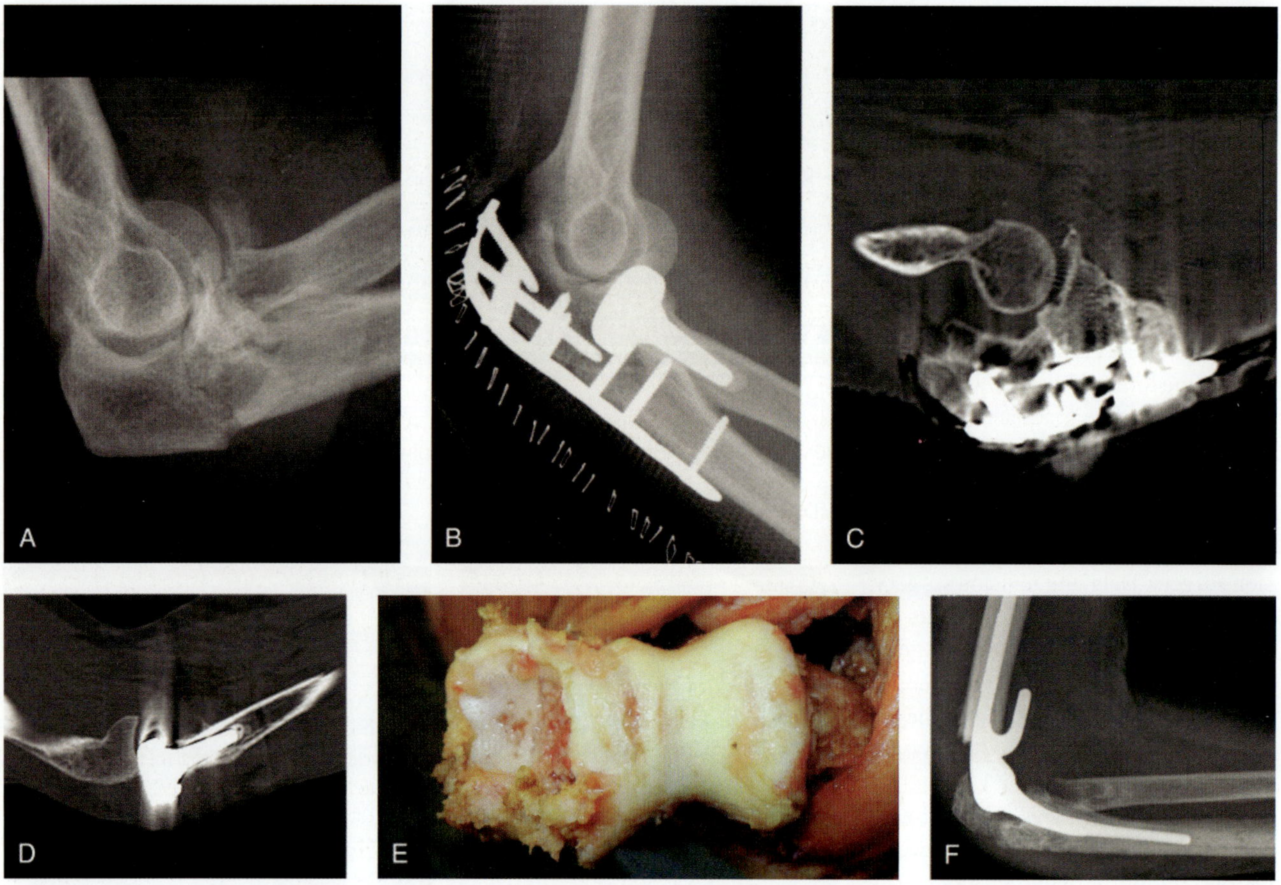

**Figure 6** Lateral radiographs (**A** and **B**) and sagittal CT scans (**C** and **D**) of the elbow from a 77-year-old patient who fell while playing tennis and underwent attempted open reduction internal fixation of the elbow joint and fractures. The patient had limited motion and pain 1 year postinjury. Previous attempts to restore the architecture of and reduce the elbow joint were unsuccessful. **E,** Intraoperative photograph shows the appearance of the elbow joint at the time of revision surgery. **F,** Lateral radiograph of the elbow obtained after the patient underwent total elbow replacement, which allowed for excellent results during light activities. The patient quit playing tennis and golf to reduce the risk for loosening. (Copyright Robert Hotchkiss, MD, New York, NY.)

because a pin-tract infection usually will delay TEA as a result of concern for losing the entire joint arthroplasty to infection.

Revision surgery for additional stabilization, often in the form of external fixation in younger patients, may be necessary and should help eliminate the risk for refractory dislocation; however, stiffness, pin-tract problems, and the complexity of revision surgery may be problematic. TEA in older patients usually offers a definitive treatment; however, patients will be subject to the activity restrictions and lifting limits currently recommended for elbow implants.

## Treatment of Refractory Dislocation: Saving the Cartilage

If an elbow has slipped into a dislocated position more than 2 to 3 weeks after the initial injury, fibrosis usually has occurred, resulting in a stiff and dislocated elbow. An attempt at closed reduction is unwise because of the risk for additional injury to the elbow joint. It is much safer to perform revision surgery to systematically mobilize the soft tissues, remove the intra-articular fibrous tissue that blocks reduction, preserve the ligaments for repair, and reduce the joint. A full contracture release, repair of the ligaments and fractures, and perhaps the use of external fixation is required to protect the repairs (**Figure 7**). A reduced joint that has even a small amount of motion may become stiff; however, the cartilage can and may survive. Stiffness can be addressed with the use of a contracture release that can be performed at a later date if necessary.

## The Effect of Time From Initial Injury

If joint dislocation has persisted for a period between 6 and 12 weeks, the contracture is well established and more extensive excision of capsule is required. Identification and mobilization of the ulnar, median, and radial nerves may be necessary. The triceps tendon will be adherent to the posterior distal humerus and require elevation from the humerus. Usually, the biceps and brachialis are tight but not adherent and the joint surfaces are damaged but usable. The patient should be warned that the future of the joint cartilage may remain unknown for several years.

Often, the greatest obstacle to durable, stable motion between 6 and 12 weeks after initial treatment is an unreduced or absent medial coronoid. In patients in whom the medial coronoid is missing or simply has been resorbed, the use of substitutes has been reported. However, an exact match is a challenge. An alternative that should be considered is to limit the degree of extension permitted. A planned flexion contracture of 30° to 40° can permit a stable, 100° arc of motion and averts the need for a coronoid reconstruction.

Refractory dislocations that are managed 4 to 6 months after injury seldom have viable cartilage and, depending on the age of the patient, will likely require interposition arthroplasty or TEA. If the subchondral bone is intact without deep erosions or cavitation, interposition arthroplasty may be successful, providing the elbow with limited motion but a reduced capacity for loading and strength. Even if treatment is successful within the first 3 to 5 years, the future outlook is guarded. Often, patients learn to reduce the load on the elbow and tolerate less demanding use as long as they have elbow stability and function sufficient for activities of daily living.

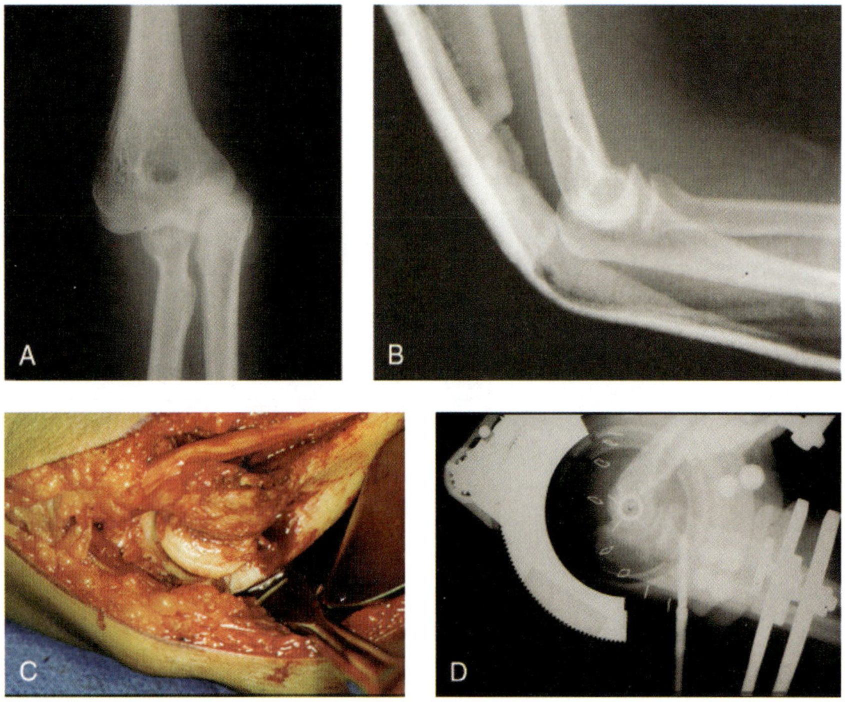


**Figure 7** AP (**A**) and lateral (**B**) radiographs of the elbow from a 56-year-old woman who fell while skiing demonstrate a medial elbow dislocation. After several attempts at closed reduction, the elbow was splinted in a dislocated position for 6 weeks. **C,** Intraoperative photograph of the elbow after open reduction with complete capsular excision and removal of interposed tissue in the joint. **D,** Lateral radiograph of the elbow demonstrates hinged external fixation, which was used to stabilize the elbow joint and permit motion. (Copyright Robert Hotchkiss, MD, New York, NY.)

## Contraindications

Contraindications to surgical repair of refractory elbow dislocation include medical or psychiatric conditions preventing surgical management or the required postoperative rehabilitation. Severe joint destruction is a relative contraindication to an open relocation without interposition or TEA.

## Alternative Treatments

The only alternative treatment is observation and pain management.

## Results

Although most case studies of patients who have long-standing subluxation or dislocation involve small and heterogeneous populations, they make several key points. Open management is necessary to mobilize and clear scar tissue from the elbow joint. Many of the patients in these studies underwent prior surgical treatment. Most patients in these studies achieved elbow stability with a functional ROM. Although adverse events are common postoperatively, most are minor (**Table 1**).

## Techniques

### Setup/Exposure

- General or regional anesthesia is used.
- In patients in whom the use of a hinged external fixator is planned, the patient is placed in either the lateral decubitus position with the affected side up or in the prone position with the affected limb on a hand table. Either of these positions allows for the application of an external fixator with greater ease compared with the supine position (**Figure 8**).

**Table 1** Results of Treatment for Refractory Elbow Dislocation[a]

| Author(s) (Year) | Number of Patients | Procedure or Approach | Mean Patient Age in Years (Range) | Mean Follow-up in Months (Range) | Results |
|---|---|---|---|---|---|
| Krishnamoorthy et al (1976) | 26 | No fixator was used<br>Elbow was splinted at 90° for 2-4 wk postoperatively | NR (6-60) | NR (3-102) | 12 of the 23 patients from whom follow-up ROM data were obtained regained >130° of flexion<br>Mean delay in treatment, 7 wk; 12 cases were dislocated for 1-4 wk (5 of these were dislocated for only 1-2 wk) |
| Jupiter and Ring (2002) | 5 | Open reduction in all patients; reattachment of LCL in 3 patients<br>Hinged external fixation in all patients | 49 (30-59) | 38 (12-98) | Mean maximum flexion, 136°<br>Mean flexion contracture, 13°<br>Mean delay in treatment, 11 wk |
| Devnani (2004) | 9 | Open reduction | 30 (9-60) | 48 (12-138) | The elbow was held in reduction with the use of 1.6- or 2-mm Kirschner wires from the humerus to the radius; the wires were removed 4-5 wk postoperatively<br>2 patients achieved >130° of flexion<br>Mean delay in treatment, 8 mo |
| Ring et al (2004) | 13 | Open reduction, radial head repair or replacement, LCL repair, hinged external fixation, and ulnar nerve transposition; 6 patients underwent coronoid reconstruction with radial head autograft | 45 (26-74) | 57 (NR) | Mean maximum flexion, 124°<br>Mean flexion contracture, 24°<br>Mean delay in treatment, 2 mo |
| Mahaisavariya and Laupattarakasem (2005) | 24 | Open reduction, repair of the ligaments, and triceps lengthening | 24.6 (7-60) | 48.3 (12-132) | Elbows were pinned for 2-3 wk postoperatively<br>Mean maximum flexion, 122°<br>Mean flexion contracture, 40°<br>Mean delay in treatment, 7.9 mo<br>10 patients had elbow dislocations for <2 wk |

LCL = lateral collateral ligament, NR = not reported, ROM = range of motion.

[a] All studies are level IV evidence.

- In patients in whom no external fixation is planned, the supine position may be used.
- Often, a single posterior skin incision is used. This incision allows for both medial and lateral access to the elbow joint after skin flaps are developed on the appropriate side.
- Medial or lateral approaches to the elbow are used, depending on the site of the pathology that needs to be addressed.
- In most patients, the ulnar nerve is identified, freed from scar tissue, and transposed.

## Instruments/Equipment/ Implants Required

- Long right-angled retractors, large Bennett retractors, and large Gelpi retractors are helpful.
- No. 3-0 nylon suture, which is used to tie skin edges back for retraction, is often helpful.

 

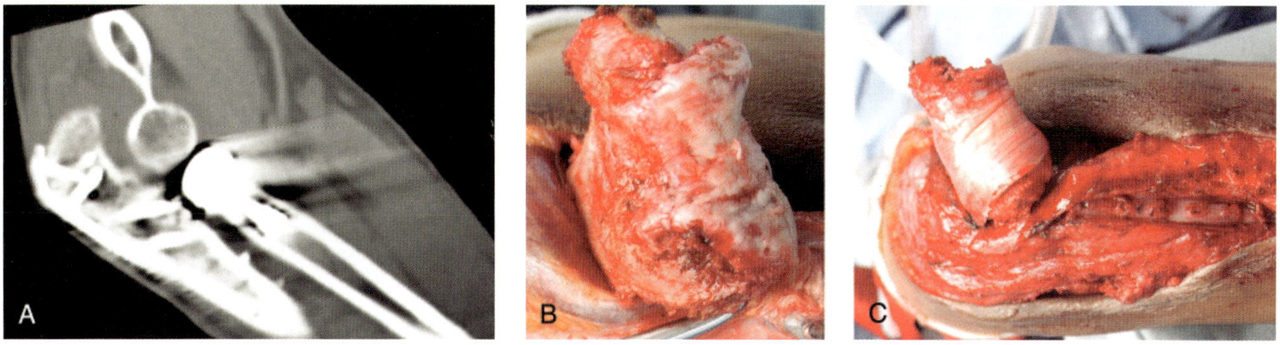


**Figure 8** Images of the elbow from a 24-year-old man who sought treatment for stiffness and pain 9 months after open reduction and internal fixation of a complex proximal ulnar fracture and replacement of a prosthetic radial head. **A,** Sagittal CT scan demonstrates subluxation of the ulnohumeral joint into a coronoid defect. **B,** Intraoperative photograph shows severe deterioration of the articular cartilage. **C,** Intraoperative photograph shows that interposition arthroplasty was performed, and that the distal humerus was resurfaced with the use of an Achilles tendon allograft. Postoperatively, a hinged external fixator was used to maintain reduction for 6 weeks. (Copyright Robert Hotchkiss, MD, New York, NY.)

- A Kerrison rongeur is useful for decompression if perineural heterotopic bone is present around the ulnar nerve.
- A headlight is helpful.
- A high-speed 3-mm burr is useful for making drill holes for collateral ligament reconstruction.
- The authors of this chapter always have a hinged external fixator set available. The authors prefer to use a Compass hinge with half rings because of the worm gear, which allows for a passive externally applied stretch.
- Fibrin sealant helps decrease postoperative bleeding and is used for deep wound closure.

## Procedure

### SURGICAL APPROACH: LATERAL SIDE

- The authors of this chapter typically approach the elbow joint at the midaxis of the radiocapitellar joint. This approach preserves the LCL. A traditional Kocher approach may put the LCL at risk of being cut. Great care is taken to avoid direct exposure of the posterolateral corner, which is defined as the entire soft-tissue sleeve posterior to the midaxis of the radiocapitellar joint, because this tissue is important for preserving elbow stability and can be used to reinforce the LCL repair.
- If dissection extends distal to the proximal radioulnar joint along the lateral side of the elbow, the posterior interosseous nerve is identified and protected.
- If dissection extends proximal to the lateral supracondylar ridge, the radial nerve proper is identified between the brachialis and brachioradialis muscles and traced across the elbow joint for protection.
- The lateral approach is used for removal, repair, or replacement of the radial head; repair or reconstruction of the LCL; or repair of other lateral structures.

### SURGICAL APPROACH: MEDIAL SIDE

- On the medial side, the authors of this chapter use the over-the-top approach.
- The ulnar nerve is identified and traced proximally and distally.
- The first few small posterior nerve branches are cut to achieve adequate length for the transposition. Often, the ulnar nerve has been dissected during prior surgical treatment and is encased in scar tissue or bone.
- The ulnar nerve is mobilized sufficiently to allow transposition into the anterior subcutaneous tissues at the conclusion of the procedure.
- The flexor-pronator mass is split in the middle, of which the proximal/anterior one-half along with the brachialis muscle is elevated off the elbow joint, the elbow capsule is incised, and the elbow joint is entered.
- One-half of the flexor-pronator origin is available on the medial epicondyle for repair.
- The medial approach can be used to repair the tip of the coronoid.
- To expose the medial coronoid, the ulnar nerve is dissected and transposed, and the split in the flexor carpi ulnaris at the ulnar nerve runs is opened distally. To expose the insertion of the medial collateral ligament onto the sublime tubercle and the medial coronoid, the muscle is elevated bluntly with the use of an elevator.

### SURGICAL APPROACH: LONG-STANDING DISLOCATIONS

- Long-standing elbow dislocation distorts the anatomy.
- Care is taken to avoid injury to the collateral ligaments by staying within safe intervals and re-creating the avulsion injury of the ligaments from the epicondyles to gain better exposure.

- Usually, the collateral ligaments will heal back to the epicondyles and stabilize the elbow as long as the elbow is located for at least 1 month postoperatively.
- Tendon grafts are not necessary to restore stability unless there is loss of ligament substance resulting from débridement or injury.
- The elbow joint is cleared of fibrous tissue and relocated.
- The radial head and medial coronoid facet are repaired or reconstructed.
- The LCL is reattached to the lateral epicondyle with the use of suture anchors or suture that is passed through drill holes. The authors of this chapter prefer to use a braided nonabsorbable No. 2 running locked suture.
- Three 3.0-mm burr holes are placed in the lateral epicondyle in an inverted triangle fashion.
- The suture ends are passed into the apical hole, with one suture arm pulled through each of the base holes.
- The two ends of the suture are tied over the bone bridge with the elbow positioned in 45° of flexion.
- The radial head is excised, repaired, or replaced.
- After these repairs, if the elbow demonstrates congruent ROM from 70° to full flexion with no gapping and no gross instability, the wound is closed in layers, and the elbow is splinted in 110° of flexion.
- Tenuous fixation of the medial coronoid and a tendency for residual subluxation are managed with supplementary static or hinged external fixation.

#### SURGICAL APPROACH: EXTERNAL FIXATORS

- It is easier to apply a static external fixator than a hinged external fixator. Static external fixation requires exposure proximal to the lateral supracondylar ridge.
- The radial nerve is at risk for injury at the location at which it crosses from posterior to anterior, approximately 14 cm proximal to the lateral epicondyle.
- Two lateral pins are placed proximally in the humerus and two are placed on the lateral side of the ulna diaphysis.
- A static external fixator is applied to the pins with the elbow positioned in approximately 90° of flexion.
- Alternatively, a hinged external fixator can be applied (**Figures 2**, 7, and **8**). Several hinged external fixators are available.
- The key to all external fixation devices is the appropriate placement of the axis pin directly in the center of rotation of the elbow joint, which is accomplished most easily with both the lateral and medial epicondyles exposed and with the use of fluoroscopic imaging. The axis pin is in the correct position if it appears as a single dot in the center of the circle created by the capitellum on lateral fluoroscopic imaging.
- The flexor-pronator origin and the lateral extensor muscles are reattached to the epicondyles with the use of No. 2 braided nonabsorbable suture.
- The ulnar nerve is transposed and maintained anteriorly with the use of a strip of medial intermuscular septum or subcutaneous fat.

### Wound Closure

- The wounds are closed in layers using standard techniques.

## Postoperative Regimen

Beginning at the time of the surgery, the authors of this chapter administer 8 mg of dexamethasone intravenously every 8 hours to most patients who undergo complex elbow procedures, including those who undergo elbow contracture releases, acute fracture fixation, and delayed treatment of subluxated elbows. Although the authors believe that the administration of dexamethasone may help decrease postoperative swelling and improve postoperative ROM, no published evidence exists to support this belief. A postoperative drain is kept in place until less than 20 mL of drainage exists in an 8-hour period. Patients remain hospitalized for 1 or 2 days postoperatively. Often, indwelling brachial plexus catheters are used for pain relief.

The elbow is immobilized in a posterior splint if external fixation was not used. Formal physical therapy is routinely prescribed to assist with stretching exercises. The importance of stretching exercises is emphasized both before and after surgery. Patients in whom external fixation was used should be instructed on proper pin care.

Patients should attend physical therapy two or three times a week for the first 2 weeks postoperatively. Physical therapy sessions allow for repeated evaluations, and the patient may benefit from observing other patients in various stages of recovery. For most patients, weekly radiographs should be obtained in the first 4 weeks postoperatively to ensure concentric reduction. If an external fixator was used, it should be removed between 3 and 6 weeks postoperatively.

## Limiting Adverse Events

Adverse events are common. Notable cartilage damage may be best managed with interposition arthroplasty or TEA (**Figure 4**). Damage to the radial nerve from proximal pin placement can be reduced with the use of direct visualization of the bone and, perhaps, the radial nerve. Ulnar nerve dysfunction is common after dissection and mobilization. Usually, the ulnar nerve recovers after many months; however, recovery may be incomplete.

Pin-tract infections are common and often can be treated with oral antibiotics alone. Postoperative seroma may develop in patients with posterior incisions and large skin flaps. Infection of a seroma is uncommon; however, the authors of this chapter monitor for seroma infection until a seroma resolves. Large seromas may require aspiration. The authors of this chapter prefer to treat patients with the use of oral antibiotics until wounds cease all drainage. Occasionally, a postoperative hematoma may require surgical treatment. A deep infection can be managed with one or more surgeries to débride and irrigate the wound as well as with the use of intravenous antibiotics.

## Bibliography

Arafiles RP: Neglected posterior dislocation of the elbow: A reconstruction operation. *J Bone Joint Surg Br* 1987;69(2):199-202.

Bruce C, Laing P, Dorgan J, Klenerman L: Unreduced dislocation of the elbow: Case report and review of the literature. *J Trauma* 1993;35(6):962-965.

Devnani AS: Outcome of longstanding dislocated elbows treated by open reduction and excision of collateral ligaments. *Singapore Med J* 2004;45(1):14-19.

di Schino M, Breda Y, Grimaldi FM, Lorthioir JM, Merrien Y: Surgical treatment of neglected elbow dislocations: Report of 81 cases. *Rev Chir Orthop Reparatrice Appar Mot* 1990;76(5):303-310.

Jupiter JB, Ring D: Treatment of unreduced elbow dislocations with hinged external fixation. *J Bone Joint Surg Am* 2002;84(9):1630-1635.

Krishnamoorthy S, Bose K, Wong KP: Treatment of old unreduced dislocation of the elbow. *Injury* 1976;8(1):39-42.

Lyons RP, Armstrong A: Chronically unreduced elbow dislocations. *Hand Clin* 2008;24(1):91-103.

Mahaisavariya B, Laupattarakasem W: Neglected dislocation of the elbow. *Clin Orthop Relat Res* 2005;(431):21-25.

Naidoo KS: Unreduced posterior dislocations of the elbow. *J Bone Joint Surg Br* 1982;64(5):603-606.

Ring D, Hannouche D, Jupiter JB: Surgical treatment of persistent dislocation or subluxation of the ulnohumeral joint after fracture-dislocation of the elbow. *J Hand Surg Am* 2004;29(3):470-480.

Ruch DS, Triepel CR: Hinged elbow fixation for recurrent instability following fracture dislocation. *Injury* 2001;32(suppl 4):SD70-SD78.

Schreiber JJ, Paul S, Hotchkiss RN, Daluiski A: Conservative management of elbow dislocations with an overhead motion protocol. *J Hand Surg Am* 2015;40(3):515-519.

Tan V, Daluiski A, Capo J, Hotchkiss R: Hinged elbow external fixators: Indications and uses. *J Am Acad Orthop Surg* 2005;13(8):503-514.

# Chapter 27
# Nonunion of the Distal Humerus

*Peter Kloen, MD, PhD*
*David L. Helfet, MD*

**Learning Objectives**

- Gain a thorough understanding of the techniques of débridement and release of a distal humeral nonunion in order to maximize postoperative range of motion.
- Gain an improved understanding of the technique of modified locking fixation in areas of altered or compromised bone stock associated with a distal humeral nonunion.

## Indications

Distal humeral nonunion usually is located at the supracondylar level. Mobility at the nonunion site typically causes disabling pain and instability. Implants eventually break or loosen, often with a windshield-wiper effect of the screws in the bone, leading to further bone loss and further complicating internal fixation. Scar tissue often compresses the ulnar nerve. Ultimately, the patient will be unable to use the arm for loading activities and/or position the forearm and hand against gravity. Factors commonly associated with distal humeral nonunions are multiple failed surgeries, smoking, infection, poor bone quality, and obesity.

Nonunions are classified radiographically as hypertrophic, oligotrophic, or atrophic per the criteria established by Weber and Čech. In addition, the nonunions can be subclassified on the basis of location, whether supracondylar, transcondylar, intercondylar, unicondylar (medial or lateral), or osteochondral. It can be difficult to accurately measure the size of the distal fragment based on evaluation of the AP radiograph alone because the fragment is often flexed on that view. CT helps determine the actual size of the distal fragment (**Figure 1**).

Associated infection must be considered in any nonunion, even if the patient does not exhibit clear symptoms such as fever, drainage, or wound problems. Therefore, nonunions could be further classified as aseptic, presumed aseptic, or septic. Some nonunions are associated with a malunion.

The authors of this chapter prefer to manage most distal humeral nonunions with open reduction and internal fixation (ORIF). Fixation is similar to that used to manage acute distal humeral fractures. However, surgical techniques for nonunion place greater emphasis on preoperative planning, careful surgical exposure, release, and bone grafting. During preoperative planning, the surgeon should scrutinize all previous surgical notes and carefully assess the patient's neurovascular status, scars, and condition of the soft tissues. A preoperative drawing outlining the surgical tactic will help anticipate and prevent intraoperative complications (**Figure 2**).

## Contraindications

A distal humeral nonunion often leads to a flail and painful arm. Because of the resulting disability, there are very few contraindications to surgical management of nonunion. The only salvage procedure is a total elbow arthroplasty (TEA). Contraindications for internal or external fixation are infirmity, advanced age and low activity demand, severe distal humeral bone loss, and irreversible damage to the articular surface of the ununited segment.

---

*Dr. Helfet or an immediate family member serves as an unpaid consultant to OHK Medical Devices, HealthpointCapital, and Tri-Medics, and has stock or stock options held in OHK Medical Devices and FxDevices. Neither Dr. Kloen nor any immediate family member has received anything of value from or has stock or stock options held in a commercial company or institution related directly or indirectly to the subject of this chapter.*

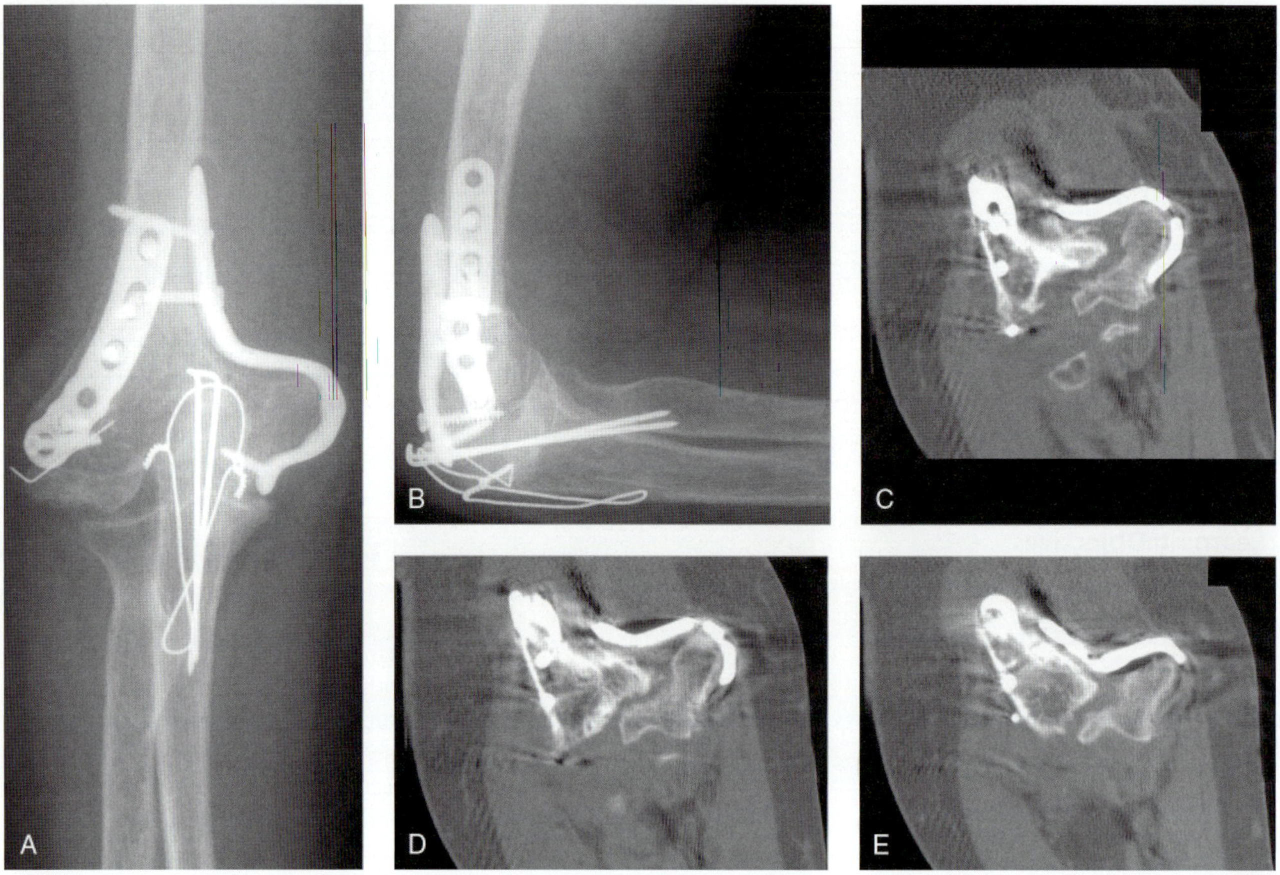


**Figure 1** Images of the elbow from a 60-year-old woman who sought treatment for pain at the fracture site and limited range of motion 8 months after undergoing open reduction and internal fixation of a right-side distal humeral fracture. AP (**A**) and lateral (**B**) radiographs and coronal CT scans (**C, D,** and **E**) demonstrate nonunion and loss of fixation with plate breakage (medial side).

## Alternative Treatments

Surgical alternatives to ORIF have included fusion, distraction arthroplasty, allograft, prosthetic replacement, and the Ilizarov technique. Historically, an elbow arthrodesis was considered an alternative for a flail, nonreconstructible elbow joint. However, obtaining bone fusion is difficult when bone stock is limited. Daily activities are limited with a fused elbow, and few patients elect to undergo this salvage procedure.

Limited data are available on the use of elbow allograft. A report on a series of 10 cadaver elbow transplants for various elbow conditions described four patients with distal humeral nonunion who were treated with cadaver elbow allograft. Patients were followed for 1 to 6 years. Indications were disabling elbow joint symptoms in patients who refused an arthrodesis or were not candidates for prosthetic replacement because of excessive bone loss or young age. The patients in that series had substantial complications. It is noteworthy that in these cadaver elbows, degenerative joint changes increased with time, as with neuropathic joints. Risk of nonunion of the allograft-host junction, allograft resorption, and disease transmission are concerns with this treatment method. Because of these concerns, elbow allograft should be considered a salvage procedure.

Elbow replacement is a good salvage procedure in low-demand, often elderly (older than 70 years) patients. Its drawbacks are a limited lifespan of the prosthesis, component wear, loosening, and subsequent need for revision. Results of prosthetic elbow replacement as a salvage procedure after trauma are inferior and less predictable than results after primary elbow replacement. However, satisfactory results can be obtained if complications are avoided. Heavy lifting is discouraged after TEA. Young, active patients might not accept these limitations. A previous infection is a relative contraindication for TEA. Goals of prosthetic replacement are a functional range of motion (ROM) with relief of pain. Indications for replacement rather than internal fixation are a distal humerus that is either too osteopenic or comminuted for reduction and fixation and the presence of extensive articular

 

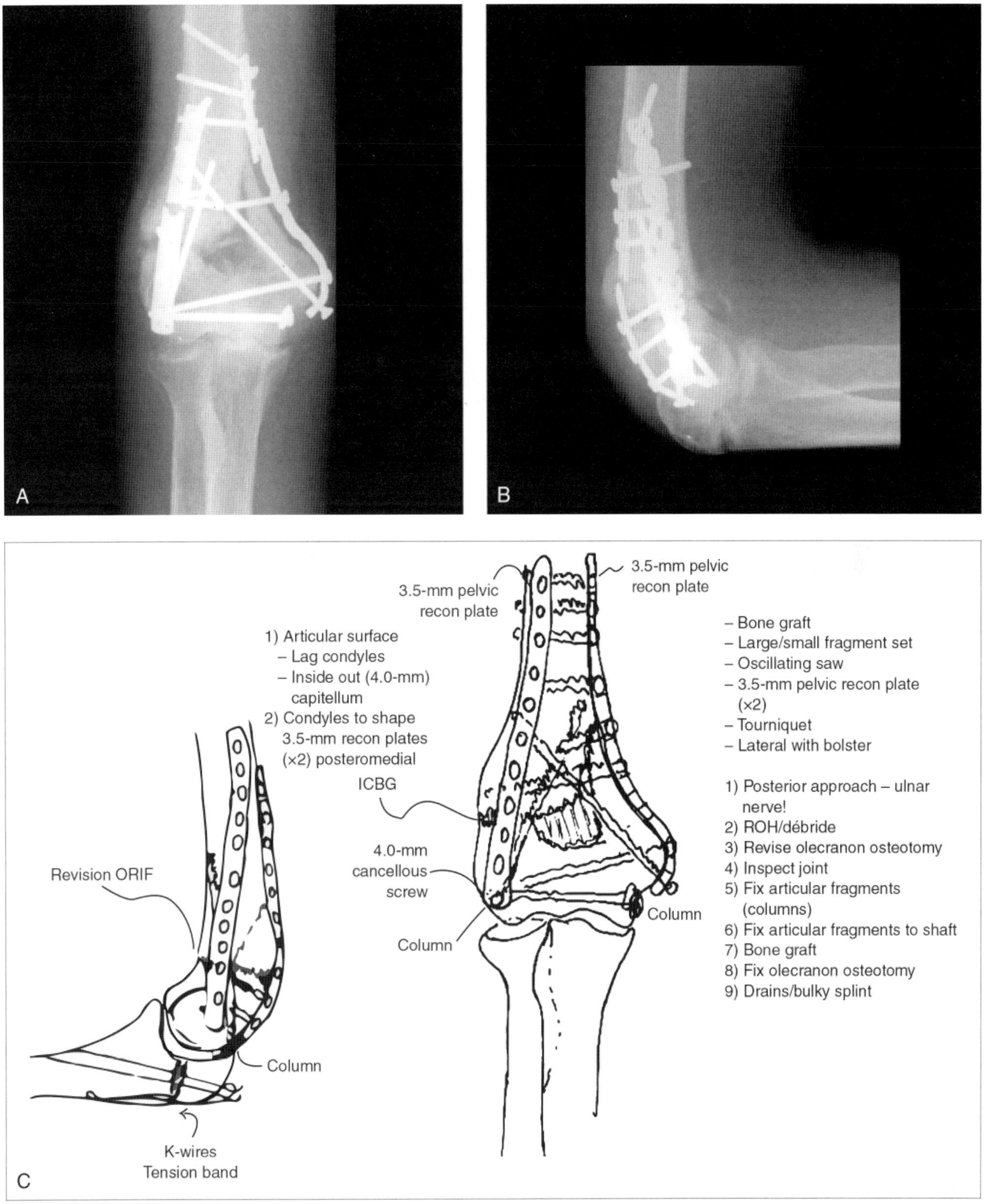


**Figure 2** Preoperative AP (**A**) and lateral (**B**) radiographs demonstrate distal humeral nonunion 6 months after previous open reduction and internal fixation. **C,** Illustration of the preoperative plan shows the stepwise surgical details needed to achieve 40° anterior angulation of the distal humerus. ICBG = iliac crest bone graft, K-wires = Kirschner wires, ORIF = open reduction and internal fixation, recon = reconstruction, ROH = removal of hardware.

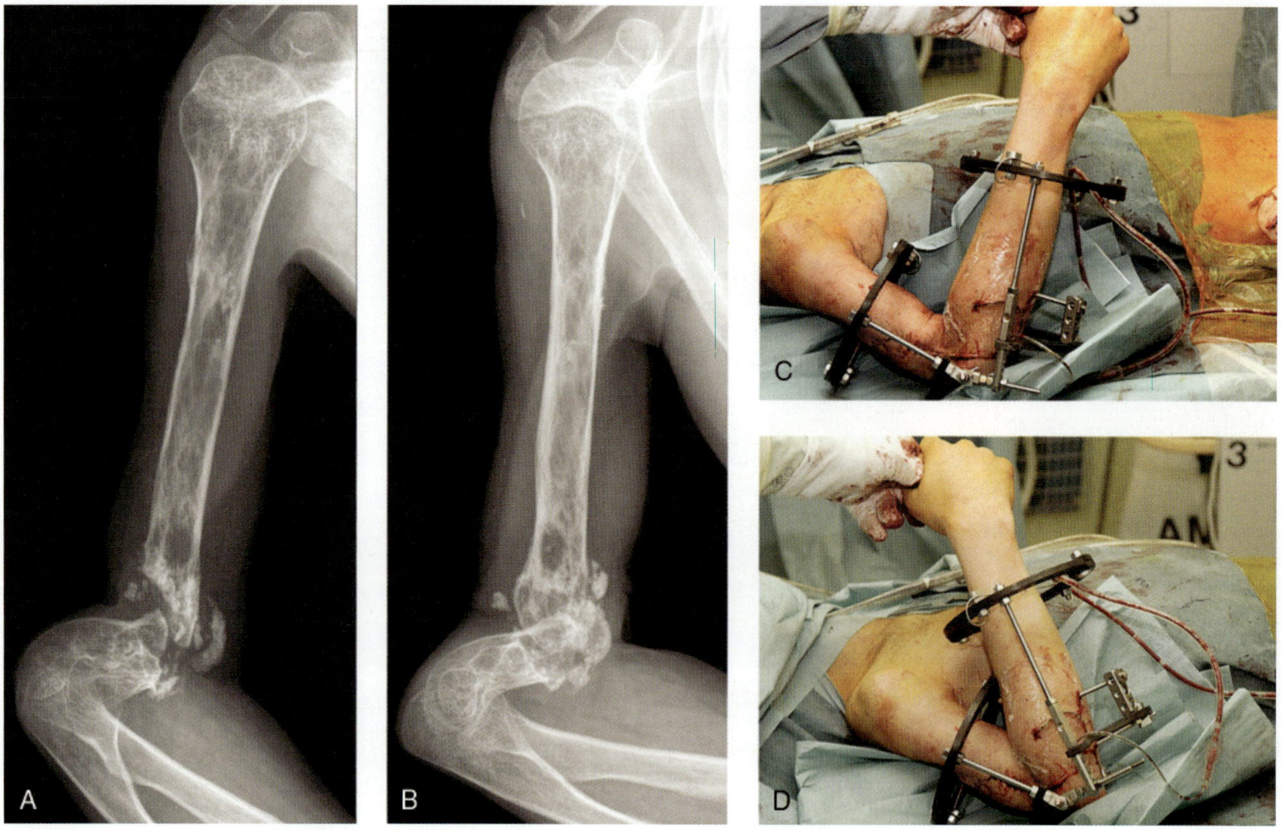


**Figure 3** Images from a 26-year-old man who underwent the Ilizarov technique to manage distal humeral nonunion. **A** and **B,** Lateral radiographs demonstrate the nonunion and stiff elbow joint. Motion was limited to the nonunion site. **C** and **D,** Intraoperative photographs show the Ilizarov frame with an elbow hinge after the nonunion was débrided and an intramedullary nail placed as an internal strut. These images also show the maximum extension (**C**) and flexion (**D**) possible with the frame in place.

disease such as rheumatoid arthritis, posttraumatic arthritis, or ankylosis. The ideal surgical candidate is an older patient with good soft tissues and no prior infection who will comply with postoperative rehabilitation and restrictions.

Small case series have reported use of the Ilizarov technique to manage infected nonunions. An infected distal humeral nonunion often presents after multiple failed surgeries with loss of bone stock, capsular contracture, compromised soft tissues, and ulnar nerve symptoms. Because bone healing depends on eradicating the infection while maintaining a stable fixation and alignment, theoretically the Ilizarov technique might be ideal for patients with this complex presentation. However, the learning curve for performing the technique properly is steep, and patients must be motivated because the frame is cumbersome. In addition, thorough preoperative planning is essential to optimize the surgical procedure. The first of two small series published in the English-language literature showed an 80% union rate in five patients; however, each patient required more than one procedure. The second series presented a single-stage procedure with débridement, release, shortening, Ilizarov frame fixation, and bone grafting, which resulted in healing in all six patients treated.

The authors of this chapter have limited experience with the Ilizarov technique. A 26-year-old man sustained a distal humeral nonunion. At age 8 years, he had undergone chemotherapy and radiation (65 Gy in 60 fractions) to manage a Ewing sarcoma of his humerus. At age 12 years, he sustained a distal humeral fracture and wore a cast for 2 years. Numerous surgeons were consulted during that 2-year period, but surgery was thought to be too risky because the patient's upper arm had remained much the same size as when he was 8 years old, with a thickened, stiff skin and a soft-tissue cuff around the nonunion. He functioned reasonably well and entered medical school anticipating a career in plastic surgery. During medical school, he experienced increasing pain and instability of the arm and sought treatment. Motion was limited to the nonunion site, with a stiff elbow joint (**Figure 3**, **A** and **B**). Treatment with ORIF was not an option. The patient was referred to an expert in the Ilizarov technique, who agreed to operate in a combined procedure with the authors of this chapter.

 

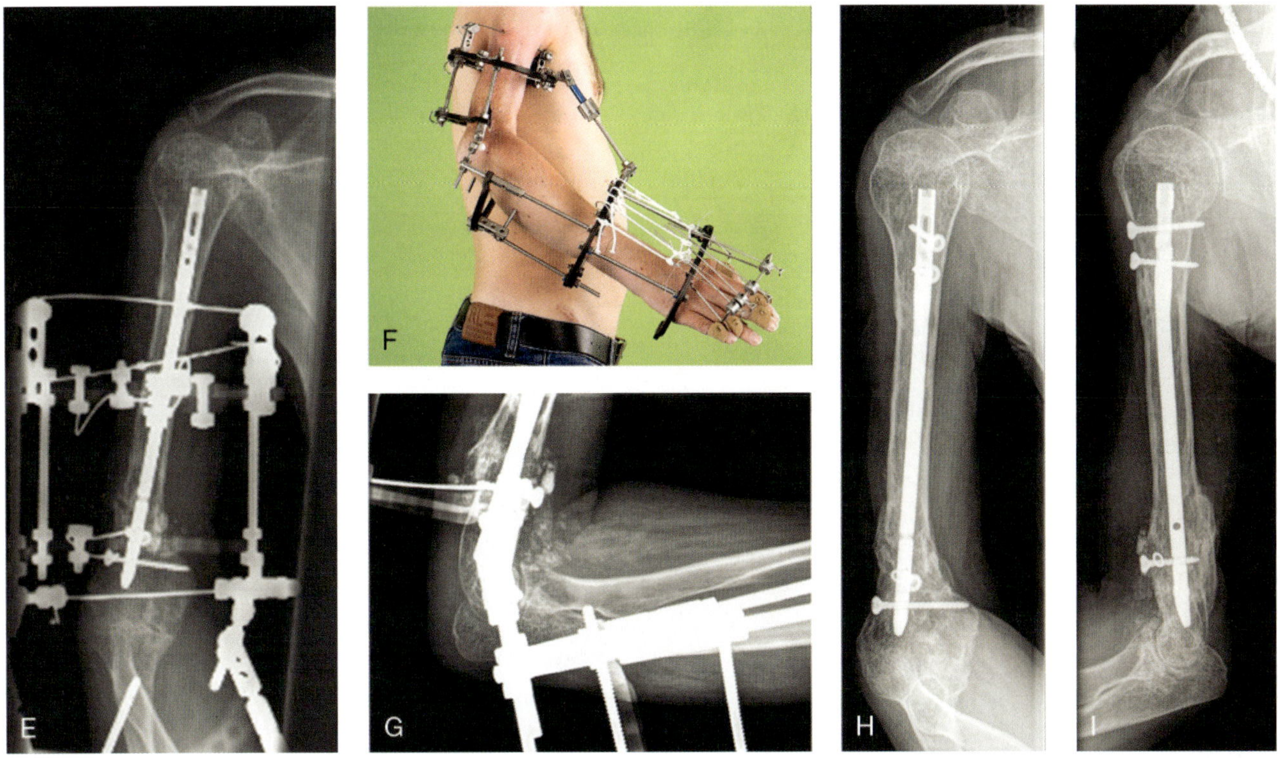


**Figure 3** *(continued)* Images from a 26-year-old man who underwent the Ilizarov technique to manage distal humeral nonunion. AP radiograph (**E**), photograph (**F**), and lateral radiograph (**G**) obtained 6 months postoperatively. Additional bone graft was placed at 6 months. At that time, the Ilizarov frame was removed and the nail was locked proximally. AP (**H**) and lateral (**I**) radiographs obtained 5 years postoperatively demonstrate a healed nonunion. The median nerve fully returned to function, but the radial nerve deficit remained complete.

Using a minimal approach, the nonunion was débrided and an intramedullary nail was placed as an internal strut, after which an Ilizarov frame with an elbow hinge was placed (**Figure 3, C** through **G**). Autologous bone graft was added locally. During the first 24 hours postoperatively, increasing swelling as well as median and radial nerve deficits developed, likely because of anasarca caused by compromised lymph outflow. Exploration of the median and radial nerves was done on postoperative day 2. The median nerve recovered within days but the radial nerve did not recover. Additional bone graft was added 6 months postoperatively, at which time the Ilizarov frame was removed and the nail was locked proximally. The nonunion healed (**Figure 3, H** and **I**). The median nerve returned to full function, but the complete radial nerve deficit persisted. Ten years and 6 months postoperatively, the patient was pleased with the outcome despite the radial nerve deficit. There was no pain, and his elbow was stable. At the time this chapter was written, the patient was working as a radiologist and had returned to all athletic activities, including downhill skiing.

## Results

Since the early 1980s, fewer than 20 reports specifically regarding the treatment of distal humeral nonunions have been published in the English-language literature (**Tables 1** and **2**). Most series reported on internal fixation, although two small subgroups used TEA or Ilizarov fixation. ORIF is described in this chapter.

## Techniques

### Setup/Exposure

- Surgery can be done with the patient placed prone or in the lateral decubitus position. The authors of this chapter prefer the lateral decubitus position because setup time is less and enables the anesthesiologist to more easily monitor the patient.
- Prone positioning is preferred in surgeries in which a large quantity of autologous bone graft is necessary and previous harvesting has depleted anterior iliac crest graft.
- For an osteochondral shearing type nonunion, a lateral approach might be best, with the patient positioned supine with the surgical arm abducted on an arm table.
- Positioning the patient in the lateral decubitus position can be

**Table 1** Results of Nonarthroplasty Management of Nonunion of the Distal Humerus[a]

| Authors (Year) | No. of Patients | Procedure or Approach | Mean Patient Age in Years (Range) | Mean Follow-up in Months (Range) | Success Rate (%) | Results |
|---|---|---|---|---|---|---|
| Mitsunaga et al (1982) | 25 | ORIF and grafting via a posterior or lateral approach (23)<br>ORIF via a posterior or lateral approach followed by external fixation (2) | 43 | 29 (12-72) | 88 | Mean ROM, 71°<br>Mean pain score, 1.3 on a 4-point scale<br>6 patients required multiple surgeries |
| Ackerman and Jupiter (1988) | 20 | ORIF (17), distal humerus allograft (2), immobilization in (1) | 40 (20-70) | 43.2 (13-108) | 94 | Mean ROM, 76° (range, 30°-130°)<br>Jupiter scores were excellent in 1 patient, good in 6, fair in 7, and poor in 6<br>1 patient was treated with a custom total elbow implant |
| Sanders and Sackett (1990) | 5 | Posterior approach, decortication, ORIF, and graft | 56.2 (22-81) | 40 (24-65) | 100 | Mean ROM, 86° (range, 38°-124°)<br>Modified Cassebaum score was good in 2 patients, fair in 2, and poor in 1 |
| Jupiter and Goodman (1992) | 6 | Posterior approach, débridement, release, ORIF, graft | 68 (55-85) | 18 (12-30) | 100 | Mean ROM, 102° (range, 90°-110°)<br>Broberg-Morrey scores were good in 5 patients and fair in 1<br>HSS scores were excellent in 2 patients, good in 3, and fair in 1 |
| McKee et al (1994) | 13 | Posterior or lateral approach, débridement, ORIF, graft | 39.7 (17-62) | 25 (12-60) | 100 | Mean ROM, 97° (range, 55°-125°)<br>Mean Morrey and Bryan score, 83 (range, 60-97): excellent in 2 patients, good in 8, and fair in 3 |
| Ring et al (1999) | 5 | Thin wire fixation, débridement, vascularized graft | 40.2 (15-67) | 43.2 (24-72) | 80 | At the time of surgery, 4 patients had infected elbows and 1 had a contaminated elbow<br>Mean ROM, 94° (range, 90°-100°)<br>All 4 patients who were successfully treated underwent a second operation |
| Paramasivan et al (2000) | 8 | Transolecranon, arthrolysis, IM nail antegrade, graft | 40.7 (20-62) | 32.1 (22-41) | 88 | Mean ROM, 94° (range, 10°-130°) |
| Helfet et al (2003) | 52 | Posterior approach, release, débridement, ORIF, graft | 47 (16-88) | 33 (3-198) | 98 | Mean ROM, 94° (range, 10°-145°)<br>Preoperatively 13 patients had delayed union and 39 had nonunion |

ASES = American Shoulder and Elbow Surgeons; DASH = Disabilities of the Arm, Shoulder and Hand; HSS = Hospital for Special Surgery; IM = intramedullary; MEPI = Mayo Elbow Performance Index; MEPS = Mayo Elbow Performance Score; ORIF = open reduction and internal fixation; QALY = quality-adjusted life year; ROM = range of motion; SF-12 = Medical Outcomes Study 12-Item Short Form.

[a] All studies are level IV evidence.

 

**Table 1** Results of Nonarthroplasty Management of Nonunion of the Distal Humerus[a] (*continued*)

| Authors (Year) | No. of Patients | Procedure or Approach | Mean Patient Age in Years (Range) | Mean Follow-up in Months (Range) | Success Rate (%) | Results |
|---|---|---|---|---|---|---|
| Ring et al (2003) | 15 | Posterior, débridement, ORIF, graft (2 vascularized) | 60 (26-75) | 51 (24-130) | 80 | Mean ROM, 95° (range, 60°-130°)<br>MEPI result was excellent in 2 patients, good in 9, and fair in 1<br>Although 12 nonunions healed, 5 of those patients underwent additional procedures<br>The 3 nonunions that did not heal were managed with total elbow arthroplasty |
| Ali et al (2005) | 16 | Posterior approach, débridement, ORIF, graft | 47 (19-82) | 39 (8-69) | 100 | Mean ROM, 96° (range, 45°-130°)<br>Mean MEPS score, 88 (range, 50-100)<br>MEPS score was excellent in 11 patients, good in 2, fair in 2, and poor in 1<br>1 patient underwent additional grafting |
| Beredjiklian et al (2005) | 5 | Posterior approach, release, débridement, ORIF, vascularized graft | 48 (29-70) | 15.2 (9-24) | 80 | Average ROM arc 94° (80°-110°)<br>1 failure resulting from articular collapse was managed with a prosthesis |
| Ring and Jupiter (2006) | 3 | ORIF | 35 (18-47) | 33.6 (27-46) | 100 | All 3 patients had osteochondral nonunion<br>Mean ROM, 100° (range, 90°-115°)<br>Mean MEPI score, 85 (range, 80-95)<br>Mean DASH score, 19.5 (range, 4-35)<br>Mean ASES score, 90 (range, 80-95) |
| Brinker et al (2007) | 6 | Débridement, shortening via Ilizarov, graft | 49.9 (33-77) | 49.2 (24-84) | 100 | All 6 distal humeral nonunions were infected at the time of surgery<br>Mean ROM, 81° (range, 70°-100°)<br>Mean DASH score, 77 (range, 50-93)<br>Mean SF-12 score, 44.8 (range, 33.8-53.4)<br>Mean QALY improvement, 3.8 |
| Allende and Allende (2009) | 24 | Posterior or lateral approach, release, débridement, ORIF, graft | 45 (19-73) | 46 (18-108) | 100 | At the time of surgery, 6 patients had an active infection<br>Mean ROM, 98° (range, 65°-125°)<br>Mean DASH score, 16 (range, 0-36) |

ASES = American Shoulder and Elbow Surgeons; DASH = Disabilities of the Arm, Shoulder and Hand; HSS = Hospital for Special Surgery; IM = intramedullary; MEPI = Mayo Elbow Performance Index; MEPS = Mayo Elbow Performance Score; ORIF = open reduction and internal fixation; QALY = quality-adjusted life year; ROM = range of motion; SF-12 = Medical Outcomes Study 12-Item Short Form.

[a] All studies are level IV evidence.

accomplished with a beanbag with anterior and posterior padding.

- A large roll of sterile gowns is made and placed on the patient's chest, and the surgical arm is positioned over the chest roll.
- The bed is tilted slightly so that the patient rolls forward slightly. This allows for gravity to assist in stabilizing the arm.
- A sterile tourniquet is preferred to increase the surgical field.

**Table 2** Results of Total Elbow Arthroplasty[a]

| Authors (Year) | No. of Patients | Procedure or Approach | Mean Patient Age in Years (Range) | Mean Follow-up in Months (Range) | Results |
|---|---|---|---|---|---|
| Mitsunaga et al (1982) | 7 | Total elbow arthroplasty | 60 | 29 (12-72)[b] | Mean ROM, 103°<br>Mean pain score, 1.8 on a 4-point scale<br>29% of patients underwent revision |
| Figgie et al (1989) | 14 | Semiconstrained elbow replacement | 65 (31-77) | 60 (24-144) | Mean ROM, 100° (range, 65°-120°)<br>Mean HSS score, 84 (range, 57-100)<br>Results were excellent in 6 patients, good in 2, fair in 3, and poor in 3<br>3 patients underwent revision |
| Ramsey et al (1999) | 14 | Semiconstrained elbow replacement | 66 (52-81) | 77 (25-128) | Mean ROM, 108° (range, 60°-140°)<br>MEPI score was excellent in 9 patients, good in 3, and fair in 2<br>2 patients underwent revision |
| Cil et al (2008) | 91 (92 elbows) | Semiconstrained elbow replacement | 65 (22-84) | 78 (6-243.6) | Mean ROM, 113°<br>MEPS score was excellent in 35 elbows, good in 37, fair in 12, and poor in 8<br>5 patients developed deep infections, 5 had component fractures, 4 had periprosthetic fractures, and 12 developed aseptic loosening |

HSS = Hospital for Special Surgery, MEPI = Mayo Elbow Performance Index, MEPS = Mayo Elbow Performance Score, ROM = range of motion.
[a] All studies are level IV evidence.
[b] Follow-up included patients who underwent open reduction and internal fixation.

Alternatively, the patient's arm can be placed on an elevated arm board or arm holder. The contralateral arm is placed on an arm board in abduction, making sure that it does not block intraoperative AP imaging.

- The C-arm is placed parallel to the long axis of the patient's body and perpendicular to the arm to allow AP and lateral views of the arm.
- A sterile stockinet is placed over the hand and forearm.
- All previous incisions are marked with a sterile pen. If there is any doubt regarding safety of incisions, a preoperative consultation with a plastic surgeon is recommended.
- No antibiotics are administered until at least five cultures are obtained (**Figure 4**).
- Ideally, a posterior approach is used. This approach allows elevation of medial and lateral skin flaps as well as an olecranon osteotomy. The incision should be superficial to the fascia over the flexor/pronator mass and to the anconeus muscle.
- If a TEA is considered, the surgical approach needs to be adjusted. A triceps-reflecting anconeus pedicle approach might be better for performing TEA.
- The ulnar nerve is identified first. It is generally easiest to find it proximally; the authors of this chapter do not use loupe magnification.
- With careful dissection, the ulnar nerve is traced toward the elbow and released from scar tissue. Distally, the nerve enters the flexor carpi ulnaris muscle. The first branch of the ulnar nerve is to the joint; this branch can be sacrificed without complication, and its absence might decrease pain if arthritis develops later.
- After the ulnar nerve is freed from the cubital tunnel and scar tissue, the intramuscular septum is removed proximally for approximately 3 to 4 cm.
- Distally, the fascia over the entry point into the flexor carpi ulnaris (Osborne bands) is incised. The nerve is freed up to 7 cm after the flexor pronator mass is entered and is protected during the remainder of the procedure with a vessel loop. The authors of this chapter do not use a clamp on the vessel loop because it increases the risk of inadvertent pull on the nerve.
- If ulnar nerve symptoms such as pain, weakness, or a positive Tinel sign over the nerve were present preoperatively, an external neurolysis is done.
- Typically, all implants are removed unless they are stable and not preventing planned reconstruction.

 

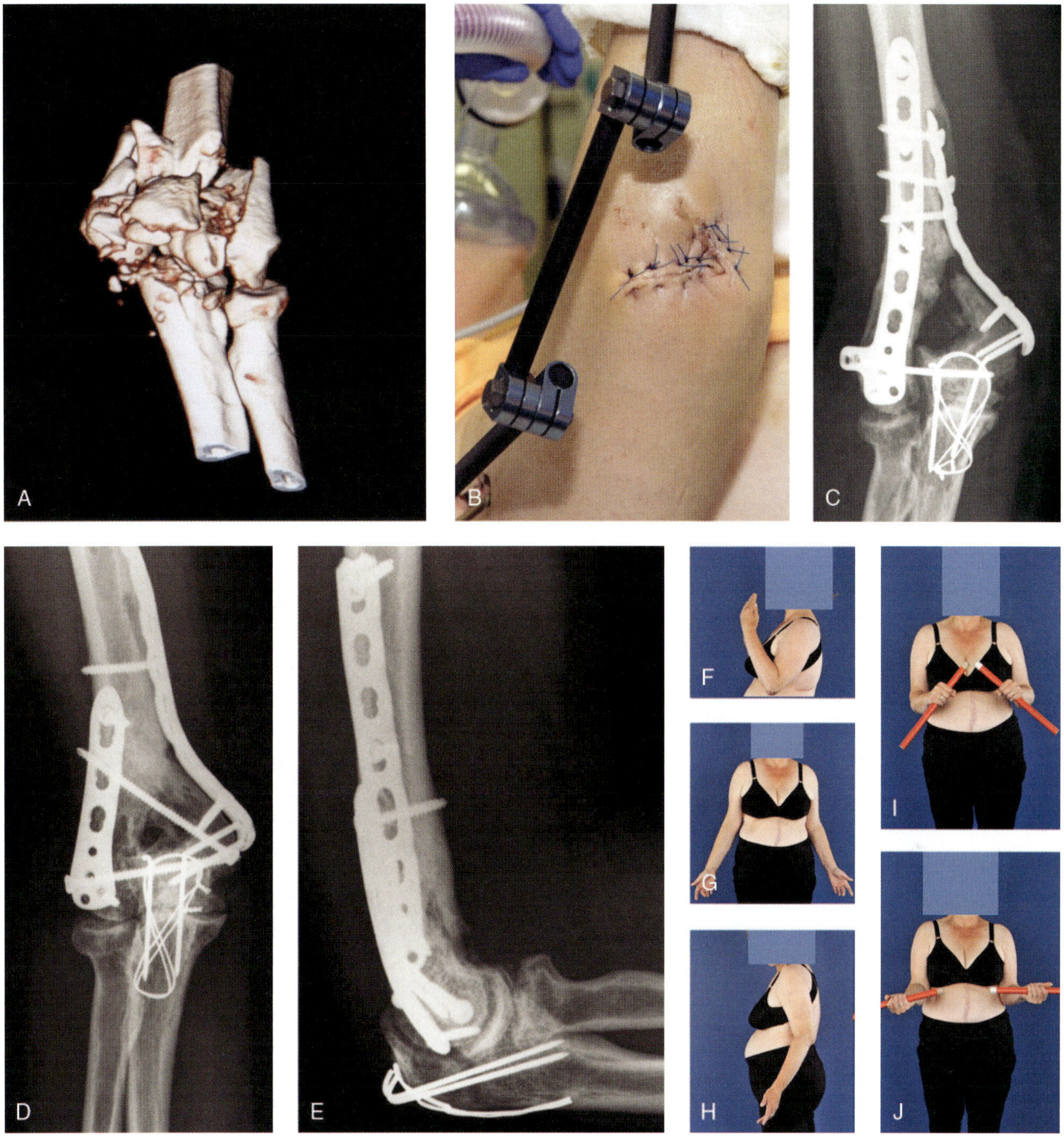


**Figure 4** **A,** CT reconstruction of the elbow of a 47-year-old woman who fell from a height of 15 m and sustained a comminuted (AO type C3), Gustilo type II open fracture of the right distal humerus in addition to other injuries. **B,** Clinical photograph of the elbow after irrigation and débridement of the open elbow fracture and placement of a spanning external fixator. Osteosynthesis of the radius was performed on postinjury day 3, followed by open reduction and internal fixation (ORIF) of the olecranon and distal humerus on postinjury day 14. **C,** AP radiograph obtained 6 months after ORIF demonstrates no sign of healing of the distal humerus. AP (**D**) and lateral (**E**) radiographs obtained 22 months after revision ORIF via an olecranon osteotomy that included a thorough débridement of the nonunion, release of the capsule and ulnar nerve, and autologous bone grafting demonstrate a healed distal humerus. Although there had not been clear signs of infection preoperatively, routine intraoperative cultures obtained before administration of antibiotics showed *Enterobacter cloacae,* which was treated with oral ciprofloxacin. Clinical photographs demonstrate 130° of elbow flexion with an extension deficit of 30° (**F**, **G**, and **H**) as well as 45° of pronation (**I**) and 80° of supination (**J**). There was no sign of infection. At the time of this follow-up, the patient had no pain and was working full-time as a home health nurse.

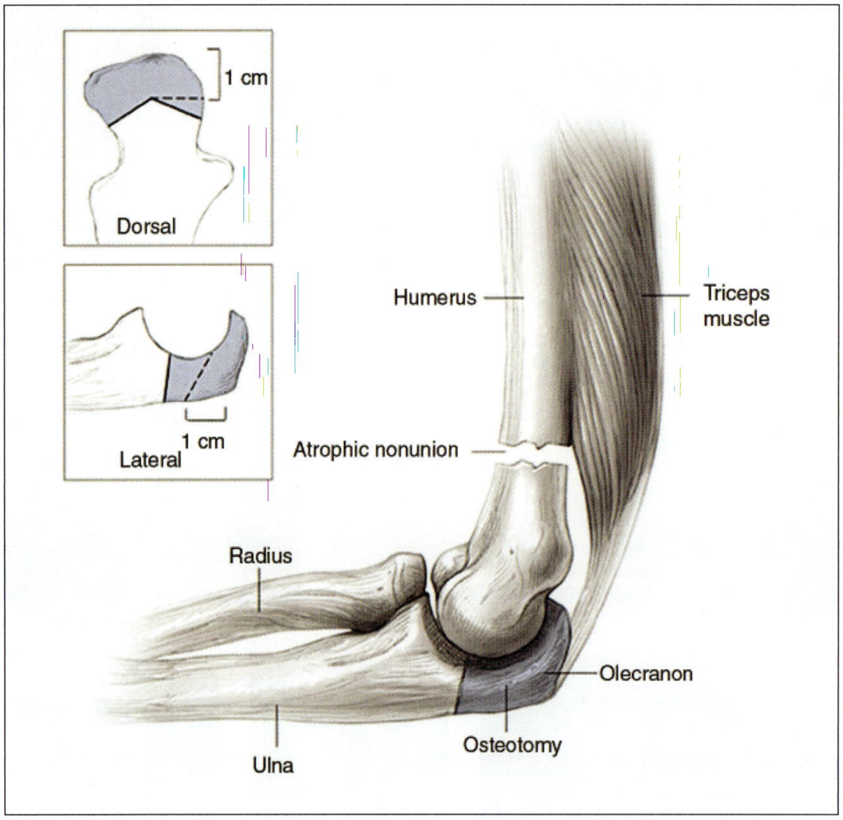


**Figure 5** Illustration of an elbow shows olecranon osteotomy. The insets show the angulation of the osteotomy from the dorsal and lateral aspects. This angulation forms an apex to facilitate reduction and provides additional rotational stability for fixation. (Reproduced with permission from Helfet DL, Kloen P, Anand N, Rosen HS: ORIF of delayed unions and nonunions of distal humeral fractures: Surgical technique. *J Bone Joint Surg Am* 2004;86[suppl 1, pt 1]:18-29.)

- Deep cultures are always obtained. At least five cultures are obtained, one of which is a screw. There is some evidence that the use of sonication to remove tissue from implants can increase culture yield. Only if gross signs of infection are present (pus) would the authors of this chapter consider staging the surgery. In that case, aggressive débridement would be performed and an external fixator placed, with revision surgery performed 6 weeks later.
- Soon after intravenous antibiotics are administered, the tourniquet is deflated briefly to allow circulation of the antibiotic into the arm.
- Even if a previous olecranon osteotomy was done, there should be no difficulty performing a second osteotomy. The authors of this chapter always perform an olecranon osteotomy for intra-articular nonunions, transcondylar nonunions, and low distal humeral nonunions. The superb exposure and ability for extensile releases cannot be provided by other approaches around the elbow.
- For supracondylar distal humeral nonunion, a triceps-split, triceps-elevation, or paratricipital approach can be considered.
- In patients with unicondylar nonunion, a medial or lateral approach can be sufficient. Alternatively, a paratricipital approach can be attempted; if sufficient exposure cannot be achieved, the approach can easily be converted to include an olecranon osteotomy.
- Prior to the olecranon osteotomy, the optimal localization is determined by visualizing the medial and lateral gutter of the elbow joint. The medial joint is visualized after releasing the flexor carpi ulnaris off the olecranon, and the lateral joint is visualized by releasing the anconeus muscle off the lateral olecranon.
- Gauze can be placed from medial to lateral through the ulnohumeral joint to protect the articular surface when the osteotomy is made.
- The olecranon osteotomy is a chevron type with the apex positioned distally. A microsagittal saw under cooling is used to prevent unnecessary bone loss, and the osteotomy is completed with a thin osteotome to allow for controlled fracture of the volar subchondral bone. The osteotomy is made at the apex of the semilunar notch, where the cartilage of the olecranon is thinnest (**Figure 5**).
- After the osteotomy is complete, the proximal fragment of the olecranon is retracted proximally. The articular surface of the olecranon can be adherent to the trochlea, and its surface can become separated. Careful elevation of the proximal fragment with an elevator will prevent this articular separation.
- The triceps is adherent to the posterior cortex but typically can be elevated off the bone with a rasp or via finger dissection (**Figure 6**). Depending on the level of the nonunion or hardware, the triceps is usually peeled off the posterior cortex for up to 10 cm (4 inches).
- Laterally, the radial nerve is at risk approximately 12 to 14 cm

 

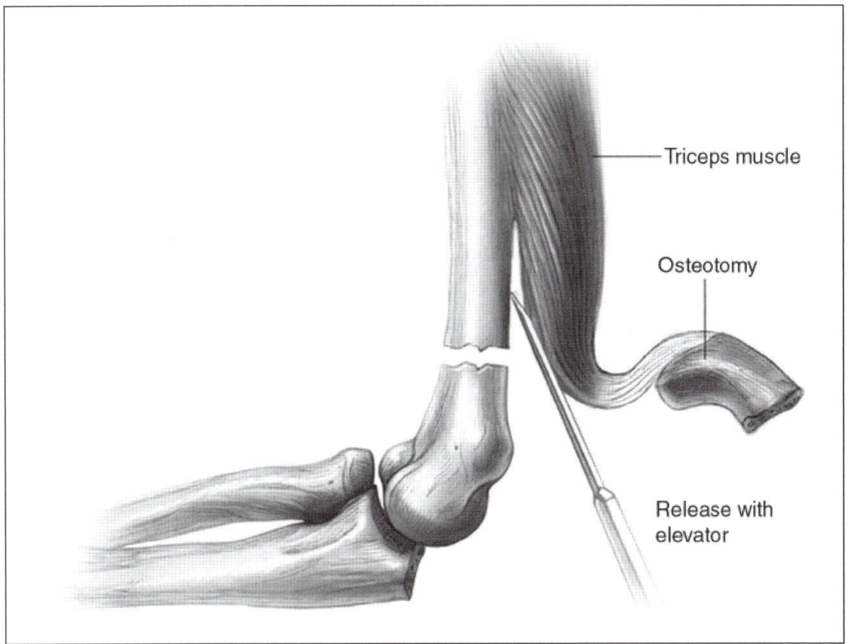


**Figure 6** Illustration of an elbow shows the triceps released from the nonunion and the distal part of the shaft via periosteal dissection after the osteotomy is complete. (Reproduced with permission from Helfet DL, Kloen P, Anand N, Rosen HS: ORIF of delayed unions and nonunions of distal humerus fractures: Surgical technique. *J Bone Joint Surg Am* 2004;86[suppl 1, pt 1]:18-29.)

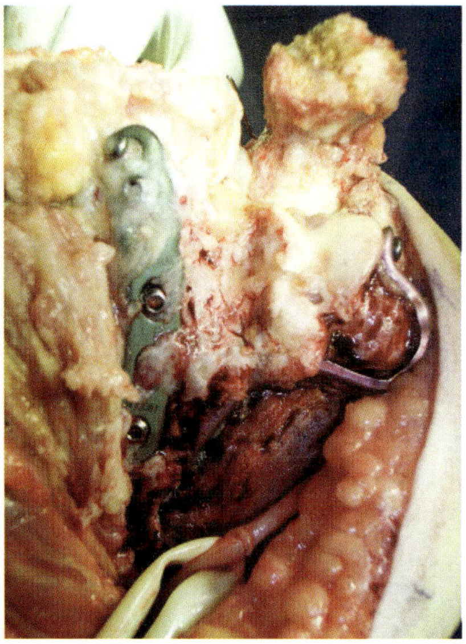

**Figure 7** Intraoperative photograph of the elbow from the same patient discussed in Figure 1. The ulnar nerve has been identified, and the olecranon osteotomy is complete. The hardware is from a previous surgery.

proximal to the lateral epicondyle. Excessive traction on the triceps should be prevented.

- Suturing the reflected olecranon and triceps and covering them with a moist sponge to the proximal soft tissues will tidy the surgical field and prevent desiccation.

## Instruments/Equipment/ Implants Required

- A sterile stockinet, tourniquet, and gowns or drapes to make the chest roll are used.
- Anatomic forceps and dissection scissors are used for nerve release.
- A vessel loop; microsagittal saw; lamina spreader; and thin, sharp osteotomes are used.
- Drill bits measuring 3.5, 2.5, and 2.0 mm are used.
- Various plates are used, including locking and nonlocking plates measuring 3.5, 2.7, and 2.4 mm.
- Headless screws, Kirschner wires (K-wires), and tension-band wires are used.
- Pointed reduction clamps (large and small Weber clamps) are used.
- Bone graft harvesting instruments are used.

## Procedure

- Ideally, all unstable implants are removed. Broken, embedded screws are left in situ if removal would cause excessive bone loss (**Figure 7**).
- Nonunion tissue, including the synovial tissue in a true synovial pseudarthrosis, is removed with a curet or rongeur. Although nonunion tissue might have regenerative potential, the authors of this chapter prefer débriding the nonunion down to bleeding bone to optimize bone-on-bone contact with the reconstruction. Tissue removal is performed by opening the intramedullary canal and making small petals (bone cuts) with a chisel on both sides of the nonunion.
- After the scar tissue and posterior capsule are cleared, the surgery proceeds through the nonunion toward the anterior aspect, where the anterior capsule can be released, thereby allowing increased mobilization of the joint (**Figure 8**). The distal aspect of the nonunion can be extended by using a bone hook to pull it into extension.
- If motion is still limited, osteotomy of the lateral collateral ligament of the lateral epicondyle can be performed. The joint can then be hinged open on the medial ligamentous structures. After reconstruction, the lateral collateral ligament complex can be reconstructed with use of bone anchors or transosseous sutures.
- The medial and lateral muscular attachments to the epicondyles should be preserved because they provide the vascular supply to the distal segments.

- With good access to both ends of the nonunion, a 2.0-mm drill bit is used to open the medullary canal on both sides. There is often a fibrous or sclerotic end cap that seals off the medullary canal. Making multiple passes through this cap allows for blood to egress from the canal. If the nonunion is very distal, there is no medullary canal.
- Realignment and reduction in the presence of distorted anatomy, bone loss, or both can be facilitated by creating a trough in the distal fragment in which the shaft is impacted.
- Position of the distal segment in relation to the shaft is carefully checked. Excessive flexion, extension, varus, valgus, or malrotation of the distal segment will compromise the final outcome. Care must be taken to restore the 15° carrying angle as well as the 40° flexion of the condyles relative to the shaft.
- Using Weber clamps placed in unicortical drill holes will facilitate reduction.
- K-wires will provisionally hold reduction. Definitive plate position should be anticipated when the K-wires are placed so that they do not obstruct the plate positioning.

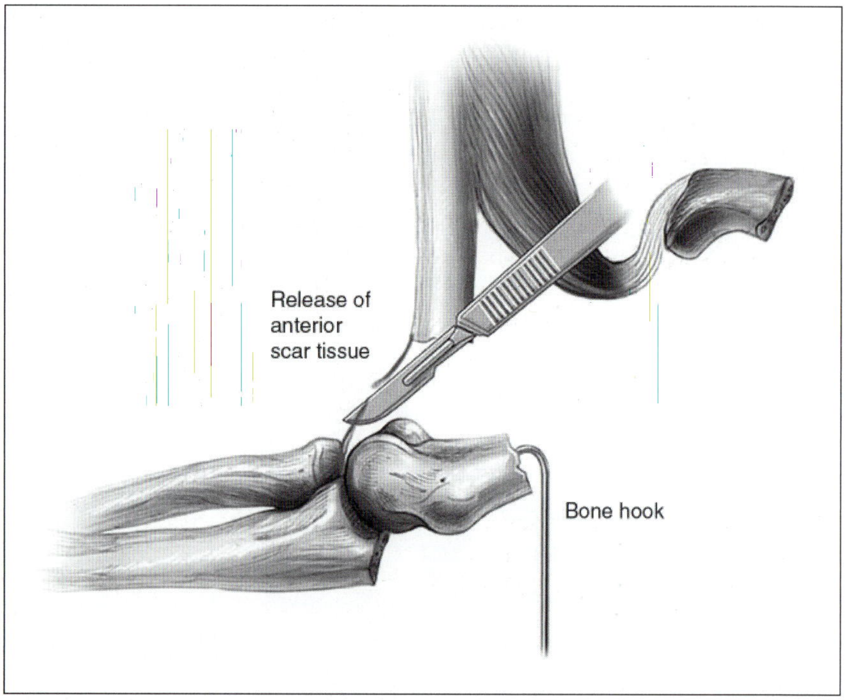


**Figure 8** Illustration of an elbow shows release of the anterior capsule and scar tissue through the nonunion site from posterior to anterior by means of a knife. (Reproduced with permission from Helfet DL, Kloen P, Anand N, Rosen HS: ORIF of delayed unions and nonunions of distal humeral fractures: Surgical technique. *J Bone Joint Surg Am* 2004;86[suppl 1, pt 1]:18-29.)

**FIXATION**

- Typically, the nonunion is extra-articular and the condylar block is one piece. In rare patients, a malunion of the condyles is present that can impede motion. A corrective osteotomy can be done to realign the intra-articular component.
- In the patient with an intra-articular nonunion or an osteotomized intra-articular malunion, the fragments are reduced temporarily with small 1.6- or 2.0-mm K-wires, after which the condylar block is reduced to the shaft with two crossed K-wires (**Figure 9, A**). The reconstruction is verified radiographically.

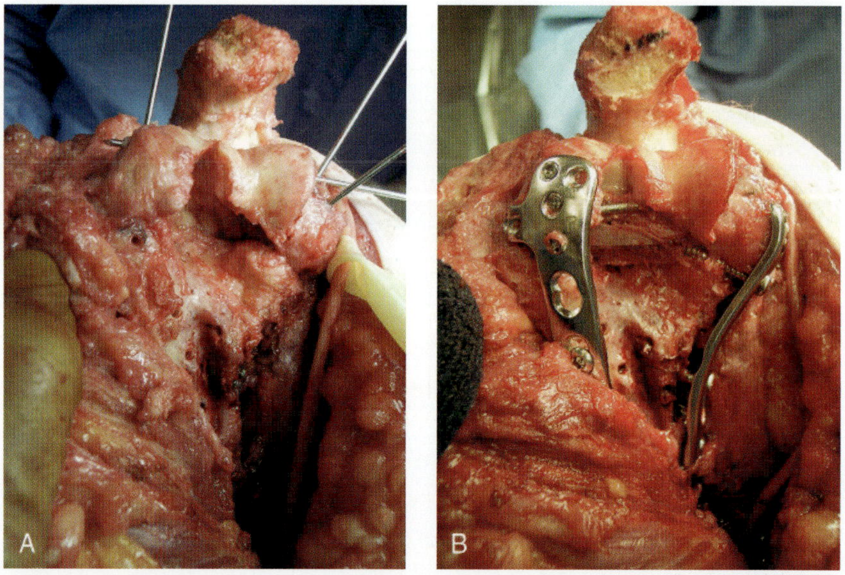


**Figure 9** Intraoperative photographs of the elbow from the same patient discussed in Figure 1. **A,** After extensile release was performed, the hardware was removed and the nonunion/articular surface was provisionally reduced using four Kirschner wires. **B,** Two locking compression plates were placed (one medially, one laterally) with screws that included a crossing interfragmentary lag screw. This exposure provides excellent visualization of the articular surface and allows confirmation of reduction.

 

- Plates and screws are used to achieve definitive fixation. The altered anatomy often precludes the use of anatomic plates, and fixation must be customized. The authors of this chapter typically use 3.5-mm plates. Although locking plates are not obligatory, they offer the benefit of distal locking, albeit with higher implant costs. In the opinion of the authors of this chapter, these plates allow better and more versatile fixation (**Figure 9, B**).
- Recently, plates with 3.5-mm screws along the shaft and metaphysis and 2.7-mm screws close to the joint were introduced into the market. These new plates with holes along the shaft allow for placement of more screws distally, which is helpful in managing small osteopenic distal fragments.
- The medial plate should cradle the medial epicondyle to increase stability.
- There is no evidence whether orthogonal (90°-90°) or parallel plating is best (**Figure 10**).

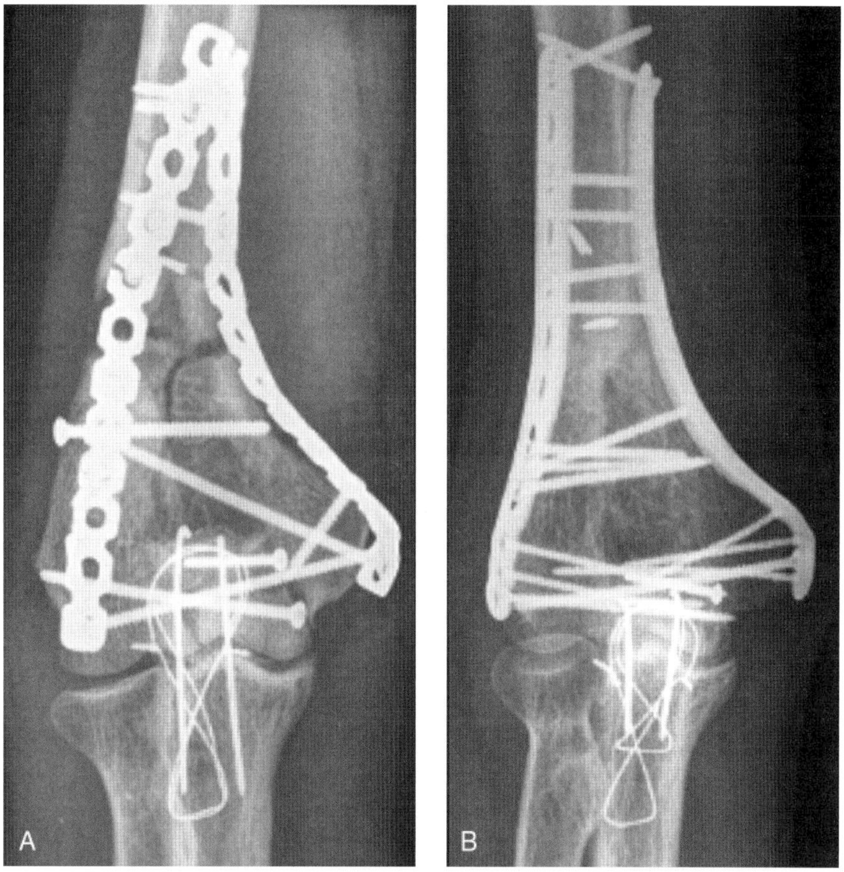


**Figure 10** **A** and **B,** AP radiographs of an elbow obtained 3 months after standard 90°-90° plating for a grade 1 open distal humerus fracture demonstrate delayed union and hardware failure. This patient later underwent a salvage procedure, during which all hardware was removed and the elbow was managed with débridement, fixation with parallel plates, and bone graft. Healing was uneventful after the salvage procedure.

- Cross-threading of screws, whether done intentionally or unintentionally, increases their holding power. To maximize stability of fixation, the authors of this chapter prefer to place two 3.5-mm-long screws from the distal aspect of the epicondyle through the plates crossing from medial to lateral and from lateral to medial.
- Use of tension-band wiring relies on muscle and ligament attachment to the bone and only slightly on bone quality. This technique can augment fixation in osteopenic bone fragments.

## BONE GRAFTING

- Autologous bone graft is the preferred graft material. One author of this chapter (D.L.H.) uses mostly demineralized bone graft, and the other author (P.K.) prefers autologous cancellous graft.
- Local autologous bone can be harvested from the olecranon tip. Most often, however, the authors of this chapter harvest bone from the patient's iliac crest. It is important to roughen an area measuring approximately 2 cm on each side of the nonunion site. A small chisel can be used to make small bone cuts, retaining as much soft-tissue attachment as possible. Roughening each side of the nonunion and making small bone cuts increases the area with which the bone graft or demineralized matrix will have contact and also causes microfractures and a renewed local healing response.
- Vascularized bone graft can be a viable and useful addition in patients with severe bone loss.

## FIXATION OF OLECRANON OSTEOTOMY

- With the aid of two large, pointed reduction clamps, the olecranon osteotomy is closed with the elbow in extension.
- Two 1.8-mm K-wires are placed from the tip of the olecranon through the volar cortex of the ulna as close to the joint as possible but not into the joint. One or two 18-gauge (1-mm) wires are placed in a figure-of-8 fashion around the proximal ends of the K-wire under the triceps and through a drill hole in the ulna.

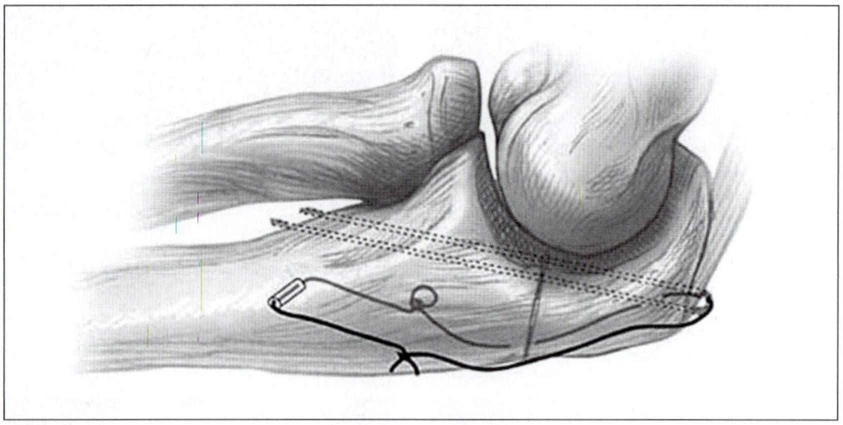

**Figure 11** Illustration of the elbow joint shows fixation of the olecranon osteotomy via a tension-band construct. (Reproduced with permission from Helfet DL, Kloen P, Anand N, Rosen HS: ORIF of delayed unions and nonunions of distal humerus fractures: Surgical technique. *J Bone Joint Surg Am* 2004;86[suppl 1, pt 1]:18-29.)

- The two loops in the figure-of-8 tension band are tightened sequentially with pliers.
- The K-wires are withdrawn 1 cm, bent 180°, and cut. The K-wires are then tapped back in place, making sure that the hooks of the K-wires are around the tension band (**Figure 11**).
- The elbow is gently moved through ROM to check mobility, stability of fixation, and presence of crepitus.
- Alternately, fixation may be performed with a 3.5-mm intramedullary screw with a washer and tension band or with a tension-band plate.

### Wound Closure

- Before closure, the tourniquet is deflated and hemostasis is obtained.
- A deep drain is placed at the discretion of the surgeon.
- In a patient with preoperative symptoms of the ulnar nerve or in whom the nerve cannot be replaced in its normal position without impingement on the new implants, the authors of this chapter leave the nerve in an anterior subcutaneous position.

## Postoperative Regimen

The elbow is splinted in 90° flexion and neutral rotation for 2 days postoperatively. After wound inspection on postoperative day 2, the patient is fitted with either a hinged elbow brace or a removable splint. Gentle active and active-assisted ROM exercise is started under the guidance of a physical or occupational therapist. The patient is allowed to use the arm for light functional activities as pain allows. The authors of this chapter do not prescribe continuous passive motion.

If the results of intraoperative cultures are positive, consultation with an infectious disease specialist is obtained and antibiotics are generally administered (2 weeks of intravenous antibiotics, followed by 4 weeks of oral antibiotics). Hardware is removed only if it is loose, and graft is removed if it does not incorporate. No preoperative or postoperative radiation or other form of heterotopic ossification prophylaxis (for example, indomethacin) is used. It has been clearly shown that radiation around the elbow to prevent heterotopic bone formation compromises bone healing.

Radiographs are obtained 2 days postoperatively and again at 6 and 12 weeks postoperatively. Healing is generally attained by 12 weeks, and no further radiographs are needed. After the nonunion is healed, the patient is allowed unrestricted activities (**Figure 12**).

## Limiting Adverse Events

A nonunion in an open fracture will often be infected. Even in the absence of wound healing problems or clinical symptoms such as fever or redness, every nonunion should be presumed septic. Obtaining at least five representative cultures before administering intravenous antibiotics is essential to rule out infection or to identify the organism (**Figure 4**).

Inadequate débridement will compromise bone healing. Both ends of the nonunion should be viable, with good bone-on-bone contact. It is more important to obtain bone-on-bone contact than to preserve length. Shortening of the humerus is tolerated up to 4 to 5 cm. Biology should be optimized by providing sufficient bone graft. The preferred standard is autologous cancellous bone.

The elbow joint should be released to provide maximum motion. Residual stiffness of the elbow will cause increased forces on the nonunion site, where most of the motion takes place. Bone healing is more important than motion at this stage. If fixation is thought to be less than optimal, then postoperative exercises are delayed.


## Acknowledgment

The authors wish to thank Dror Paley, MD, for joining with the authors of this chapter to perform the Ilizarov technique in the patient discussed in this chapter.


 

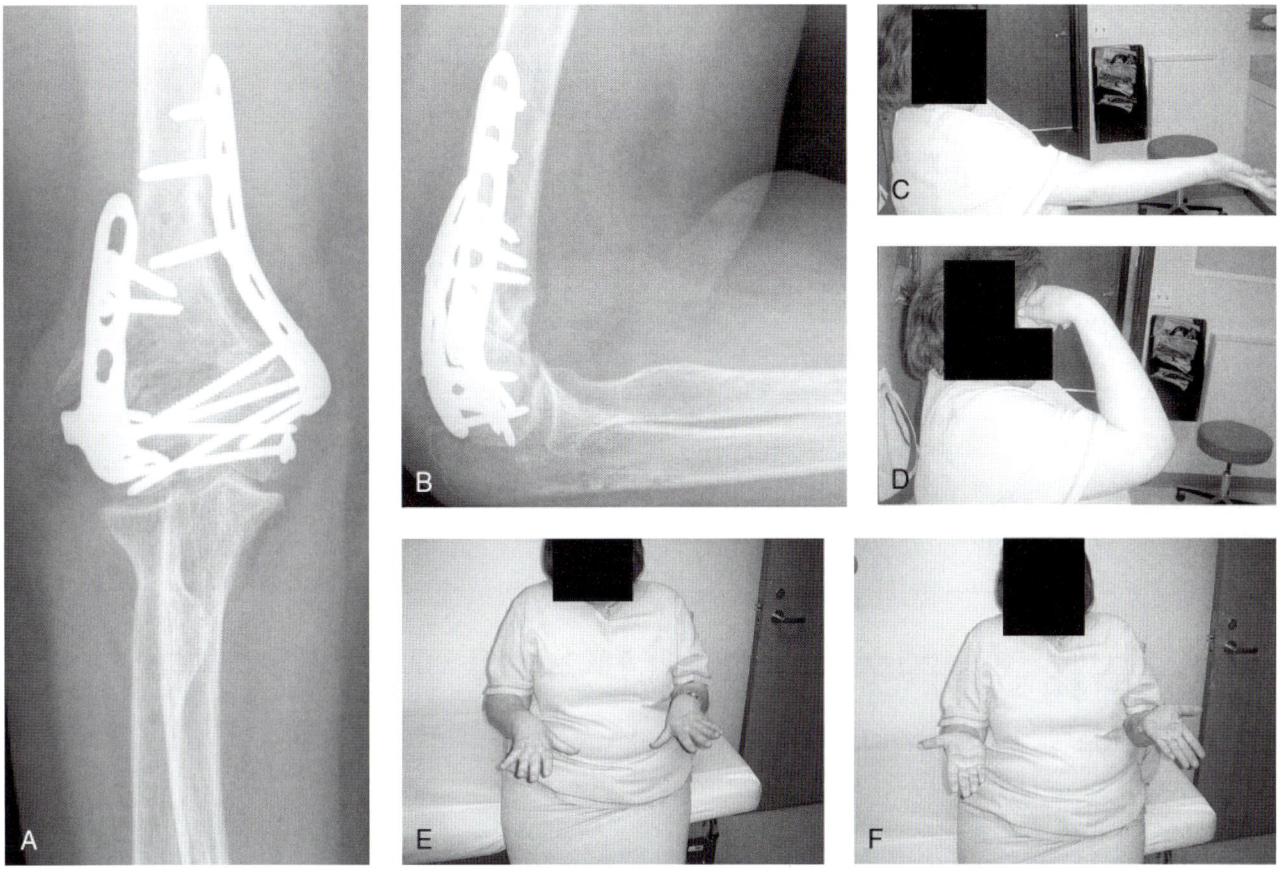


**Figure 12** Images from the same patient as shown in Figure 1. AP (**A**) and lateral (**B**) radiographs obtained 5 months postoperatively demonstrate a healed distal humeral nonunion. The patient returned to preinjury activity status with a restoration of her elbow function and motion: extension (**C**), flexion (**D**), pronation (**E**), and supination (**F**).

## Bibliography

Ackerman G, Jupiter JB: Non-union of fractures of the distal end of the humerus. *J Bone Joint Surg Am* 1988;70(1):75-83.

Ali A, Douglas H, Stanley D: Revision surgery for nonunion after early failure of fixation of fractures of the distal humerus. *J Bone Joint Surg Br* 2005;87(8):1107-1110.

Allende C, Allende BT: Post-traumatic distal humerus non-union: Open reduction and internal fixation. Long-term results. *Int Orthop* 2009;33(5):1289-1294.

Beredjiklian PK, Hotchkiss RN, Athanasian EA, Ramsey ML, Katz MA: Recalcitrant nonunion of the distal humerus: Treatment with free vascularized bone grafting. *Clin Orthop Relat Res* 2005;(435):134-139.

Brinker MR, O'Connor DP, Crouch CC, Mehlhoff TL, Bennett JB: Ilizarov treatment of infected nonunions of the distal humerus after failure of internal fixation: An outcomes study. *J Orthop Trauma* 2007;21(3):178-184.

Cil A, Veillette CJ, Sanchez-Sotelo J, Morrey BF: Linked elbow replacement: A salvage procedure for distal humeral nonunion. *J Bone Joint Surg Am* 2008;90(9):1939-1950.

Figgie MP, Inglis AE, Mow CS, Figgie HE III: Salvage of non-union of supracondylar fracture of the humerus by total elbow arthroplasty. *J Bone Joint Surg Am* 1989;71(7):1058-1065.

Gallay SH, McKee MD: Operative treatment of nonunions about the elbow. *Clin Orthop Relat Res* 2000;(370):87-101.

Helfet DL, Kloen P, Anand N, Rosen HS: Open reduction and internal fixation of delayed unions and nonunions of fractures of the distal part of the humerus. *J Bone Joint Surg Am* 2003;85(1):33-40.

Jupiter JB: The management of nonunion and malunion of the distal humerus: A 30-year experience. *J Orthop Trauma* 2008;22(10):742-750.

Jupiter JB, Goodman LJ: The management of complex distal humerus nonunion in the elderly by elbow capsulectomy, triple plating, and ulnar nerve neurolysis. *J Shoulder Elbow Surg* 1992;1(1):37-46.

McKee M, Jupiter J, Toh CL, Wilson L, Colton C, Karras KK: Reconstruction after malunion and nonunion of intra-articular fractures of the distal humerus: Methods and results in 13 adults. *J Bone Joint Surg Br* 1994;76(4):614-621.

Mitsunaga MM, Bryan RS, Linscheid RL: Condylar nonunions of the elbow. *J Trauma* 1982;22(9):787-791.

Paramasivan ON, Younge DA, Pant R: Treatment of nonunion around the olecranon fossa of the humerus by intramedullary locked nailing. *J Bone Joint Surg Br* 2000;82(3):332-335.

Ramsey ML, Adams RA, Morrey BF: Instability of the elbow treated with semiconstrained total elbow arthroplasty. *J Bone Joint Surg Am* 1999;81(1):38-47.

Ring D, Jupiter JB: Operative treatment of osteochondral nonunion of the distal humerus. *J Orthop Trauma* 2006;20(1):56-59.

Ring D, Jupiter JB, Toh S: Salvage of contaminated fractures of the distal humerus with thin wire external fixation. *Clin Orthop Relat Res* 1999;(359):203-208.

Ring D, Gulotta L, Jupiter JB: Unstable nonunions of the distal part of the humerus. *J Bone Joint Surg Am* 2003;85(6):1040-1046.

Sanchez-Sotelo J: Distal humeral nonunion. *Instr Course Lect* 2009;58:541-548.

Sanders RA, Sackett JR: Open reduction and internal fixation of delayed union and nonunion of the distal humerus. *J Orthop Trauma* 1990;4(3):254-259.

Urbaniak JR, Black KE Jr: Cadaveric elbow allografts: A six-year experience. *Clin Orthop Relat Res* 1985;(197):131-140.

 

# Chapter 28
# Malunion of the Distal Humerus

*Thomas R. Duquin, MD*

**Learning Objectives**

- Understand the normal anatomy of the distal humerus and the typical deformity associated with distal humeral malunion.
- Understand how to evaluate patients with distal humeral malunions, including how to assess for associated pathology (tardy ulnar nerve palsy, posterolateral rotatory instability, and arthritis).
- Understand the indications and the surgical technique options for corrective distal humeral osteotomy.
- Understand the components of preoperative planning for corrective distal humeral osteotomy, including three-dimensional CT.
- Understand the technique of a step-cut closing wedge osteotomy for distal humeral malunion.

## Indications

Distal humerus fractures have a bimodal distribution that peaks in children and elderly individuals. In children, malunion of the distal humerus is typically the sequela of a supracondylar humerus fracture. Some studies report cubitus varus in more than 50% of nonsurgically managed patients. The deforming forces in distal humerus fractures typically result in varus, extension, and internal rotation malunion of the distal humerus. The cubitus varus deformity is often considered a cosmetic deformity without functional consequences; however, severe deformities may be associated with pain, posterolateral rotatory instability, posttraumatic ulnar nerve dysfunction, and associated shoulder pathology. The cosmetic appearance of an elbow deformity can cause patient distress, which some patients may report as physical pain. Surgeons should proceed with caution in the treatment of patients with pain that does not have a clear explanation as well as with patients who have substantial symptoms of depression or ineffective coping strategies. The author of this chapter performs corrective distal humeral osteotomy in patients with a relatively severe distal humeral deformity who are willing to undergo the surgical risks of the procedure despite the associated discomforts and inconveniences, are willing to trade a deformity for a scar, and believe that surgery will result in more long-term benefits rather than harm.

Most distal humeral malunions are largely asymptomatic and aesthetic. Osteotomy is considered only in distal humeral malunions with a varus carrying angle greater than 15°. The indication for corrective distal humeral osteotomy is a symptomatic, substantial malunion with a healthy articular surface of the elbow joint. The role of prophylactic osteotomy in children with a severe distal humeral deformity is not clear but is considered in some patients (**Figure 1**). If malunion occurs before skeletal maturity, there may be secondary developmental deformities of the elbow joint and surrounding soft tissues. Preoperative planning for associated procedures, including ulnar nerve decompression, lateral ulnar collateral ligament reconstruction, capsular release, removal of loose bodies or osteophytes, and deepening of the olecranon or coronoid fossae, may be required to achieve a successful outcome.

## Contraindications

The benefits of distal humeral osteotomy for the treatment of distal humeral malunion rarely balance the risks. Alternative treatment options should be considered in patients who have advanced arthritic changes or intra-articular malunions. The presence of an active infection is an absolute contraindication to distal humeral osteotomy. Relative contraindications to distal

*Dr. Duquin or an immediate family member is a member of a speakers' bureau or has made paid presentations on behalf of, serves as a paid consultant to, and has received research or institutional support from Zimmer Biomet.*

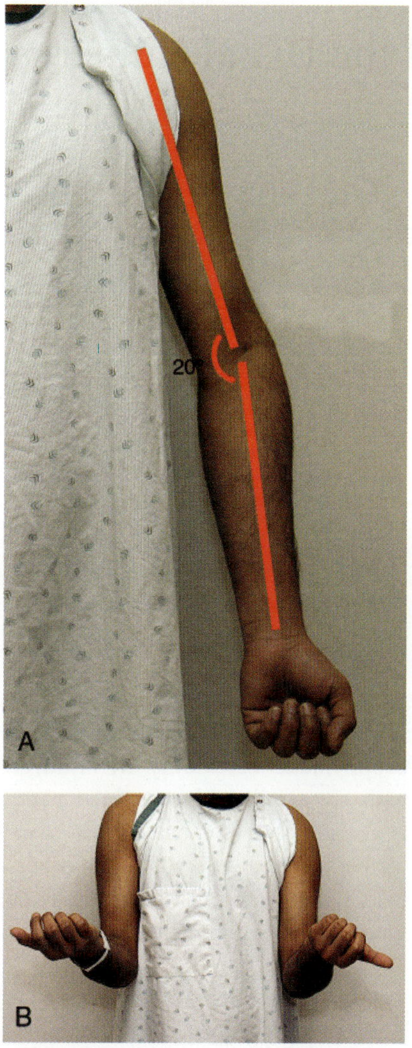


**Figure 1** Clinical photographs of a patient who has a cubitus varus deformity with a 20° varus carrying angle (**A**) and hypersupination deformity of the left elbow (**B**).

humeral osteotomy include advanced age, poor bone quality, tobacco use, metabolic bone disease, and inability to participate in postoperative rehabilitation. The presence of psychological factors, including substantial symptoms of depression and ineffective coping strategies, can result in dissatisfaction with the correction of a distal humeral deformity; therefore, such factors should be addressed before any surgical procedure is considered.

## Alternative Treatments

Patients who have advanced arthritic changes of the elbow joint or elderly patients who have poor bone quality are not candidates for distal humeral osteotomy. Alternative treatment options include total elbow arthroplasty or elbow arthrodesis. In patients who have mild distal humeral deformity or isolated sagittal plane deformity, alternative procedures including deepening of the olecranon or coronoid fossa and contracture release with ulnar nerve decompression may be considered. Recontouring of the olecranon or coronoid fossae can be performed using open or arthroscopic techniques to prevent bone impingement in flexion or extension without the need for a formal osteotomy. Intra-articular malunions cannot be managed with standard extra-articular distal humeral osteotomy techniques. Depending on the quality of the joint and patient characteristics, intra-articular osteotomy, allograft joint reconstruction, interposition arthroplasty, total elbow arthroplasty, and arthrodesis have been used for the management of intra-articular malunion.

## Results

Most studies on distal humeral osteotomy for the correction of cubitus varus are case series of children who were treated with a variety of techniques. Most of these case studies report good or excellent outcomes in more than 85% of patients (**Table 1**).

## Techniques

### Preoperative Planning

- Radiographs used for preoperative planning should include AP, lateral, and radial head (45° oblique lateral of the radiocapitellar joint) views of the elbow as well as radiographs of the entire affected upper extremity and the contralateral upper extremity (from the shoulder to the wrist with the elbow fully extended and the forearm supinated; **Figure 2**).
- The degree of varus deformity can be measured on radiographs of the entire affected upper extremity and compared with those of the contralateral upper extremity.
- Advanced imaging can aid in appreciating the distal humeral deformity. At the institution of the author of this chapter, a three-dimensional (3D) CT reconstruction is obtained preoperatively (**Figure 3**).
- In many patients, deformity exists in more than one plane, with the most common deformity in varus and extension. A biplanar osteotomy often helps correct both coronal and sagittal plane deformities.
- Internal rotation deformity also is common in patients who have distal humeral malunion. The value of correcting an internal rotational deformity is controversial.
- Many different osteotomies for the management of distal humeral deformity have been described, including a simple closing wedge osteotomy, an oblique closing wedge osteotomy, a step-cut closing wedge osteotomy, a step-cut translational osteotomy, and dome osteotomy, each of which has a varying degree of complexity and results in a varying degree of correction. Currently, the author of this chapter prefers to use a step-cut closing wedge osteotomy to manage distal humeral deformity.
- The osteotomy is planned using tools standard to most image-viewing software or, if digital radiographs are unavailable, tracing paper (**Figure 4**). The planned osteotomy should correct all deformity, with slight overcorrection preferred to undercorrection.

 

**Table 1** Results of Distal Humeral Osteotomy to Manage Malunion of the Distal Humerus[a]

| Authors (Year) | No. of Patients | Procedure or Approach | Mean Patient Age in Years (Range) | Mean Follow-up in Months (Range) | Success Rate (%) | Results |
|---|---|---|---|---|---|---|
| Cobb and Linscheid (1994) | 3 | Intra-articular derotational opening wedge osteotomy with bone graft | 29 (26-36) | 91.2 (36-152.4) | NA | Significant pain relief<br>1 fibrous ankylosis developed; managed with interposition arthroplasty |
| McKee et al (1994) | 13 | Osteotomy, ORIF with or without bone graft | 39.7 (17-62) | 25 (12-60) | 50 | Mean arc of motion: 97°<br>MEPS: 2 excellent, 2 good, and 8 fair<br>1 trochlear osteonecrosis noted radiographically but did not progress during the follow-up period |
| O'Driscoll et al (2001) | 21 | Osteotomy, LCL reconstruction, arthroplasty | 34 (13-70) | 36 (12-96) | 86 | MEPS: 13 excellent, 6 good, 1 fair, and 2 poor<br>Complications: 1 wound infection, 1 nonunion, 1 compartment syndrome, and 1 transient ulnar neuropathy |
| Chung and Baek (2003) | 23 | 3D osteotomy | 26 (17-47) | 22 (12-36) | 96 | Complications: 4 radial nerve palsies, 1 myositis ossificans |
| Kim et al (2005) | 32 | Step-cut translation osteotomy | 23 (13-43) | 3 (NA) | 100 | Modified criteria of Oppenheim: 26 excellent and 6 good<br>Complications: 6 tardy ulnar nerve palsies requiring transposition and 2 hypertrophic scars |
| Hahn et al (2009) | 19 | Dome osteotomy | 31 (16-50) | 41 (36-95) | 100 | 13 excellent and 6 good |
| Moradi et al (2013) | 13 | Spike translation, step-cut osteotomy | 19 (9-31) | 27 (16-43) | 100 | Modified criteria of Oppenheim: 11 excellent and 2 good<br>2 hypertrophic scars developed |
| Takeyasu et al (2013) | 30 | 3D osteotomy with custom surgical template | 15 (4-49) | 23.1 (12-53) | 93 | Hahn criteria: 27 excellent and 3 good<br>1 loss of correction with recurrent cubitus varus and 1 hardware failure developed |

3D = three-dimensional, LCL = lateral collateral ligament, MEPS = Mayo Elbow Performance Score, NA = not available, ORIF = open reduction and internal fixation.

[a] All studies are level IV evidence.

- In patients who have complex or severe distal humeral deformities, a 3D printer can be used to create a 3D model of the patient's distal humerus or custom cutting guides. The use of these 3D models helps ensure accurate correction.

## Setup/Exposure

- The patient is positioned supine with a bump under the surgical shoulder.
- The surgical arm is draped over the patient's chest to allow full access to the distal humerus.
- The patient's arm is abducted to allow for fluoroscopic imaging from the lateral side of the surgical table.
- After standard preparation and draping, a sterile tourniquet is applied to the patient's upper arm.
- Appropriate antibiotics are administered 30 minutes before the tourniquet is inflated.

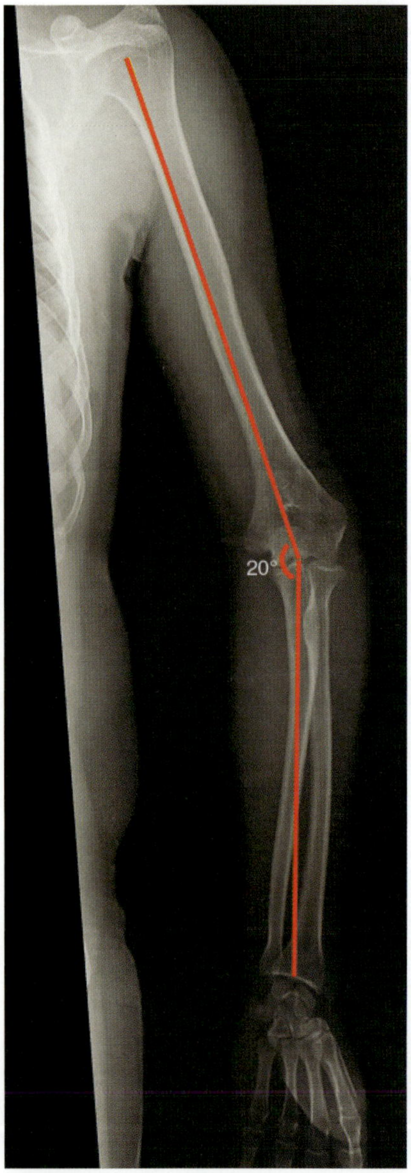


**Figure 2** AP radiograph of an upper extremity demonstrates a 20° varus deformity of the distal humerus. Inclusion of the shoulder and wrist is necessary to determine the degree of deformity.

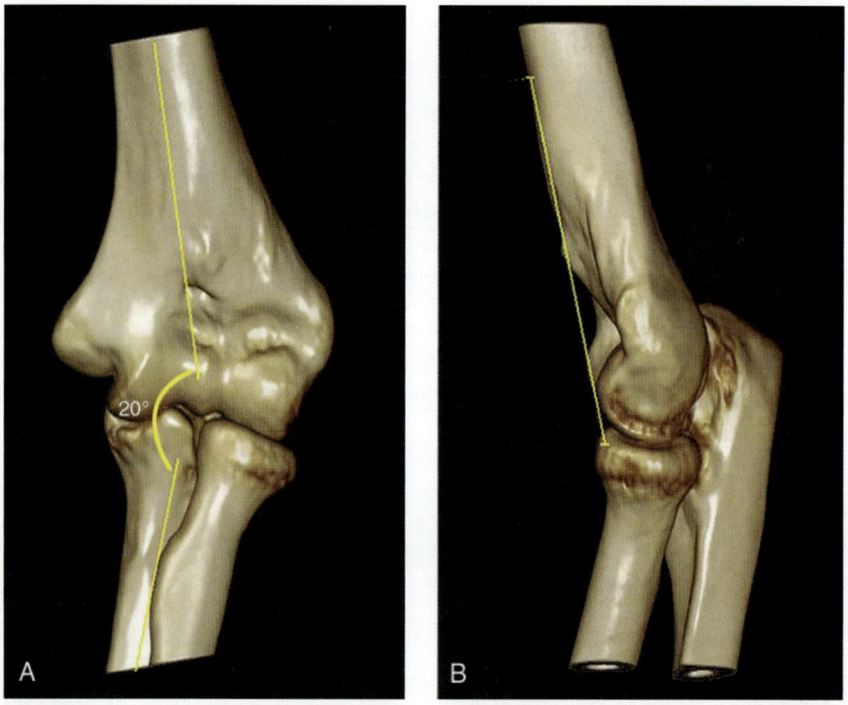


**Figure 3** Three-dimensional CT reconstructions of an elbow with a distal humeral malunion. **A,** AP view demonstrates a 20° varus deformity in the supracondylar region of the distal humerus. **B,** Lateral view demonstrates an extension and posterior translation deformity (yellow line) of the supracondylar malunion.

## Instruments/Equipment/Implants Required

- Standard surgical instruments and retractors should be available.
- Bone reduction clamps, Steinmann pins, and a sterile goniometer are used.
- A system for internal fixation with precontoured distal humeral locking plates is used.
- A C-arm is used for intraoperative imaging.
- Allograft or autograft tendon is necessary if ligament reconstruction is to be performed.

## Procedure

- Corrective osteotomy can be performed via multiple surgical approaches, including triceps-sparing, triceps-splitting, or triceps-reflecting approaches, or via an olecranon osteotomy. The author of this chapter prefers to use a triceps-sparing approach and perform distal humeral osteotomy through windows on the medial and lateral columns.
- A single posterior skin incision with mobilization of flaps can be made to allow access to the medial and lateral columns; however, this results in more soft-tissue mobilization, which may affect wound healing, causing seroma or hematoma formation. The author of this chapter prefers to use two separate incisions to allow access to the medial and lateral columns (**Figure 5**).
- The lateral incision is begun 5 to 8 cm proximal to the lateral epicondyle and extends distally to the level of the elbow joint.
- The intermuscular plane between the triceps and the brachioradialis muscles is identified.
- The radial nerve is not routinely identified but is at risk if dissection extends more than 10 cm proximal to the lateral epicondyle.
- The medial incision is begun 5 to 8 cm proximal to the medial epicondyle and extended to the level of the joint.
- The plane between the triceps and the brachialis muscles is identified.
- The ulnar nerve is identified on the medial border of the triceps tendon and carefully mobilized until

 

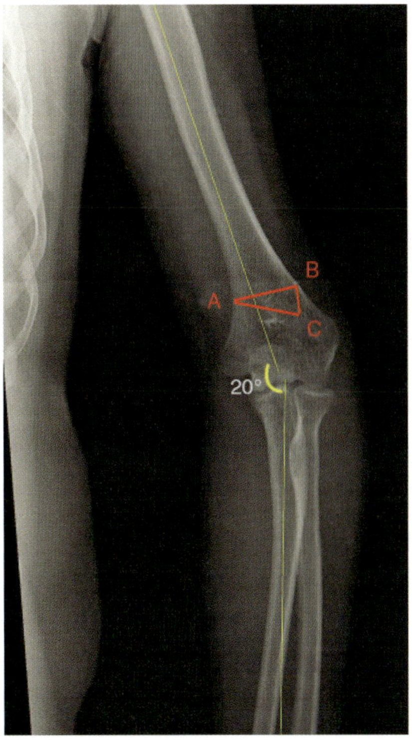


**Figure 4** AP radiograph of an elbow with a 20° cubitus varus deformity demonstrates preoperative templating for a step-cut closing wedge osteotomy. The planned osteotomy site (triangle) is located in the metaphyseal region just above the superior margin of the olecranon fossa. Correction to approximately 10° of valgus should be performed. Point A represents the location of the osteotomy on the medial column. Point B represents the location of the osteotomy along the lateral column. Point C represents the point that completes the wedge of bone to be removed for the correction of the deformity. The angle created by the points BAC represents the degree of correction desired for the osteotomy. The length of the segment AB should equal the length of the segment AC.

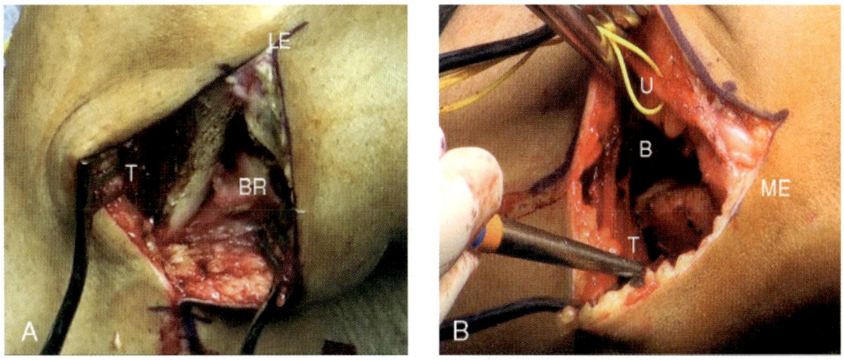


**Figure 5** Intraoperative photographs of an elbow show exposure of the lateral (**A**) and medial (**B**) columns for distal humeral osteotomy. The medial and lateral exposures are connected anteriorly and posteriorly to fully expose the distal humerus at the site of the osteotomy. B = brachialis, BR = brachioradialis, LE = lateral epicondyle, ME = medial epicondyle, T = triceps, U = ulnar nerve.

it enters the flexor carpi ulnaris muscle. This allows for retraction of the ulnar nerve without tension during the procedure.

- The triceps is elevated from the humerus posteriorly, and the brachialis and brachioradialis muscles are elevated anteriorly. Subperiosteal elevation of these muscles helps protect the radial and median nerves anteriorly.
- The joint capsule can be left intact in patients without joint contracture.
- The preoperative template is consulted, and the location of the osteotomy is identified based on landmarks, including the medial and lateral epicondyles.
- The osteotomy is created in the metadiaphyseal junction just above the olecranon fossa. Maintaining the olecranon and coronoid fossae allows maximal bone contact for healing and avoids loss of range of motion (ROM).
- The use of intraoperative fluoroscopy helps ensure that the osteotomy matches the preoperative template.
- Steinmann pins can be used as guides for the osteotomy cuts. The first Steinmann pin is placed perpendicular to the humeral shaft. A second Steinmann pin is placed at an angle that matches the degree of correction desired. The use of a sterile goniometer helps ensure the appropriate degree of correction (**Figure 6, A**).
- A saw is used to create the osteotomy, with careful retraction used to prevent injury to the surrounding neurovascular structures.
- The distal cut is created at the angle of the desired correction. The depth of the cut should be equal to the width of the humeral shaft at the location of the proximal cut, which is made perpendicular to the humeral shaft. It may be helpful to mark the saw blade with a pen at the desired depth of the cut.
- After the distal cut is made, the proximal cut is made.
- The wedge osteotomy is completed by making a vertical cut that connects the proximal cut to the end of the distal cut. In patients who have biplanar deformity, the proximal cut should be made with angulation in the sagittal plane to correct the extension deformity (**Figure 6, B**).
- The proximal and distal fragments are reduced and provisional fixation is obtained with a Steinmann pin.
- Appropriate correction in the coronal and sagittal planes and appropriate rotational alignment are confirmed clinically and via fluoroscopic imaging.
- A 3.5-mm screw is placed through the lateral spike in the distal fragment to attain initial fixation of the osteotomy, after which the osteotomy is fixed definitively with medial and lateral plates.
- The use of precontoured distal

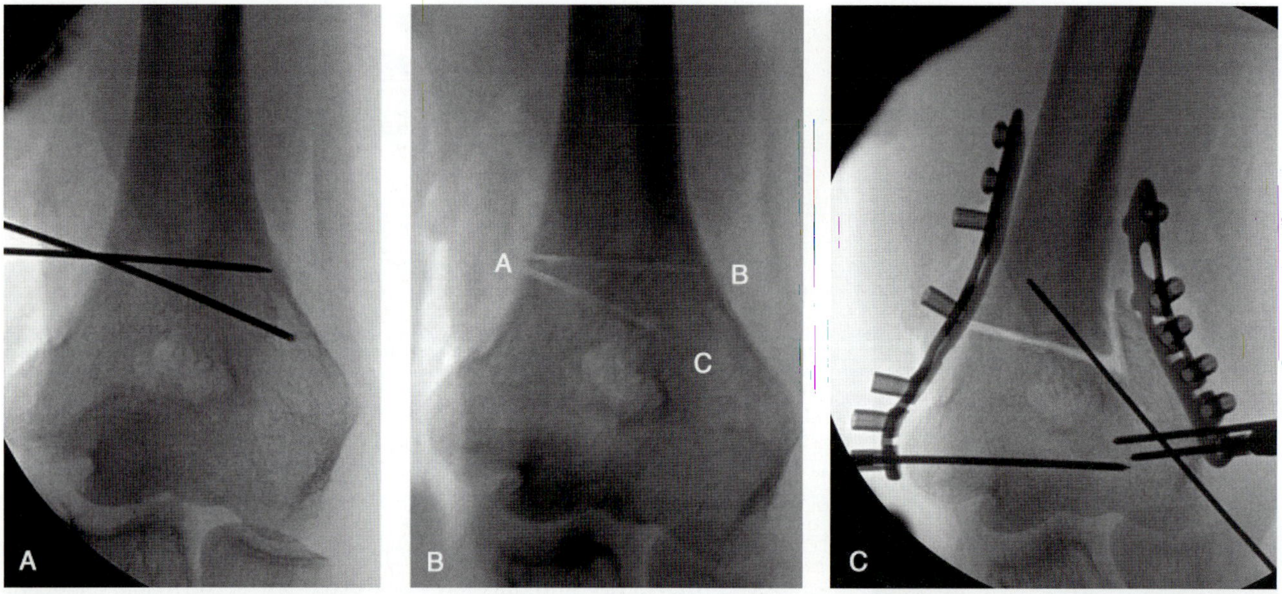


**Figure 6** Intraoperative AP fluoroscopic images of an elbow show the creation and fixation of a distal humeral osteotomy. **A,** Steinmann pins, which serve as cutting guides for the osteotomy, are placed with the aid of a goniometer under fluoroscopic visualization. **B,** Initial saw cuts are made for the osteotomy (from point A to point B and from point A to point C) with the proper angle of correction. The osteotomy is completed by cutting from point B to point C. **C,** Compression of the osteotomy is achieved with provisional fixation and the placement of plates on the medial and lateral columns.

humeral plates can be helpful; however, modification of precontoured plates is often necessary because of the altered distal humeral anatomy.

- Compression of the osteotomy is performed by fixing the plates distally and placing compression screws into the proximal aspect of the medial and lateral plates. Rigid fixation with plates on both the medial and lateral columns increases the load sharing of the bone, making early active motion more secure (**Figure 6, C**).
- In children, fixation can be attained with pins or limited internal fixation.
- The patient's arm is examined to ensure full ROM and stability of the elbow. If limited ROM is present in flexion or extension, the osteotomy should be checked to ensure appropriate correction of the sagittal plane deformity.
- If the alignment is good, a capsular release should be considered. The capsule can be released by extending the lateral incision distally and exposing the joint capsule laterally via a columnar approach.
- The capsule is isolated and excised, and the joint surfaces are examined.
- Persistent limitations in flexion or extension after capsular release are typically caused by the olecranon, the coronoid fossae, or impinging osteophytes. Removal of osteophytes or deepening of the olecranon or coronoid fossae with a burr may be required to create adequate space and achieve full ROM.
- If the patient's arm is unstable, a lateral ligament repair or reconstruction should be considered.
- The lateral incision can be extended distally via the Kocher approach to expose the lateral ligament complex.
- The interval between the anconeus and extensor carpi ulnaris muscles is developed, and the lateral ulnar collateral ligament is exposed.
- Ligament repair with advancement or plication of the ligament tissue can be performed if adequate tissue quality is present. In most patients, the ligament tissue is attenuated and augmentation with a ligament reconstruction is preferred.
- Many techniques for lateral ulnar collateral ligament reconstruction have been described. Surgeons should select the technique with which they are most comfortable. The author of this chapter prefers to use an allograft hamstring reconstruction with bone tunnels in the ulna and a docking technique in the humerus.

## Wound Closure

- The tourniquet is released, and hemostasis is attained before closure.
- In most patients, the ulnar nerve is placed back in its anatomic position. However, if the plate on the medial side narrows the area available for the ulnar nerve or if the nerve subluxates over the medial epicondyle during flexion, the

 

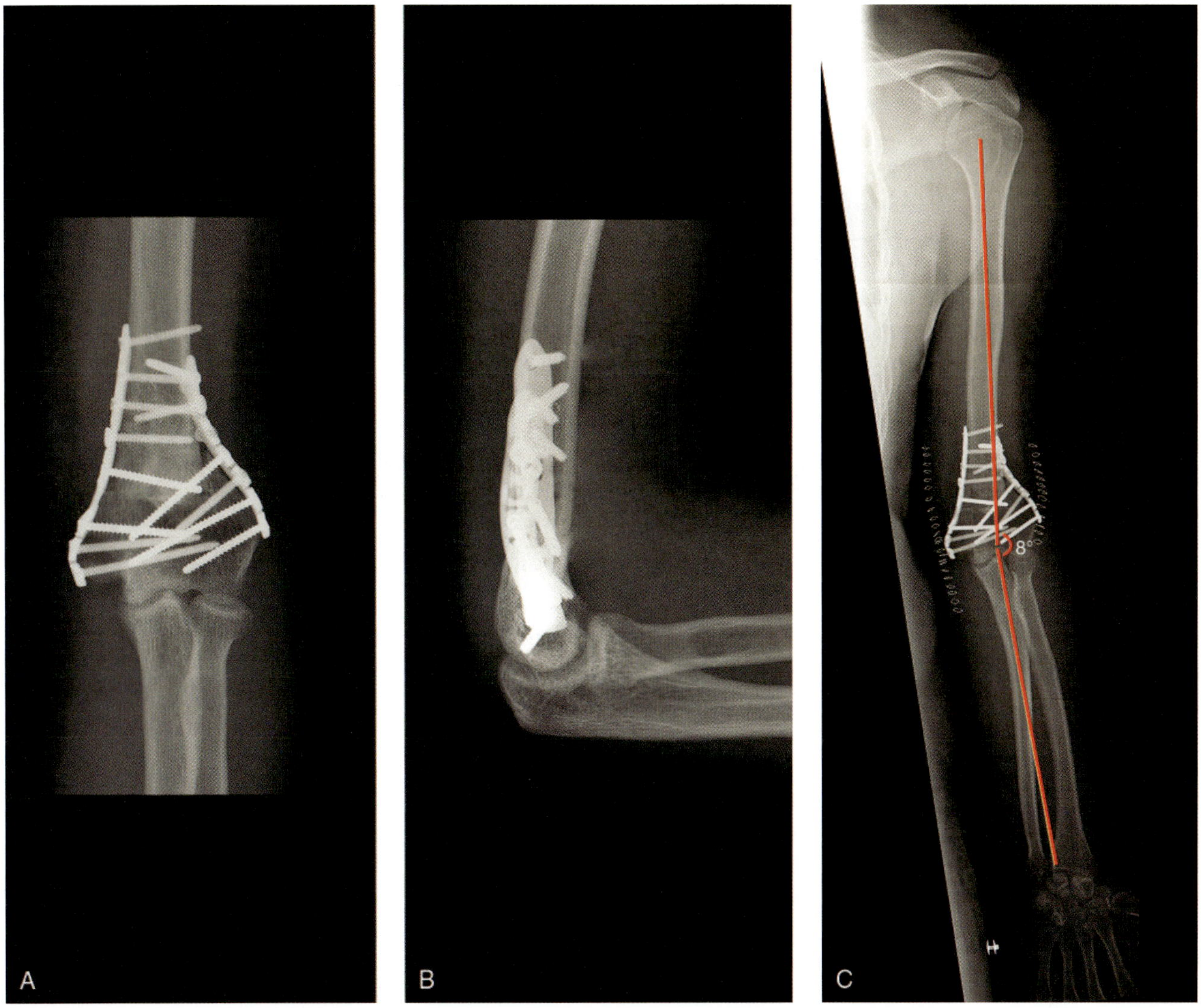


**Figure 7** Postoperative radiographs of an elbow demonstrate a healed distal humeral osteotomy. **A,** AP radiograph demonstrates healing of the osteotomy. **B,** Lateral radiograph demonstrates correction of an extension malunion. **C,** Upper extremity radiograph demonstrates correction of a varus malunion to normal alignment with 8° of valgus.

author of this chapter performs an anterior subcutaneous ulnar nerve transposition.

- The fascial layers over the medial and lateral columns are closed with the use of interrupted absorbable sutures.
- The skin is closed in a layered fashion with the use of absorbable subcutaneous sutures and skin staples.
- A bulky dressing is applied, and the surgical arm is splinted in 60° of flexion and neutral rotation.

## Postoperative Regimen

The patient is admitted to the hospital overnight for pain control and neurovascular monitoring and is discharged from the hospital the next day. The patient returns to the office between 1 and 2 weeks postoperatively for splint removal and a wound check. The elbow is kept in a sling to prevent weight bearing, and gravity-assisted flexion and extension ROM exercises are initiated. The patient returns of the office 4 weeks postoperatively to ensure appropriate gains in ROM and to be assessed for radiographic signs of healing. Active and active-assisted ROM is initiated; however, patients are instructed to not use the arm for daily activities until 6 weeks postoperatively. Healing typically occurs 10 to 12 weeks postoperatively. Patients are allowed to increase activity as tolerated after clinical and radiographic healing has occurred (**Figure 7**).

## Limiting Adverse Events

Preoperative assessment of the distal humeral anatomy and malunion helps ensure a successful osteotomy. A preoperative 3D CT reconstruction helps determine the extent of the distal humeral deformity and the degree of correction desired. The use of 3D custom cutting guides or a 3D model of the patient's distal humerus can help in planning the osteotomy in patients who have complex deformities. An evaluation for associated pathology, including tardy ulnar nerve palsy and posterolateral rotatory instability, is an important part of the preoperative assessment.

A triceps-preserving approach is preferred because it allows for adequate exposure of the distal humeral osteotomy site. Careful mobilization of the ulnar nerve and subperiosteal dissection anteriorly are essential to prevent nerve injury. Many configurations for corrective osteotomy have been described, and surgeons should select the technique with which they are most comfortable. Rigid fixation with medial and lateral column plates ensures stability and allows for early elbow ROM. Identification and management of associated pathology, including ulnar nerve palsy, joint contracture, and instability, are essential to ensure successful outcomes.

## Bibliography


Beuerlein MJ, Reid JT, Schemitsch EH, McKee MD: Effect of distal humeral varus deformity on strain in the lateral ulnar collateral ligament and ulnohumeral joint stability. *J Bone Joint Surg Am* 2004;86(10):2235-2242.

Chung MS, Baek GH: Three-dimensional corrective osteotomy for cubitus varus in adults. *J Shoulder Elbow Surg* 2003;12(5):472-475.

Cobb TK, Linscheid RL: Late correction of malunited intercondylar humeral fractures: Intra-articular osteotomy and tricortical bone grafting. *J Bone Joint Surg Br* 1994;76(4):622-626.

Cohen MS, Jupiter JB: Intra-articular osteotomy for malunited articular fractures of the distal end of the humerus. *J Shoulder Elbow Surg* 2014;23(4):579-585.

Hahn SB, Choi YR, Kang HJ: Corrective dome osteotomy for cubitus varus and valgus in adults. *J Shoulder Elbow Surg* 2009;18(1):38-43.

Husband JB, Hastings H II: The lateral approach for operative release of post-traumatic contracture of the elbow. *J Bone Joint Surg Am* 1990;72(9):1353-1358.

Kawanishi Y, Miyake J, Kataoka T, et al: Does cubitus varus cause morphologic and alignment changes in the elbow joint? *J Shoulder Elbow Surg* 2013;22(7):915-923.

Kim HT, Lee JS, Yoo CI: Management of cubitus varus and valgus. *J Bone Joint Surg Am* 2005;87(4):771-780.

Labelle H, Bunnell WP, Duhaime M, Poitras B: Cubitus varus deformity following supracondylar fractures of the humerus in children. *J Pediatr Orthop* 1982;2(5):539-546.

McKee M, Jupiter J, Toh CL, Wilson L, Colton C, Karras KK: Reconstruction after malunion and nonunion of intra-articular fractures of the distal humerus: Methods and results in 13 adults. *J Bone Joint Surg Br* 1994;76(4):614-621.

Moradi A, Vahedi E, Ebrahimzadeh MH: Surgical technique: Spike translation. A new modification in step-cut osteotomy for cubitus varus deformity. *Clin Orthop Relat Res* 2013;471(5):1564-1571.


 

O'Driscoll SW, Spinner RJ, McKee MD, et al: Tardy posterolateral rotatory instability of the elbow due to cubitus varus. *J Bone Joint Surg Am* 2001;83(9):1358-1369.

Piggot J, Graham HK, McCoy GF: Supracondylar fractures of the humerus in children: Treatment by straight lateral traction. *J Bone Joint Surg Br* 1986;68(4):577-583.

Sanchez-Sotelo J: Nonunion and malunion of distal humerus fractures, in Morrey BF, ed: *The Elbow and Its Disorders*, ed 4. Philadelphia, PA, Saunders Elsevier, 2009, pp 349-358.

Solfelt DA, Hill BW, Anderson CP, Cole PA: Supracondylar osteotomy for the treatment of cubitus varus in children: A systematic review. *Bone Joint J* 2014;96(5):691-700.

Stans AA, Maritz NG, O'Driscoll SW, Morrey BF: Operative treatment of elbow contracture in patients twenty-one years of age or younger. *J Bone Joint Surg Am* 2002;84(3):382-387.

Takagi T, Takayama S, Nakamura T, Horiuchi Y, Toyama Y, Ikegami H: Supracondylar osteotomy of the humerus to correct cubitus varus: Do both internal rotation and extension deformities need to be corrected? *J Bone Joint Surg Am* 2010;92(7):1619-1626.

Takeyasu Y, Oka K, Miyake J, Kataoka T, Moritomo H, Murase T: Preoperative, computer simulation-based, three-dimensional corrective osteotomy for cubitus varus deformity with use of a custom-designed surgical device. *J Bone Joint Surg Am* 2013;95(22):e173.

Zhang YZ, Lu S, Chen B, Zhao JM, Liu R, Pei GX: Application of computer-aided design osteotomy template for treatment of cubitus varus deformity in teenagers: A pilot study. *J Shoulder Elbow Surg* 2011;20(1):51-56.

# Chapter 29

# Nonunion of the Proximal Ulna

*Neal C. Chen, MD*

*Jesse B. Jupiter, MD*

**Learning Objectives**

- Understand the indications for surgical management of nonunited fractures.
- Learn surgical tactics for managing nonunion of the proximal ulna.

## Indications

Nonunion of the proximal ulna is uncommon. Like most fractures, a proximal ulnar fracture is considered a nonunion if it exhibits no clinical or radiographic signs of union after 6 months postinjury. Nonunion is often recognized in the setting of hardware loosening or breakage.

A nonunited proximal ulnar fracture can be painful and unstable. The goals of surgery are to achieve bony union, a stable ulnohumeral joint, and proper forearm alignment. Postoperative exercises help optimize range of motion (ROM). The following factors should be considered before planning surgery: patient symptoms, patient infirmity, function of the limb distal to the fracture, patient demands, status of the soft-tissue envelope, status of the extensor mechanism, size and condition of the proximal fracture fragment containing the triceps attachment, status of the articular cartilage, existing implants, colonization or infection, and capsular contracture and heterotopic ossification.

## Contraindications

Surgical treatment is contraindicated for patients who have medical comorbidities that preclude surgery. In some patients, radiographic nonunion may be stable due to the presence of a nonossified, fibrous connection. In some patients, function is good even in the setting of a widely displaced nonunion. In such patients, if the nonunion is asymptomatic and forearm alignment is acceptable, surgery may not be warranted. In a patient in whom the nonunion is infected, the infection should be addressed before attempts to achieve union are begun.

Relative contraindications are patient unwillingness or inability to comply with postoperative protocols. Patients with a heavy smoking history are encouraged to stop smoking, if possible. If the patient has an infected nonunion, it may be necessary to delay fixation until the infection is eradicated with débridement and parenteral antibiotics.

## Alternative Treatments

Triceps advancement has been described for the treatment of small proximal olecranon nonunions in which the bone may not be able to support implants. Triceps advancement should not be performed if less than 50% of the articular surface is available for reconstruction.

## Results

The authors of limited case series have described the treatment of proximal ulnar nonunion with rigid plating and autogenous bone grafting (**Table 1**). The available data are retrospective, and the injuries and techniques of treatment are heterogeneous. In most patients, treatment resulted in bony union; however, final ROM was decreased. Reported complications include heterotopic bone, ulnar neuropathy, hardware irritation, and arthrosis.

---

*Dr. Chen or an immediate family member serves as a board member, owner, officer, or committee member of the American Association for Hand Surgery. Dr. Jupiter or an immediate family member is a member of a speakers' bureau or has made paid presentations on behalf of Synthes; serves as a paid consultant to or is an employee of Aptis Medical and OHK Medical Devices; serves as an unpaid consultant to Synthes and TriMed; has stock or stock options held in OHK Medical Devices; has received research or institutional support from AO Foundation; and serves as a board member, owner, officer, or committee member of the American Association for Hand Surgery, American Shoulder and Elbow Surgeons, and the American Society for Surgery of the Hand.*

**Table 1** Results for the Treatment of Nonunion of the Proximal Ulna and Olecranon[a]

| Authors (Year) | Number of Patients | Procedure or Approach | Mean Patient Age (yr) | Mean Follow-up (mo) | Success Rate (%) | Results |
|---|---|---|---|---|---|---|
| Danziger and Healy (1992) | 5 | ORIF to manage olecranon nonunion | 18 | 36 | 100 | Union was achieved in all patients |
| Papagelopoulos and Morrey (1994) | 24 | 16 ORIF with graft, 3 TEAs, 1 excision, and 4 distraction arthroplasties to manage olecranon nonunion | 42 | 18 | 100 | Union was achieved in 15 of the nonunions that were managed with ORIF |
| Ring et al (2003) | 10 | ORIF with graft to manage atrophic ulnar nonunion (8 patients also had bony defects) | 46.5 | 39 | 100 | Union was achieved in all patients at 3-mo follow-up |
| Rotini et al (2008) | 12 | ORIF with graft to manage olecranon nonunion | 41 | 27 | 91 | Union was achieved in 11 patients |
| Khalil et al (2010) | 21 | ORIF with graft (18 patients) or without graft (3 patients) | 41.7 | 22 | 90 | Union was achieved in 19 patients |

ORIF = open reduction and internal fixation, TEA = total elbow arthroplasty.
[a] All studies are level IV evidence.

# Techniques

## Preoperative Planning

- In patients in whom the fracture alignment is not easily understood, contralateral forearm radiographs are obtained to determine ulnar length intraoperatively. If necessary, CT helps clarify fracture morphology.
- Preoperative laboratory studies may include an erythrocyte sedimentation rate, C-reactive protein level, and a white blood cell count with differential to evaluate for underlying infection.

## Setup/Exposure

- Patients may be placed in the prone, supine, or lateral decubitus position.
- For supine positioning, an arm holder attached to the contralateral side of the table can be helpful; if used, adequate access to the ulnar shaft must be ensured. If the arm holder is prohibitive, a bump can be placed over the chest; a nonpenetrating clip can be used to hold the elbow to the patient; and a small, stout bump can be placed along the humerus.
- If an arm holder is used, any compression wraps used must be applied loosely to avoid elevating compartment pressures in the forearm.
- The C-arm can be moved in from the contralateral side as well. The radiology technician should obtain sample radiographs to ensure adequate images can be obtained.
- For lateral decubitus positioning, the patient is positioned over a bean bag.
- An arm holder or bump is placed before the patient is prepped and draped. The arm holder is at the level of the chest to place the affected shoulder in 90° of forward flexion. If an arm holder is not available, a rolled blanket can be used as a bump.
- Regardless of approach, a sterile tourniquet is used intraoperatively.

## Instruments/Equipment/Implants Required

- Instruments that may be used include threaded and smooth Kirschner wires (K-wires) in sizes up to 0.062 inches, Steinmann pins, a small or medium external fixator, a laminar spreader or articulated tensioning device, and an anterior cruciate ligament tibial guide.
- Equipment used includes a fluoroscope or mini C-arm, an arm holder, and a sterile tourniquet.
- The following implant hardware is used: olecranon plate with corresponding screws; cannulated screws; 22-gauge wire, if necessary; hand/digital plates and screws; and bone graft or bone graft substitute, if necessary.

## Procedure

- An Esmarch bandage is used to exsanguinate the limb.
- The tourniquet is inflated to 250 mm Hg.
- A posterior elbow incision is made.

 

- The triceps fascia tendon is identified proximally. This indicates the depth at which the flap can be elevated medially and laterally.
- The ulnar nerve is identified proximally and traced distally.
- The Osborne ligament is released.
- The superficial and deep heads of the flexor carpi ulnaris are released. It helps to release the nerve approximately 6 to 8 cm proximal and 6 to 8 cm distal to the medial epicondyle.
- A 0.25-inch Penrose drain or a vessel loop is passed around the nerve to help with manipulation, and the nerve is released from its bed using Stevens scissors for dissection and bipolar electrocautery. Nerve transposition at the end of the procedure is performed based on the surgeon's preference.
- The fracture nonunion site often can be identified by sliding a closed Adson forceps along the intact bone while applying gentle pressure. Often, the forceps will fall into the nonunion site.
- A pseudarthrosis can express fluid. If unanticipated infection is a concern, tissue should be sent for culture and pathology, and then surgery is staged.
- The edges of the fracture are identified using a No. 15 blade to remove tissue at the edges of the bone. The area around the bone is prepared via osteoperiosteal petalling.
- The interposed tissue between the fracture edges is removed using a curet and a rongeur. A reamer can be passed into the ulna distally to help recannulate the bone.
- In some patients in whom radial head injury exists, the radial head can be addressed through the proximal ulnar fracture.
- In many nonunion cases, open reduction and internal fixation of the radial head may not be possible and arthroplasty may be necessary. Occasionally, a separate lateral approach using a lateral skin flap and a Kaplan or Kocher interval approach can help expose the radial neck to fully evaluate or manage the radial head injury.
- The radial head is excised using a sagittal saw or osteotome at the level of the radial neck.
- The radial head is sized and the radial neck is broached.
- Prosthetic trials are inserted to estimate the actual prosthesis fit. For nonunited fractures, traditional methods used to evaluate overstuffing are limited; however, the goal is to keep the prosthetic radial head level with the cartilage of the lateral coronoid facet.
- The radial head fragments are preserved to be used for potential reconstruction of any bony deficiency of the coronoid.
- If the radiocapitellar joint is incongruent, congruity is restored via proper alignment of the ulnar fracture.
- If the coronoid is fractured, this fracture is treated first. Any large coronoid fragments can be stabilized using bicortical screws to secure the coronoid to the ulnar shaft. Smaller fragments can be captured with threaded K-wires.
- For patients in whom there is large comminution or poor bone quality, a medial split of the flexor-pronator mass or an approach through the bed of the ulnar nerve can be used to place a plate to buttress the coronoid anteriorly. If approaching through the ulnar nerve bed, the nerve may be tethered by the first posterior branch to the flexor carpi ulnaris. Some surgeons have described transecting this branch to improve access through the bed.
- If the coronoid is insufficient and the native radial head is available, the radial head can be used to reconstruct the coronoid. The radial head is contoured to fit the coronoid. The radial head graft can be secured with screws passed either anterior-to-posterior or posterior-to-anterior.
- If possible, two screws are preferred to help control rotation.
- If cannulated screws are passed from posterior to anterior, an anterior cruciate ligament tibial guide can help with guidewire placement.
- If preferred by the treating surgeon, fixation can be reinforced by passing a size 0 polydioxanone suture through the cannulated hole in each screw to relay a nonresorbable high-caliber suture through the screws. The suture is tied over an ulnar bone bridge.
- After the coronoid and collateral ligament elements are repaired, the proximal ulna is plated. Plating can be difficult in the setting of nonunion because achieving proper alignment and length of the ulna is a challenge. Two methods used to attain proper alignment are the push-pull screw technique (**Figure 1**) and placement of an external fixator (**Figures 2** and **3**).
- The push-pull screw technique begins with securing the plate to the proximal ulna, either by placing locked screws into the proximal fragment or by placing K-wires into the proximal fragment. Correct alignment of the plate is difficult because angular and rotational malalignment of long plates is magnified distally.
- After the proximal fragment is secured, the plate is provisionally secured to the distal fragment using a Verbrugge clamp.
- A screw is placed distal to the plate, and, depending on the fracture configuration, a laminar spreader or a clamp is used to distract or close the fracture fragments relative to the plate.
- With small amounts of malrotation

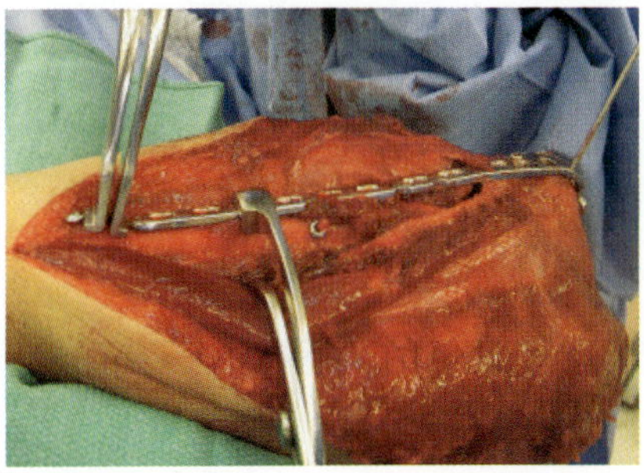

**Figure 1** Intraoperative photograph of an elbow shows a push-pull technique used to manage an acute proximal ulna fracture. The plate is secured to the olecranon with screws and Kirschner wires, and the distal plate is held to the ulnar shaft with a Verbrugge clamp. As the laminar spreader is opened, the ulnar fracture is brought to the proper length and the plate secured with screws. (Copyright Massachusetts General Hospital, Boston, MA.)

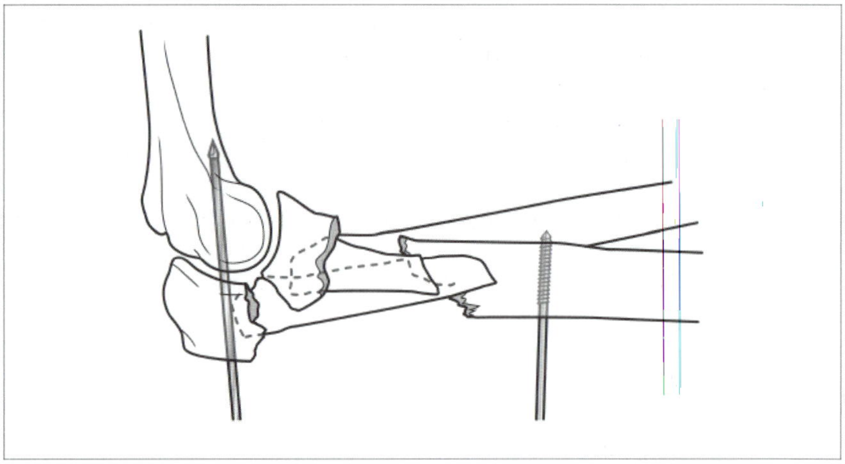

**Figure 2** Illustration of an elbow shows an external fixator used to align a proximal ulna fracture.

or malalignment, the plate can be bent in situ; however, if more malrotation or malalignment is present, it may be necessary to reapply the plate proximally.

- For the external fixator technique, a pin is placed through the proximal fragment and advanced into the distal humerus.
- A plate is selected and aligned to ensure engagement of one of the proximal holes at the location of the external fixator pin.
- An external fixator pin is placed into the ulnar shaft at a position that will not interfere with plate placement.
- Distraction and alignment are obtained and provisionally maintained using the external fixator. Although this can be ideally obtained via a single external fixator bar that links the proximal and distal pins, imperfect alignment can be improved by using additional external fixator joints that allow additional rotational and angular freedom.
- After obtaining acceptable alignment of the nonunion, the plate can be secured and, if preferred, bone graft added (**Figure 4**).
- In the setting of an ulnohumeral joint with tenuous stability or gross instability, supplemental fixation using an external fixator, internal hinge, or transjoint pinning should be considered. Currently, the authors of this chapter favor hinged external fixation.
- In general, an axis pin is placed into the axis of the distal ulna. The best way to achieve this is by acquiring a perfect lateral image of the distal humerus by using a mini C-arm.
- The center of the trochlea should be in the center of the image intensifier and the arm should be as close to the image intensifier as possible. The axis guide pin is aligned to the axis of the source and the intensifier, then advanced. Axis pins are placed proximally and distally after the primary wounds are closed. The fixator is assembled based on the axis pin. After the fixator is secured, the axis pin is removed.

## Wound Closure

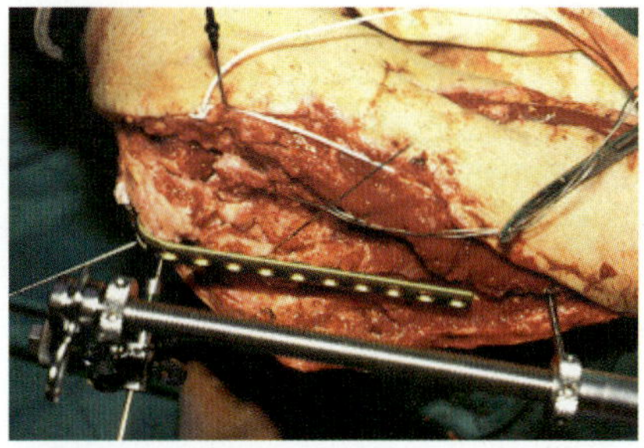

**Figure 3** Intraoperative photograph of an elbow shows an external fixator/distractor used to repair a proximal ulna nonunion. The device location is designated to avoid interference with plate placement. This device allows gradual distraction to help limit soft-tissue stripping. (Reproduced from Jupiter JB, Mudgal CS: Reconstruction of delayed unions and nonunions of the proximal ulna and olecranon, in Yamaguchi K, King GJ, McKee MD, O'Driscoll SW: *Advanced Reconstruction: Elbow.* Rosemont, IL, American Academy of Orthopaedic Surgeons, 2007, pp 375-386.)

- Muscular intervals are closed by using resorbable sutures.
- Any ligament origins that have been damaged can be reattached using suture anchors.
- When a hinged fixator is used, lateral suture anchors are placed after the axis pin has been placed.
- In the setting of ulnar nerve transposition, the course of the nerve should be checked for any undue tension. A 1-cm-wide slip of the

 

flexor-pronator fascia can be used as a sling to maintain the transposed position. Alternatively, the subcutaneous fat or a free slip of the intermuscular septum can be used.

- Hemostasis is attained and the wound is closed in layers over a negative suction drain.
- If possible, skin staples are used, but nylon sutures may be preferable if the skin is friable.

## Postoperative Regimen

Active ROM is begun as soon as possible postoperatively, beginning with gentle active ROM exercises. ROM with the patient in a supine position with the shoulder at 90° of forward flexion can be helpful if there are concerns regarding ulnohumeral joint instability. The patient wears a long arm posterior orthoplast splint for comfort for the first 2 weeks postoperatively, but the patient is gradually weaned from the splint for protection in public after this interval. A hinged fixator used to treat ulnohumeral instability can be removed 4 weeks postoperatively; however, a hinged fixator used to manage tenuous fixation is removed after early signs of radiographic healing are observed. Gentle passive ROM can begin at 4 weeks postoperatively. Active, self-assisted ROM is encouraged, but forceful pushing is avoided until there is evidence of radiographic healing. Static progressive splinting is suggested if patients experience stiffness and have trouble performing the stretches on their own. Resistance and strengthening exercises are begun only after there is radiographic evidence of union (**Figure 5**).

## Limiting Adverse Events

The thickest possible soft-tissue envelope should be maintained on the posterior elbow during dissection. In revision surgery, if the skin envelope is insufficient, it is preferable to achieve improved soft-tissue coverage with either a local or a distant flap and wait for tissue homeostasis before treating the

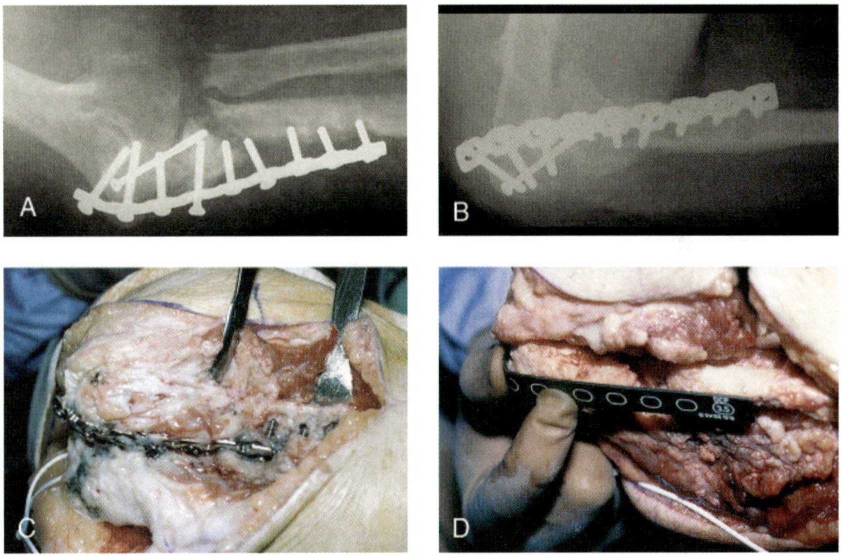

**Figure 4** AP (**A**) and lateral (**B**) radiographs of an elbow demonstrate an atrophic olecranon nonunion. **C,** Intraoperative photograph shows nonunion exposed via a prior posterior incision. **D,** Intraoperative photograph shows a metal template used to model the fixation plate contour. (Copyright Massachusetts General Hospital, Boston, MA.)

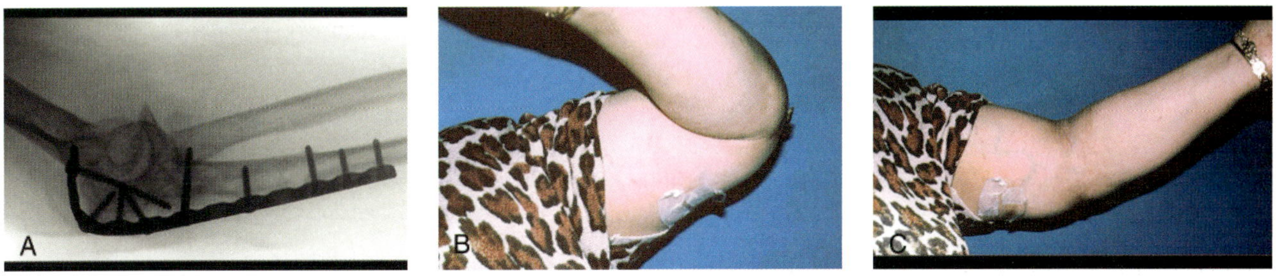

**Figure 5** **A,** Postoperative lateral AP radiograph of an elbow demonstrates healed nonunion after plating. Postoperative photographs show elbow flexion (**B**) and extension (**C**). (Panel A reproduced from Jupiter JB, Mudgal CS: Reconstruction of delayed unions and nonunions of the proximal ulna and olecranon, in Yamaguchi K, King GJ, McKee MD, O'Driscoll SW: *Advanced Reconstruction: Elbow*. Rosemont, IL, American Academy of Orthopaedic Surgeons, 2007, pp 375-386; panels B and C copyright Massachusetts General Hospital, Boston, MA.)

nonunion. In addition, ulnar neuropathy can contribute to elbow pain, and subcutaneous transposition is strongly considered in patients with symptoms or signs of ulnar nerve dysfunction. During revision surgery, devascularization of fracture fragments should be avoided, especially during mobilization. If the fracture has shortened, an external fixator can be used to stretch soft tissues to better preserve vascularity to fragments than can additional soft-tissue dissection.

Plate selection is important. A limited contact–dynamic compression plate may be preferable to locked plating in some patients. In cases of nonunion, the goal is to achieve bony healing via secondary bone healing. Some concern exists that locked plating may be too stiff to allow the micromotion needed for callus formation. But if bone quality is poor and screw purchase may be compromised, locked plating can be useful.

## Bibliography

Danziger MB, Healy WL: Operative treatment of olecranon nonunion. *J Orthop Trauma* 1992;6(3):290-293.

Jupiter JB, Leibovic SJ, Ribbans W, Wilk RM: The posterior Monteggia lesion. *J Orthop Trauma* 1991;5(4):395-402.

Khalil A, Elsayed M, Seleem O: Contoured plating for proximal ulna nonunion: An improved technique. *Int Orthop* 2010;34(3):441-445.

Modabber MR, Jupiter JB: Reconstruction for post-traumatic conditions of the elbow joint. *J Bone Joint Surg Am* 1995;77(9):1431-1446.

O'Driscoll SW, Jupiter JB, Cohen MS, Ring D, McKee MD: Difficult elbow fractures: Pearls and pitfalls. *Instr Course Lect* 2003;52:113-134.

Papagelopoulos PJ, Morrey BF: Treatment of nonunion of olecranon fractures. *J Bone Joint Surg Br* 1994;76(4):627-635.

Ring D, Jupiter JB, Gulotta L: Atrophic nonunions of the proximal ulna. *Clin Orthop Relat Res* 2003;409:268-274.

Ring D, Tavakolian J, Kloen P, Helfet D, Jupiter JB: Loss of alignment after surgical treatment of posterior Monteggia fractures: Salvage with dorsal contoured plating. *J Hand Surg Am* 2004;29(4):694-702.

Rotini R, Antonioli D, Marinelli A, Katusi D: Surgical treatment of proximal ulna nonunion. *Chir Organi Mov* 2008;91(2):65-70.

 

# Chapter 30
# Interposition Arthroplasty for the Elbow

*Robert N. Hotchkiss, MD*

**Learning Objectives**

- Appreciate the technical challenges and objectives of interposition arthroplasty.
- Reconsider the indications for and limitations of interposition arthroplasty.

## Indications

Interposition arthroplasty of any joint seldom, if ever, results in outcomes as good as those of a well-designed implant arthroplasty, at least with regard to short-term (2- to 3-year) outcomes. In the lower extremity, specifically the hip and knee, the interposition of tissue was never a serious alternative after Charnley and implant arthroplasty of the hip and the continued successful evolution of metal-plastic implants. Although several total elbow arthroplasty implants have been developed over the past three decades, none can withstand moderate postoperative daily demands (lifting of >15 to 20 lb), provide immediate and stable function, and deliver predictable durability (>10 years). Active, healthy patients who have loss of cartilage, limited motion, and disabling pain in combination with an expectation of moderate postoperative demands may not be optimal candidates for total elbow arthroplasty with the use of a linked cemented implant.

The optimal indications, technique, and patient selection for interposition arthroplasty have changed in the past 20 years. Before the introduction of biologic agents, inflammatory arthritis, typically rheumatoid arthritis, caused considerable destruction to most joints in the upper extremity. As a result, patients with hand and shoulder impairment placed fewer and lower demands on the elbow, both in peak load and in the duration of use. With improved life expectancy of patients with rheumatoid arthritis and with fewer joints affected or destroyed, the nature of the destruction of the affected joints is often less profound, with greater preservation of periarticular bone. Whereas historically a painful arthritic elbow was subjected to lower demands in a patient with a disabled hand and shoulder, the healthier patients of today place greater physical demands on the joint and have an expectation of higher activity demands.

Interposition elbow arthroplasty does not necessarily provide reliable pain relief and long-term durability. In the upper extremity, load bearing across the joint can be effectively controlled with position and activity modification, without resulting in complete loss of function. Patients who lift an object with the shoulder in no (zero) abduction place less contact pressure on medial bearing surfaces; however, as shoulder abduction increases toward 90°, a substantial varus load develops, and any loss of lateral ligament integrity or erosion of the load-bearing surface on the medial coronoid/humeral surface makes lifting and holding an object a formidable challenge. Disease progression, especially with resorption of bone, will lead to instability, pain, and marked loss of function. Larsen class 3 rheumatoid arthritis (narrowing of joint space only) may be managed with interposition arthroplasty (**Figure 1**). However, interposition arthroplasty is not recommended to manage Larsen class 4 rheumatoid arthritis (major defect).

In the absence of erosion, interposition arthroplasty can provide pain relief and improved function. Behavioral and lifting modifications as well as biologic and disease-modifying antirheumatic drug therapies play an essential role in obtaining a successful outcome. Although the Larsen classification was intended only for use in patients with rheumatoid arthritis, the distinction between class 3 and 4 rheumatoid arthritis can be extended to the evaluation of posttraumatic patients. That is, interposition arthroplasty likely will be unsuccessful if substantive defects extend into the subchondral surface in the ulnohumeral articulation or if bone is missing as a result of injury.

*Dr. Hotchkiss or an immediate family member has received research or institutional support from Auxilium Pharmaceuticals, now a division of Endo Pharmaceuticals.*

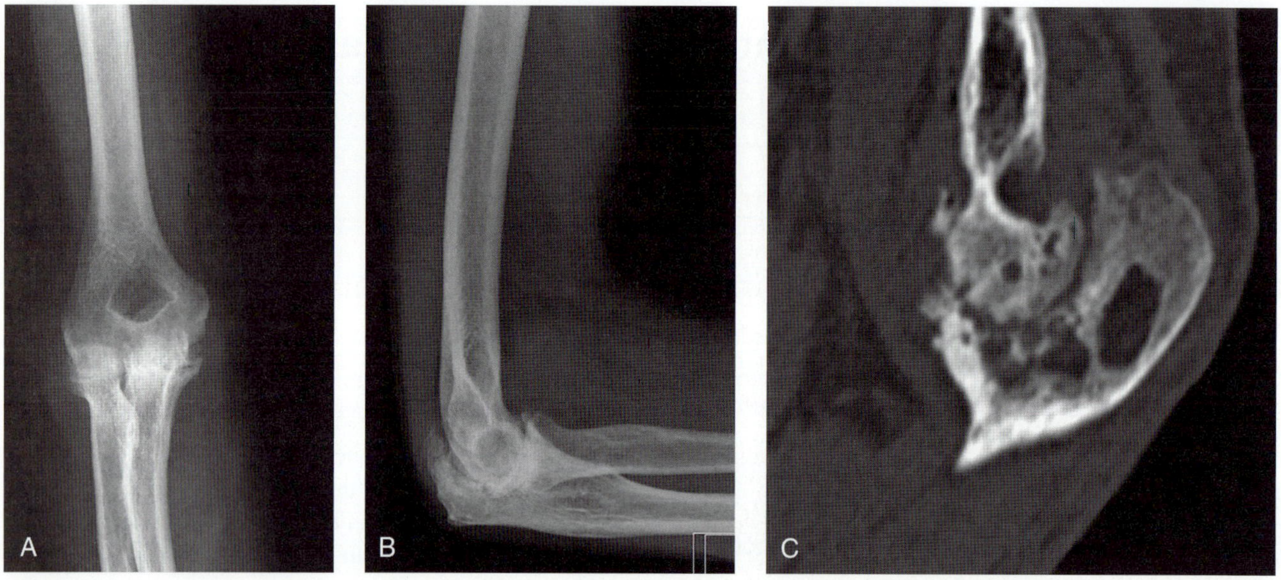


**Figure 1** AP (**A**) and lateral (**B**) radiographs of an elbow with Larsen class 3 rheumatoid arthritis (narrowing without major defects). **C,** Sagittal CT scan of an elbow with Larsen class 4 rheumatoid arthritis (major defect). (Copyright Robert Hotchkiss, MD, New York, NY.)

Many patients with painful inflammatory arthritis are well informed and are wary of undergoing implant arthroplasty. Similarly, most patients with painful rheumatoid arthritis have neither heard of nor been offered interposition arthroplasty as a treatment option. The decision to proceed with interposition arthroplasty often requires more than one preoperative visit and discussion. Patients who have undergone interposition arthroplasty are an excellent resource and are often willing to discuss their experience, whether good or bad, with a patient who is deciding whether to undergo interposition arthroplasty. Such peer-to-peer discussion should be encouraged. Patients also should be encouraged to obtain a second opinion from a surgical colleague.

Most patients who undergo interposition arthroplasty are unable to achieve full extension postoperatively, and no patients who undergo interposition arthroplasty describe having a normal elbow postoperatively. The goals of interposition arthroplasty are to decrease pain, increase mobility, improve function, and allow for several years of durability. In general, all of these goals can be achieved; however, surgeons must have a frank discussion with patients with regard to the possibility of continued pain, either in the short term (the first 6 months) or in subsequent years.

Interposition elbow arthroplasty may be performed to manage severe cartilage loss, limited motion, and disabling pain in a healthy, active patient with inflammatory or posttraumatic arthritis. Interposition arthroplasty offers select patients with inflammatory or posttraumatic arthritis a treatment option that does not preclude later total implant arthroplasty that can be quite durable. Although it is usually possible to perform total elbow arthroplasty after failed interposition arthroplasty, interposition arthroplasty cannot be performed after failed total elbow arthroplasty.

The ideal patient for interposition elbow arthroplasty is younger than 60 years, has a healthy and strong upper extremity (shoulder, wrist, and hand), Larsen class 2 or 3 rheumatoid arthritis of the elbow, inflammatory arthritis that is actively managed and monitored by a rheumatologist, and the capacity to make an informed decision. Such patients may experience years of improved function postoperatively. Subchondral cavitary bone loss is common after elbow trauma, and patients with subchondral bone loss are less likely to have successful outcomes after interposition elbow arthroplasty. Nonetheless, interposition arthroplasty should be considered, albeit with caution, in younger patients with intact subchondral surfaces who have elbow cartilage damage as a result of trauma.

## Contraindications

Interposition arthroplasty is not recommended to manage Larsen class 4 rheumatoid arthritis (deep erosion into the subchondral bone) or posttraumatic injury with subchondral defects because the arthroplasty is likely to be unstable. Interposition arthroplasty also is contraindicated in patients who are older than age 60 years, have poor upper extremity health, are not under active treatment by a rheumatologist, and cannot make an informed decision or adhere to postoperative activity restrictions.

 

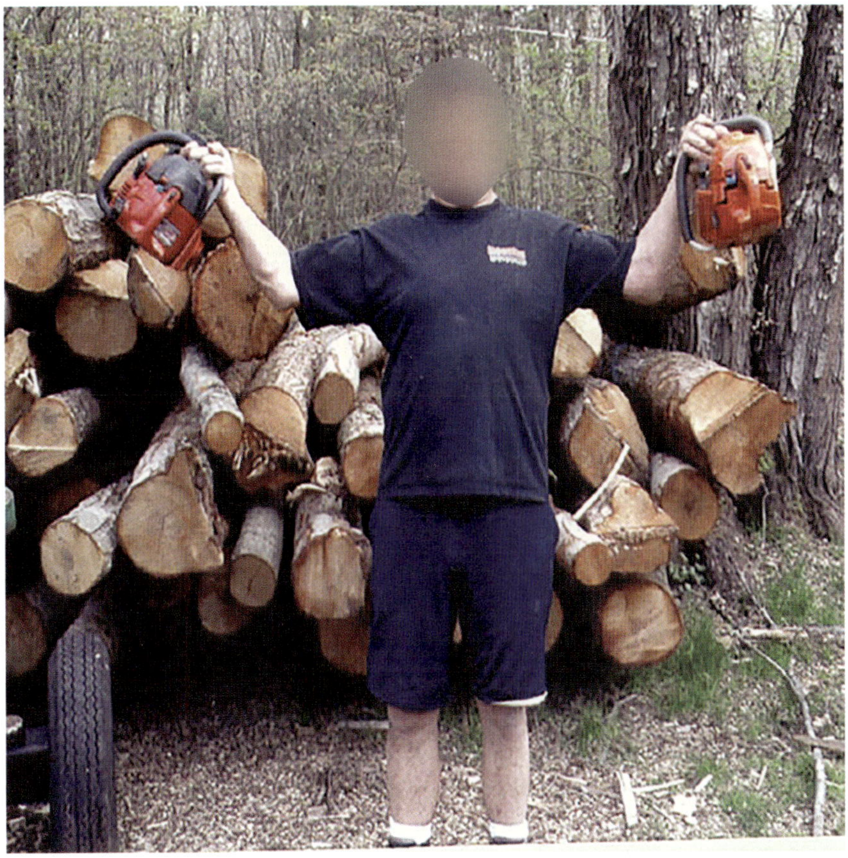

**Figure 2** Photograph of a 55-year-old man holding chainsaws in the air after having undergone interposition arthroplasty of the right elbow 5 years earlier and of the left elbow 4 years earlier. (Copyright Robert Hotchkiss, MD, New York, NY.)

## Alternative Treatments

Total elbow arthroplasty is an alternative to interposition arthroplasty.

## Results

In his own practice, the author of this chapter observed improved pain at rest and with moderate activity in the first 15 patients on whom he performed interposition arthroplasty. Many of those patients resumed high-demand activities postoperatively, including carpentry, plumbing, electrical work, sport fishing, and golf (**Figure 2**). A small number of patients chose to undergo interposition arthroplasty for the contralateral elbow at a later date. Since performing those first interposition arthroplasties, the author of this chapter has performed an additional 25 such surgeries, with results not much different from those of the first 15. Interposition arthroplasty is unlikely to offer patients a long-term solution for an arthritic elbow. Currently, interposition arthroplasty provides patients with the opportunity to postpone implant arthroplasty, attain pain relief lasting several years, and achieve relatively high function without activity restrictions.

The surgical technique for interposition arthroplasty has changed considerably over time. Studies have described joint dislocation in which the collateral ligaments were divided to interpose and secure the interposition material on both sides of the joint, after which the ligaments were reattached, repaired, or reconstructed. When this technique was used, the ligament repair and reconstruction was protected with the use of a hinged external fixator.

The use of various interposition materials, ranging from fascia lata (autograft) to Achilles tendon allograft and other materials, has been reported. The material used for interposition does not seem to have a substantial influence on outcomes. The author of this chapter switched from the use of fascia lata autograft to Achilles tendon allograft without a detectable change in outcomes. This switch in interposition material was made because the donor site for fascia lata autograft often was uncomfortable for patients for many months postoperatively.

The necessity of hinged external fixation and/or joint distraction has been questioned. In the first 6 weeks postoperatively, it is necessary to maintain joint stability during motion with no subluxation or dislocation; however, if the ligaments, especially those on the lateral side, are preserved during interposition arthroplasty, hinged external fixation and/or distraction of the joint may not be necessary. The role and effect of joint distraction, which separates the surfaces by a few millimeters for a few weeks during mobilization, is unknown. Because of the infrequency of interposition arthroplasty and patient variability, a clinical trial to determine the role of joint distraction is not feasible. The practical value of joint distraction is observed in patients in whom the axis pin is slightly off center and the joint is starting to bind; 3 to 4 mm of joint distraction can help reduce the effect of this small error and allow for motion.

## Techniques

### Setup/Exposure

- The patient is placed in the prone or lateral position to allow access

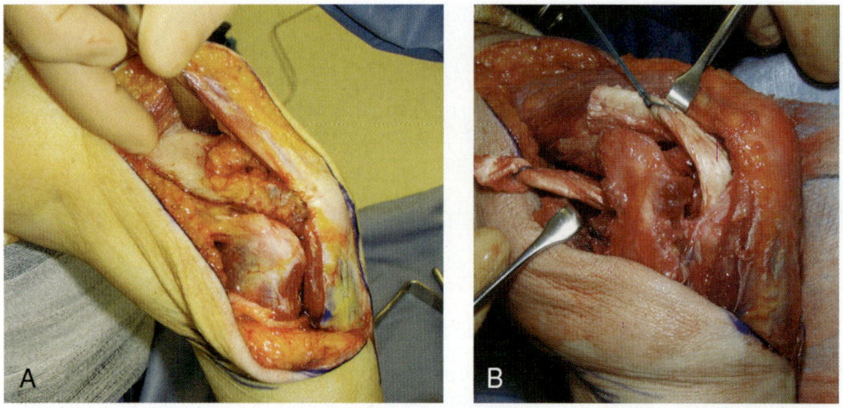

**Figure 3** Intraoperative photographs of the elbow of a patient placed in the prone position, which allows for excellent access to the joint during interposition arthroplasty. **A,** The medial side of the joint is exposed first. **B,** The graft is passed from posterior to anterior, taking care to preserve the medial collateral ligament. (Copyright Robert Hotchkiss, MD, New York, NY.)

to the elbow, with the arm draped over a holder. Often, the prone position is easier for the anesthesiologist because he or she can position the patient in a manner similar to that of a patient undergoing a spinal procedure, adding a regional block with an indwelling infraclavicular catheter before intubation. The lateral position also can be used; however, that position provides the anesthesiologist less access to the patient's airway if the patient is not intubated, which may be a problem because interposition arthroplasty can last several hours. The prone and lateral positions both allow for access to the entire arm and elbow.

- Before draping, the patient's arm is prepared all the way to the axilla. Depending on the type of external fixator used, if any, access to the upper one-third of the humerus usually is necessary.
- In general, a long posterior skin incision, which can be used in combination with flaps raised on either side, is preferred to gain access to the medial and lateral sides of the joint (**Figure 3, A**). If skin incisions from previous surgery are present, separate medial and lateral incisions or an extension of a medial incision that curves back toward the posterior midline both proximally and distally may be used.
- The use of a tourniquet is not required but can aid in the speed of dissection, especially of the ulnar nerve. A single-use tourniquet is narrower and allows for greater length of access to the humerus compared with a reusable, inflatable tourniquet.

## Instruments/Equipment/ Implants Required

- A regional block is necessary.
- An indwelling infraclavicular catheter is required.
- A fluoroscope is necessary.
- An Achilles tendon allograft is required.
- Either an axis-based hinged external fixation system or a plane-based external fixation system may be necessary.
- A single-use tourniquet may be used but is not required.

## Procedure

- The ulnar nerve is carefully dissected and mobilized so it is not under tension and can be protected throughout the procedure. Dissection of the ulnar nerve can be time-consuming, especially in patients who have undergone previous surgery.
- Ulnar nerve mobilization of 20 cm is common. In most patients, the ulnar nerve is left in the transposed position, anterior to the joint.
- If an external fixation system is used, pins should be placed along the medial side of the humerus, posterior to the transposed ulnar nerve, to avoid tension on the transposed ulnar nerve.
- Complete exposure of the joint without dislocation is crucial to success and may be the most important difference in the technical evolution of interposition arthroplasty.
- The capsule and synovium at both the anterior and posterior aspects of the joint must be completely excised. Most patients who undergo interposition arthroplasty lack motion; therefore, surgical approaches for contracture release are directly applicable.
- The medial over-the-top approach used to expose the medial side of the joint is almost identical to the approach used for contracture release. The medial over-the-top approach allows for full exposure of the ulnar nerve and access to the anterior and posterior joint for a near-complete synovectomy and capsular excision. The anterior medial collateral ligament is protected during the approach.
- A long posterior skin incision is made to expose the lateral side of the joint. This exposure allows for completion of the capsulectomy and synovectomy with preservation of the lateral collateral ligament.
- Usually in interposition arthroplasty, the radial head is excised because of deformity of the radial head and to improve pronation and supination.

 

- After the capsulectomy is complete, the tip of the olecranon (at least 1 cm) is removed. The surgeon should visualize olecranon tip excision from the medial and lateral perspectives.
- At this point, the surgeon should gently move the joint through a range of motion (ROM) to determine the extent of the contracture release. The ligaments in a very stiff elbow may exhibit limited pliability.
- A portion of each collateral ligament may begin to fail as the joint is gently moved from flexion to extension. There may be a tradeoff between full extension and loss of ligamentous integrity. The author of this chapter thinks that 20° to 25° of flexion contracture is preferable to instability and purposely accepts this limitation.
- A partial release of the medial side of the joint is preferable to detaching the lateral side of the joint. Even if both ligaments are partially or completely detached, repair of the tissue, including the medial flexor-pronator mass and the lateral extensor origin, back to the humerus will assist in healing of the underlying tissue and attaining ultimate stability. In these patients, an external fixation device usually will be necessary. Full extension is rarely achieved; however, 20° to 140° of motion is a goal for most patients.
- To insert the graft, the ulnohumeral joint must be distractible enough to allow for a graft with a thickness of 2 to 3 mm. Gentle manipulation of the joint with traction and rolling of the joint, alternating between varus and valgus, can aid in graft insertion.

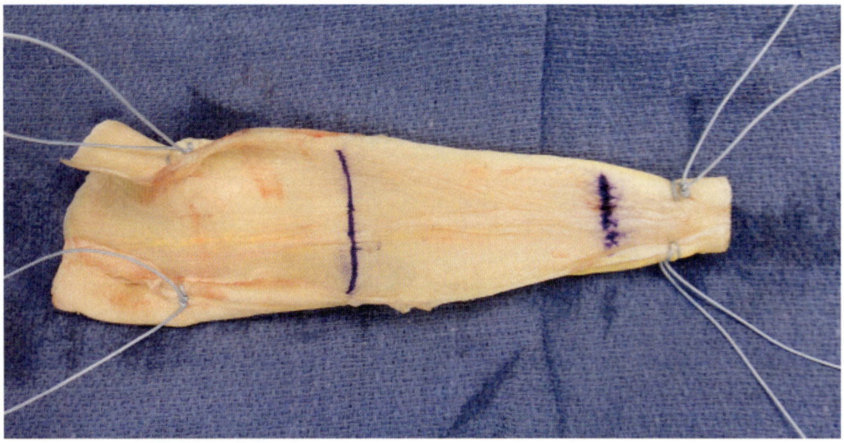

**Figure 4** Photograph shows an Achilles tendon allograft (OHK Medical Devices) that has been prepared for insertion into a joint. Suture tags are used to grasp the corners of the allograft during insertion. The lines marked in ink indicate the boundaries of the typical area of graft with the optimal thickness for interposition. (Copyright Robert Hotchkiss, MD, New York, NY.)

## GRAFT PREPARATION AND INSERTION

- The Achilles tendon allograft is thawed and inspected for continuity. Usually, the thicker portion of the Achilles graft, approximately 4 cm from the insertion, is the ideal location to center the graft on the distal humerus; typically, the allograft is approximately 10 cm long (**Figure 4**).
- The corners of the allograft are sutured with No. 2 braided suture.
- Using a long curved clamp, the corners of the allograft typically are passed from posterior to anterior. The medial side of the allograft is passed first, after which the lateral side of the allograft is passed (**Figure 3, B**).
- Usually, the joint needs to be flexed and extended with gentle tension on the allograft corner of choice as the allograft is passed. Gentle manipulation of the joint with traction and rolling of the joint, alternating between varus and valgus, can assist in the passage of the graft to cover the ulnohumeral articulation.
- The surgeon should inspect the coverage of the distal humerus at the ulnohumeral joint. After the graft is well centered, bone anchors can be placed in the supracondylar ridge to tether the corners of the allograft on the medial and lateral sides.
- If the joint has been completely dislocated, graft placement is much simpler (**Figure 5**).

## EXTERNAL FIXATOR FOR STABILITY AND DISTRACTION

- External fixation should be used if exposure and mobilization of the elbow necessitated detachment of the ligaments for exposure (**Figure 6**).
- If the joint was almost ankylosed, a hinged fixator can be advantageous for the application of passive mobilization and incremental displacement. The control provided by a hinged fixator can gradually stretch the soft tissues, including the biceps/brachialis, without risk for dislocation or subluxation.
- The application of 3 to 4 mm of joint distraction also may be useful in patients with a joint that was almost ankylosed. Distraction can help reduce the risk for impingement during motion if axis placement is slightly (a few millimeters only) off center.
- If the joint moves easily and smoothly in the planned ROM and does not subluxate or dislocate,

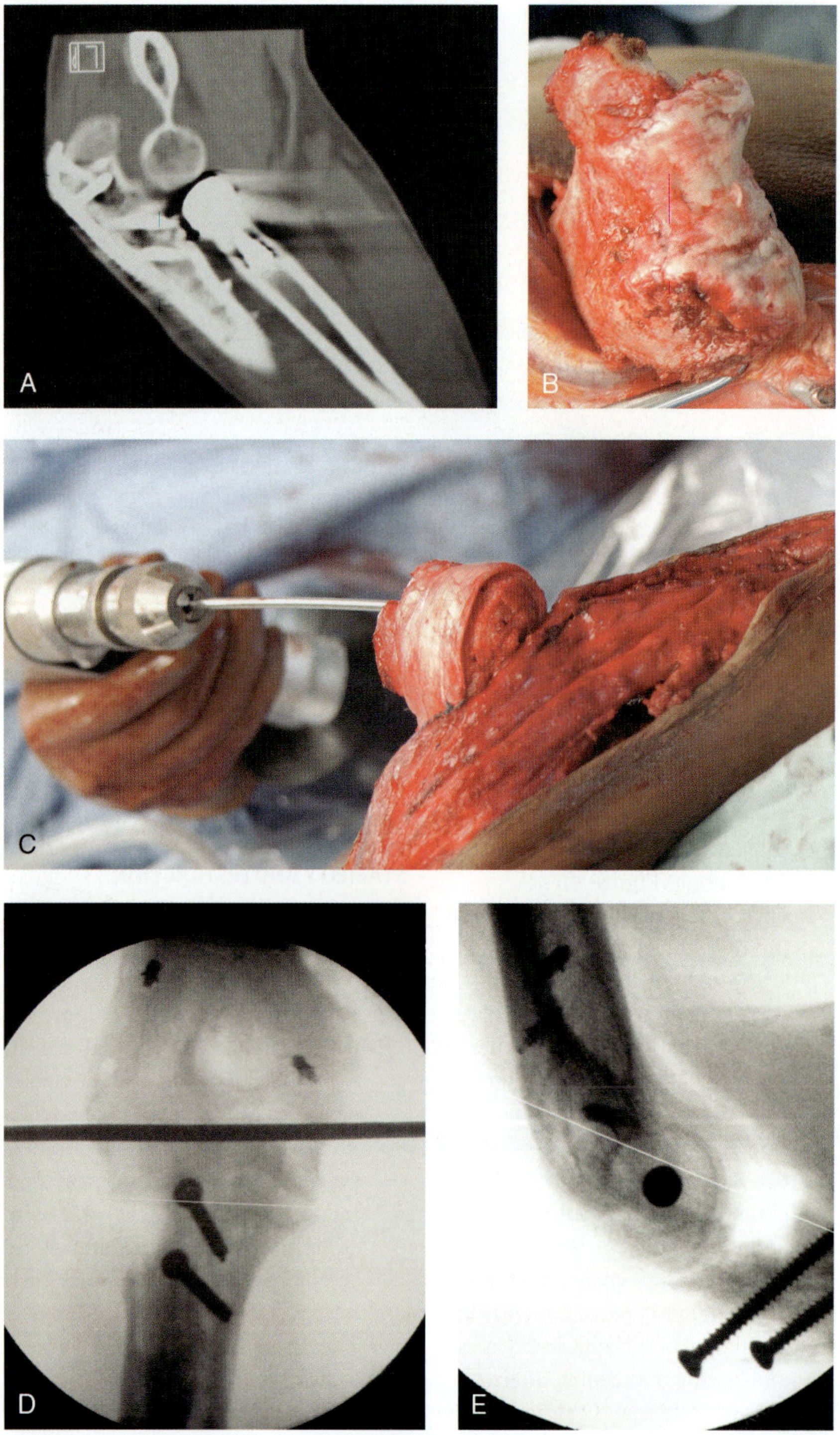

**Figure 5** Images of the elbow of a 24-year-old patient several months after injury and primary attempted fixation. **A,** Sagittal CT scan demonstrates loss of articulation and subluxation of the joint. Intraoperative photographs show complete loss of cartilage (**B**) and placement of a graft and a temporary axis pin in the completely dislocated joint (**C**). Intraoperative PA (**D**) and lateral (**E**) fluoroscopic views demonstrate accurate placement of the axis pin for subsequent application of a hinged fixator. (Copyright Robert Hotchkiss, MD, New York, NY.)

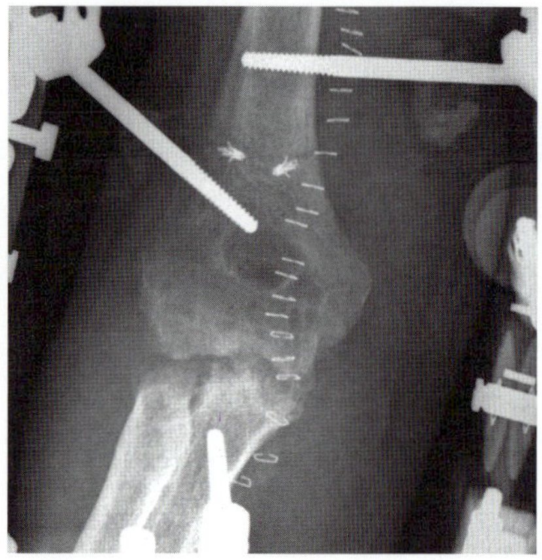

**Figure 6** AP radiograph of the elbow of the same patient shown in Figure 5 obtained 10 days postoperatively. An external fixation frame is in place, and 3 to 4 mm of distraction is applied. (Copyright Robert Hotchkiss, MD, New York, NY.)

use of an external fixator is not required. In the absence of an external fixator, the surgeon should observe the joint for signs of stiffness or instability, especially within the first 3 weeks postoperatively.

- If an external fixator is applied, the type of external fixator selected should be based on the experience and training of the surgeon. Each external fixator model has different features, complexity, and challenges. Regardless which fixator is used, the surgeon must locate the center of rotation of the joint under intraoperative fluoroscopic visualization.
- After the external fixator is in place, the joint must be checked to ensure that the external fixation frame allows for a nearly complete ROM (**Figure** 7).
- Regardless of the type of external fixation frame used, conical hydroxyapatite-coated pins should be used to decrease the incidence of premature pin loosening.
- A plane-based external fixator is an alternative to an axis-based external fixator. For plane-based external fixators, pin fixation of the ulna

is accomplished first, after which the plane of motion is identified and the humeral pins are applied with overlapping rings or plates. Plane-based external fixators allow the external fixation frame to be unlocked at the site of the overlapping rings or plates during rehabilitation and then relocked in the same position. Plane-based external fixators allow for supervised and careful mobilization without the risk for dislocation if the external fixator is locked. Currently, no plane-based external fixators are commercially available; however, they can be assembled by surgeons who have experience with external fixation devices and techniques (**Figure 8**).

- Suction drains that are 0.18-inch in diameter are placed to allow for drainage of both the anterior and posterior joint compartments. Sutures are used to hold the suction drains in place. If the suction drains dislodge within the first 12 to 24 hours postoperatively, a hematoma may develop, which can prevent mobilization of the joint. Should the suction drain dislodge, the patient may require another operation to replace it to its correct position.
- At the end of the procedure but before wound closure, the surgeon must assess whether the joint is stable and articulating properly throughout the range of flexion and extension, whether the interposition graft shears with motion or has moved out of place during external fixation frame placement, and whether forearm pronation and supination is smooth and unimpeded.
- If an external fixation frame was used, the surgeon also must determine whether the joint appears evenly distracted via inspection or fluoroscopy, the external fixation pins are at the proper length and depth, the suction drains are securely situated at the anterior and posterior aspects of the joint, and all of the connections on the external fixation frame are tight.

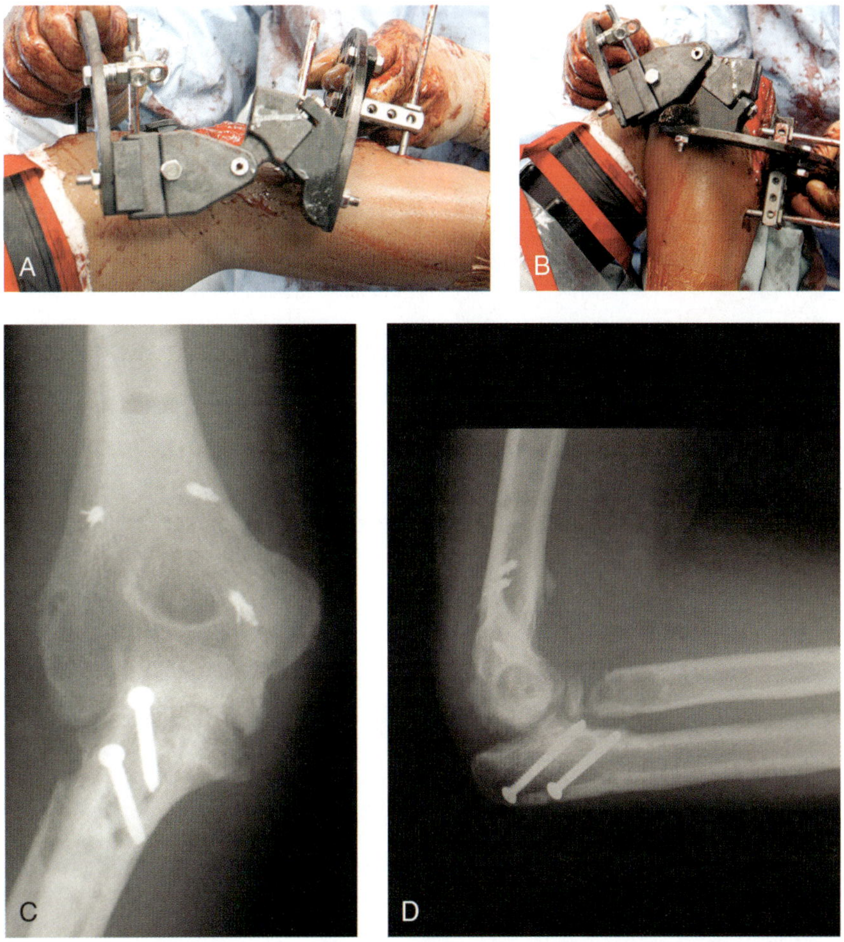


**Figure 7** Intraoperative photographs show confirmation of free movement of the elbow joint from extension (**A**) to flexion (**B**) with an external fixator in place. AP (**C**) and lateral (**D**) radiographs demonstrate the appearance of the joint approximately 2 years after interposition arthroplasty. (Copyright Robert Hotchkiss, MD, New York, NY.)

### Wound Closure

- The use of a straight posterior incision allows wound closure even in the presence of external fixation pins.
- Typically, the proximal and distal extent of the wound is more easily closed with an absorbable subcutaneous suture followed by skin staples.
- The thinner skin over the olecranon tip may require a more delicate technique with the use of 4-0 polypropylene alone. As the joint is flexed, the surgeon should pay close attention to skin perfusion near the olecranon tip. If this blanches under tension, the elbow should be positioned in greater extension for 4 to 5 days postoperatively before initiating joint flexion.

## Postoperative Regimen

Little need for motion exists in the first 24 hours postoperatively, but pain control and minimizing the amount of

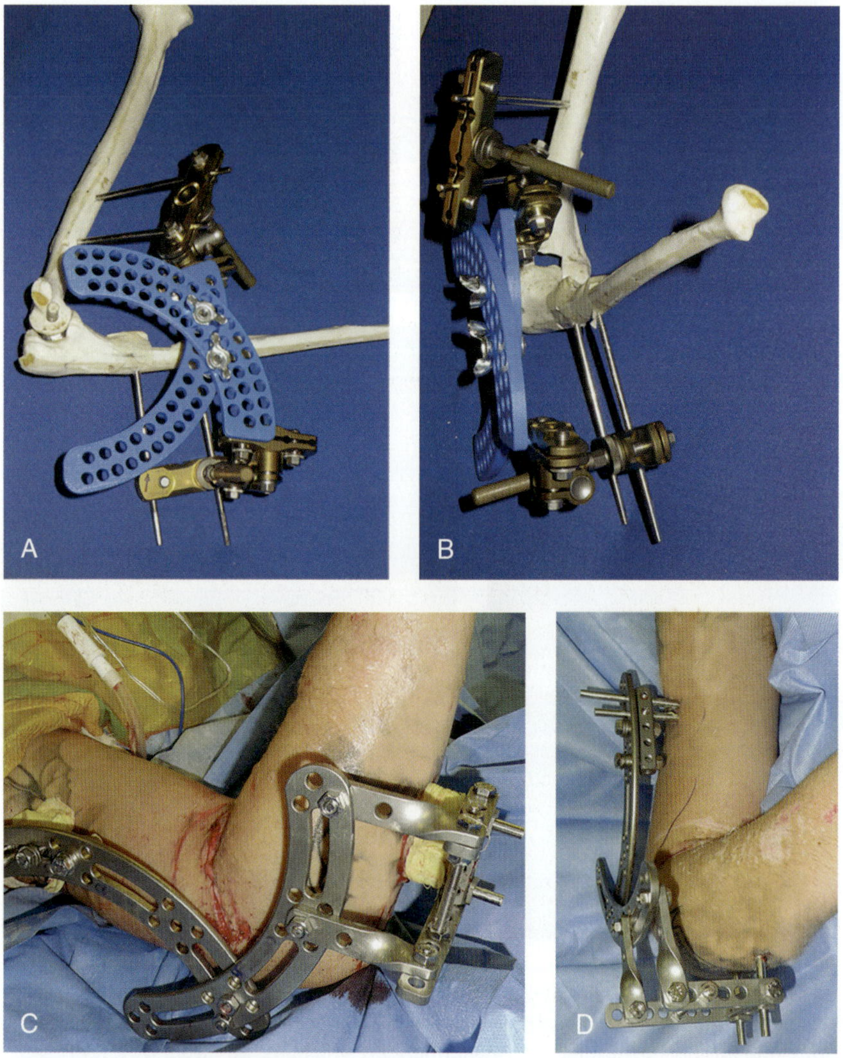


**Figure 8** Lateral (**A**) and AP (**B**) view clinical photographs and lateral (**C**) and AP (**D**) view intraoperative photographs show examples of a plane-based external fixator. The two bolts that link the two partial rings can be loosened to allow for protected overhead motion and then relocked in the same position to protect the reduction. (Copyright Robert Hotchkiss, MD, New York, NY.)

swelling is important. The use of dexamethasone (8 mg administered intravenously every 8 hours) can help minimize immediate edema for 48 hours postoperatively. On postoperative day 2, a program of active and passive motion begins, as tolerated. Redosing of the regional anesthetic block, if still in place, or the indwelling infraclavicular catheter, if operational, can assist in mobilization. If an external fixation frame was used, additional patient education will be necessary. On postoperative day 2, patients are taught how to use the external fixation frame based on the manufacturer's recommendations. Some patients will need to learn how to operate the drive mechanism as well as how to release the lock and begin active motion. The suction drains are left in place for the first 2 days postoperatively.

ROM is gradually increased during the first 3 weeks postoperatively to achieve the same (or better) ROM that was observed at the end of the procedure. Often, at the beginning of postoperative weeks 2 and 3, there is a tendency for the patient's elbow to gel and temporarily lose the ROM achieved in the first few days postoperatively. There are many explanations for this; however, regardless of the reason, vigilance is crucial. If an external fixation frame is in place, the pin sites can become irritated and superficial infection can develop. This is especially true in patients with more mobility, because more excursion is required of the soft tissues and skin. The surgeon should check all of the external fixation frame connections and the alignment of the external fixation frame via visual inspection and radiographic evaluation.

If there are no obvious and correctable causes of the decreased motion, the surgeon should consider performing an examination and manipulation under regional anesthesia. In general, if flexion past 90° is impossible, the distal triceps may be adherent to the posterior distal humerus. Gentle manipulation under regional anesthesia in an ambulatory setting may be helpful. Removal of the external fixator, which usually occurs at 4 weeks postoperatively, is usually performed under regional anesthesia, after which the elbow is gently moved through a ROM. No splint is applied.

In postoperative weeks 4 through 15, the patient is encouraged to begin using the upper extremity as tolerated. Supervised physical therapy and rehabilitation is often prescribed; however, the duration and frequency is individualized to each patient and should be reassessed at 4-week intervals. Return to sports such as swimming can begin at 6 weeks postoperatively. Return to more demanding activities is determined on a patient-by-patient basis.

Unlike patients who undergo implant arthroplasty, patients who undergo interposition arthroplasty do not require monitoring postoperatively. The author of this chapter typically recommends an annual radiographic assessment (**Figures 9** and **10**).

 

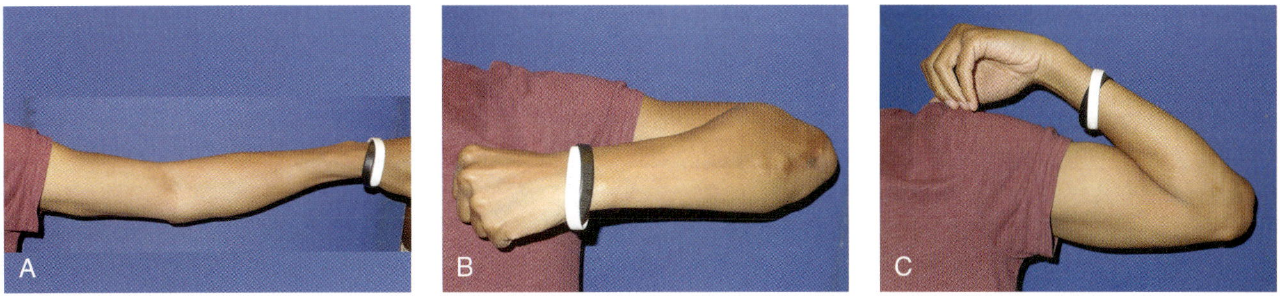

**Figure 9** Clinical photographs of the elbow of the same patient shown in Figures 5 and 6 taken approximately 5 years after interposition arthroplasty show extension to 20° (**A**), stability in varus (**B**), and flexion to 145° (**C**) without pain. At the time the photographs were taken, the patient was participating in physical activities such as basketball but avoided push-ups and bench presses. (Copyright Robert Hotchkiss, MD, New York, NY.)

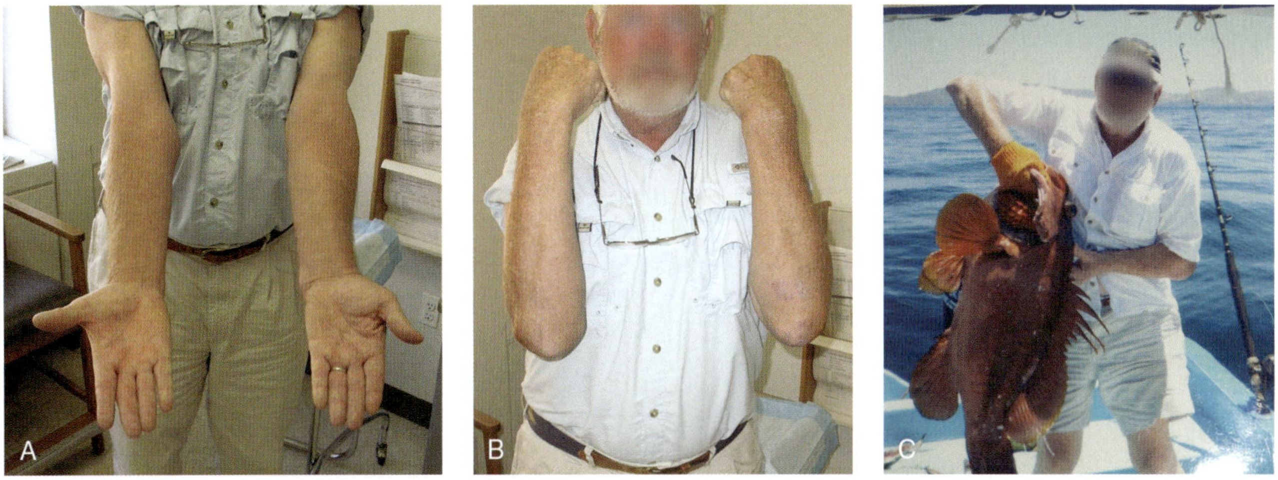

**Figure 10** Photographs of a 60-year-old man after interposition arthroplasty of the right elbow 5 years earlier and of the left elbow 7 years earlier. Clinical photographs show bilateral extension (**A**) and flexion (**B**). **C,** Photograph shows the patient's ability to participate in sport fishing. (Copyright Robert Hotchkiss, MD, New York, NY.)

## Limiting Adverse Events

Adverse events, including pin-tract infection, excessive swelling, ulnar nerve dysfunction, and unexpected stiffness are all common but unpredictable. Some patients who experience such adverse events require weekly clinical visits for the first 6 weeks to receive oversight of their postoperative care. In addition, joint position must be evaluated radiographically and under direct examination.

## Bibliography

Aldridge JM III, Lightdale NR, Mallon WJ, Coonrad RW: Total elbow arthroplasty with the Coonrad/Coonrad-Morrey prosthesis: A 10- to 31-year survival analysis. *J Bone Joint Surg Br* 2006;88(4):509-514.

Blaine TA, Adams R, Morrey BF: Total elbow arthroplasty after interposition arthroplasty for elbow arthritis. *J Bone Joint Surg Am* 2005;87(2):286-292.

Callhoff J, Weiß A, Zink A, Listing J: Impact of biologic therapy on functional status in patients with rheumatoid arthritis: A meta-analysis. *Rheumatology (Oxford)* 2013;52(12):2127-2135.

Chauhan A, Palmer BA, Baratz ME: Arthroscopically assisted elbow interposition arthroplasty without hinged external fixation: Surgical technique and patient outcomes. *J Shoulder Elbow Surg* 2015;24(6):947-954.

Chen DD, Forsh DA, Hausman MR: Elbow interposition arthroplasty. *Hand Clin* 2011;27(2):187-197, vi.

Cheng SL, Morrey BF: Treatment of the mobile, painful arthritic elbow by distraction interposition arthroplasty. *J Bone Joint Surg Br* 2000;82(2):233-238.

Er en A, Demirhan M, Atalar AC, Salduz A, Tunalı O: Stiff elbow: Distraction interposition arthroplasty with an Achilles tendon allograft. Long-term radiological and functional results. *Acta Orthop Traumatol Turc* 2014;48(5):558-562.

Fernandez-Palazzi F, Rodriguez J, Oliver G: Elbow interposition arthroplasty in children and adolescents: Long-term follow-up. *Int Orthop* 2008;32(2):247-250.

Fox RJ, Varitimidis SE, Plakseychuk A, Vardakas DG, Tomaino MM, Sotereanos DG: The Compass Elbow Hinge: Indications and initial results. *J Hand Surg Br* 2000;25(6):568-572.

Husband JB, Hastings H II: The lateral approach for operative release of post-traumatic contracture of the elbow. *J Bone Joint Surg Am* 1990;72(9):1353-1358.

Kasparyan NG, Hotchkiss RN: Dynamic skeletal fixation in the upper extremity. *Hand Clin* 1997;13(4):643-663.

Lee DH: Posttraumatic elbow arthritis and arthroplasty. *Orthop Clin North Am* 1999;30(1):141-162.

Ljung P, Jonsson K, Larsson K, Rydholm U: Interposition arthroplasty of the elbow with rheumatoid arthritis. *J Shoulder Elbow Surg* 1996;5(2 pt 1):81-85.

Mansat P: Surgical treatment of the rheumatoid elbow. *Joint Bone Spine* 2001;68(3):198-210.

Morrey BF: Posttraumatic stiffness: Distraction arthroplasty. *Orthopedics* 1992;15(7):863-869.

Nolla J, Ring D, Lozano-Calderon S, Jupiter JB: Interposition arthroplasty of the elbow with hinged external fixation for post-traumatic arthritis. *J Shoulder Elbow Surg* 2008;17(3):459-464.

Pennig D, Heck S, Mader K: Distraction arthroplasty for treatment of posttraumatic elbow stiffness (German). *Orthopade* 2011;40(4):329-338.

Regan WD, Reilly CD: Distraction arthroplasty of the elbow. *Hand Clin* 1993;9(4):719-728.

Sears BW, Puskas GJ, Morrey ME, Sanchez-Sotelo J, Morrey BF: Posttraumatic elbow arthritis in the young adult: Evaluation and management. *J Am Acad Orthop Surg* 2012;20(11):704-714.

Shi LL, Zurakowski D, Jones DG, Koris MJ, Thornhill TS: Semiconstrained primary and revision total elbow arthroplasty with use of the Coonrad-Morrey prosthesis. *J Bone Joint Surg Am* 2007;89(7):1467-1475.

 

Vancabeke M, Lamraski G, Berthe JV, Coessens BC: One-stage elbow interposition arthroplasty with a fasciocutaneous distally planned lateral arm flap. *Acta Orthop Belg* 2002;68(4):392-395.

Volkov MV, Oganesian OV: Restoration of function in the knee and elbow with a hinge-distractor apparatus. *J Bone Joint Surg Am* 1975;57(5):591-600.

# Index

Page numbers with *f* indicate figures;
page numbers with *t* indicate tables

## A



## B

## R



## S



 

## V



## W